Malignant Melanoma

Malignant Melanoma

Alfred W. Kopf, M.D.

Professor, Department of Dermatology,
New York University School of Medicine;
Head, Oncology Section, Skin and Cancer Unit,
University Hospital, New York University Medical Center

Robert S. Bart, M.D.

Associate Professor, Department of Dermatology,
New York University School of Medicine;
Associate Head, Oncology Section, Skin and Cancer Unit,
University Hospital, New York University Medical Center

René S. Rodríguez-Sains, M.D.

Teaching Assistant, Department of Medicine,
New York University School of Medicine

A. Bernard Ackerman, M.D.

Professor, Departments of Dermatology and Pathology,
New York University School of Medicine;
Consultant in Dermatopathology, Department of Pathology,
Memorial Sloan Kettering Cancer Center

Masson Publishing USA, Inc
New York • Paris • Barcelona • Milan • Mexico City • Rio de Janeiro

This book represents information obtained from authentic and highly regarded sources. A wide variety of references is listed. Every reasonable effort has been made to give reliable data and information, but the authors and the publisher cannot assume responsibility for the validity of all materials or for the consequences of their use.

Copyright © 1979, by Masson Publishing USA, Inc.

All rights reserved. No part of this book may be reproduced in any form, by photostat, microfilm, retrieval system, or any other means, without the prior written permission of the publisher.

ISBN 0-89352-040-3

Library of Congress Catalog Number: 78-71687

Printed in the United States of America

Foreword

AWARENESS OF A new or changing skin lesion with a gray or blue-black hue will often prompt a person to consult a dermatologist or his primary physician, who in turn may refer the patient to a dermatologist. Thus the dermatologist, more often than any other physician, is placed in the singularly responsible position of diagnosing early-stage melanomas and of having to help decide upon their ensuing management. This is a heavy responsibility that can be fulfilled only if he or she is completely conversant with current knowledge concerning clinical and histologic features and management of this tumor, one of the most biologically malignant in man.

Should the biopsy be incisional or excisional? Which portion of the lesion should be biopsied? How should the biopsy scar be positioned? These are all seemingly simple questions, but the answers to them have significant bearing upon the subsequent management.

Statistics reveal that in the United States alone about 9,000 persons annually are afflicted with malignant melanomas. Despite significant advances in its diagnosis, staging, and management, approximately 3,000 patients succumb each year to malignant melanoma, while only 1,500 die of all other forms of skin cancer from among the 300,000 persons who annually develop them.

In view of all this, a complete and thorough text devoted to an intensive exploration of malignant melanomas, using, to some extent, an approach from the dermatologist's viewpoint, is a most helpful adjunct to the collection of writings on the subject.

Doctors Kopf and Bart are particularly suited to deal with this task, because of their extensive experience with the clinical variants of malignant melanoma, modulated by close collaboration with experts in the fields of surgery, radiology, chemotherapy, pathology, and immunology. Actually it is the clinical, histologic, laboratory, therapeutic, and computer-oriented approaches utilized in the Skin Tumor Conference and Pigmented Lesion Conference of the Skin and Cancer Unit, developed in cooperation with the Melanoma Cooperative Group at this institution, that to a great extent have influenced this work. Together with the above authors, Dr. Rodriguez-Sains carried out an extensive review of the melanoma literature. Of special interest also is the comprehensive section on the histology of malignant melanomas written by Dr. Ackerman, a highly experienced worker in this field, in collaboration with Dr. Su.

The clarity and conciseness with which the subject is presented, enhanced by exceptionally fine clinical and microscopic photographs, mark this volume as a most valuable and timely contribution to the literature concerning cutaneous neoplasia.

Rudolf L. Baer, M.D.

Preface

THIS BOOK HAS grown from our review article published in the January–February 1977 issue of the *Journal of Dermatologic Surgery and Oncology*. In that review we attempted to emphasize practical aspects of diagnosis and treatment of malignant melanomas. For this book the material has been expanded and updated and a comprehensive chapter on histopathology of malignant melanomas has been added. This chapter is unique in that it provides guidelines for histopathologic diagnosis that stress architectural rather than cytologic features.

We do not mean this book to be a manual on how to treat malignant melanomas. Such a manual would presume that there are complete answers to the many questions that arise concerning the management of malignant melanomas. For example, it is virtually impossible at present to make firm recommendations about immunotherapy for malignant melanomas, based on what has been written in the literature. This is so despite the fact that a substantial portion of the current literature concerning malignant melanomas deals with immunology and immunotherapy. Another telling example is uncertainty about making absolute statements with regard to elective lymph-node dissections, the value of which is currently being vigorously debated.

Looking to the future, we are sure that the therapy of malignant melanomas will have to change if significant improvement in survival rates of patients with advanced malignant melanomas is to occur. For the present, the best hope for reduction in the morbidity and mortality from malignant melanomas is their early diagnosis and prompt treatment.

What we have tried to do, relying primarily on an extensive review of the recent literature and on our own experience, is to bring to the reader what we believe to be important in the present state of knowledge about the clinical aspects, epidemiology, classification, histopathology, and treatment of cutaneous malignant melanomas. We hope that this book will also serve as a stimulus to others to study, to observe, and to publish their experiences toward the ultimate goal of prevention or cure of every type of cutaneous malignant melanoma.

Alfred W. Kopf, M.D.
Robert S. Bart, M.D.
René Rodríguez-Sains, M.D.
A. Bernard Ackerman, M.D.

Contents

	Foreword	v
	Preface	vii
	Illustrations	xi
1.	Incidence and Mortality Rates	1
2.	Sunlight and Malignant Melanoma	4
3.	Classification and Clinical Diagnosis of Cutaneous Malignant Melanomas	7
4.	Histopathology of Cutaneous Malignant Melanoma	25
5.	Familial Malignant Melanoma	148
6.	Malignant Melanomas in Children	152
7.	Congenital Nevocytic Nevi and Malignant Melanomas	154
8.	Multiple Primary Malignant Melanomas	157
9.	Subungual Malignant Melanoma	159
10.	Leukoderma and Malignant Melanomas	162
11.	Occult Primary Malignant Melanomas and Spontaneous Regression of Malignant Melanomas	166
12.	Extra-regional Metastases from Malignant Melanomas	169
13.	Staging of Malignant Melanomas	170
14.	Prognostication of Behavior of Malignant Melanoma	172
15.	Biopsy of Malignant Melanoma	177
16.	Surgical Management of Malignant Melanomas	179
17.	Elective Lymph Node Dissection for Malignant Melanoma	183
18.	Chemotherapy	187
19.	Radiotherapy for Malignant Melanoma	197
20.	Survival Rates in Malignant Melanoma	200
21.	Immunologic Aspects of Malignant Melanoma	204
22.	Miscellaneous Aspects of Malignant Melanomas	206
	Appendix	214
	General Bibliography	218
	Index	235

21.	Immunologic Aspects of Malignant Melanoma	204
22.	Miscellaneous Aspects of Malignant Melanomas	206
	Appendix	214
	General Bibliography	218
	Index	235

Illustrations
(*Italics indicate Photomicrographs*)

Figure number		Page
1A	Mortality due to cutaneous malignant melanomas, geographic variations	2
1B	Non-melanoma skin cancer mortality rates, geographic variations	2
2–4	Lentigo maligna	7–8
5–6	*Lentigo maligna melanoma*	*8*
7–8	Superficial spreading malignant melanoma	9
9–11	*Superficial spreading malignant melanoma*	*9–10*
12	Nodular malignant melanoma	10
13	Amelanotic malignant melanoma	10
14	*Nodular malignant melanoma*	*10*
15–16	Acral-lentiginous malignant melanoma	11
17	*Acral-lentiginous malignant melanoma*	*11*
18–19	Levels of invasion in malignant melanoma	12
20	Thickness of malignant melanomas	13
21–25	Superficial spreading malignant melanoma	17
26–30	Lentigo maligna melanoma	18
31–34B	Nodular malignant melanoma	19–20
35A–37	Acral-lentignous malignant melanoma	20–21
38	Malignant melanoma, scalp	21
39–42	Satellitosis and in-transit metastases	22
43	Diagram dipicting malignant melanoma as one pathological process	35
44	*Lentigo maligna*	*36*
45	*Acral-lentiginous malignant melanoma*	*37*
46	*Superficial spreading malignant melanoma*	*38*
47	*Nodular malignant melanoma*	*40*

Figure number		Page
48	*Involvement of adnexa by malignant melanoma*	*41*
49–52	*Lentigo maligna*	*42–44, 46*
53–54	Acral-lentiginous malignant melanoma	48, 49
55–56	*Superficial spreading malignant melanoma*	*50, 52, 53*
57–58	Superficial spreading and nodular malignant melanoma	54, 55
59	*Malignant melanoma, unclassified*	*56*
60	Inflammatory-cell infiltrate with malignant melanoma	57
61	*Desmoplastic malignant melanoma*	*58–59*
62	Lamellar fibrosis in malignant melanoma	60
63–64	*Epidermal collarette in malignant melanoma*	*61–62*
65	*Verrucous malignant melanoma*	*63*
66	*Malignant melanoma with ulceration*	*64*
67–71	Malignant melanomas associated with melanocytic nevus	65–68, 70–71
72	*Melanoma cells in epidermis*	*72*
73	Inflammatory-cell infiltrate prior to regression of malignant melanoma	73
74–80	*Spontaneous regression of malignant melanoma*	*74–78, 80–82*
81	Technique of total excision biopsy	86
82	*Crucial zone for histologic diagnosis of malignant melanomas (diagram)*	*88*
83–84	*Spitz's nevus*	*89–91*
85	*Failure of maturation of melanocytes in malignant melanoma*	*92*
86	*Marked variation in size and shape of nests of atypical melanocytes in malignant melanomas*	*93*
87	*Malignant melanoma involving eccrine duct*	*94*
88	*Halo nevus*	*95*
89	*Cytologic atypia in malignant melanoma*	*96–97*
90	*Necrosis in malignant melanoma*	*98*
91	*Mitoses in malignant melanoma*	*99*
92	*Prominent nucleoli in malignant melanoma*	*100*

Figure number		Page
93	*Intranuclear vacuoles in malignant melanoma*	*101*
94	*Multinucleated melanocytic giant cells in malignant melanoma*	*102*
95	*Traumatized compound melanocytic nevus*	*103*
96	*Ulcerated melanocytic nevus*	*104–105*
97	*Spitz's nevus*	*106*
98	*Halo nevus*	*107–108*
99–100	*Pseudomelanoma*	*109–110*
101	*Pagetoid Bowen's disease*	*111*
102–103	*Paget's disease of breast*	*112, 114–115*
104	*Unusual melanocytic nevus with Spitz-like features*	*116*
105	*Spitz's nevus with nodule*	*117–118*
106	*Lentigo maligna in association with an intradermal nevocytic nevus*	*119*
107	*Desmoplastic melanoma masquerading as a blue nevus*	*120*
108	*Mycosis fungoides*	*121*
109	*Epidermotropically metastatic malignant melanoma*	*122*
110	*Malignant melanoma metastatic to dermis*	*123*
111	*Metastatic malignant melanoma cells in a vein*	*124*
112	*Metastatic malignant melanoma simulating angiosarcoma*	*125*
113	*Satellitosis in malignant melanoma*	*126*
114	*In-transit metastases in malignant melanoma*	*127*
115	*Satellitosis in malignant melanoma*	*128*
116	*Superficial spreading malignant melanoma with extensive melanosis*	*129*
117	*Sessile malignant melanoma*	*130*
118	*Cells of malignant melanoma intermingling with cells of melanocytic nevus*	*131–132*
119	*Basal-cell carcinoma*	*133*
120	*Malignant melanoma contiguous with basal-cell carcinoma*	*134*
121	*Unusual proliferation of melanocytes, in situ*	*136–137*

Figure number		Page
122	*Focal acantholytic dyskeratosis in association with malignant melanoma*	*138*
123	*Specimen of malignant melanoma removed by shave excision*	*139*
124–125	*Shave excision biopsy of a malignant melanoma*	*140–141*
126	*Proper sectioning of a lesion suspected of being malignant melanoma*	*142*
127	*Malignant melanoma in association with an intradermal nevus*	*142–144*
128	Multiple primary malignant melanomas (familial)	149
129	Congenital malignant melanoma	152
130	Malignant melanoma arising in a congenital nevocytic nevus	155
131	Giant nevocytic nevus (before and after excision)	155
132–133	Subungual malignant melanomas	160
134	*Subungual malignant melanoma*	*160*
135	Leukoderma associated with malignant melanoma	163
136	Nodal metastasis of malignant melanoma	170
137	*Malignant melanoma metastatic to lymph node*	*170*
138	The cell cycle (diagram)	188

Malignant Melanoma

Chapter 1

Incidence and Mortality Rates

The Third National Cancer Survey (1975) was based on surveying a population of approximately 20 million inhabitants of the United States. It was conducted in ten geographically separated areas of the country in order to include representative groups from all socioeconomic and racial strata. From the preliminary report the following data concerning malignant melanoma can be extracted:

(a) The age-adjusted annual incidence for the United States is 4.2 per 100,000 population (males, 4.3; females, 4.1).
(b) Blacks have a much lower age-adjusted annual incidence (0.8 per 100,000) than whites (4.5 per 100,000).
(c) The highest age-adjusted annual incidence in whites (7.7 per 100,000) is in the South (e.g., Dallas-Ft. Worth) and the lowest (3.2 per 100,000) in the North (e.g., Iowa).
(d) The older the age of whites, the greater the annual incidence (e.g., at age 5 it is 0.1 per 100,000; at age 85, 17.6 per 100,000).
(e) The total number of cases in whites is greatest in the 40- to 49-year-old age group.

In the United States there is a steadily rising incidence of all primary cutaneous malignancies including melanomas (Lee, 1973), although some regional exceptions may occur (Ressequie et al., 1977). Malignant melanomas account for most of the deaths from skin cancers. The mean age of those dying from melanomas is less than that of those dying from other skin cancers. In the United States, for the years 1967–1968, there were about 2,850 deaths from melanoma and 1,530 deaths from other skin cancers in Caucasians. Thus, nearly two-thirds of deaths from skin cancer were caused by melanomas. Other important facts are: a) the survival rate of treated melanomas is improving; b) the absolute number of deaths from malignant melanoma is rising largely because of increase in population; c) loss of expected years of life per million population due to deaths from malignant melanomas is 498 for white men and 390 for white women; comparable figures for all other skin cancers are 175 and 98, respectively.

From England and Wales (Lee and Carter, 1970), Norway (Magnus, 1973), Australia, Canada, Denmark and Sweden (Ellwood and Lee, 1975; Davis, 1976) a considerable increase in incidence and mortality from malignant melanomas has also been reported. These increases cannot be explained solely on the basis of better reporting. They may be related to the increased tendency of people to expose large areas of their skins to sunlight for prolonged periods.

DISCUSSION AND SUMMARY

Annually, in the United States, with a population of over 210,000,000, approximately 9,000 individuals develop cutaneous malignant melanomas, 300,000 develop other skin cancers, and 600,000 develop cancers of all other organs exclusive of skin (Scotto et al., 1974). Thus, approximately one of three new cancers of man is a cancer of the skin and one of a hundred is a malignant melanoma.

The incidence and mortality rates of malignant melanomas are rising more rapidly than any other cancer except, in some countries, lung cancers (Elwood et al., 1974).

The incidence (i.e., new cases per 100,000 population) of malignant melanoma is constantly rising in various parts of the world. This rise cannot be explained by better record keeping alone, but implies greater exposure to the causative factors responsible for this form of cutaneous cancer.

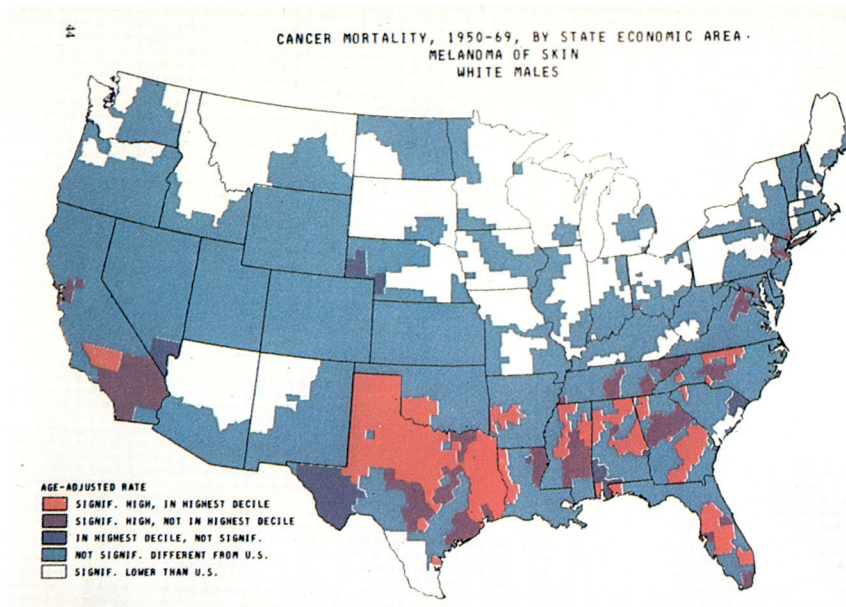

FIGURE 1A. **Mortality due to cutaneous melanomas, 1950–1969, by state economic areas in white men.** *The areas in red show the highest prevalence of deaths due to malignant melanomas. It should be noted that these occur mostly in the southern half of the United States where sun exposure is greatest. (Figures 1A & 1B reproduced with permission from Mason, T. J., et al., "Atlas of Cancer Mortality for U.S. Counties: 1950–1969," DHEW publication #(NIH) 75-780, 1975.)*

FIGURE 1B. **Non-melanoma skin cancer mortality in white men.** *The distribution of deaths due to non-melanoma skin cancer mimics that of melanoma suggesting the possibility of a common causative factor, such as sunlight.*

N.B. White women have a similar geographic distribution of mortality due to melanomas and non-melanoma skin cancers.

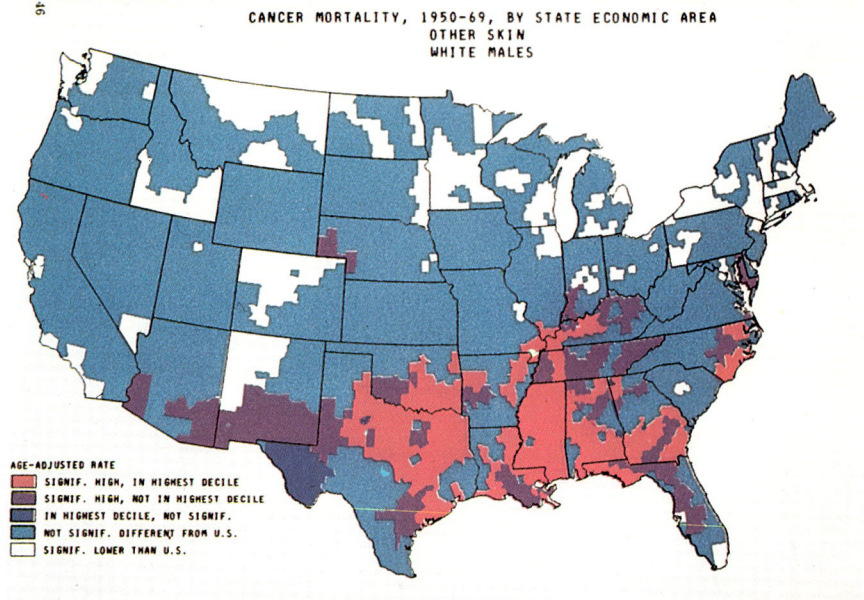

The mortality rate in the United States from malignant melanoma is approximately 3,000 patients per year (Lee, 1973). In contrast, the annual mortality rate for all other types of skin cancer is only 1,500. Thus, approximately two-thirds of deaths from skin cancers are caused by malignant melanomas, but only 3% of all cancers of the skin are melanomas.

In the United States the number of deaths due to melanoma among whites rose from 9.3 per million in 1950 to 16 per million in 1967; comparable figures for England and Wales are 5.1 and 10.2 per million (Cosman et al., 1976). Despite the increased deaths, there has been a progressive improvement in five-year survival rates for treated malignant melanoma, the increase being from 41% in 1940–49 to 67% in 1965–69 (Cutler et al., 1975). Presumably this reflects a real improvement in outlook from treatment and not entirely a statistical artifact resulting from earlier diagnosis.

There are suggestions in the literature, however, that melanomas are being diagnosed earlier. For example, Cady et al. (1975) report that the mean maximum diameter of melanomas in their patients seen before 1949 was 2.5 cm, whereas it was 1.2 cm for those seen since 1949. Thus, education of the public and of the medical profession about melanomas would probably result in great benefits, since early diagnosis often means cure.

REFERENCES

Cady, B., Legg, M. A., and Redfern, A. B. Contemporary treatment of malignant melanoma. Am. J. Surg. 129:472–482, 1975.

Cosman, B., Heddle, S. B., and Crikelair, G. F. The increasing incidence of melanoma. Plast. Reconstr. Surg. 57:50–56, 1976.

Cutler, S. J., and Young, J. L. Third National Cancer Survey: Incidence Data, N.C.I. Monograph 41, DHEW Publication No. (NIH) 75-787, March, 1975.

Cutler, S. J., Myers, M. H., and Green, S. B. Trends in survival rates of patients with cancer. N. Engl. J. Med. 293:122–124, 1975.

Davis, N. C. Cutaneous melanoma. The Queensland experience. Curr. Probl. Surg. 13:1–63, 1976.

Elwood, J. M., and Lee, J. A. H. Recent data on the epidemiology of malignant melanoma. Semin. Oncol. 2:149–154, 1975.

Elwood, J. M., Lee, J. A. H., Walters, S. D., Mo, T., and Green, A. E. S. Relationship of melanoma and other skin cancer mortality to latitude and ultraviolet radiation in the United States and Canada. Int. J. Epidemiology 3:325–332, 1974.

Lee, J. A. H. Current evidence about the causes of malignant melanoma. Prog. Clin. Cancer 6:151–161, 1975.

Lee, J. A. H. The trend of mortality from primary malignant tumors of skin. J. Invest. Dermatol. 59:445–448, 1973.

Lee, J. A. H., and Carter, A. P. Secular trends in mortality from malignant melanoma. J. Natl. Cancer Inst. 45:91–97, 1970.

Macdonald, E. J. Epidemiology of melanoma. Prog. Clin. Cancer 6:139–149, 1975.

Magnus, K. Incidence of malignant melanoma of the skin in Norway, 1955–1970. Cancer 32:1275–1286, 1973.

Mason, T. J., et al. Atlas of Cancer Mortality for U.S. Counties: 1950–1969. DHEW Publication No. (NIH) 75-780, 1975.

Milton, G. W., McGovern, and Lewis, M. G. Malignant Melanoma of the Skin and Mucous Membrane. Edinburgh, London, and New York, Churchill Livingston, 1977.

Resseguie, L. J., Marks, S. J., Winkelmann, R. K., and Kurtland, L. T. Malignant melanoma in the resident population of Rochester, Minnesota. Mayo Clin. Proc. 52:191–195, 1977.

Scotto, J., Kopf, A. W., and Urbach, F. Non-melanoma skin cancer among caucasians in four areas of the United States. Cancer 34:1333–1338, 1974.

Third National Cancer Survey: Incidence Data. National Cancer Institute Monograph 41. U.S. Department of Health, Education and Welfare, Public Health Service, National Institutes of Health, National Cancer Institute, Bethesda, Maryland. DHEW Publication No. (NIH) 75-787, 1975.

Chapter 2

Sunlight and Malignant Melanoma

Epidemiologic data implicating sunlight as a cause of basal- and squamous-cell carcinomas of the skin is convincing (Brodkin et al., 1969; Scotto et al., 1974; Daniels, 1975; Mason et al., 1975). Many studies and reviews show a direct correlation between the amount of sun exposure and the incidence or prevalence of epithelial carcinomas of the skin. The carcinogenicity of ultraviolet light has been demonstrated in experimental animal models, particularly in the hairless mouse (Winkelmann, 1963; Epstein et al., 1969; Snyder and May, 1975; Chopra, 1976).

Recent reports suggest that not only are epithelial cutaneous cancers related to sun exposure but that malignant melanomas are also. However, the relationship of malignant melanomas to sun exposure is not as clear cut (Davis, 1976). The principal evidence that malignant melanomas in man may sometimes be caused by sun exposure is based on epidemiologic studies. Those areas of the world (e.g., Australia, Israel) in which light-skinned Caucasians are exposed to large amounts of solar radiation have high incidences of malignant melanoma (Davis, 1976). Furthermore, in those countries which extend over many latitudes, the incidence of malignant melanomas among Caucasians is greatest in those individuals who reside closest to the equator. From Australia, Lancaster (1956) and Lee and Merrill (1970) reported an inverse correlation between incidence of malignant melanoma and latitude. In Norway, Magnus (1973) found an almost three-fold greater incidence of melanoma in the southern part of the country compared to the northern part. In Israel, Movshovitz and Modan (1973), in a nationwide survey of melanomas, found the highest incidence in native-born Israelis of European extraction. Rates were intermediate in veteran foreign-born Europeans and lowest in recent European-born immigrants. Thus, the longer the exposure to the intense sun of Israel the greater the age-adjusted incidence of malignant melanomas. Anaise et al. (1978) also studied malignant melanomas in Israelis. They report a significantly higher incidence of melanoma in (1) European born Jews than those born in Africa or Asia, (2) those European-born Jews of same age and ethnic background who stayed in Israel 20 to 30 years compared to those who stayed only 2 to 5 years, and (3) those who worked on agricultural Kibbutzes compared to those in the cities.

In the United States, Mason et al. (1975) plotted skin cancer deaths (1950 to 1969) by county and demonstrated that the highest age-adjusted mortality rates in whites occurred in the southern half of the nation (Fig. 1).

Several authors have also pointed out the markedly lower incidence of malignant melanomas in non-Caucasian groups, and in Caucasians with darkly pigmented skins (Lewis, 1967; Movshovitz and Modan, 1973; Third National Cancer Survey, 1975). The report of the Third National Cancer Survey indicates that in the United States, the age-adjusted incidence of melanoma in blacks is 0.8 per 100,000 population compared to 4.5 per 100,000 population in whites. The implication is that pigment protects from the sun's damaging rays. This does not completely exclude other hypotheses such as that of a destructive effect of excessive pigment on melanoma cells (Pawelek, 1976).

Per contra, some observers raise questions about the role of sunlight in inducing melanoma. For example, they point out that the incidence of malignant melanomas is not greater in sun-exposed areas of the skin, the distribution of them is different from that of basal- or squamous-cell carcinomas which are cogently thought to be caused by solar factors, and there is a lack of significant elastosis in many patients with melanomas, which bespeaks little sun damage. These discrepancies have led Lee and Merrill (1970) to postulate a "solar circulating factor" as the agent responsible for the high incidence of malignant melanomas on unexposed sites. This "factor" is further postulated to be a product of sun-irradiated skin that travels via the bloodstream and acts at distant sites to stimulate malignant transformation of melanocytes.

The following observations support an association between sun exposure and malignant melanomas:

(1) Patients who develop malignant melanomas are much more likely to have light-colored eyes (blue, green, grey), light complexions, light hair-color, and to sunburn more readily than individuals who do not develop malignant melanomas (Gellin et al., 1969). This correlation parallels the findings in patients who develop basal-cell carcinomas in that they have similar phenotypic and sunburning characteristics (Gellin et al., 1965). In both studies cited, despite the fact that patients with skin cancer tended toward light complexions and sunburned easily, they spend more time outdoors than did individuals in the control groups.

(2) Patients afflicted with xeroderma pigmentosum, in which sunlight induces numerous cutaneous tumors (solar keratoses, basal-cell carcinomas, keratoacanthomas and squamous-cell carcinomas), have a much higher risk of developing malignant melanomas. Moore and Robinson (1954), in a review of the literature, found that 3% of 360 cases of xeroderma pigmentosum developed malignant melanomas. In a study of 15 patients with xeroderma pigmentosum at the National Institutes of Health, seven (47%) were found to have malignant melanomas.

(3) Malignant melanomas rarely occur on "doubly clothed" areas (bathing suit area in men and women and breasts of women) according to the data gathered by the Malignant Melanoma Clinical Cooperative Group (Fitzpatrick et al., 1975).

(4) More malignant melanomas develop on the legs of women than on those of men. The legs of women are more exposed to sunlight from their habit of dress than are those of men (McLeod, 1971). Bodenham (1968) speculated that the sharp rise of malignant melanomas on the legs of women following the Second World War could be attributed to the fact that sheer nylon stockings permit more of the sun's ultraviolet light to reach the skin whereas the pre-war stockings offered a higher level of protection.

(5) Scotto, Fears and Gori (1976) using a "sunburning-ultraviolet meter," that measures the effectiveness of ultraviolet in producing erythema of the skin, took recordings at half-hourly intervals for one year in ten geographically widespread locations in the United States. The incidence of skin cancer (including basal-cell carcinomas, squamous-cell carcinomas, and malignant melanomas) correlated positively with the ultraviolet intensity. Thus, we have for the first time, actual measurements which support the theory that ultraviolet radiation causes skin cancers (including malignant melanomas) in man.

In further studies Fears et al. (1976) have devised a mathematical formula to calculate the relative increase in skin cancers associated with increase in erythema-producing ultraviolet light (UVL), e.g., due to depletion of atmospheric ozone from supersonic transports or chlorofluoromethanes. These authors calculate that increases of 30% of erythema-producing UVL could double the incidence of melanoma and increase deaths due to melanomas by 45%. Also, the National Research Council has reported recently that fluorocarbon gases used as propellants for spray products also deplete the ozone layer.

(6) Artificial sources of ultraviolet light in combination with topically applied carcinogen (dimethyl benzanthracene) in hairless mice has resulted in the induction of metastasizing malignant melanomas (Epstein et al., 1967).

(7) The location on the face of the most cases of lentigo maligna and lentigo maligna melanoma strongly suggests connection with exposure to sunlight.

(8) Malignant melanomas in eyes do not show the strong North-South increasing incidence seen in cutaneous malignant melanomas (Scotto, Fraumeni and Lee, 1976).

DISCUSSION AND SUMMARY

The role of ultraviolet light in the induction of malignant melanomas in man has received considerable attention recently in discussions on the impact of supersonic aircraft on the environment. It has been estimated that a 5% reduction of the ozone shield, which as it is now constituted filters out much of carcinogenic ultraviolet light that reaches the surface of the earth, by a fleet of commercial supersonic aircraft, would result in at least 8,000 more cases of skin cancer a year in the white population of the United States and about 300 more deaths from cancers of the skin inclusive of malignant melanomas (Booker et al., 1975).

If malignant melanomas are in fact induced by sunlight, prevention by the use of topical or systemically administered sunscreens becomes a possibility. Public education programs, such as those conducted in Australia, on the importance of reducing sun exposure and on early diagnosis of malignant melanoma should also prove useful.

REFERENCES

Anaise, D., Steinitz, R., and Ben Hur, N. Solar radiation: A possible etiological factor in malignant melanoma in Israel. Cancer 42:499–504, 1978.

Bodenham, D. C. A study of 650 observed malignant melanomas in the south-west region. Ann. R. Coll. Surg. Engl. 43:218–239, 1968.

Booker, H. G., et al. Environmental Impact of Stratospheric Flight: Biological and Climatic Effects of Aircraft Emissions in the Stratosphere, National Academy of Sciences, 1975, pp. 177–221.

Brodkin, R. H., Kopf, A. W., and Andrade, R. Basal-cell epithelioma and elastosis: a comparison of distribution. In: Urbach, F., ed. The Biologic Effects of Ultraviolet Radiation: With Emphasis on the Skin. New York, Pergamon, 1969, pp. 581–618.

Chopra, D. P. Ultraviolet light carcinogenesis in hairless mice. J. Invest. Dermatol. 66:242–247, 1976.

Daniels, F. Sunlight. In: Schottenfeld, D., ed. Cancer Epidemiology and Prevention: Current Concepts. Springfield, Charles C. Thomas, 1975, pp. 126–152.

Davis, N. C. Cutaneous Melanoma. The Queensland experience. Cur. Probl. Surg. 13:1–63, 1976.

Elwood, J. M., Lee, J. A. H., Walter, S. D., Mo, T., and Green, A. E. S. Relationship of melanoma and other skin cancer mortality to latitude and ultraviolet radiation in the United States and Canada. Int. J. Epidemiology 3:325–332, 1974.

Epstein, J. H., Epstein, W. L., and Nakai, T. Production of melanomas from DMBA-induced "blue nevi" in hairless mice with ultraviolet light. J. Natl. Cancer Inst. 38:19–30, 1967.

Epstein, J. H., Fukuyama, K., and Dobson, R. L. Ultraviolet light carcinogenesis. In: Urbach, F., ed. The Biologic Effects of Ultraviolet Radiation: With Emphasis on the Skin. New York, Pergamon, 1969, pp. 551–568.

Fears, T. R., Scotto, J., and Schneiderman, M. A. Skin cancer, melanoma, and sunlight. Am. J. Public Health 66:461–464, 1976.

Fitzpatrick, T. B., Sober, A., and Pearson, B. Early Diagnosis of Malignant Melanoma. Exhibit at the 1975 Meeting of the American Academy of Dermatology, San Francisco, December 6–11, 1975.

Gellin, G. A., Kopf, A. W., and Garfinkel, L. Basal cell epithelioma: a controlled study of associated factors. Arch. Dermatol. 91:38–45, 1965.

Gellin, G. A., Kopf, A. W., and Garfinkel, L. Malignant melanoma: a controlled study of possible associated factors. Arch. Dermatol. 99:43–48, 1969.

Lancaster, H. O. Some geographical aspects of mortality from melanoma in Europeans. Med. J. Aust. 1:1082–1087, 1956.

Lee, J. A., and Merrill, J. M. Sunlight and the etiology of malignant melanomas: a synthesis. Med. J. Aust. 2:846–851, 1970.

Lewis, M. G. Malignant melanoma in Uganda. Br. J. Cancer 21:483–495, 1967.

London, D. A., Carter, D. M., and Condit, E. S. Effect of pigment on photomediated production of thymine dimers in cultured melanoma cells. J. Invest. Derm. 67:261–264, 1976.

Magnus, K. Incidence of malignant melanoma of the skin in Norway 1955–1970: variations in time and space and solar radiation. Cancer 32:1275–1286, 1973.

Mason, T. J., et al. Atlas of Cancer Mortality for U.S. Counties: 1950–1969. DHEW Publication No. (NIH) 75-780, National Institutes of Health, Bethesda, Maryland, pp. 44–47 and 91–92.

McLeod, G. R., Beardmore, G. L., Little, J. H., Quinn, R. L., and Davis, N. C. Results of treatment of 361 patients with malignant melanoma in Queensland. Med. J. Aust. 1:1211–1216, 1971.

Moore, C., and Iverson, P. C. Xeroderma pigmentosum: showing common skin cancers plus melanocarcinoma controlled by surgery. Cancer 7:377–382, 1954.

Movshovitz, M., and Modan, B. Role of sun exposure in the etiology of malignant melanoma: epidemiologic inference. J. Natl. Cancer Inst. 51:777–779, 1973.

Pawelek, J. M. Factors regulating growth and pigmentation of melanoma cells. J. Invest. Dermatol. 66:201–209, 1976.

Robbins, J. H., Kraemer, K. H., Lutzner, M. A., Festoff, B. W., and Coon, H. G. Xeroderma pigmentosum: an inherited disease with sun sensitivity, multiple cutaneous neoplasms, and abnormal DNA repair. Ann. Intern. Med. 80:221–248, 1974.

Scotto, J., Kopf, A. W., and Urbach, F. Non-melanoma skin cancer among Caucasians in four areas of the United States. Cancer 34:1333–1338, 1974.

Scotto, J., Fears, T. R., and Gori, G. B. Measurements of Ultraviolet Radiation in the United States and Comparisons with Skin Cancer Data. National Cancer Institute, Division of Cancer Cause and Prevention, National Institutes of Health, DHEW No. (NIH) 76-1039, 1976.

Scotto, J., Fraumeni, J. F., and Lee, J. A. H. Melanomas of the eye and other noncutaneous sites: epidemiologic aspects. J. Natl. Cancer Inst. 56:489–491, 1976.

Snyder, D. S., and May, M. Ability of PABA to protect mammalian skin from ultraviolet light-induced skin tumors and actinic damage. J. Invest. Dermatol. 65:543–546, 1975.

Third National Cancer Survey: Incidence Data. National Cancer Institute Monograph 41. U.S. Department of Health, Education and Welfare, Public Health Service, National Institutes of Health, National Cancer Institute, Bethesda, Maryland. DHEW Publication No. (NIH) 75-787, 1975.

Chapter 3

Classification and Clinical Diagnosis of Cutaneous Malignant Melanomas

PART ONE

Classification of Primary Cutaneous Malignant Melanomas

Primary malignant melanomas can be classified in several principal ways: A) by the clinico-histologic type; B) by the level of invasion; and C) by the thickness of the lesion.

A. CLINICO-HISTOLOGIC TYPES

In recent years, a very useful clinico-histologic classification has been developed (Clark, 1967; McGovern et al., 1967; Clark et al., 1969, 1977; Clark and Mihm, 1969; Mihm et al., 1971; McGovern et al., 1973) which includes the following types of malignant melanomas:

(*1*) *Lentigo Maligna Melanoma*. This type of melanoma begins as a preinvasive lesion that is designated lentigo maligna, circumscribed precancerous melanosis (Dubreuilh), or melanotic freckle (Hutchinson). Such lesions usually occur in the elderly (Fig. 2), but we have seen a patient in his twenties with the condition (Fig. 3). Most melanotic freckles are on the face, but they may occur in any area of the cutaneous surface where there has been excessive sun exposure.

Lentigo maligna usually begins as a small, tan, macular lesion that may easily be confused with an ordinary solar lentigo. Through the years the size of the lesion gradually increases (the so-called "radial-growth phase") and the margins become very irregular. The color modifies so that there are areas of tan and brown and black, and areas of regression occur which may be pinkish or white in color. We have seen at least one instance in which a pink color preceded hyperpigmentation. When dermal invasion, also known as the "vertical-growth phase" occurs, the involved area generally becomes slightly elevated and, on occasion,

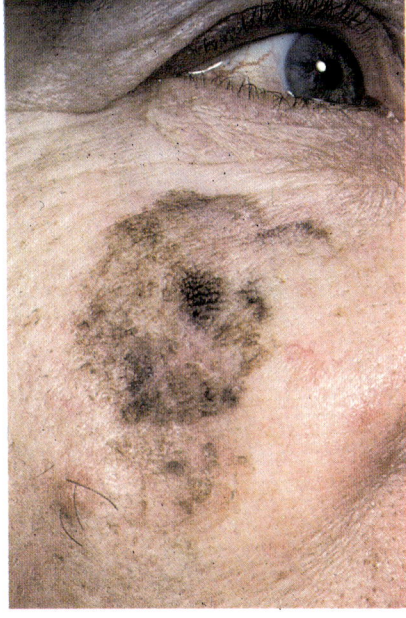

FIGURE 2. *Lentigo maligna* in an elderly person. In addition to tans and browns there is a faint pink background that is especially visible in those areas where partial spontaneous regression has taken place.

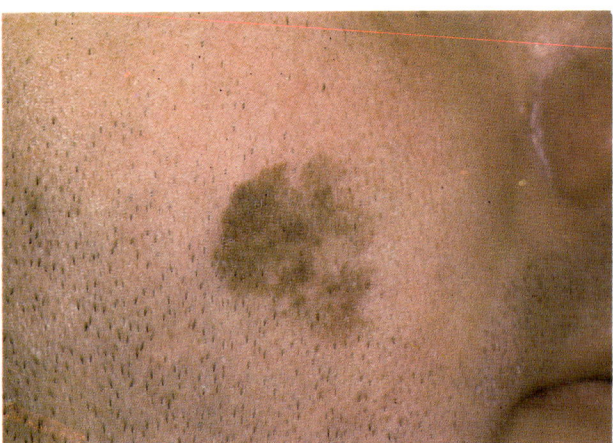

FIGURE 3. **Lentigo maligna** in a 28-year-old man. This lesion was of at least three years' duration. Note the play of colors, particularly the tans and browns, and irregular outline. (Reproduced by permission of Arch. Dermatol. 106:189, 1972). Copyright 1972, American Medical Association.

papular or nodular (Fig. 4). The elevated portion may be darker or lighter than the surrounding non-invasive area.

Histologically, during the lentigo maligna phase, there is an increased number of atypical melanocyic cells individually and/or in clusters in the basal-cell layer of the epidermis (Fig. 5) and in the epithelium of adnexal structures (Fig. 6). Once invasion of the dermis occurs, the lesion acquires the capacity to metastasize and is termed lentigo maligna melanoma. Often the invading malignant melanomatous cells are spindle-shaped.

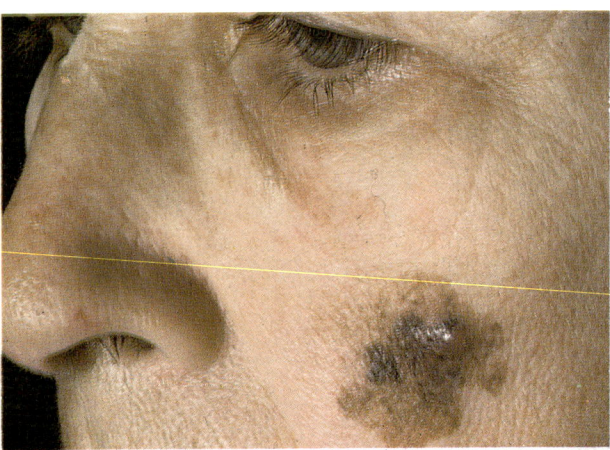

FIGURE 4. **Lentigo maligna melanoma.** Superimposed on this macular, mulicolored, irregularly outlined patch is an elevated papule on the upper-outer quadrant. The histologic features of the papule were those of malignant melanoma of the spindle-cell variety. The histologic features of the radial-growth portion of the rest of this lesion were typical of lentigo maligna.

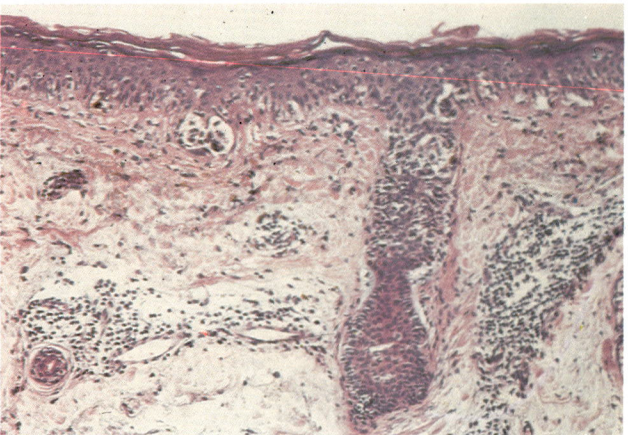

FIGURE 5. Radial-growth component of **lentigo maligna melanoma**. Note the proliferation of atypical melanocytes, singly, and in nests, at the dermoepidermal junction. The atypical cells are also in the walls of the pilar apparatus. H & E stain.

(2) *Superficial Spreading Malignant Melanoma.* This type of malignant melanoma tends to occur in persons younger than those who develop lentigo maligna melanoma. It may develop anywhere on the body but most character-

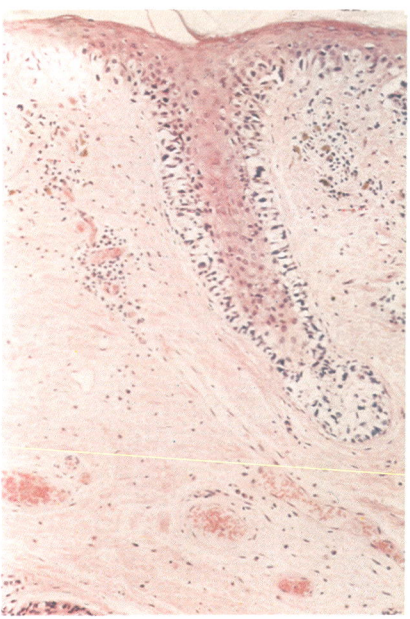

FIGURE 6. **Lentigo maligna.** There is a profusion of atypical melanocytes ("clear cells") at the dermal-epidermal junction and in the peripheral portions of hair follicles. Such melanocytes are precancerous and may extend deeply into the dermis in association with pilar and sweat gland units. H & E stain.

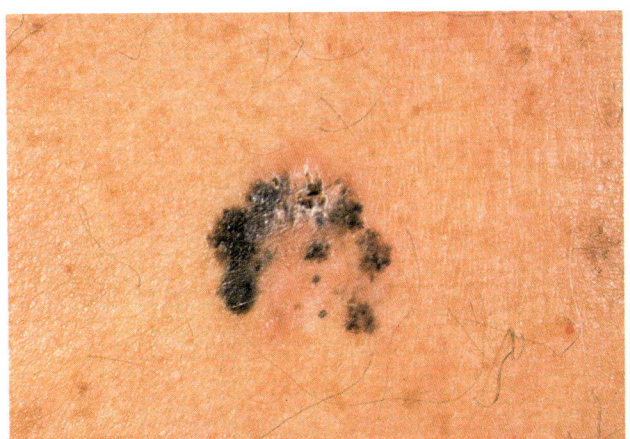

FIGURE 7. **Superficial spreading melanoma.** *This lesion was 2.2 cm in its largest diameter. It shows a combination of features which are typical for superficial spreading melanoma. The edges are barely elevated. There is a play of colors, including shades of tan and brown, and also a combination of red, white, and blue. The edges are irregular in outline and the borders are notched.*

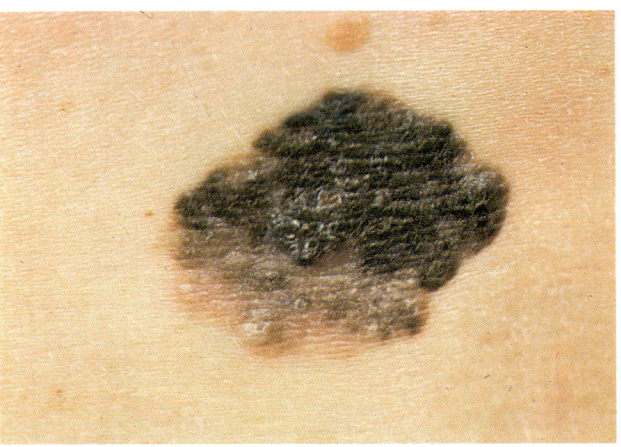

FIGURE 8. **Superficial spreading melanoma.** *This irregularly elevated plaque has some areas of light pigmentation and others in which the hyperpigmentation is quite dark. Unlike most superficial spreading melanomas, this lesion has a regular outline. The largest diameter of this lesion was 3.5 cm.*

istically appears on the upper back in both sexes and on the legs in women. Superficial spreading melanomas tend to be somewhat less irregular in outline than lentigo maligna melanomas. Not infrequently, however, the borders are notched. They tend to be multicolored with shades of brown (tan, light brown, dark brown), grey and black, and combinations of red, white and blue (Fig. 7). Early in their evolution, these lesions may be barely palpable. When they evolve to the vertical-growth phase, papules and nodules appear clinically (Figs. 8 and 9). The epidermal component of these lesions consists of atypical melanocytes similar in their distribution and appearance to the intraepidermal tumor cells found in mammary and extramammary Paget's disease (Fig. 10). The purely intraepidermal phase of such lesions is often preferentially signed out by some pathologists as "atypical melanocytic hyperplasia" rather than malignant melanoma (Fig. 11).

(3) *Nodular Malignant Melanoma.* Such lesions do not have a discernible radial-growth phase, such as is found in lentigo maligna melanoma and superficial spreading malignant melanoma, and therefore there is no so-called "surround component," that is, no intraepidermal growth phase without associated dermal invasion (Fig. 12). Clinically, these lesions appear as nodules or plaques (Fig. 13). Most commonly they are dark brown or black in color, often with a greyish or a bluish cast. Occasionally they are amelanotic (Fig. 14).

(4) *Acral-Lentiginous Melanomas.* These lesions (Mihm et al., 1976; Reed, 1976) occur on the palms, soles,

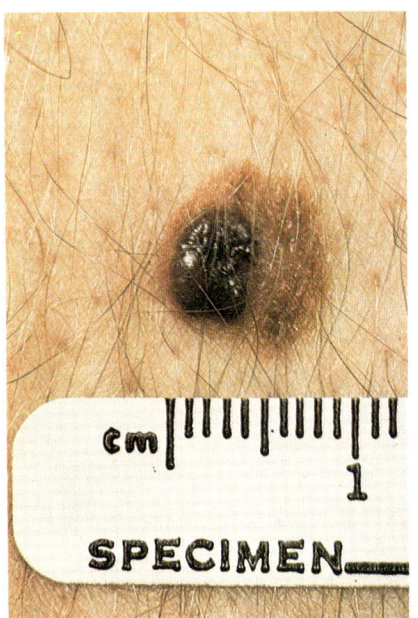

FIGURE 9. **Superficial spreading melanoma.** *This lesion is only 8 mm in its largest diameter. It has both a radial- and vertical-growth phase clinically. It should be emphasized that there are no clinical features that establish or rule out the diagnosis of malignant melanoma. For example, this lesion does not have the colors of red, white and blue typical of superficial spreading melanoma.*

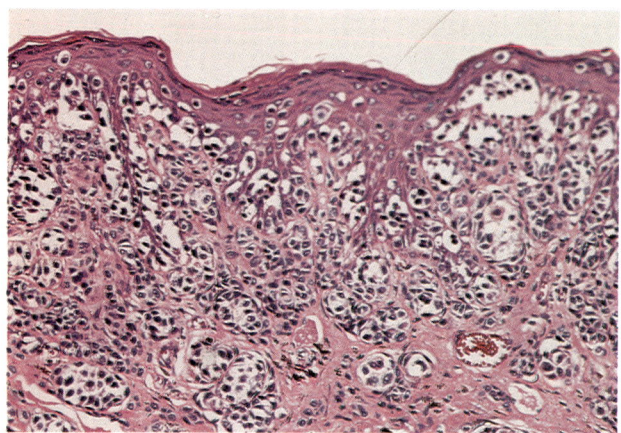

FIGURE 10. **Superficial spreading melanoma, level II.** Note the pagetoid character of the malignant melanoma cells dispersed in the epidermis and morphologically similar cells invading the thickened papillary layer of the cutis. H & E stain.

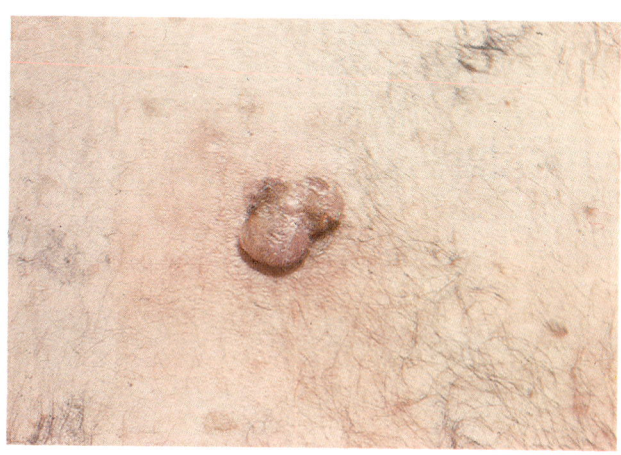

FIGURE 13. **Amelanotic nodular malignant melanoma.** The nature of this lesion is often not discerned clinically because these tumors are not pigmented.

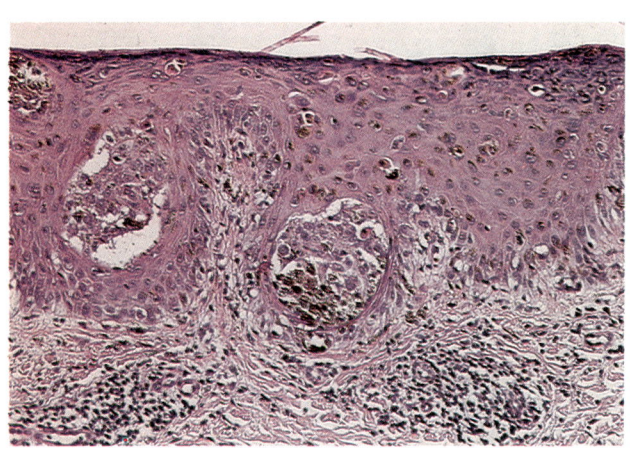

FIGURE 11. Radial-growth component of **superficial spreading melanoma, level I.** Note atypical melanocytes, singly, and in nests, at epidermal-dermal junction as well as in the upper layers of the epidermis. H & E stain.

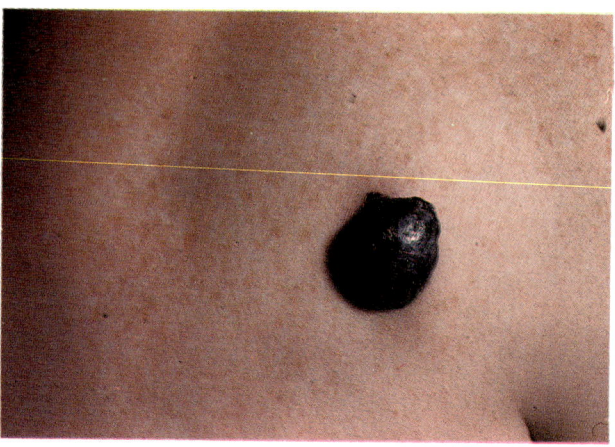

FIGURE 12. **Nodular melanoma.** This lesion appeared on the scapular area in a pregnant woman. Note that there is no "surround component," that is, no radial-growth phase.

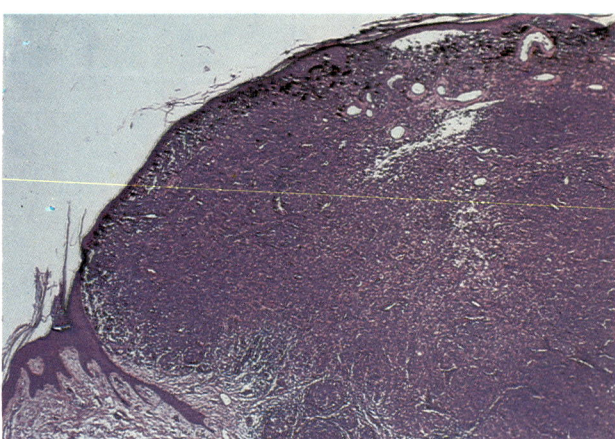

FIGURE 14. **Nodular melanoma.** There is no radial-growth component at the periphery of the specimen. H & E stain.

and terminal phalanges (Fig. 15). In cases involving the digits, lesions may occur peri- and subungually and may be associated with a hyperpigmented and/or distorted nail plate. In the early preinvasive intraepidermal phase of involvement, these lesions may be histologically disarming (Fig. 16). Biopsies from some parts of the lesion may be interpreted by pathologists as "melanocytic hyperplasia, benign" and biopsies from other portions of the lesion as indubitable malignant melanoma (Fig. 17). Sometimes it is only after several biopsies or total excision of the clinically visible lesion that the true nature of such a lesion is determined histologically. Clinically, these neoplasms have features in common with lentigo maligna melanoma, that is, they have similar variations in color and may be entirely macular (Rippey et al., 1975). Like lentigo maligna melanoma and superficial spreading malignant melanoma, acral-lentiginous melanomas eventually develop an invasive vertical-growth phase.

(5) *Malignant Melanomas on Mucous Membranes.* According to Mihm et al. (1975), such lesions occur more frequently in blacks and orientals than in whites, have a worse prognosis than do melanomas occurring in the skin because they are often not diagnosed until they have entered the vertical-growth phase, and have a histologic picture similar to that of lentigo maligna melanoma of the skin, but a biologic behavior similar to that of superficial spreading malignant melanoma. These melanomas may occur in the mouth, nasal cavity, sinuses, vagina or anus. Anorectal melanomas may have histologic features similar to lentigo maligna melanoma, but they behave very aggressively, and the five-year survival rate is less than 10% (Husa and Hockerstedt, 1974).

Bernardino et al. (1976) have recently reviewed 23 conjunctival melanomas using the Clark classification and conclude that the three most common forms of melanoma in the skin (i.e., lentigo maligna melanoma, superficial

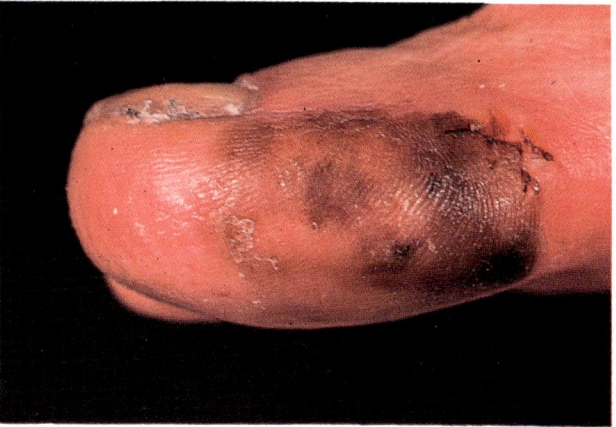

FIGURE 15. **Acral-lentiginous melanoma.** *Several biopsies had to be taken from this lesion before this diagnosis could be established. (For further details see Bart and Kopf, 1977)*

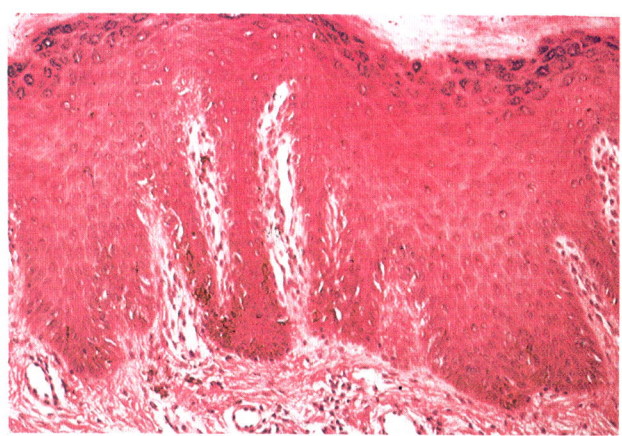

FIGURE 16. **Acral-lentiginous melanoma.** *This photomicrograph illustrates the disarming histologic features of this disorder. Only slight increase in the number of melanocytes at the dermal-epidermal junction is seen. See Figure 15 for the clinical photo.*

FIGURE 17. **Acral-lentiginous melanoma.** *Another biopsy of the same lesion as in Figures 15 and 16 showing nests of atypical melanocytes at the dermal-epidermal junction and in higher levels of the epidermis. Repeated biopsies are important if prior specimens fail to show melanoma in conditions that are still suspicious.*

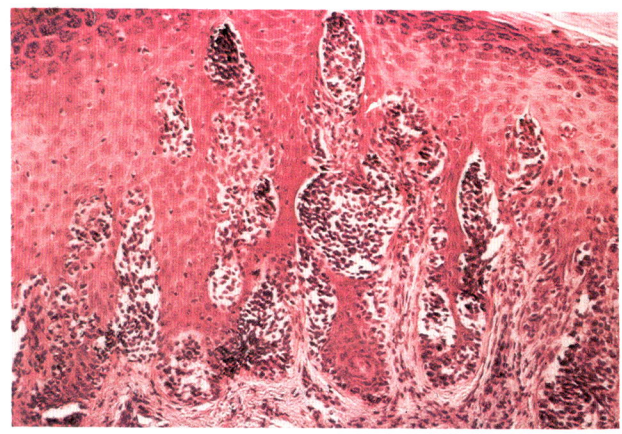

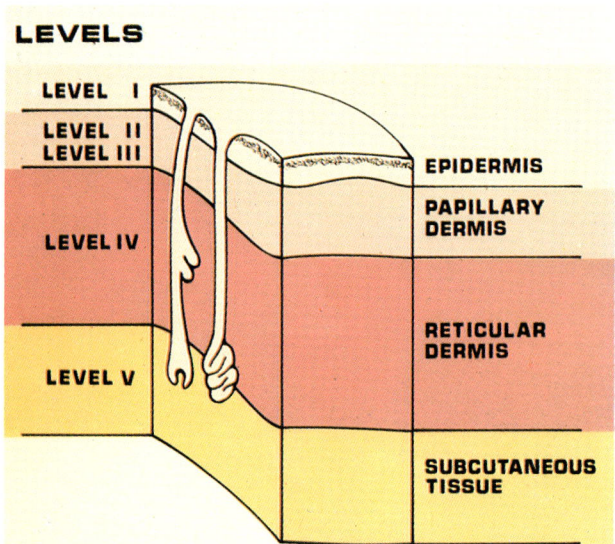

FIGURE 18. *The anatomic landmarks used in the Clark classification of levels of invasion of melanomas are (1) the epidermo-dermal junction, (2) the interface between the papillary and reticular dermis, and (3) the interface between the reticular dermis and the subcutis.*

Level I tumors are entirely intraepidermal, i.e., above the epidermal-dermal junction; level II tumors penetrate into the relatively loosely woven papillary dermis; level III tumors fill the papillary dermis and press on the reticular dermis; level IV tumors penetrate into the reticular dermis; level V tumors invade the subcutis.

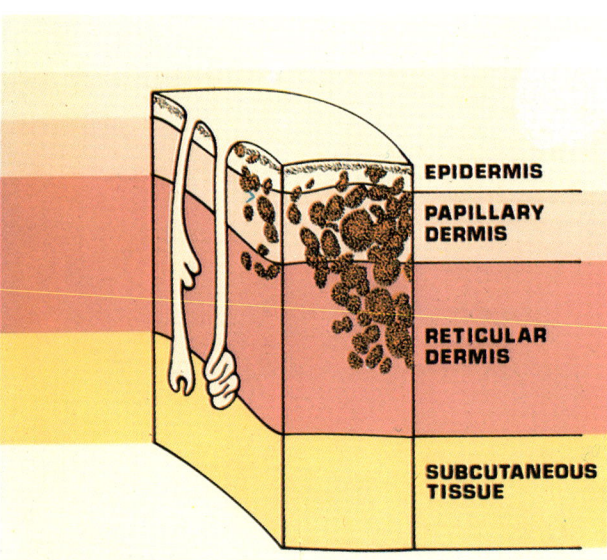

FIGURE 19. *Schematic representation of a level IV melanoma, i.e., the malignant melanoma cells have penetrated the reticular dermis.*

spreading melanoma, and nodular melanoma) can be recognized on conjunctival mucous membranes. Thus, the term "cancerous melanosis," widely used in the ophthalmologic literature (Reese, 1963), is no longer justified. In another publication the same authors (Naidoff et al., 1976) report that lesions involving the eyelid skin and ocular conjunctivae retain the same pathology on both surfaces, i.e., if the cutaneous lesion is a superficial spreading melanoma, so is the conjunctival tumor.

Konigsberg and Gray (1976) reviewed the literature concerning penile melanomas. Of a total of 47 melanomas of penile skin and 13 arising in the urethra, only 6 patients survived longer than 5 years after the diagnosis was made.

Chung et al. (1975) report that malignant melanoma of the vulva is associated with a poor prognosis.

(6) *Miscellaneous.* This group includes malignant melanomas that arise in blue nevi, in congenital and giant nevocytic nevi, in the dermal component of acquired compound and intradermal nevi, in the central nervous system, and in the viscera.

B. LEVEL OF INVASION

The method of Clark depends on using histologic landmarks in order to "level" the depth of invasion (Lund and Ihnen, 1955, Mehnert and Heard, 1965; Clark et al., 1969; Mihm et al., 1971; McGovern et al., 1973; Hermanek et al., 1976; Suffin et al., 1977). Thus, according to the Clark classification, level I designates intraepidermal involvement only, level II designates invasion of the papillary dermis, level III designates filling of the papillary dermis with abutment upon the reticular dermis, level IV designates invasion of the rectricular dermis, and finally, level V designates invasion of the subcutaneous tissues (Figs. 18 and 19).

If one considers only the first three types of malignant melanomas (lentigo maligna melanoma, superficial spreading melanoma, and nodular melanoma), there is not enough information to indicate whether or not there is a difference in prognosis among these types of malignant melanomas *for the same levels of invasion.* It is commonly believed that lentigo maligna melanoma has a better prognosis, level for level, than do the other types of malignant melanomas, but there is so far insufficient data to substantiate this clinical impression. There is sufficient data, however, to support the importance of depth of invasion in the prognosis of malignant melanoma (See Section on Prognosticiation of Behavior of Malignant Melanomas).

The distribution of malignant melanomas by type and by level of invasion in the records of the Malignant Mela-

TABLE 1
Frequency of Various Types of Melanomas*

	Number	Percent
Lentigo Maligna Melanoma	52	4.7
Superficial Spreading Melanoma	777	69.6
Nodular Melanoma	175	15.7
Other	113	10.0
Total	1117	100

*Data from Malignant Melanoma Clinical Cooperative Group, see Appendix.

noma Clinical Cooperative Group as of December 1977 are summarized in Tables 1 and 1A.

C. GREATEST THICKNESS

Another method of classifying the degree of invasion utilizes the greatest thickness of a lesion measured downward from the top of the granular layer of the epidermis to the deepest melanoma cells in the dermis (Breslow, 1970; Hansen and McCarten, 1974; Breslow, 1975, Wanebo et al., 1975; Tonak et al., 1976; Greehoed et al., 1977) (Fig. 20).

In order to properly utilize the Breslow method of classification by thickness of the lesion, step-sections (i.e., multiple blocks cut throughout the primary lesion) are required. Breslow (1976) summarizes the problem as follows, when step-sections are not available:

TABLE 1A
Frequency of Clark's Levels of 1117 Melanomas (%)*

	Lentigo Maligna Melanoma	Superficial Spreading Melanoma	Nodular Melanoma
Level II	46.2	33.2	0.0
Level III	25.0	32.9	33.7
Level IV	17.3	29.6	44.0
Level V	7.7	3.6	20.6
Unknown	3.8	0.6	1.7

*Data from Malignant Melanoma Clinical Cooperative Group, see Appendix.

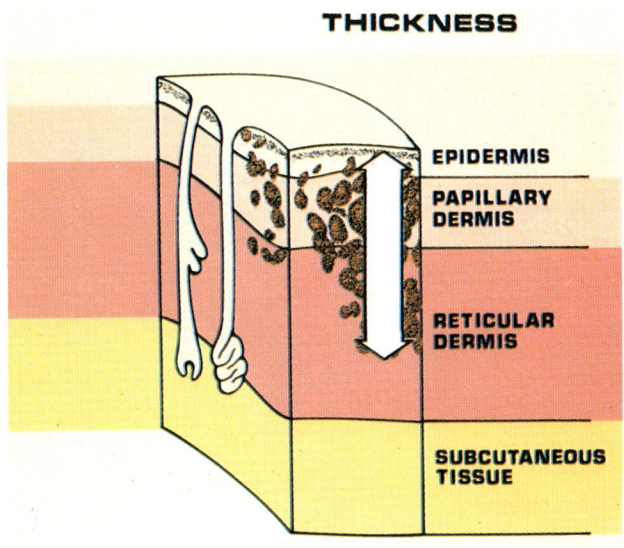

FIGURE 20. *Method used to measure thickness of melanomas. The white double-headed arrow indicates that the measurement is made from the top of the granular layer of the epidermis to the deepest melanoma cells.*

"If it is not possible to obtain all of the tumor, including slides, paraffin blocks and unembedded fixed tissue, the pathologist can only study what is available and indicate that the examination was incomplete. If the tumor is more than 1.50 millimeters thick, there is no problem since the prognosis is poor. If, however, the tumor appears to be thin, there is an insoluble problem and such measurements should not be used to guide treatment."

There is increasing evidence that the two methods of classifying depth of invasion i.e., level and thickness, may be complementary to each other. For example, thick level III lesions have a worse prognosis than thin level III lesions (Breslow, 1975).

Caveats in using thickness as a guide to prognosis include the following: (1) One cannot use this system of measurement for melanomas that show histologic signs of regression (i.e., lesions with areas of normal-appearing epidermis overlying a thickened fibrotic stroma devoid of tumor cells but containing melanophages, lymphocytes, and neovascularization) (Gromet et al., 1978); (2) one must use the thickest portion of the tumor, which means step-sections throughout the lesion; (3) one must avoid processing artifacts (e.g., stretching of tissues during cutting of very thin sections); and (4) one must beware of reading slides which have been cut at a significant angle away from perpendicular to the surface of the skin. For example, a 45° angle off perpendicular can cause a 41% increase in thickness. Nonetheless, using routine histologic material the Breslow method of measuring the thickness of malignant melanomas has greater significance than any other parameter so far determined for stage I malignant melanomas. Currently our pathologists report both level and thickness for all primary melanomas.

In 1976, Hermanek and co-workers published a study of 139 malignant melanomas. They classified the tumors according to histologic types, i.e., lentigo maligna melanomas (12%), superficial spreading malignant melanomas (35%), and nodular melanomas (53%). The melanomas were also classified according to depth of invasion (Clark) and greatest thickness (Breslow). Their conclusion, concerning survival, from this relatively small group of patients (considering the many subclassifications) was that "among tumors of equal depth of invasion the type of melanoma has little prognostic impact. The depth of invasion is decisive for the prognosis." Although the conclusion of these authors may prove to be correct, it is probably premature to assume that the type of melanoma has no prognostic significance, since the number of patients in their study was small.

D. DEGREE OF INFLAMMATORY RESPONSE

Some workers have found that dense lymphocytic infiltration under a malignant melanoma tends to correlate with a better prognosis (Mehnert and Heard, 1965; Little, 1972; Hansen and McCarten, 1974). However, it is not entirely clear whether this somewhat subjective factor might correlate with more objectively measurable factors, such as level of invasion or lesion thickness.

E. OTHER FEATURES USED TO CLASSIFY MALIGNANT MELANOMAS

Additional features which may have prognostic importance are histologic features of the lesion such as vascular involvement, mitoses and polymorphism (polyclonism); clinical features such as color, ulceration, diameter of the lesion, anatomical location; and characteristics of the patient such as age, sex, race and family history of melanoma. (See chapters on Staging and Prognostication of Behavior of Melanomas and on Histology.)

REFERENCES

Bart, R. S., and Kopf, A. W. Tumor Conference #10. A darkly pigmented lesion of the great toe (Acral lentiginous melanoma). J. Derm. Surg. Oncol. 3:158–159, 1977.

Bernardino, V. B., Naidoff, M. A., and Clark, W. H. Malignant melanomas of the conjunctiva. Am. J. Ophthal. 82:383–394, 1976.

Breslow, A. Thickness, cross-sectional areas and depth of invasion in the prognosis of cutaneous melanoma. Ann. Surg. 172:902–908, 1970.

Breslow, A. Tumor thickness, level of invasion and node dissection in stage I cutaneous melanoma. Ann. Surg. 182:572–575, 1975.

Breslow, A. In search of thin lethal melanomas. Surg., Gynec., and Obstet. 143:799, 1976.

Breslow, A. Problems in the measurement of tumor thickness and level of invasion of cutaneous melanoma. Human Path. 8:1–2, 1977.

Chung, A. F., Woodruff, J. M., and Lewis, J. L. Malignant melanoma of the vulva. Obstet. Gynecol. 45:638–646, 1975.

Clark, W. H. A classification of malignant melanoma in man correlated with histogenesis and biological behavior. In Montagna, W., and Hu, F., eds., Advances In Biology of Skin—Volume VIII. The Pigmentary System. Oxford and New York, Pergamon Press, 1967, pgs. 621–647.

Clark, W. H., Jr., From, L., Bernardino, E. H. and Mihm, M. C. The histogenesis and biolgoic behavior of primary human malignant melanomas of the skin. Cancer Res. 29:705–727, 1969.

Clark, W. H., Mestrangelo, M. J., Ainsworth, A. M., Berd, D., Bellet, R. E., and Bernardino, E. A. Current concepts of the biology of human cutaneous malignant melanoma. Adv. Cancer Res. 24:267–338, 1977.

Clark, W. H., and Mihm, M. C. Lentigo maligna and lentigo-maligna melanoma. Am. J. Path. 55:39–67, 1969.

Geehoed, G. W., Breslow, A., and McCune, W. S. Malignant melanoma: Correlation of long-term follow-up with clinical staging, level of invasion and thickness of the primary tumor. Am. Surgeon 43:77–85, 1977.

Gromet, M. A., Sagebiel, R. W., and Epstein, W. L. The regressing thin malignant melanoma: A distinctive lesion with metastatic potential. Cancer 42:2282–2292, 1978.

Hansen, M. G., and McCarten, A. B. Tumor thickness and lymphocytic infiltration in malignant melanoma of the head and neck. Am. J. Surg. 128:557–561, 1974.

Hermanek, P., Hornstein, O. P., Tonak, J., and Weidner, F. Malignant Melanoma. Depth of invasion and histologic typing, Beitr, Pathol. Bd. 157:269–282, 1976.

Husa, A., and Hockerstedt, K. Anorectal malignant melanoma. Acta Chir. Scand. 140:68–72, 1974.

Konigsberg, H. A., and Gray, G. F. Benign melanosis and malignant melanoma of penis and male urethra. Urology 7:323–326, 1976.

Little, J. H. Histology and prognosis in cutaneous malignant melanoma, In: McCarthy, W. H., ed. Melanoma and Skin Cancer, Proceedings of the International Cancer Conference, Sydney, 1972. Sydney, V. C. N. Blight, 1972, pp. 107–120.

Lund, R. H., and Ihned, M. Malignant melanoma. Surgery 38:652–659, 1955.

McGovern, V. J. Malignant Melanoma: Clinical and Histological Diagnosis. New York, Wiley, 1976.

McGovern, V. J., Caldwell, R. A., Duncan, C. A., Finlay-Jones, L. R., Hardy, E. G., Hicks, J. D., Little, J. H., and Quinn, R. L. Moles and malignant melanoma: terminology and classification. Med. J. Aust. 1:123–125, 1967.

McGovern, V. J., and Lane Brown, M. The Nature of Melanoma. Springfield, Illinois, Charles C Thomas, 1969.

McGovern, V. J., Mihm, M. C., Jr., Bailly, C., et al. The classification of malignant melanoma and its histologic reporting. Cancer 32:1446–1457, 1973.

Mehnert, J. H., and Heard, J. L. Staging of malignant melanoma by depth of invasion: a proposed index of prognosis. Am. J. Surg. 110:168–176, 1965.

Mihm, M. C. Jr., Clark, W. H., Jr., and From, L. The clinical diagnosis, classification and histogenetic concepts of the early stages of cutaneous malignant melanoma. N. Engl. J. Med. 284:1078–1082, 1971.

Mihm, M. C. Jr., Clark, W. H. Jr., and Reed, R. J. The clinical diagnosis of malignant melanoma. Semin. Oncol. 2:105–118, 1975.

Mishima, Y., and Matsunaka, M. Pagetoid premalignant melanosis and melanoma: Differentiation from Hutchinson's melanotic freckle. J. Invest. Derm. 65:434–440, 1975.

Naidoff, M. A., Bernardino, V. B., and Clark, W. H.: Melanocytic lesions of the eyelid skin. Am. J. Ophthal. 82:371–382, 1976.

Reed, R. J. Acral lentiginous melanoma. In: New Concepts in Surgical Pathology of the Skin. New York, Wiley, 1976, pp. 89–90.

Reese, A. B. Tumors of the Eye, ed. 2, New York, Harper and Row, 1963, pg. 335–345.

Rippey, J. J., Rippey, E., and Giraud, R. M. A. Pathology of malignant melanoma of the skin in black Africans. South Afr. Med. J. 49:789–792, 1975.

Suffin, S. C., Waisman, J., Clark, W. H., and Morton, D. L. Comparison of the classification by microscopic level (stage) of malignant melanoma by three independent groups of pathologists. Cancer 40:3112–3114, 1977.

Tonak, J., Hermanek, P., Hornstein, O. P., and Weidner, F. Therapie des malignen Melanomes der klinischen Stadien I und II. Dtsch. Med. Wochenschr. 101:435–440, 1976.

Wanebo, H. J., Woodruff, J. and Fortner, J. G. Malignant melanoma of the extremities: a clinicopathologic study using levels of invasion (microstage). Cancer 35:666–676, 1975.

PART TWO
Clinical Diagnosis of Cutaneous Malignant Melanomas

The diagnosis of primary cutaneous malignant melanoma is suggested by the appearance of the lesion, together with a history of change in a preexisting nevus or in a newly acquired pigmented lesion. Suspicious changes include changes in color, size, shape, surface characteristics, surrounding skin, and consistency, and the development of symptoms. Tables 2 and 2A summarize these changes.

In order to help make the diagnosis of malignant melanoma early, Mihm and Fitzpatrick (1976) stress a systematic approach to examination of the entire cutaneous surface, specifically the scalp, head and neck, visible mucosal surfaces, extremities, interdigital spaces, palms and soles, nails, trunk, genitalia and intertrigenous areas. Davis et al. (1976) suggest examining each lesion carefully with a magnifying lens in a good light, especially since minute appearance is often highly suggestive even when the patient reports no obvious change in a lesion to his observation. Primary cutaneous malignant melanoma occurs in several principal forms, namely, superficial spreading melanoma (SSM), lentigo maligna melanoma (LMM), nodular melanoma (NM), and acral-lentiginous melanoma. Superficial spreading melanoma is the most common type and may occur anywhere on the body. Nodular melanoma is less

TABLE 2*
Color, Border and Surface Changes That May Be Found In Primary Malignant Melanomas

Color
Irregularities of color with various shades of tan, brown and black, plus

Red	White	Blue
Reddish-blue (purple)	Whitish-gray	Blue
Reddish-brown	Whitish-pink	Bluish-red (violaceous)
		Bluish-gray
		Bluish-black

Border
Irregularities of the border
Notching or indentation
Pigment streaming from edge of lesion

Surface
Irregularities of surface elevations
 Loss of skin markings
 Hyperkeratosis (various degrees)
 Erosions and ulcerations

* Adapted from Mihm et al. (1973, 1975).

TABLE 2A*

Danger Signals Suggestive of Malignant Transformation in Pigmented Nevi

(a) *Change in color:* Especially red, white and blue; sudden darkening, especially shades of dark brown or black; spread of pigmentation from the periphery into previously apparently normal skin.
(b) *Change in size:* Especially sudden enlargement.
(c) *Change in surface characteristics.* Especially scaliness, erosion, oozing, crusting, bleeding, ulceration or development of a mushrooming mass on the surface of the lesion.
(d) *Change in consistency:* Especially softening or friability.
(e) *Change in symptomatology:* Especially a sense of pruritus, tenderness or pain.
(f) *Change in shape:* Especially rapid elevation from a previously flat condition.
(g) *Change in surrounding skin:* Especially signs of inflammation with redness or swelling or appearance of satellite pigmentations.

* From Gumport et al. (1974).

TABLE 3*

Anatomical Distribution of Cutaneous Melanomas by Sex

Site	Males (%)	Females (%)
Head and Neck	21.0	17.9
Face	11.1	11.1
Neck	4.2	6.0
Ear	2.7	0.3
Scalp	3.1	0.5
Trunk	47.0	19.3
Chest	7.6	3.2
Back	35.6	15.1
Buttock	0.6	0.5
Abdomen	3.3	0.6
Lower Extremity	19.3	38.7
Thigh	7.8	6.9
Leg	9.2	28.5
Foot:	0.8	2.0
Dorsum		
Plantar	1.1	0.8
Subungual	0.4	0.5
Upper Extremity	12.7	24.2
Arm	8.4	16.4
Forearm	3.3	6.6
Hand:	0.6	0.5
Dorsum		
Palm	0.0	0.3
Subungual	0.4	0.5

* Adapted from Davis et al. (1976).

common: it too may occur anywhere on the skin. Lentigo maligna melanoma is uncommon and is found most frequently on sun-exposed areas of the body (especially the face) of elderly individuals. Acral-lentiginous melanomas are rare palmar, plantar, and periungual lesions (Mihm et al., 1975; Davis et al., 1976). The anatomical distribution of malignant melanomas differs somewhat in the sexes. Males usually show a preponderance of such lesions on the trunk whereas females have more of them on the lower extremities. Table 3 summarizes the anatomical distribution of malignant melanomas in more than 1500 patients studied in Queensland.

Primary malignant melanomas of the superficial spreading and lentigo maligna types have characteristic biphasic growth patterns. The initial radial-growth (horizontal) phase is usually prolonged (up to four decades in the case of lentigo maligna) and is rarely, if ever, associated with metastases. Ideally, it is during this phase that these neoplasms should be diagnosed, because surgical cure is then more likely. When they become more deeply invasive (vertical-growth phase) a significant propensity for the development of metastases supervenes (Clark et al., 1975). Acral-lentiginous melanoma is a special biologic form of the disease also characterized by a radial-growth phase followed by a vertical-growth phase with great potential for metastases (Clark et al., 1975).

Superficial spreading melanoma usually begins as a small, brown, mole-like lesion with eventual irregular, variegated coloration in shades of red, white and/or blue within and about a brown or a black lesion (Figs. 21 and 22).

Nordlund (1975) states that the reddish hues are indicative of vascular dilation secondary to the inflammation which often accompanies melanomas and/or to high concentrations of phaeomelanins. The appearance of a gray-white area within the center of a pigmented lesion should arouse strong suspicion, as should the finding of an irregular, asymmetrical, leukodermatous halo surrounding a pigmented lesion. Irregularities or notching in the border, which became more marked as the lesion increases in size, are characteristic. Irregularities in the surface are accentuated by side lighting and may be marked by focal or diffuse hyperkeratosis. Absence of normal skin markings may also be found (Mihm et al., 1973, 1975; Mihm and Fitzpatrick, 1976). Eventually, one or more papules or nodules appear on the surface heralding the vertical-growth phase (Figs. 23, 24, and 25).

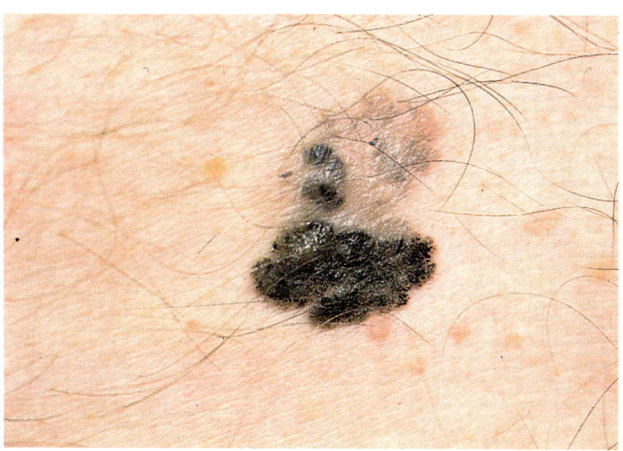

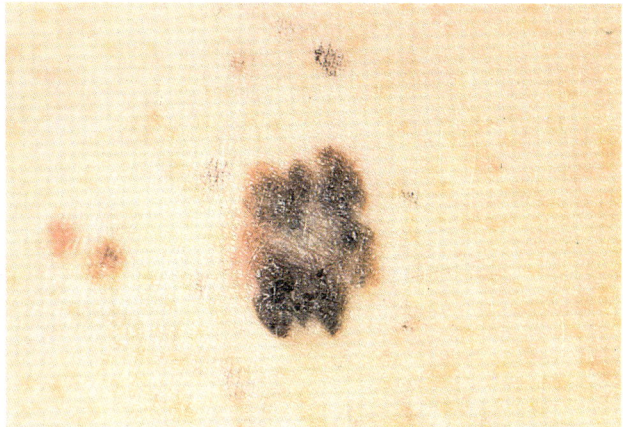

FIGURE 23. **Superficial spreading melanoma** with a large area of spontaneous partial regression. The play of colors helps in making this diagnosis.

FIGURE 21. **Superficial spreading melanoma.** This lesion shows the typical notched border, central spontaneous involution and shades of tan and dark brown. There was no distinct erythema in this lesion.

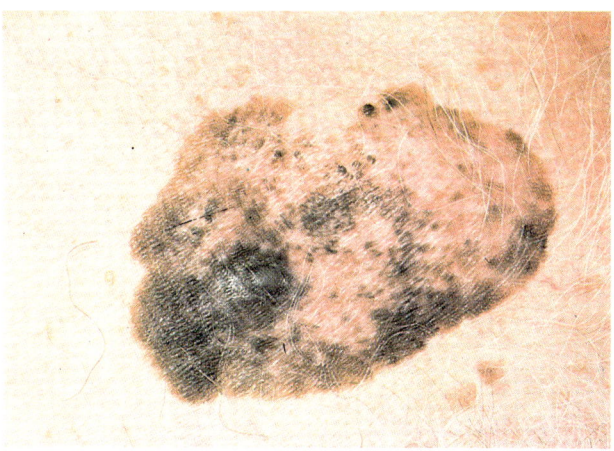

FIGURE 24. **Superficial spreading melanoma.** The largest diameter of this lesion was 8 cm. Note the radial-growth phase with the play of colors and erythematous blush. There is a notched border and the edges are barely elevated. A bluish nodule is present near the left edge.

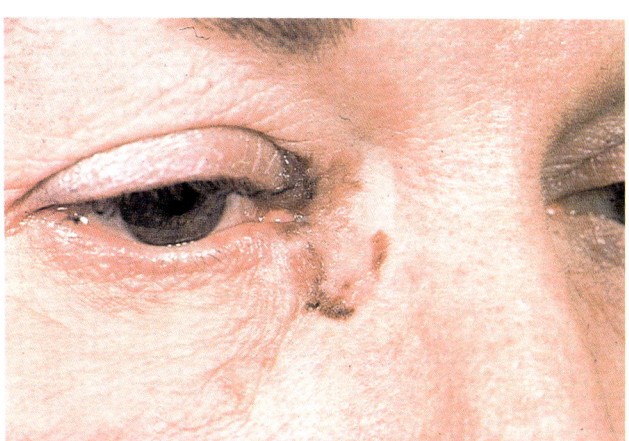

FIGURE 22. **Superficial spreading melanoma** in an inner canthus. This lesion is a difficult therapeutic problem because of its anatomic location.

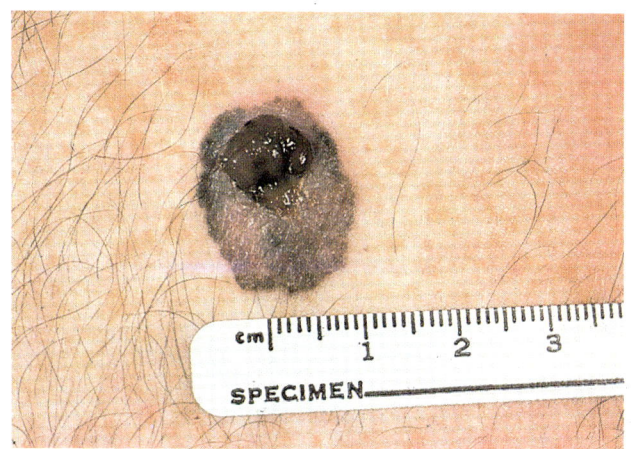

FIGURE 25. **Superficial spreading melanoma.** Once again, note the play of colors including red and various shades of tan, brown and blue. It is the combination of growth patterns, colors, surface characteristics, and symptomatology which leads the physician to make the clinical diagnosis of malignant melanoma.

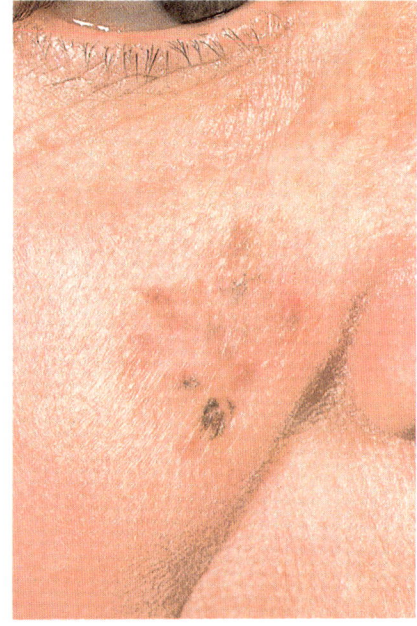

FIGURE 26. **Early lentigo maligna.** This lesion most often occurs on the cheek. There are some areas of spontaneous regression scattered throughout this pigmented patch.

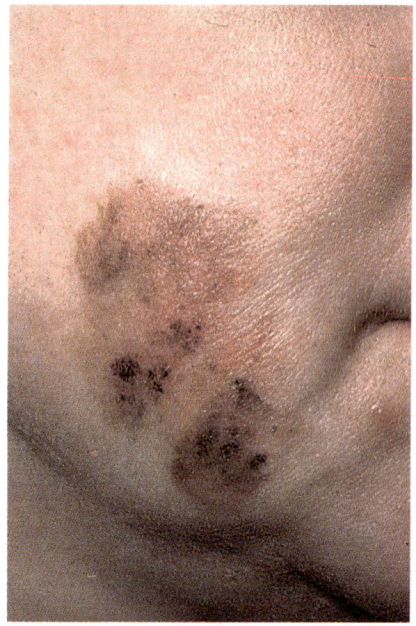

FIGURE 27. **Lentigo maligna.** The erythematous component in this lesion is more developed than in Fig. 26. Once again, notice the irregular outline and the play of colors.

Lentigo maligna, the precursor of lentigo maligna melanoma, begins as a flat, tan, to dark brown lesion, usually macular, and resembling a stain on the skin. A play of colors is usual even in small lesions (Figs. 26, 27, 28 and 29). It is found almost exclusively on sun-exposed surfaces of the body, especially on the face in elderly persons. After a radial-growth phase of many years (often decades) during which time the lesion usually increases in size progressively and may exhibit irregularities in color, one or more papules or nodules develop, which may be brown, black, blue-black or, rarely, amelanotic, signifying the clinical onset of invasive melanoma, i.e., lentigo maligna melanoma (Fig. 30). The surface overlying these nodules may be scaly, shiny, hyperkeratotic, eroded or ulcerated (Sulzberger et al., 1959;

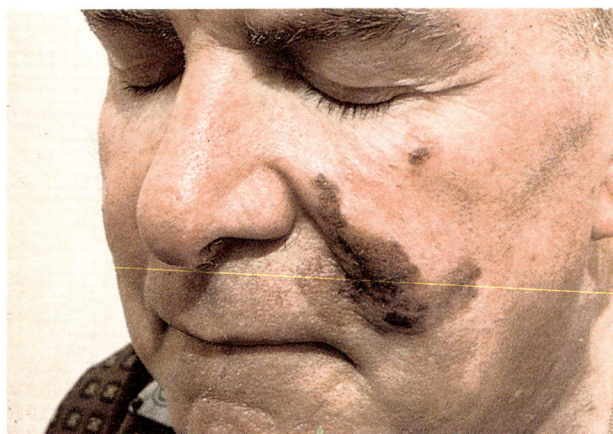

FIGURE 28. **Lentigo maligna.** This lesion was one of many years' duration. No papules or nodules had developed on the surface of this lesion at the time this photograph was taken. Histologically, the atypical melanocytic hyperplasia was confined to the dermal-epidermal junction and to the periphery of the adnexal structures.

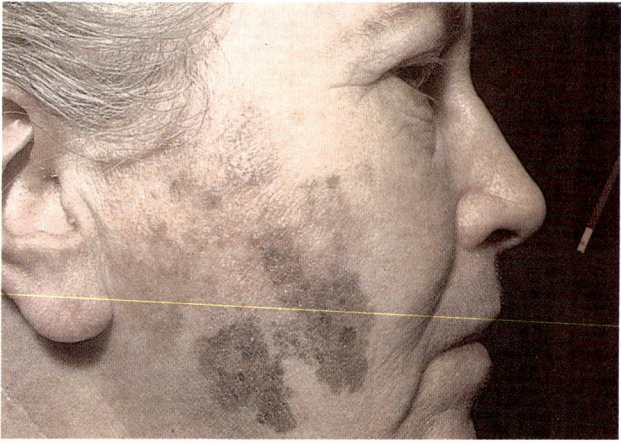

FIGURE 29. **Lentigo maligna melanoma.** Multiple biopsies of this tumor were performed. Only one showed dermal invasion (in the scaly area on the malar region). Reprinted from Arch. Dermatol. 106:189, 1972. Copyright 1972, American Medical Association.

FIGURE 30. *This large* **lentigo maligna melanoma** *shows a play of colors including tans, dark browns and pinks with areas of spontaneous regression resulting in leukodermatous patches. On the lower medial quadrant there is a raised nodule with a bloody crust on its surface.*

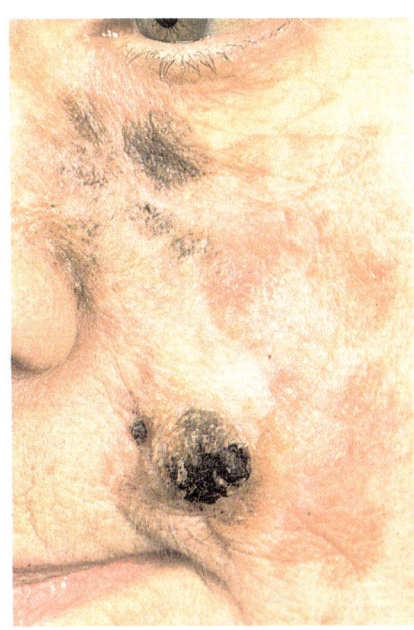

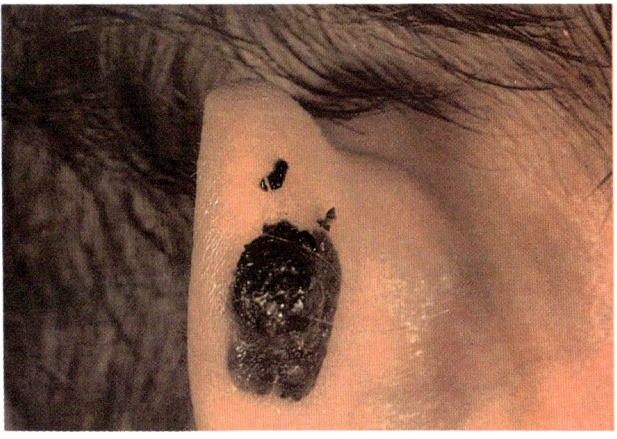

FIGURE 31. **Nodular melanoma** *with a satellite on the posterior aspect of the pinna.*

Mihm et al., 1975; Mihm and Fitzpatrick, 1976). However, Gromet (1977) points out that clinically lentigo maligna melanoma can present as a completely macular lesion.

Nodular melanoma has no clinically discernible radial-growth phase but is first observed as a reddish-blue or blue-black papule, or nodule which enlarges rapidly (Fig. 31). Amelanotic nodular melanoma may be completely free of pigment but often exhibits a tinge of grayish-blue or blue-black or flecks of black at its base. It may also present itself as a blue-black raised plaque (Figs. 32 and 33). It is usually dome-shaped but may have a polypoidal shape (Fig. 34). The surface may be perfectly smooth or may be eroded or ulcerated. The lesion may arise in association with a

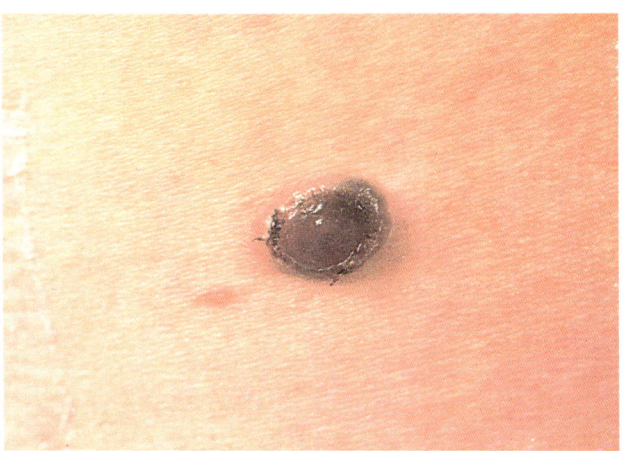

FIGURE 32. **Nodular melanoma.** *The surface of this lesion is denuded and has bled. Bleeding is an important clue to invasive malignant melanoma.*

FIGURE 33. **Nodular melanoma.** *This large lesion has an ulcerated surface. Note the deeply melanotic and the amelanotic portions of this tumor.*

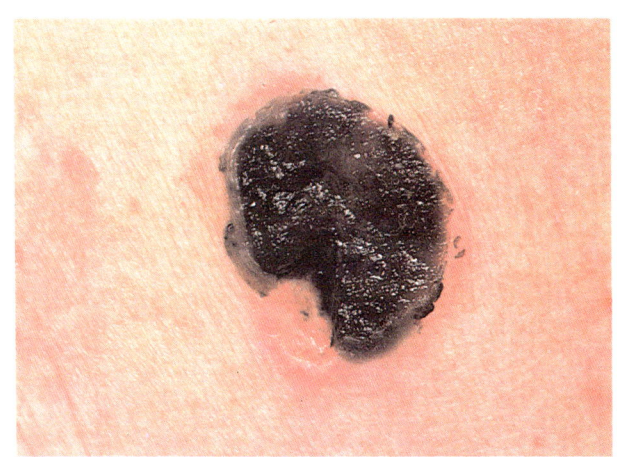

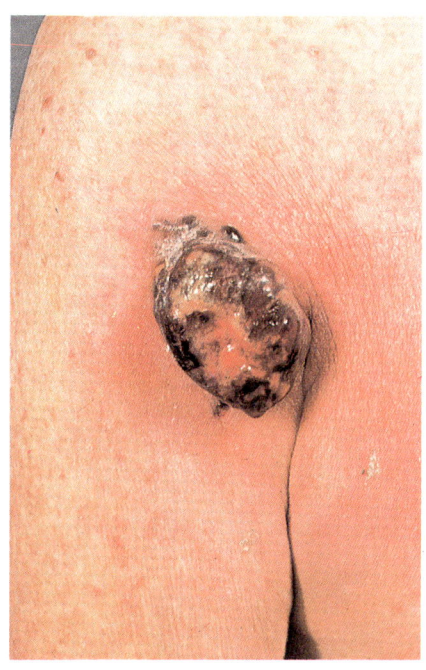

FIGURE 34A. **Nodular melanoma.** *This is an advanced lesion with poor prognosis.*

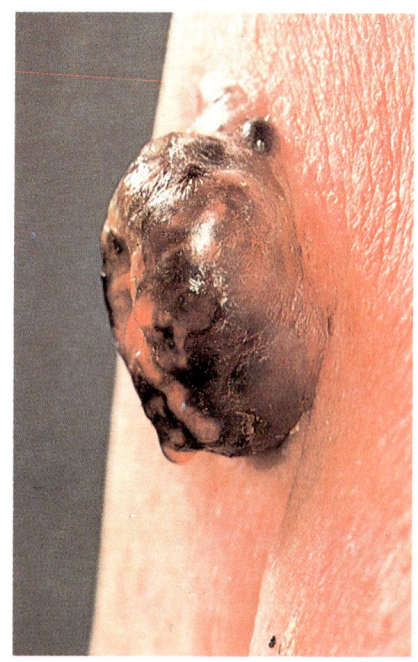

FIGURE 34B. **Nodular melanoma.** *Side view of Fig. 34A to show the marked elevation of this sessile mass.*

preexistent mole, but, in most instances, begins in normal-appearing skin (Mihm et al., 1975; Mihm and Fitzpatrick, 1976; Davis et al., 1976).

Melanomas of the palms and soles also display the characteristic color changes and irregularities of surface already mentioned (Figs. 35 and 36). On the soles, melanomas may exhibit only slight elevation and hyperkeratosis, may be barely palpable, and yet be deeply invasive. In blacks, the palms and soles are favored sites for melanomas (Giraud et al., 1975). Subungual melanomas usually appear as streaks of hyperpigmentation (tan, brown, blue-black) beneath the nail plate (Fig. 37). At times they may also appear as deformed or split nails or as paronychias. (See chapter on Subungual Melanoma for further details.)

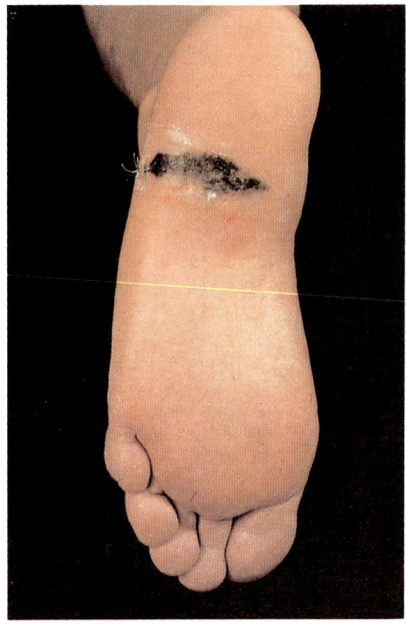

FIGURE 35A. **Acral - lentiginous melanoma.** *This lesion presents a difficult therapeutic problem.*

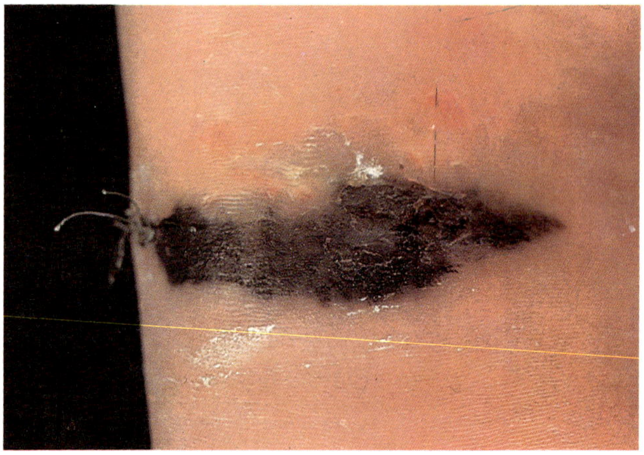

FIGURE 35B. **Acral-lentiginous melanoma.** *An incisional biopsy was performed from the edge of this lesion.*

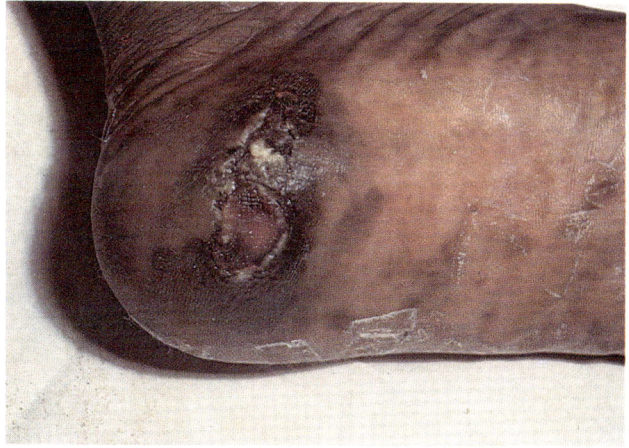

FIGURE 36. **Acral-lentiginous melanoma.** *The sole is a common site for primary malignant melanomas in blacks.*

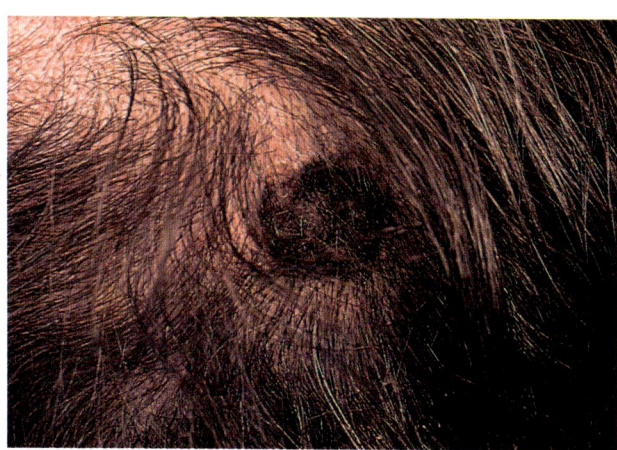

FIGURE 38. **Malignant melanoma on the scalp.** *Lesions in this site are often diagnosed late because they are obscured by the hair.*

With regard to the sizes of these lesions, lentigo maligna may attain diameters of 5 to 7 cm before the vertical-growth phase begins. Superficial spreading melanomas average about 2.5 cm in diameter by the time patients seek medical attention. Nodular melanomas may be of almost any size. Mihm and Fitzpatrick (1976) state that acquired pigmented moles usually attain a diameter of less than 10 mm. Any acquired lesion exceeding that width should alert the physician to the possibility of a malignant melanoma. Clark (1976) comments that any pigmented lesion that can be covered by the unused eraser of an ordinary pencil is likely to be benign or is a curable form of melanoma (except for the uncommon nodular malignant melanoma). He believes more attention should be paid to those lesions larger than such an eraser (7 mm). All investigators agree, however, that if question or suspicion exists concerning any lesion, regardless of size, a biopsy should be performed.

Malignant melanomas on the scalp often go unnoticed because they are obscured by the hair (Fig. 38). Examination of the scalp for pigmented lesions should be a routine part of the physical examination of every patient since such lesions have a poor prognosis.

Malignant melanoma metastases may be regional and/or extraregional. Regional metastasis is defined as the spread of the malignancy from the primary site to the lymph nodes draining the area or to tissues between the primary site and the regional lymph nodes. Extraregional metastasis is defined as the spread of the malignancy beyond the draining nodes. At the N.Y.U. Medical Center other terms used to indicate persistent disease are: *local recurrence,* the malignant process reappearing at the primary site or in the scar of its excision or graft; *satellitosis,* a cutaneous or subcutaneous spread of the malignant process within 5 cm (some say 3 cm) of the primary site or surgical scars of excision of lesions; *in-transit metastasis,* a cutaneous or subcutaneous spread of malignancy more than 5 cm beyond the primary site or local surgical scars in the direction of but not beyond the regional lymph nodes.

Examples of metastases of malignant melanomas are shown in Figs. 39 to 42.

Rarely, the entire cutaneous surface can become diffusely hyperpigmented in patients who have undiagnosed metastatic malignant melanoma (Silberberg et al., 1968).

For a discussion of sites of extraregional metastases of malignant melanomas, the reader is referred to Chapter 12.

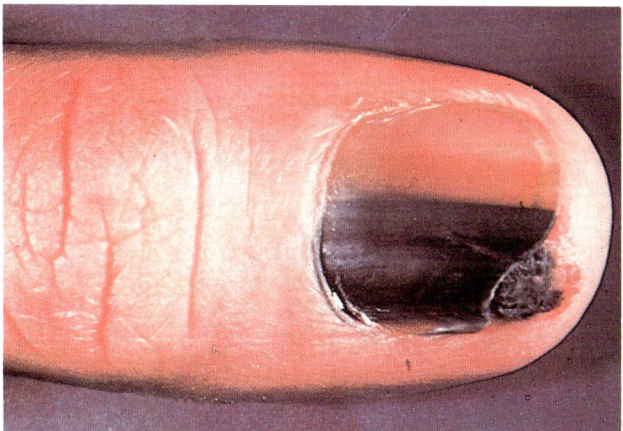

FIGURE 37. **Subungual malignant melanoma.** *Notice the spread of pigment onto the fingertip. Periungual spread of pigment is called Hutchinson's sign. This sign aids in the differential diagnosis between this condition and subungual nevocytic nevi.*

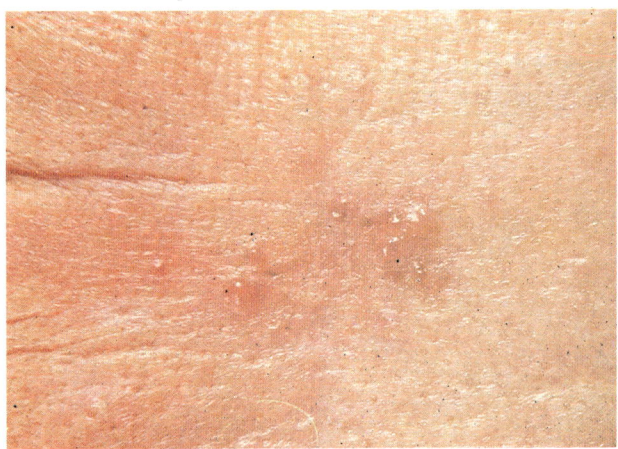

FIGURE 39. *Local recurrence and early satellitosis of amelanotic malignant melanoma of forehead.* Lesions are confined to the primary site and to a zone of skin less than 5 cm in diameter about the primary site.

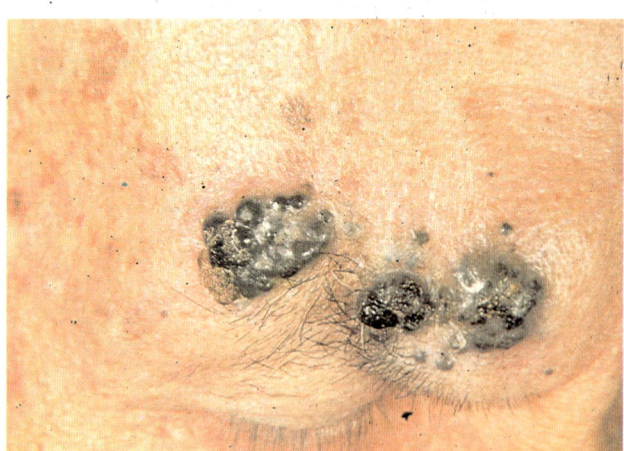

FIGURE 40. *Local recurrence of malignant melanoma with satellitosis.*

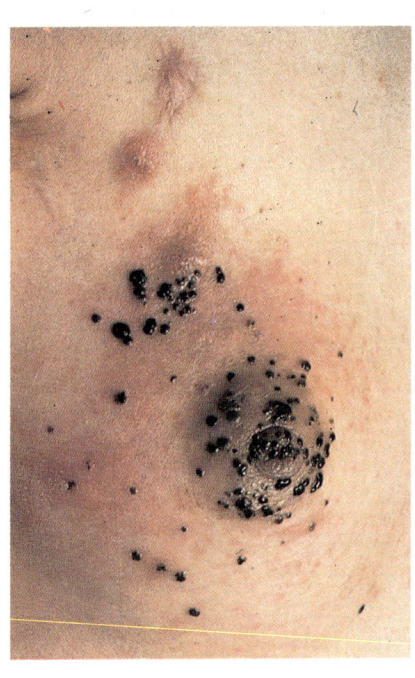

FIGURE 41. *Malignant melanoma mestastatic to the breast.* There are numerous deeply pigmented metastases involving the nipple, areola and surrounding mammary tissue. Note the marked inflammatory reaction to the tumor.

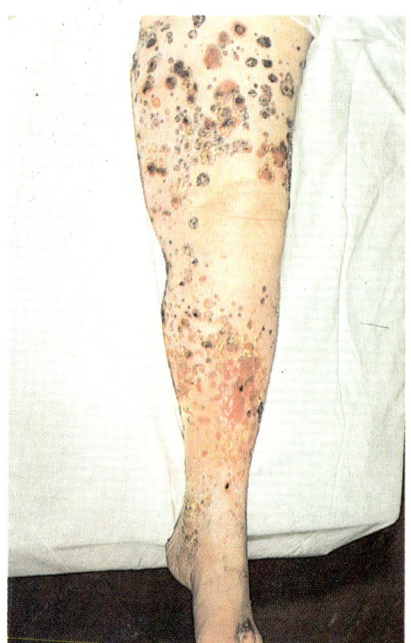

FIGURE 42. *In-transit metastatic malignant melanoma.* Note the diffuse involvement of the lower limb.

DIFFERENTIAL DIAGNOSIS

The differential diagnosis of malignant melanoma includes many benign pigmented lesions and several premalignant and malignant lesions. Junction nevi, compound nevi, intradermal nevi, benign juvenile melanomas (Spitz), halo nevi and blue nevi are all benign lesions that can mimic malignant melanomas. Recently the neologism "pseudomelanoma" has been suggested to describe a recurrent nevocytic nevus following its partial removal (Kornberg and Ackerman, 1975). The clinical and histologic features of such lesions can mimic malignant melanomas. It is essential that the original biopsy specimen be reexamined in all recurrent nevi since we are unaware of a previously, histologically proved, benign nevocytic nevus that subsequently gave rise to a malignant melanoma. The difference between benign pigmented lesions and malignant pigmented lesions can be summarized according to Mihm et al. (1975) by noting that malignant pigmented lesions exhibit disorder and benign pigmented ones usually show order in color, symmetry of border, and uniformity of surface characteristics. As noted above, benign acquired pigmented nevi usually have a maximum diameter of less than 10 mm.

Pigmented basal-cell carcinomas may appear very similar to both superficial spreading melanomas and nodular melanomas. Side-lighting of such basal-cell carcinomas may reveal a peripheral ring of small nodules that are not found in melanomas. Careful inspection will usually reveal telangiectasia over and between the nodules. Solidly pigmented basal-cell carcinomas are rare in light-eyed individuals; melanomas occur in persons of any eye color (Bart and Schnall, 1973). A solidly pigmented malignant lesion in a patient with blue, gray or green eyes, is more likely to be a malignant melanoma than a basal-cell carcinoma. Sometimes only the biopsy will yield the correct diagnosis (Mihm et al., 1975; Kopf et al., 1975; Davis et al., 1976).

Pigmented seborrheic keratosis may resemble any type of malignant melanoma. These lesions usually appear waxy and may have comedo-like keratin plugs. Their colors range from light to dark brown. The lesions often have a "stuck-on" appearance and are friable, allowing them to be "picked off." This latter feature is important; melanomas do not feel as if they can be "picked off" the skin, but seem to be an intrinsic part of it (Mihm et al., 1975; Davis et al., 1976).

Pigmented actinic keratoses can be differentiated from lentigo maligna or lentigo maligna melanoma because the surface of an actinic keratosis feels rough due to the associated hyperkeratosis. The borders of actinic keratoses are usually not as irregular as in lentigo maligna (Mihm et al., 1975).

Granuloma pyogenicum may have to be differentiated from amelanotic nodular melanoma. A granuloma pyogenicum may grow more rapidly than melanoma. However, it does not exhibit the blue-black flecks usually found at the base of an amelanotic nodular melanoma (Mihm et al., 1975; Davis et al., 1976).

Capillary hemangiomas, dermatofibromas and hemorrhage into a cyst, nevus or nail bed may also present a problem in diagnosis (Kopf et al., 1975). Solar lentigo may be difficult to differentiate from lentigo maligna. Usually the color is more uniform and the perimeter more regular in a solar lentigo.

At times the differential diagnosis between pigmented Bowen's disease (especially in the genital and perianal areas) and malignant melanoma can be difficult clinically.

SUMMARY AND DISCUSSION

To diagnose malignant melanoma clinically one must have a high index of suspicion about any pigmented lesion, and be aware of the colors, irregularities in border, and surface characteristics associated with malignant melanomas, especially if seen in acquired lesions greater than 10 mm in diameter.

Biopsy, preferably excisional, should be performed on all suspicious pigmented lesions displaying variegated colors (especially shades of red, white, and blue, including blue-black, blue-gray, blue-red) particularly if there is also an irregular border, and/or an irregular surface.

The differential diagnosis includes both benign and malignant lesions. Biopsy should be performed if any question exists as to the clinical diagnosis.

All physicians should develop a high degree of suspicion for cutaneous malignant melanoma since such lesions are usually curable in their early phases of development. Suspicion should be translated into action for any lesion suggestive of malignant melanoma. It is highly likely that the death rate from malignant melanomas could be substantially lowered if the medical profession and the public were made aware of the clinical features suggesting early melanoma.

REFERENCES

Bart, R. S., and Schnall, S. Eye color in darkly pigmented basal-cell carcinomas and malignant melanomas: an aid in their clinical differentiation. Arch. Dermatol. 107:206–207, 1973.

Clark, W. H., Jr. Clinical diagnosis of cutaneous malignant melanoma. J.A.M.A. 236:484–485, 1976.

Clark, W. H., Jr., Ainsworth, A. M., Barnardino, E. A., Yang, C. H., Mihm, M. C., Jr., and Reed, R. J. The developmental biology of primary human malignant melanomas. Semin. Oncol. 2:83–103, 1975.

Davis, N. C., McLeod, G. R., Beardmore, G. L., Little J. H., Quinn, R. L., and Holt, J. Primary cutaneous melanoma: a report from the Queensland melanoma project. CA 26:80–107, 1976.

Giraud, R. M. A., Rippey, E., and Rippey, J. J. Malignant melanoma of the skin in black africans. South Afr. Med. J. 49:665–668, 1975.

Gromet, M. A. Treatment of lentigo maligna. Arch. Dermatol. 113:1128, 1977.

Gumport, S. L., Harris, M. N., and Kopf, A. W. Diagnosis and management of common skin cancers. CA 24:218–228, 1974.

Kopf, A. W., Mintzis, M., and Bart, R. S. Diagnostic accuracy in malignant melanoma. Arch. Dermatol. 111:1291–1292, 1975.

McGovern, V. J. Malignant Melanoma: Clinical and Histological Diagnosis. New York, Wiley, 1976.

Mihm, M. C., Jr., and Fitzpatrick, T. B. Early detection of malignant melanoma. Cancer 37:597–603, 1976.

Mihm, M. C., Jr., Fitzpatrick, T. B., Lane Brown, M. M., Raker, J. W., Malt, R. A., and Kaiser, J. S. Early detection of primary cutaneous malignant melanoma. A color atlas. N. Engl. J. Med. 289:989–996, 1973.

Mihm, M. C., Jr., Clark, W. H., Jr., and Reed, R. J. The clinical diagnosis of malignant melanoma. Semin. Oncol. 2:105–118, 1975.

Nordlund, J. J. Yale J. Biol. Med. 48:403–407, 1975.

Silberberg, I., Kopf, A. W., and Gumport, S. L. Diffuse melanosis in malignant melanoma. Arch. Derm. 97:671–677, 1968.

Sulzberger, M. B., Kopf, A. W., and Witten, V. H. Pigmented nevi, benign juvenile melanoma and circumscribed precancerous melanosis. Postgrad. Med. 26:617–631, 1959.

Chapter 4

The Histology of Cutaneous Malignant Melanoma

A. Bernard Ackerman M.D. and W. P. Daniel Su M.D.*

I. HISTORICAL REVIEW

A. Early Literature

Pigmented malignant neoplasms of the skin have been clinically recognized since ancient times, but meaningful histologic descriptions of them have been made only recently. What follows is based mainly on our review of the English literature.

Hippocrates, in the 5th century B.C., is said to have been the first physician to mention what is now called malignant melanoma (Urteaga and Pack, 1966; Gordon and Silverstone, 1976), but examinations of some bones of Incas that are dated about 2400 years ago have revealed evidence of diffuse melanocytic metastases, especially in skulls and extremities (Urteaga and Pack, 1966). It may be safely said that malignant melanoma has been a human affliction from time immemorial. Rufus of Ephesus (?60–120 A.D.), a physician well-known in his day for gross anatomic and pathologic descriptions, alluded to several cancers of the skin, malignant melanoma among them (Urteaga and Pack, 1966). Carswell, in 1838, was the first to use the word "melanoma" to designate blackish malignant neoplasms of the skin, but Laennec had also discussed "la melanose" 100 years earlier. Virchow (1847) surmised that the black color of malignant melanomas was caused by a chemical substance made by the neoplastic cells. Eiselt (1861, 1862), like Highmore (1651), Bartholin (1677), Bonet (1679), and Henrici and Northnagel (1757) before him, dealt with the subject of pigmented neoplasms between 1860 and 1862 and described "fatal black tumors with metastases and black fluid in the body." Solley (1890) recognized the "proneness of melanoid cancers to grow first in or beneath pigmentary moles." He termed the black substance "melanin."

B. Evolution of Histopathologic Concepts About Malignant Melanoma

Unna was probably the first to give a detailed description of histopathologic findings in malignant melanoma. In his book *The Histopathology of the Diseases of the Skin,* published in 1896, Unna presented several cases of malignant melanoma, and in part, he wrote:

> The following description is chiefly taken from a faintly pigmented melano-carcinoma, half the size of an apple which I owe to the kindness of Dr. E. Fraenkel. In it there were parts of pretty much unaltered naevus, and others of primary melano-carcinoma, which, in the definiteness of their origin, left nothing to be desired.

Unna did not differentiate among various types of "melanocarcinoma" except to distinguish between primary and metastatic lesions. However, Kaposi in 1887, even before Unna, viewed malignant melanoma as a "melano-sarcoma":

> Histologically, this tumor represents a highly vascularized, round or spindle cell sarcoma, in some areas even as giant cell sarcoma, with abundant intra- and intercellular granules and diffuse pigmentation.

---

* Consultant in Dermatology, Mayo Clinic School of Medicine. Dr. Su collaborated in this study while a visiting Fellow in Dermatopathology at the New York University School of Medicine.

During the late 19th and early 20th centuries, malignant melanoma was given many different names, such as "melanocarcinoma," "melanoepithelioma," "nevocarcinoma," "nevosarcoma," and "melanosarcoma" (Table 4). These differences in terminology reflected different concepts about the origin of the abnormal melanocytes in the neoplasms. Atypical melanocytes with pigment in "alveolar" (nested) arrangement were considered to be of ectodermal origin and therefore malignant neoplasms composed of them were named "melanocarcinoma" or "melanoepithelioma." If atypical melanocytes in alveolar arrangement were devoid of pigment, the malignant neoplasms were called "nevocarcinoma." Atypical spindle-shaped melanocytes were thought to be mesodermal in origin and malignant neoplasms of them were termed "melanosarcoma" or "nevosarcoma."

Unna, writing in 1896, insisted that there could be no "nevocarcinoma," only "melanocarcinoma" and that all arose in preexisting melanocytic nevi:

> Since the melanocarcinomata of the skin always take their origin in pigmented moles, and, on the other hand, there can hardly be naevocarcinomata, completely without pigment, it is as well to describe together those two groups of tumours, which are combined by gradual transitions. And further, in every other aspect, the character of the two is the same. In all cases we are dealing with rapidly growing pigmented carcinomata, of alveolar structure, which soon lead to infection of the lymphatic glands, to more or less melanotic metastasis and a fatal termination.

Unna was also reluctant to accept the notion of some that every malignant melanoma was actually a melanosarcoma. He wrote that

> Many tumours developed from pigmented naevi have been described as solitary melanotic sarcoma. Since the pigmented naevi invariably lead to melanotic carcinoma and carcinomatous metastases, such cases are always to be accepted with caution, although I by no means deny the occurrence of melanotic sarcomata of the skin.

Gradually, the concept of ectodermal origin of all primary cutaneous malignant melanomas became so cogent that it was generally accepted and all neoplasms of the type were subsequently discussed as a single pathological process (Sutton, 1928; McCarthy, 1931; Ormsby and Montgomery, 1954). The only primary malignant melanoma that was considered to be a true nevosarcoma was the malignant pigmented neoplasm that developed in a blue nevus (McCarthy, 1931; Ormsby and Montgomery, 1954). Eventually, the term malignant melanoma was adapted universally because of its neutrality, which neither commits the neoplasm to be a carcinoma or a sarcoma.

TABLE 4
Terminology

Carcinoma melanodes (Muller)
Chromatophorom (Ribbert)
La Melanose (Laennec, Dupuytren)
Malignant degeneration of pigmented mole (MacKenna)
Melanoblastoma (Masson)
Melanocarcinoma (Virchow, Unna)
Melanocytoblastome (Lubarsch)
Melanoendothelioma (Johnson, J. C.)
Melanoepithelioma (Johnson, J. C.)
Melanoma (Carswell)
Melanoma Sarcomatodes (Borst)
Melanomalignome (Miescher)
Melanosarcoma (Kaposi)
Melanotic carcinoma (Solly)
Nevocarcinoma (Unna)

The concept that proliferation of atypical melanocytes starts within the epidermis and then is followed by penetration of the dermis by them was vaguely suggested by Unna (1896) in these words:

> We find that the first atypical growth of the surface epithelium, which, usually with the assistance of a great amount of pigment, leads to the formation of the naevi, recalls very much the later appearances of melanotic cancers. In the interval, this progressive disturbance of nutrition of the epithelium is at rest. The epithelial germs are snared off from the surface and remain dormant, in small and large groups, in the connective tissue of the upper cutis.

Becker, in 1930, described the evolution of cutaneous malignant melanoma beginning with proliferation of atypical melanocytes within the epidermis and later within the dermis in this manner:

> It may be stated that the initial process is one of increase in number and disintegration of the melanoblastic cells massed with hyperpigmentation of the epidermal cells and finally disintegration of the epidermal cell structure and penetration of the melanoblasts into the deeper dermis. When the process has definitely become malignant, the melanoblastic cells penetrate into the dermis and are also cast off with the stratum corneum.

By the time of the first edition of Lever's textbook in 1949, the idea that malignant melanoma begins in the epidermis and extends from there into the dermis had become well established. Lever wrote:

> In early malignant melanoma and at the advancing border of older lesions, one may find pathologic changes within the epidermis but little or no invasion of the corium by tumor cells. This stage may be referred to as malignant melanoma in situ... Once invasion of the corium by the malignant melanoma cells has taken place, the inflammatory reaction tends to be lesser...

Masson (1951) also noted that "When the malignant melanoblasts penetrate the basal layer and infiltrate the papillary dermis... it is no longer an organic process, 'nevogenic' so to say, but a cancerous invasion." Allen and Spitz, in 1953, recognized that pagetoid "melanocarcinoma" remained intraepithelial for years before dermal "invasion" occurred. In 1958, Lane and his co-workers emphasized "lateral junction activity" as an indication that the atypical melanocytes within the epidermis of malignant melanomas proliferated horizontally before extending perpendicularly into the dermis. In 1962, Peterson et al. divided progression of malignant melanoma into three histologic "stages." For them, Stage I represented epidermal involvement only, without invasion of the dermis; Stage II, invasion of the superficial dermis; Stage III, tumor formation with or without a "pigmented flare." Trapl et al. (1964, 1966), used the terms "horizontal" and "vertical" growth to indicate the sequence of pathological changes in malignant melanoma. They put it succinctly in these words:

> The period from initial changes to the beginning of rapid vertical growth is long and amounts to one or several years, whereas the period of vertical growth takes only some months.

Their division of the two growth phases was directed principally to the clinical aspects of malignant melanoma. In 1966, Clark et al. conceived of two growth phases of malignant melanoma clinically, histologically, and biologically. By 1975, Clark et al. wrote of a "radial-growth phase" and a "vertical-growth phase" thus:

> The radial-growth phase of malignant melanoma of the superficial spreading type consists of a lesion composed of melanoma cells within the epidermis and papillary dermis and the associated response of the host composed of inflammatory cells, fibroplasia, and new blood vessel formation. We specifically emphasize that radial-growth phase is a term used to designate a biologic stage of neoplastic development; the term is not a geometric term indicating a direction of growth of neoplastic cells.

The "vertical-growth phase" was defined by them as follows:

> After the radial-growth phase of malignant melanoma of the superficial-spreading type or of the lentigo-maligna type has existed for a variable number of years, a focal change takes place. This is characterized by a net direction of growth perpendicular to the net direction of growth of the radial-growth phase. This change in the pattern of growth involves deep extension of tumor cells to or into the reticular dermis or into the fat. Invasion to levels III, IV, and V is, by definition, the vertical-growth phase. The change in growth, regarded by us in most instances as a qualitative phenomenon, is associated with a dramatic change in the biologic potential of malignant melanoma of the superficial-spreading type.

In the same article, Clark and his co-workers advanced a concept of "intralesional transformation" by different "clones" of melanoma cells. According to them, neoplastic melanocytes penetrate less deeply into the dermis when those of the "vertical-growth phase" are the same as those of the "radial-growth phase." When, however, the vertical-growth phase is composed of two or more populations of melanoma cells, i.e., one or more sets that are cytologically different from those of the radial-growth phase ("polyclonism"), intralesional transformation is promoted and the neoplastic cells tend to invade more deeply into the skin. A typical area of such intralesional transformation shows melanoma cells with different cytologic features disposed in discrete nests. Clark also suggested that the cytologic changes have biologic significance.

> The host response to the phenomenon we have referred to as intralesional transformation is intriguing. One kind of cell may have no host response of any kind and the nest immediately adjacent to it may be permeated with lymphocytes. In fact, we have viewed this selective host response as evidence that the different cell populations in intralesional transformation are true clones.

C. Major Types of Malignant Melanoma

There are currently four commonly recognized types of primary cutaneous malignant melanomas, namely, lentigo maligna, acral lentiginous, superficial spreading, and nodular.

1. Lentigo Maligna Melanoma

What is now called lentigo maligna (and what we consider to be lentigo maligna melanoma *in situ*) was first described by Hutchinson in 1892 as follows:

Cases have been alluded illustrating a peculiar tendency to freckles in old persons, attending often with the adjacent development of cancer ... I do not suppose that more can be said as to the connection between the black stains and the development of epithelial cancer near to them, which these two cases illustrate, than that both the changes were indicative of senile disturbance of nutrition. The black stains were probably not positively sarcomatous, and in each instance the epitheliomatous ulcer was quite without pigment. Yet it remains a very remarkable fact, as seeming to imply some connection between the two conditions, that in each instance the epitheliomatous ulcer developed in close proximity to the black stain. In neither case was it, however, exactly on it.

Hutchinson subsequently reported several other similar cases and called them "infective melanotic freckle" and "lentigomelanosis" (Hutchinson, 1892, 1894, 1896). In 1894, Dubreuilh termed cases similar to those of Hutchinson "lentigo maligna des vieillards" (malignant lentigo of the aged), but he realized later that this designation was inexact because younger persons could sometimes be affected by the lesion. By 1912 Dubreuilh had collected 32 cases of this peculiar pigmented condition to which he then applied the term "melanose circonscrite precancereuse" (circumscribed precancerous melanosis). The condition has had various other titles given to it, among them "lentigo infectieux" by Bayet (1895) and "precancerose melanose" by Miescher (1933, 1936).

In the late 19th and early 20th centuries, lentigo maligna became confused with certain melanocytic nevi, especially junction nevi, and as such was named "acquired mole" by Hazen (1920), "tardive nevus" by Deckner (1931) and by Kumer and Lang (1935), "junction nevus" by Sachs (1947), and "dermo-epidermal nevus" by Allen (1948). In 1954, Becker divided junction nevi into three types: (1) quiescent, smooth pigmented nevus; (2) active, smooth, pigmented nevus; and (3) lentigo maligna. He regarded lentigo maligna as a stage of a junction nevus, advanced in the pathogenetic progression somewhere between a quiescent junction nevus and a malignant melanoma. Mishima (1960), however, considered Dubreuilh's circumscribed precancerous melanosis to be different from junction nevus in its pathogenesis and clinical characteristics. He argued that

> Dubreuilh's tumor can be considered as a precancerous non-nevoid melanocytoma which is derived from the junctional mature melanocytes and shows the segregation phenomenon of these cells. It represents an alternate pathway by which malignant melanoma can originate without the intermediate formation of nevus cells.

Klauder and Beerman (1955) noted that metastases to regional lymph nodes and beyond were delayed longer in malignant melanomas that arose from lentigo maligna than in those that developed in a junction nevus. For them, this favored the view that lentigo maligna is separate and distinct from junction nevus. Additional confusion developed when Webster et al. (1944), like Hutchinson 50 years earlier, used the term "malignant freckle" for lentigo maligna, which carried a false implication that malignant melanoma could result from conversion of an ephelis. In 1966, Ollstein et al. reviewed 23 cases of so-called malignant freckle and concluded that these lesions were so variable histologically that they could not be diagnosed with certainty by conventional microscopy. Superficial malignant melanoma was another confusing term used in the 1950s and 1960s to include all malignant melanomas, including lentigo maligna melanomas, which invaded only superficially into the dermis (Lever, 1961).

Sulzberger et al. (1959) emphasized three clinical features of the precancerous (lentigo maligna) phase of lentigo maligna melanoma, namely, its changeability, irregular outline, and unevenness of color. They also suggested that this condition be separated from other malignant melanomas that were often confused with it, such as superficial malignant melanoma (Allen and Spitz, 1953), amelanotic malignant melanoma resembling Paget's disease (Stout, 1938), and malignant melanomas arising in junction or compound nevi. Thus, lentigo maligna melanoma gradually came to be recognized as a specific type of malignant melanoma (Lund and Ihned, 1955; Mishima, 1960; Jackson et al., 1966; Davis et al., 1967; Wayte and Helwig, 1968).

The histopathology of lentigo maligna was first described by Dubreuilh in 1912. He wrote that the first stage of the disease was characterized mainly by melanosis and reported changes varying from simple epidermal pigmentation to "basal cell metaplasia." Unna (1896) did not discuss circumscribed precancerous melanosis separately from malignant melanomas in general. McCarthy, in 1931, discussed the clinical and histopathologic findings of Hutchinson's lentigo maligna in this way:

> In the beginning, these spots are simply localized areas of hyperpigmentation (lentigo). After a longer or shorter period of time they are gradually transformed into either flat, pigmented or nonpigmented, superficial scar-forming tumors or into ulcerated mushroom-like growths which sooner or later give rise to glandular metastases. In the transitional stage from the simple lentigo to the melanoma, we find that the basal cells are loaded with abnormal amounts of pigment and their normal pali-

sade arrangement is highly disturbed, i.e., individual cells or groups of cells in the form of "nests" separate themselves from the epithelium and grow down into the cutis. In addition many of the basal cells that are the forerunners of the cells growing down into the cutis appear much larger than normal and their nuclei have become much larger and paler.

In 1955, Klauder and Beerman observed that the characteristic changes of Hutchinson's melanotic freckle occur in the region of the epidermal basal cells. The individual cells of the basal layer, which seemed larger and paler to them, were said to be separated by a gap from neighboring cells and either to contain pigment or be entirely pigment-free. They found no mitoses. Costello et al., in 1959, noted that histopathologic changes in lentigo maligna ranged from simple hyperpigmentation of the melanocytes in the basal layer to true proliferation of junctional melanocytes with occasional nests of melanocytes found even in the stratum corneum and in the dermis. Mishima, in 1960, described the main histologic change of Dubreuilh's circumscribed precancerous melanosis as a neoplastic proliferation of dendritic melanocytes in the lower epidermis. By the early 1970s, Clark and his associates (1975) emphasized that "the radial growth phase (of lentigo maligna melanoma) must be divided into two developmental stages; 'non-invasive' and 'invasive' into papillary dermis."

In the absence of dermal "invasion," Clark and his colleagues did not consider the lesion to be truly malignant melanoma and therefore they called this stage simply lentigo maligna. Only when there was invasion of atypical melanocytes into the papillary dermis did Clark and co-workers call the lesion lentigo maligna melanoma.

Some sense of the evolution of histopathologic concepts about lentigo maligna and lentigo maligna melanoma can be gleaned from the several editions of Lever's textbook *Histopathology of the Skin*. In his first and second editions (1949 and 1954), Lever did not mention lentigo maligna or lentigo maligna melanoma at all. One of his photomicrographs did show atypical spindle-shaped melanocytes at the dermoepidermal junction and in the dermis, but the neoplasm was included in his general discussion of malignant melanoma. In his third edition (1961), Lever considered "melanosis circumscripta preblastomatosa" under the heading of "superficial malignant melanoma." In the fourth edition (1967), the term "melanosis circumscripta preblastomatosa" was still used by him, but for the first time it was discussed independently of the other malignant melanomas. In this same edition, Lever did acknowledge that malignant melanoma could arise from melanosis circumscripta preblastomatosa. In the fifth edition (1975), Lever employed the term "lentigo maligna" and "lentigo maligna melanoma." Both conditions were discussed in detail and separately from other types of malignant melanomas.

In our opinion, the most important contributions to the understanding of lentigo maligna and lentigo maligna melanoma were made by:

1. Hutchinson who first described the condition clinically in 1892 and subsequently added additional cases.
2. Dubreuilh who in 1894 described cases similar to those of Hutchinson, termed the condition "circumscribed precancerous melanosis" in 1912, and also gave a brief description of its histopathologic features.
3. Mishima who in 1960 described in detail the clinical and pathologic characteristics of "circumscribed precancerous melanosis" and separated it from those of a junctional nevus.
4. David et al. (1967), Wayte and Helwig (1968), Jackson et al. (1966), McGovern et al. (1967, 1970, 1973), Peterson et al. (1962), Clark et al. (1966, 1967, 1975), and several other authors who in the 1960s and 1970s gradually delineated lentigo maligna and lentigo maligna melanoma as a distinct and separate clinical, histological, and biological type of malignant melanoma.

2. Acral Lentiginous Malignant Melanoma

In 1886, Hutchinson described "melanotic whitlow," a malignant melanoma occurring on a finger that resembled an infectious whitlow, as follows:

> There is a rare form of disease of the nail-bed which is malignant, and usually takes the type of melanotic sarcoma. It is generally attributed in the first instance to injury, and its diagnosis is always missed in the early stages. Because it resembled whitlow, and is usually so named at first, I prefer to give it that name. It is, however, from the beginning, malignant. Careful observation will find at the edge of the inflamed nail a little border of coal-black colour, and this, however slightly marked, must be allowed to make the diagnosis . . .

Cases similar to Hutchinson's were subsequently reported by Jackson (1899) and Hertzler (1922). Sutton (1928) in his textbook *Disease of the Skin* printed a photomicrograph of "melanotic whitlow" of the thumb, showing atypical dendritic, heavily pigmented melanocytes at the dermoepidermal junction with a marked inflammatory-cell infiltrate in the dermis. Gibson et al. (1957) reviewed 38 cases of the condition seen at the Mayo Clinic and noted that

Factors such as cell shape, density of mitotic figures, depth of invasion, or presence or absence of melanin all varied, sometimes widely, in different parts of the same lesion. In general, practically all lesions contained both polyhedral and spindle-shaped cells...

They concluded that there is no single, practical histologic criterion for grading malignancy or predicting the outcome in individual cases of this type of malignant melanoma. Although there have been many clinical, epidemiologic, and therapeutic studies of subungual malignant melanomas, few have concerned their histological features. Such is the case of Pack and Oropeza's (1967) report of 72 cases of subungual melanoma, which has detailed epidemiologic and clinical information, but no histological data.

In 1972, Lupulescu and associates reported a clinical, histologic, and ultrastructural study of two cases of "lentigo maligna of the fingertips." These authors concluded that the lesions had the clinical and histologic characteristics of lentigo maligna. Examination by conventional and electron microscopy showed atypical melanocytes that were clearly different from those of superficial spreading malignant melanoma. However, they considered their cases of lentigo maligna of the fingertips to be different from "melanotic whitlow." They gave this explanation:

> While its [melanotic whitlow] first manifestations may be a dark, longitudinal streak in the nail plate, it soon begins to destroy the nail, which later is completely absent and replaced by a granulomatous-appearing raw surface. Histologically, melanotic whitlow belongs to the nevocytic malignant melanomas (malignant nevocytomas [Mishima]). Our cases, which started in the epidermis of the fingertip and involved the nail only secondarily without destroying it, are clinically as well as histologically different from melanotic whitlow and are to be considered as instances of lentigo maligna (premalignant melanocytosis [Pinkus and Mishima]) in an unusual localization.

Cases similar to those of Lupulescu et al. were also described by Boglino (1971) and Arao et al. (1971). Mihm and co-authors (1975, 1976) emphasized that variegation of pigmentation is the earliest clinical change of malignant melanomas of the nail bed. They wrote: "In the intact nail streaks of brown, blue, white, and tan abut one on the other."

Clark et al. in 1975 applied their concept of "radial-growth" phase of malignant melanomas to those of the palms, soles, and subungual regions as follows:

> "Abnormal melanocytes are located in the basal regions of the nail or epidermis: the cells are large or spindled and pagetoid growth is not prominent...
> The radial-growth phase is indistinguishable from that of lentigo maligna melanoma and superficial spreading melanoma. When the vertical-growth phase supervenes, the neoplasms are biologically similar to superficial spreading melanoma."

Reed (Clark et al., 1975; Reed, 1976) regarded malignant pigmented lesions that originated on palms and soles as a special variant of malignant melanoma and termed it "acral-lentiginous melanoma." He described that variant thus:

> These lesions are characterized by marked acanthosis, elongation of rete ridges, and lentiginous proliferation of atypical melanocytes in the epidermis. The lesion has a significant lateral growth phase to produce a large pigmented halo. There is usually evidence of dermal invasion in one or more areas. The tumor cells in the dermis are often spindle shaped and are arranged in fascicles. In many areas they have nevus cell characteristics with individual cells surrounded by a delicately fibrous matrix. In some of the fibrosing areas the pattern resembled that seen in blue nevi. This pattern of melanoma is histologically deceptive and may be easily misdiagnosed on small biopsies. Some of the acral melanomas are desmoplastic.

Arrington et al. (1977) reported 27 patients (18 of whom were blacks) with "plantar lentiginous melanoma" and compared the histologic features of this form of malignant melanoma with those of other malignant melanomas that have a radial-growth phase. They concluded that plantar lentiginous melanoma is a distinctive variant of cutaneous malignant melanoma. Clinically and histologically, they viewed plantar lentiginous melanoma to be characterized by a period of radial growth and often thereafter by one or more foci of regression. Eighteen of their twenty-seven patients with plantar lentiginous melanoma died of distant metastases.

In our opinion, major contributions to the understanding of acral lentiginous malignant melanoma were by:

1. Hutchinson who in 1886 described "melanotic whitlow" clinically.
2. Gibson et al. who in 1957 presented a more detailed histopathologic and clinical study of melanotic whitlow.
3. Pack and Oropeza (1967) and many other authors (Booher and Pack, 1957; Das Gupta and Brasfield, 1965; Lewis, 1967; Lewis and Kiryabwire, 1968; Graham, 1973; Leppard et al, 1974; Wanebo et al., 1975) who did clinical, epidemiologic, and therapeutic studies of subungual melanoma.

4. Reed who in 1975 suggested that "acral-lentiginous melanoma" was a separate variant of malignant melanoma.
5. Clark et al. who in 1975 applied the concept of radial-growth and vertical-growth phases to acral lentiginous melanoma.
6. Arrington et al. who in 1977 compared and contrasted histologic features of "plantar lentiginous melanoma" with those of lentigo maligna melanoma and superficial spreading melanoma and concluded that it was a distinct variant of cutaneous malignant melanoma.

3. Superficial Spreading Malignant Melanoma

Unna (1896) in describing the features of "melanocarcinoma" wrote:

> They are cubical, pale, pretty homogeneous cells, with regular oval nuclei, four or six in a cell . . . The large alveoli break up into a quantity of small ones; there is a widespread scattering of the epithelium.

Thus, Unna recognized "cubical, pale, pretty homogeneous cells" (later to be called "pagetoid cells") in some of his biopsy specimens of malignant melanoma. Stout, in 1938, reviewed seven cases of malignant melanoma and stated that they "showed intraepidermal invasion by cells resembling Paget cells." In 1939, Corsi again described large, pagetoid cells, but in lesions he thought to be circumscribed precancerous melanosis. Retrospectively, Corsi's cases were probably superficial spreading malignant melanomas rather than lentigo malignas. Allen and Spitz, in 1953, divided melanocarcinomas into superficial and deep types. They also called superficial melanocarcinoma "pagetoid" melanocarcinoma and wrote that

> These "pagetoid" melanocarcinomas may remain intraepithelial for years . . . and only slowly involved large areas of the genital or perineal region without invading the dermis until late in their course. Eventually, however, these lesions, unless completely eradicated, metastasize to regional nodes and beyond, behaving then as aggressively as the average cutaneous melanocarcinoma.

Allen and Spitz appeared to recognize that variant of malignant melanoma to be classified by Clark et al. (1966, 1967, 1975) as superficial spreading malignant melanoma more than a decade later. However, some of the lesions in the genital and perianal regions diagnosed by Allen and Spitz as pagetoid melanocarcinoma were almost certainly examples of extramammary Paget's disease. Furthermore, unlike Clark, Allen and Spitz did not discuss, and apparently did not appreciate, differences between superficial spreading malignant melanoma and lentigo maligna melanoma.

Clark, in 1966, was the first to use the term "superficial spreading malignant melanoma." He called attention to the clinical, histologic, and biologic characteristics of what he conceived to be a distinctive form of malignant melanoma. Clark discussed the histologic features in this way:

> Microscopically, the neoplasm is best described as pagetoid, as it is characterized by the presence of many large rather "clear" cells distributed in profusion throughout the various epidermal layers. The cells, which rarely show dendrites, have abundant cytoplasm stippled with finely divided, "dusty" melanin. The nuclei are large, frequently pale with infolded nuclear membranes. Such cells may be seen in the papillary dermis in several areas. Where nodules are present, they produce a microscopic picture of extension through the papillary dermis to the reticular dermis or deeper. Virtually all of the cells of superficially spreading malignant melanoma are structurally "malignant," in contrast with those of the lentigo maligna-melanoma which vary from normal to the atypical of malignancy.

"Radial-growth" and "vertical-growth" phases of superficial spreading melanoma were noted by Clark in his original publication and discussed in detail by him and his associates in 1975.

Since Clark's designation of superficial spreading melanoma, several comprehensive clinical and/or histopathologic descriptions of this form of malignant melanoma have been presented, particularly by Mihm et al. (1973, 1975), McGovern et al. (1967, 1970), and others. However, neither Clark nor any of these authors attempted to establish firm histologic criteria for the differentiation of superficial spreading malignant melanoma from unusual melanocytic nevi. Price et al., in 1976, sought to establish histologic criteria for the diagnosis of superficial spreading malignant melanoma based on proven metastatic eventuation. Their criteria included: (1) Poor circumscription of the intraepidermal melanocytic component of the lesion with individual melanocytes extending laterally within the epidermis; (2) increased numbers of single melanocytes and conglomerates of melanocytes within and above the epidermal basal-cell layer and within adnexal epithelium; (3) marked variation in size and shape of melanocytic nests and their tendency to confluence; (4) absence of maturation of melanocytes as they descend progressively into the dermis; (5) melanocytes with nuclear atypia; (6) melanocytes in mitosis; (7) necrosis of melanocytes. They agreed with the conclusions of Helwig (1963), Couperus and Rucker (1954), Caro (1953), Milne (1972), and Jackson (1971) that no single criterion could be relied upon for unequivocal histologic diagnosis of malignant melanoma, but rather that the diagnosis must be made on the basis of a combination of several criteria.

In our opinion, the major contributions to the understanding of superficial spreading malignant melanoma were by

1. Unna, Stout, and Corsi who in 1896, 1938, and 1939, recognized "pagetoid cells" in some malignant melanomas.
2. Allen and Spitz who in 1953 wrote about "superficial melanocarcinoma" and called it "pagetoid melanocarcinoma."
3. Clark who in 1966 separated superficial spreading malignant melanoma from the nodular and lentigo maligna types.
4. Clark et al. (1967, 1975), Mihm et al. (1973, 1975), and McGovern et al. (1967, 1970) who called attention to clinical and histopathologic recognition of early superficial spreading malignant melanoma enabling curative surgery to be performed.
5. Price et al., who in 1976 attempted to establish firm histologic criteria for the diagnosis of superficial spreading malignant melanoma on the basis of proven metastatic eventuation in order to differentiate superficial spreading malignant melanoma from unusual melanocytic nevi with which it would be confused.

4. Nodular Malignant Melanoma

From early in recorded medical history, malignant melanomas were described as "fatal black tumors with metastasis" (Eiselt, 1861, 1862). This simple concept obtained throughout the 19th and 20th centuries, as is evident from the descriptions of malignant melanomas by Kaposi in 1893, Jackson in 1899, Hyde in 1901, Shoemaker in 1909, Sutton in 1938, and Ormsby and Montgomery in 1954. A typical description of malignant melanoma from that era is that of Ormsby and Montgomery who wrote in their book *Diseases of the Skin* (1954) that

> Malignant melanoma usually begins as a blueblack nodule; it often causes death because of its tendency to metastasize early in its course. It is the most malignant and rapidly fatal of all cutaneous neoplasms.

By 1966, Clark had proposed the following classification of malignant melanomas:

1. Malignant melanoma arising in association with lentigo maligna.
2. Superficial spreading malignant melanoma.
3. Verrucous malignant melanoma.
4. Nodular malignant melanoma.

Verrucous malignant melanomas were at first separated from nodular melanomas by Clark and considered by him to be "a rather circumscribed form which tends to protrude deeply into the dermis with relatively little spread along the dermoepidermal interface." Later, Clark questioned the reasonableness of segregating verrucous melanoma from nodular melanoma (Clark, 1966), and in subsequent publications (Clark et al., 1967, 1975), he alluded only to nodular, and not at all to verrucous malignant melanoma. To differentiate malignant melanoma of the nodular type from malignant melanoma of the superficial spreading type, Clark et al. (1969) wrote that in nodular melanoma

> The primary tumor is characterized by being uniformly invasive. In fact, the demonstration of dermal invasion throughout the lesion, wherever there is intraepidermal growth, is nodular melanoma by definition. If this growth extends beyond the width of 3 rete ridges in any section, the tumor is classified as a superficial spreading melanoma. The intraepidermal growth overlying the invasive tumor may be so sparse as to suggest that the lesion is metastatic. The majority of nodular melanomas extend to or into the reticular dermis or into the fat, i.e., they are level III, IV, or V tumors.

In 1975, Clark et al. emphasized that

> Nodular melanomas are comprised exclusively of a vertical-growth phase. This developmental stage, which is the early stage for nodular melanoma, usually shows invasion of melanoma cells into the deeper dermis. The histology is similar to the verticalgrowth phase of superficial spreading melanoma; there may be only one cell type, but commonly two or more kinds of cells may be observed. Presumably, early in the course of evolution, the neoplasms have undergone intralesional transformation.

The view that there is only vertical-growth without any radial-growth in nodular melanoma has been widely accepted (Kopf et al., 1977; Mihm, 1977; Callen et al., 1978).

In our opinion, major contributions to the understanding of nodular malignant melanoma were made by many authors, namely, Eiselt (1861, 1862), Kaposi (1893), Jackson (1899), Hyde (1901), Shoemaker (1909), Sutton (1928), and Ormsby and Montgomery (1954). But they considered all malignant melanomas to be nodular in form. It was Clark who in 1966 differentiated nodular malignant melanoma from superficial spreading and lentigo maligna melanomas.

D. SPECIAL HISTOLOGIC FEATURES OF MALIGNANT MELANOMAS AND THEIR RELATION TO PROGNOSIS

Several histopathologic features have been said to be useful for assessing prognosis in patients with malignant melanoma, namely, depth (levels) of invasion, thickness, volume of tumor, general architecture of the neoplasm, ulceration, extent of elevation of the neoplasm above the skin surface, shape of the elevated portion (e.g., sessile, polypoid), invasion of blood and lymph vessels, cytologic atypia, mitotic figures, size of nucleoli, and density of the inflammatory-cell infiltrate.

It has long been recognized that the deeper the invasion of malignant melanoma into the skin, the worse the prognosis. As early as 1858, Pemberton advocated wide and deep excision of primary malignant melanoma, carrying the excision below the fascia and also dissecting regional lymph nodes. Allen and Spitz, in 1953, divided malignant melanomas into superficial and deep types and stated that the superficial melanocarcinomas have an appreciably better prognosis than the more deeply infiltrating ones. Peterson et al., in 1962, described a "stage one" malignant melanoma confined wholly to the epidermis and therefore incapable of producing metastasis. Many other authors have attempted to correlate the depth of invasion with prognosis (Lund and Inhed, 1955; Lane et al., 1958; Trapl et al., 1966). Mehnert and Heart, in 1965, proposed an index of prognosis by "staging" malignant melanomas according to depth of invasion as follows:

Stage 0	*In situ*
Stage 1	Superficial
Stage 2	Intradermal
Stage 3	Subcutaneous

McGovern and his associates, in 1967, suggested histologic "staging" of cutaneous malignant melanoma in this manner:

Stage i	Intraepidermal
Stage ii	Invading papillary zone of dermis
Stage iii	Invading reticular zone of dermis
Stage iv	Invading subcutaneous fat

However, in 1966, Clark and his associates had already proposed reading "levels of invasion" of malignant melanoma, a schema that in the ensuing decade gained popular acceptance. According to Clark,

Level I = All the neoplastic cells are above the epidermal basement membrane.
Level II = The neoplastic cells lie beyond the basement membrane and extend to some degree into the papillary dermis, but not quite to the reticular dermis.
Level III = The melanoma cells fill the papillary dermis and reach the interface between papillary and reticular dermis.
Level IV = The neoplastic cells extend into the reticular dermis.
Level V = The neoplastic cells extend into the subcutaneous fat.

The survival rates for patients with primary cutaneous malignant melanoma have been shown to be inversely related to the level of invasion of the neoplastic cells by many investigators, namely, Clark et al. (1967), Jones-Williams et al. (1968), Bodenham (1968, 1969), McGovern (1970), McLeod et al. (1971), Mackie et al. (1972), Huvos et al. (1973), Sinha and Buntine (1974), Wanebo et al. (1975), Franklin et al. (1975), and Davis et al. (1976).

Clark (1969) found that only 8% of patients with level II malignant melanomas died within 5 years after the diagnosis had been made and surgery performed, whereas 35% of patients with level III melanomas, 46% of those with level IV, and 52% of those with level V malignant melanomas died within 5 years. McGovern (1976) found no difference in prognosis between levels III and IV, 52% of all of these patients having died within 5 years.

Breslow, in 1970, was the first to introduce the concept of tumor thickness as an important gauge for prognosis of primary cutaneous malignant melanoma. He measures the thickness of malignant melanomas in histopathologic sections with a micrometer in the ocular of the microscope. The thickness is measured from the uppermost part of the granular layer of the epidermis to the deepest portion of the neoplasm as seen in histologic sections. Breslow reported that lesions of malignant melanoma less than 0.76 mm in thickness did not metastasize or recur, whereas lesions greater than 1.5 mm in thickness often developed metastases. The zone of thickness from 0.76 to 1.5 mm was regarded by Breslow to be a "gray area" for prognostication. It was hoped that the combination of Breslow's measurements of thickness of malignant melanoma and Clark's levels of invasion could be utilized to determine accurately prognoses of patients with malignant melanoma [Breslow (1970) and Wanebo et al. (1975)].

The type of malignant melanoma as judged histologically is regarded by many authors to be of prognostic importance. Overall, patients with nodular malignant melanoma are considered to have the worst prognoses, those with superficial spreading malignant melanoma less grave prognoses, and those with lentigo maligna melanoma, the best prognoses (Ackerman, 1948; Pack et al., 1952; Sulzberger et al.,

1959; Wayte and Helwig, 1968; Huvos et al., 1973; Wanebo et al., 1975). These differences in prognosis may depend on the rate of growth of malignant melanomas, i.e., nodular melanomas grow most rapidly and deeply, whereas lentigo malignant melanomas grow most slowly and superficially (Huvos et al., 1973).

Hermanek et al. (1976) concluded that no significant prognostic differences existed between malignant melanomas of different types and comparable levels (depths) of invasion. According to them and to Wanebo et al. (1975) a level IV superficial spreading malignant melanoma has a similar prognosis as a level IV nodular malignant melanoma. Thus, for malignant melanomas of the same thickness the rate of mortality was said by them to be the same, irrespective of the histologic type.

The amount of pigment in the melanocytic lesion was regarded by Unna (1896) as having prognostic significance:

> The pigment has evidently a favouring effect on the epithelial growth and extension; the most pigmented the nevus, the most active is the growth and deleterious the action of the new formation.

That the amount of melanin varies greatly in malignant melanoma (Lever, 1975) is generally acknowledged. Amelanotic malignant melanomas are said by Veronesi et al. (1971) and Huvos et al. (1972, 1974) to behave more aggressively and bespeak worse prognoses than their melanotic counterparts. However, Ackerman (1948), Lewis and Kirywabwire (1968), Jones-Williams et al. (1968), and MacLeod and Munde (1940) conclude that the amount of pigment in malignant melanomas bears no relationship to prognosis.

Ulceration of lesions of malignant melanoma is associated with poor prognosis according to Bodenham (1968, 1969), Veronesi et al. (1971) Mackie et al. (1972), Huvos et al. (1974), and Davis et al. (1970).

Extent of elevation of malignant melanoma above the skin surface was considered to be an important factor in severity of prognosis by Bodenham (1968, 1969) and Davis et al. (1976), but not by Huvos et al. (1974). Pedunculated lesions of malignant melanomas are said to have a grave prognosis (Niven and Lubin, 1975).

Invasion of blood vessels or lymphatics in the dermis or subcutaneous tissue by atypical melanocytes is obviously a poor prognostic sign (Mackie et al., 1972, and Huvos et al., 1974).

The number of mitoses per high-power field was considered to have predictive value by Jones-Williams et al. (1968) Mackie et al. (1972), and Schmoeckel and Braun-Falco (1978), but was regarded as insignificant by Huvos et al. (1974).

Malignant melanomas with dense lymphocytic infiltrates at their bases were thought to have a more favorable prognosis than lesions without this feature by Mehnert and Heard (1965), Cochrane (1969), Little (1972), Fitzpatrick et al., (1972), Hansen and McCarten (1974), and Huvos et al. (1974). According to Jones-Williams et al. (1968) the extent of the inflammatory-cell infiltrate has no effect on eventual course. Other authors contend that the denser the inflammatory-cell infiltrate, the better the prognosis, whereas absence of inflammatory-cell infiltrate is associated with a high incidence of mortality (Huvos et al., 1974; Bodenham, 1968, 1969; Fitzpatrick et al., 1972; Hansen and McCarten, 1972).

II. DEFINITIONS OF SOME RELEVANT TERMS

A. Melanocyte—a cell that makes melanin and is derived from the neural crest from which it migrates to the epidermis, dermis, leptomeninges, eye, etc. Melanin-making cells in the epidermis are all called melanocytes by convention.

B. Nevus cell (nevocyte)—a cuboidal or spindle-shaped melanocyte in the dermis (and rarely the subcutaneous fat) that has the capacity to make melanin, but under normal circumstances may not. These melanocytes in the dermis are called nevus cells or nevocytes by convention.

C. Atypical melanocyte—a cell that makes melanin and has a nucleus that is larger or more deeply staining than a normal melanocyte. It may have one or more prominent nucleoli, be in mitosis, or be undergoing necrosis. Atypical melanocytes tend to have plemorphic nuclei. An atypical melanocyte is not necessarily a "malignant" melanocyte.

D. Melanophage—a macrophage containing melanin.

E. Junction "activity" and "active" junction nevus—terms to be avoided because they imply motion when, in fact, only morphologic judgments can be made about tissue sections studied by conventional microscopy. Junctional "activity" presumably is intended to mean hyperplasia of atypical melanocytes within the epidermis, but it is generally used by pathologists as a euphemism for histologic findings in a melanocytic lesion that cannot be classified with certainty as a benign junction nevus or a malignant melanoma *in situ*. Cytologically, melanocytes are either typical or atypical, not inactive or active. "Active" junction nevus is also used by some pathologists for a junction nevus that is thought to be becoming a malignant melanoma. In fact, there is no evidence that melanocytes of junction nevi convert directly into neoplastic cells of malignant melanomas, and the lesion in question is either a junction nevus of some kind, a malignant melanoma *in situ*, or, exceptionally, a combination of the two.

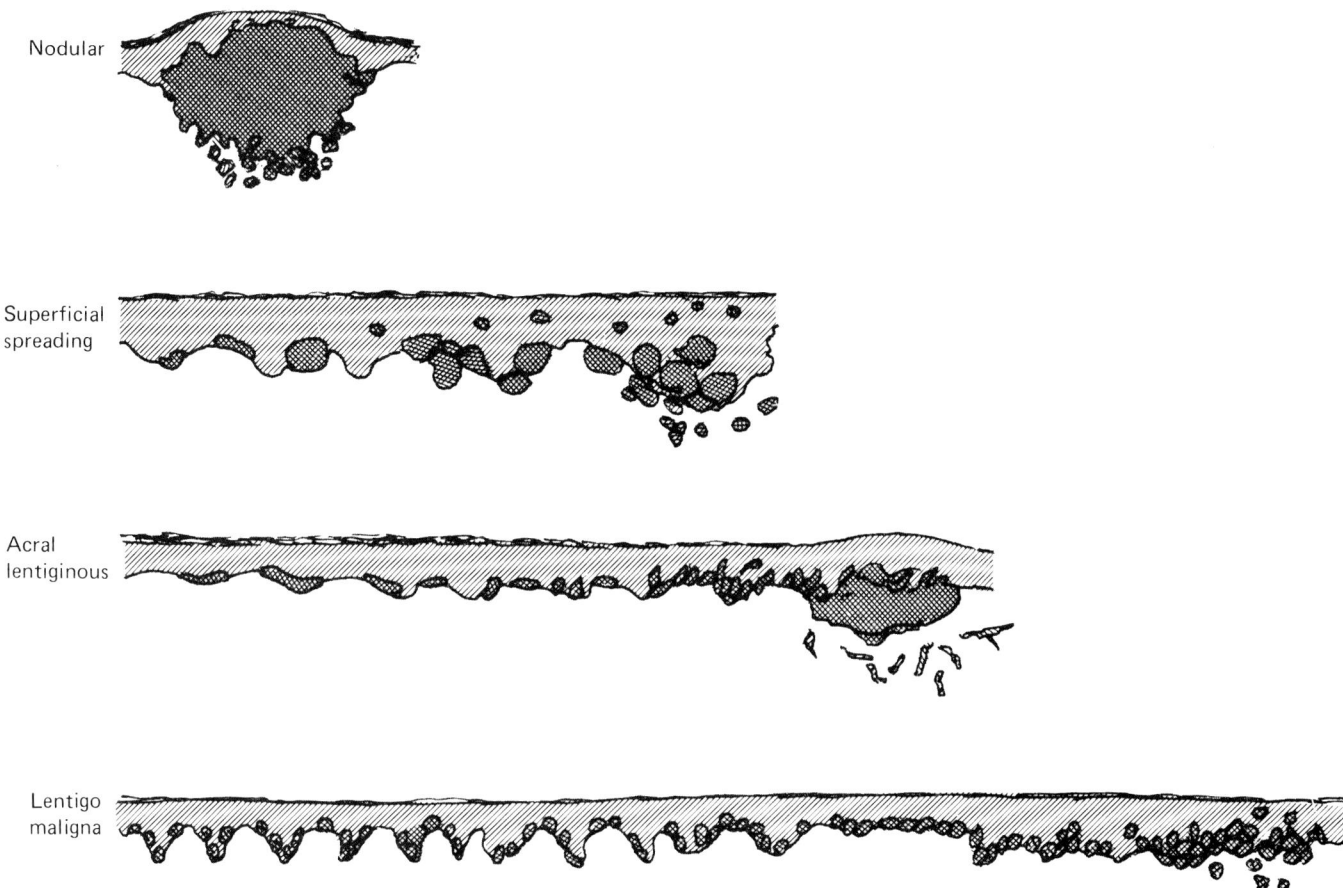

FIGURE 43. *Malignant melanoma of the skin pictured as one pathological process.* Virtually all primary cutaneous malignant melanomas begin in the epidermis with extension of melanocytes horizontally. The four common types of malignant melanoma illustrated, namely, nodular, superficial spreading, acral lentiginous, and lentigo maligna, differ mostly in the duration of proliferation of atypical melanocytes horizontally within the epidermis, i.e., shortest for nodular malignant melanoma, longest for lentigo maligna melanoma.

III. A UNIFYING CONCEPT OF CUTANEOUS MALIGNANT MELANOMA

We think that primary cutaneous malignant melanomas develop fundamentally as a single pathological process but with different clinical, histological, and biological expressions. Histologically, the various types of malignant melanomas have many more features in common than they have differences. In our view, for practical purposes, virtually all malignant melanomas that arise in skin (or in mucous membranes) begin with proliferation of melanocytes within the surface epithelium. In other words, first there is horizontal extension of melanocytes within the epidermal or mucosal epithelium and only later may there be extension into the subjacent connective tissue. In this sense, all malignant melanomas start out as "superficially spreading" (Fig. 43). That type of malignant melanoma that tends to spread superficially (i.e., horizontally within the surface epithelium) for the longest period of time is what has been designated lentigo maligna (Fig. 44). As long as the atypical melanocytes remain confined to the epidermis or epithelium of adnexa in that condition, which may be for decades if not for the lifetime of the patient, the process is truly a malignant melanoma *in situ,* analogous to squamous-cell carcinoma *in situ.* Just as every squamous-cell carcinoma *in situ* does not inevitably become an "invasive" squamous-cell carcinoma, so too, not every malignant melanoma *in situ* (e.g., lentigo maligna) will invariably become an "invasive" malignant melanoma.

The acral lentiginous is another variant of cutaneous malignant melanoma that extends horizontally within the epidermis for many years (Fig. 45). As long as the atypical

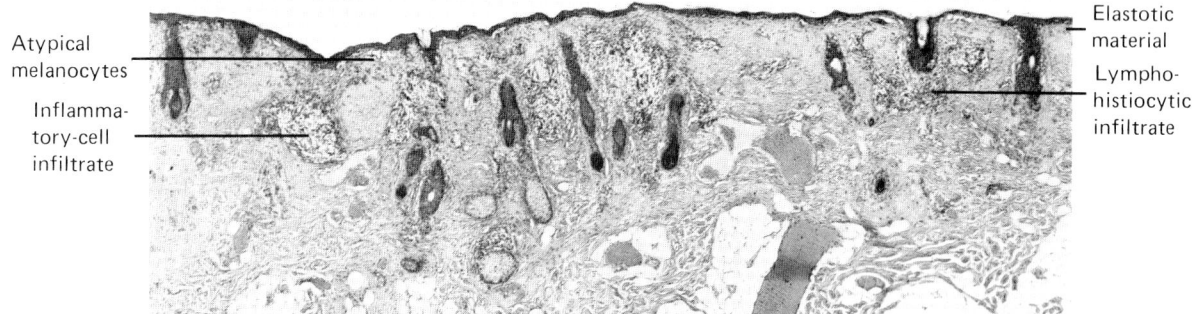

FIGURE 44A. **Lentigo maligna.** *Even under scanning power one can see an increased number of melanocytes both singly and in nests within and along the entire front of the thinned epidermis and within epithelial structures of adnexa. A moderately dense inflammatory-cell infiltrate with melanophages is present in a dermis that has been severely altered by long-standing exposure to sunlight. (Reduced from ×27)*

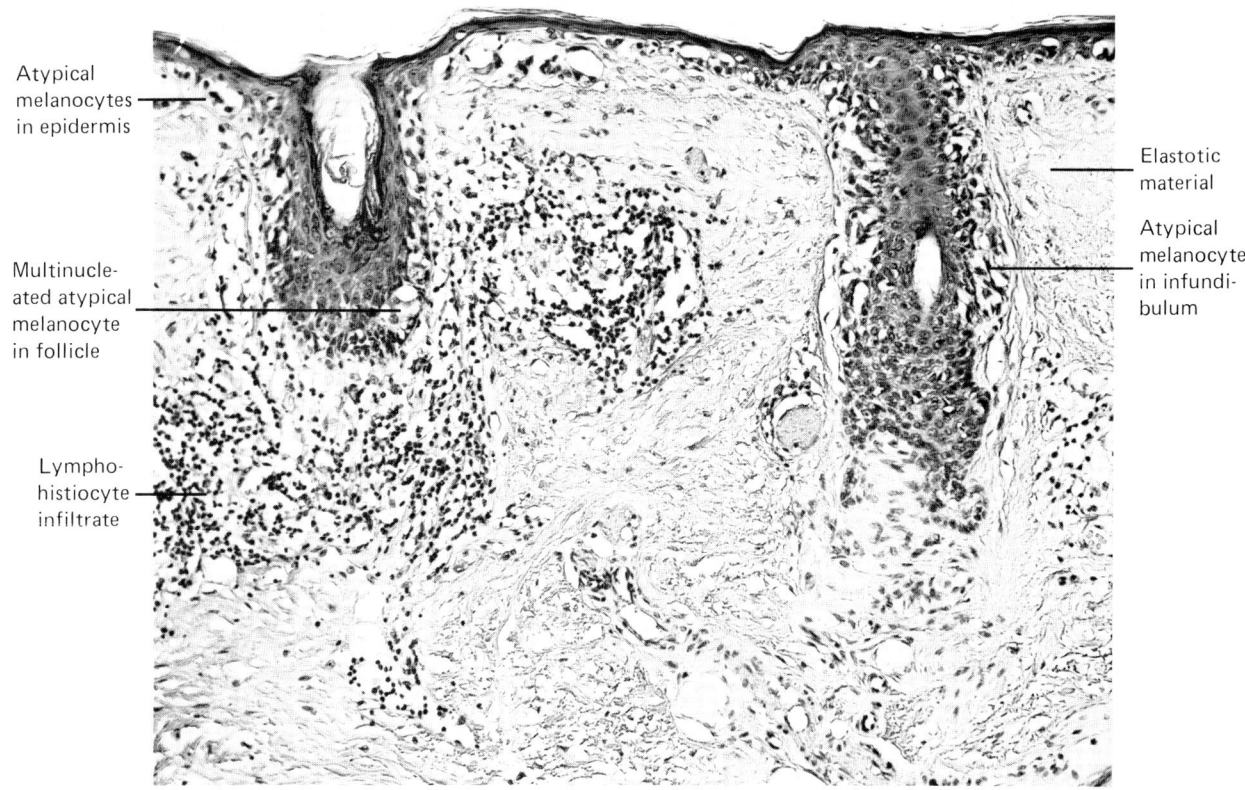

FIGURE 44B. **Lentigo maligna.** *This higher magnification of Fig. 44A shows to better advantage the atypical melanocytes within the epidermis and within the adnexal structures. Some of the melanocytes are multinucleated and some of the nests of melanocytes tend to confluence. Lentigo maligna is simply a synonym for one type of malignant melanoma in situ. (Reduced from ×155)*

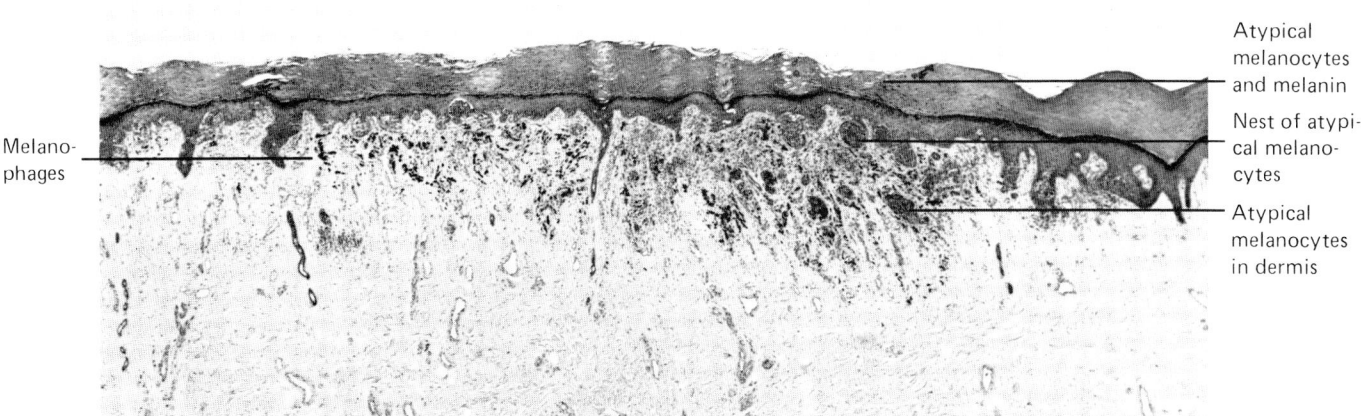

FIGURE 45A. **Malignant melanoma, acral-lentiginous type.** *With scanning magnification of this specimen from volar skin, evidenced by the compact orthokeratosis and prominent granular zone, irregularly shaped nests of atypical melanocytes may be seen to extend across the entire epidermis and into the upper part of the dermis. Many of the darkly staining cells within the dermis are melanophages. (Reduced from ×29)*

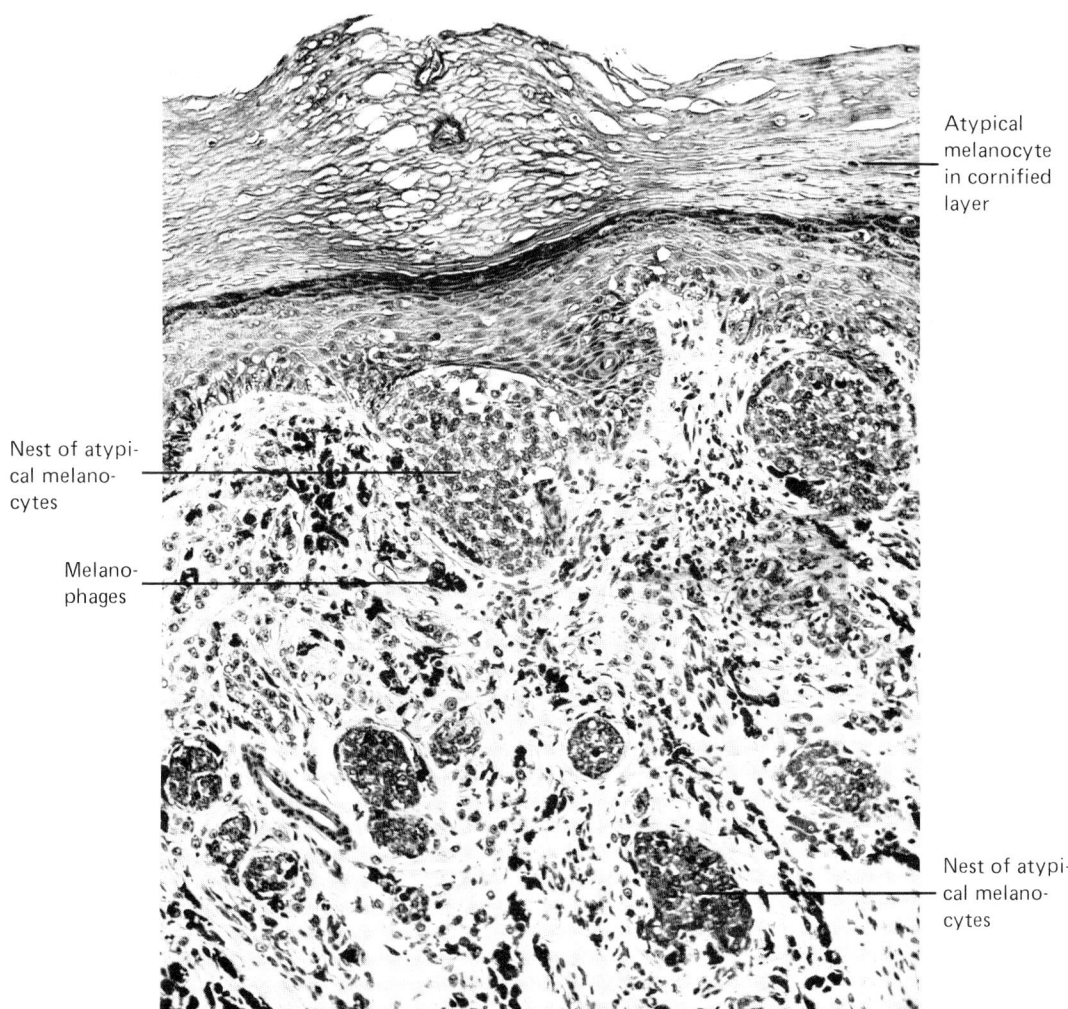

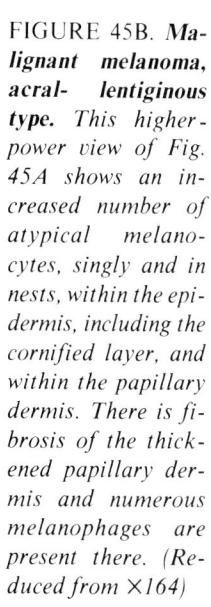

FIGURE 45B. **Malignant melanoma, acral- lentiginous type.** *This higher-power view of Fig. 45A shows an increased number of atypical melanocytes, singly and in nests, within the epidermis, including the cornified layer, and within the papillary dermis. There is fibrosis of the thickened papillary dermis and numerous melanophages are present there. (Reduced from ×164)*

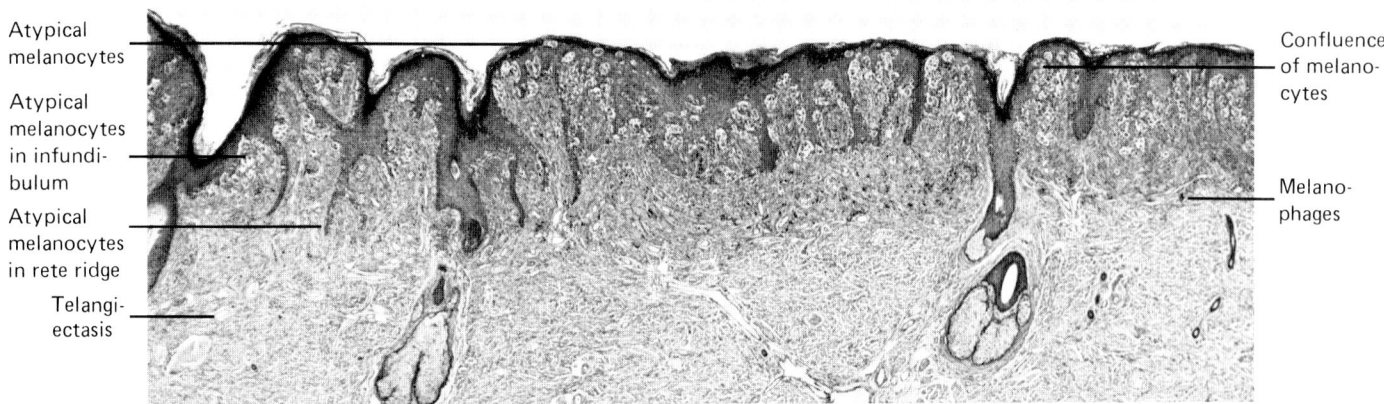

FIGURE 46A. **Malignant melanoma, superficial spreading type.** *This scanning power magnification illustrates well the horizontal extension of atypical melanocytes within the epidermis. Pagetoid melanocytes are present not only within the hyperplastic epidermis, but within the epithelium of adnexal structures. The papillary dermis is thickened by the inflammatory-cell infiltrate that contains melanophages and by fibrosis. Note the widely dilated blood vessels of the superficial plexus beneath the thickened papillary dermis. (Reduced from ×23)*

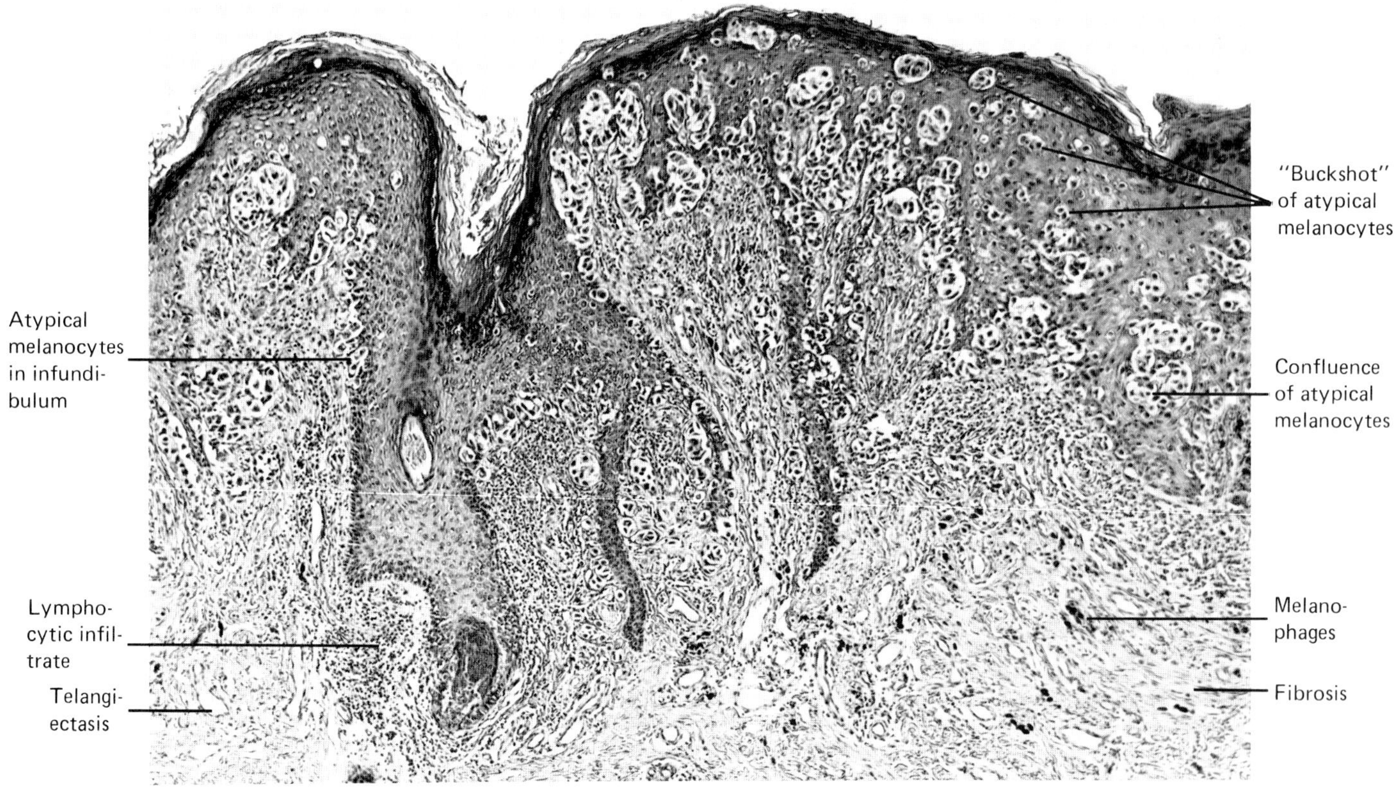

FIGURE 46B. **Malignant melanoma, superficial spreading type.** *Higher magnification of Fig. 46A showing the buckshot scatter of atypical pagetoid melanocytes throughout the epidermal and the adnexal epithelium. (Reduced from ×80)*

melanocytes are confined to the epidermis, the condition is an acral lentiginous malignant melanoma *in situ*. That variant of malignant melanoma, currently termed superficial spreading malignant melanoma, usually extends centrifugally within the epidermis for a much shorter period of time before reaching into the dermis than either the lentigo maligna or acral lentiginous types of malignant melanoma (Fig. 46). The form of malignant melanoma that remains confined to the epidermis for the shortest period of time before descending into the dermis is now called nodular malignant melanoma (Fig. 47). In the nodular type of malignant melanoma one never sees melanocytes only in the epidermis because by the time a nodule has developed, diffuse infiltration of atypical melanocytes has already occurred throughout at least the upper portion of the dermis. At one moment in time, however, the neoplastic cells of nodular malignant melanoma, like all other forms of cutaneous malignant melanoma, must have also been confined to the epidermis. In the flat clinical stages of the other three forms of malignant melanoma (the lentigo maligna, the acral lentiginous, and the superficial spreading), atypical melanocytes are restricted completely to the epidermis or epithelia of adnexal structures, none being in the dermis (Fig. 48). Surely there must also be an initial flat (macular or patch) stage in the evolution of nodular malignant melanoma where atypical melanocytes are present wholly within the epidermis. At that flat incipient stage the lesion may not be recognizable as what will become a nodular malignant melanoma because, by definition, the diagnosis of nodular malignant melanoma can only be made when nodularity has occurred. In fully developed lesions of nodular malignant melanoma, it is not uncommon to still see features (e.g., pagetoid or cuboidal melanocytes) within the epidermis overlying the nodule that are indistinguishable from those of superficial spreading malignant melanoma and even some atypical melanocytes within the epidermis at the sides of the nodule (Fig. 47).

With this concept in mind, that is, initial proliferation of melanocytes horizontally within the epidermis for varying periods of time in all types of primary cutaneous malignant melanoma, we can now begin to think about the similarities and differences among the four commonly accepted types of malignant melanoma, namely, lentigo maligna, acral lentiginous, superficial spreading, and nodular. But before doing that we are constrained to remark that the term "radial-growth phase," although denied to be meant as geometric by Clark, is confusing in its constant pairing with "vertical-growth phase," which is affirmed to be geometric in sense. In actuality, "radial-growth phase" means proliferation of melanocytes in all directions, whereas "vertical-growth phase" means extension of melanocytes downward into the dermis and/or the subcutaneous fat (with resultant elevation of the lesion, i.e., a plaque or nodule, eventually) and upward into the epidermis (with resultant alterations in color and surface, including erosion). It seems to us that "horizontal-growth phase" and "vertical-growth phase" would be more instantly and clearly understandable.

Lentigo maligna melanoma develops on severely sun-damaged skin, usually of the face of older persons. Like all other neoplastic processes in skin that develop in regions of marked solar elastosis, this melanocytic neoplasm tends to behave in a rather benign way biologically compared to those malignant melanomas that originate in regions shielded from sunlight. The same may be said for most squamous-cell carcinomas that arise in skin that has been severely injured by chronic exposure to sunlight, in contrast with squamous-cell carcinomas that arise *de novo* and in scars resulting from thermal burns, radiotherapy, or vaccination and chronic inflammatory processes like granuloma inguinale, lupus vulgaris, or discoid lupus erythematosus.

Lentigo maligna begins with an increase in number of normal-looking melanocytes in the basal layer of the epidermis. These more numerous melanocytes are not at first cytologically atypical as judged by conventional microscopy. Therefore, a lesion on sun-damaged skin which initially consists simply of individual melanocytes in greater abundance, cannot be diagnosed histologically with certainty as lentigo maligna at the early, small, macular or patch stage. In time, some of the melanocytes become slightly larger, hyperchromatic, and more pleomorphic than normal; some of them extend down along the epithelial cells of hair follicles and sweat ducts, and the hyperpigmented epidermis becomes thinned with diminution of the usual undulating pattern between rete ridges and dermal papillae (Fig. 49). At this stage the lesion can be diagnosed histologically with certainty as lentigo maligna. Still later, some of the melanocytes within the epidermis become dendritic and/or spindle-shaped and aggregated into nests that vary in size and shape (Fig. 50). The uninitiated may misdiagnose this stage of lentigo maligna as junction nevus. It is not unusual in lentigo maligna to see elongated nests of spindle-shaped melanocytes at the dermoepidermal junction aligned parallel to the surface of the skin (Fig. 50). Similar nests are also often present within the hyperpigmented epithelial structures of the adnexa. As long as the atypical melanocytes are confined to the epithelium, no matter how much of it is replaced or distorted by them, the lesion is a malignant melanoma *in situ* of the lentigo maligna type. When

40 The Histology of Cutaneous Malignant Melanoma

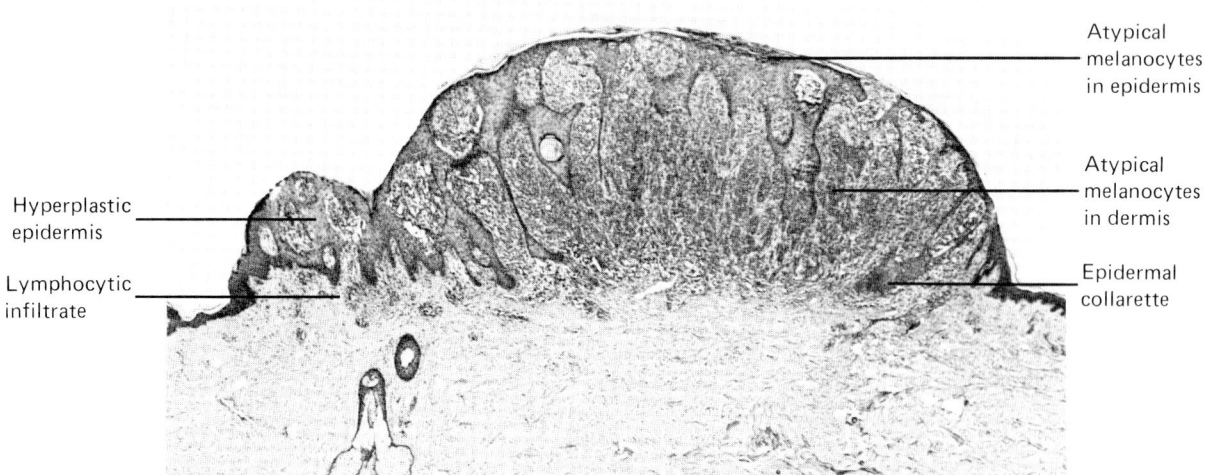

FIGURE 47A. **Malignant melanoma, nodular type.** This is a nodular melanoma according to Clark because the domed lesion is sharply circumscribed and no atypical melanocytes extend horizontally within the epidermis to the sides of the nodule. Note the tendency of the peripheral rete ridges to bend inward (arborize), a feature of a variety of benign and malignant processes that grow by pushing outward, such as pyogenic granuloma and verruca vulgaris, on the one hand, and nodular malignant melanoma on the other. (Reduced from ×27)

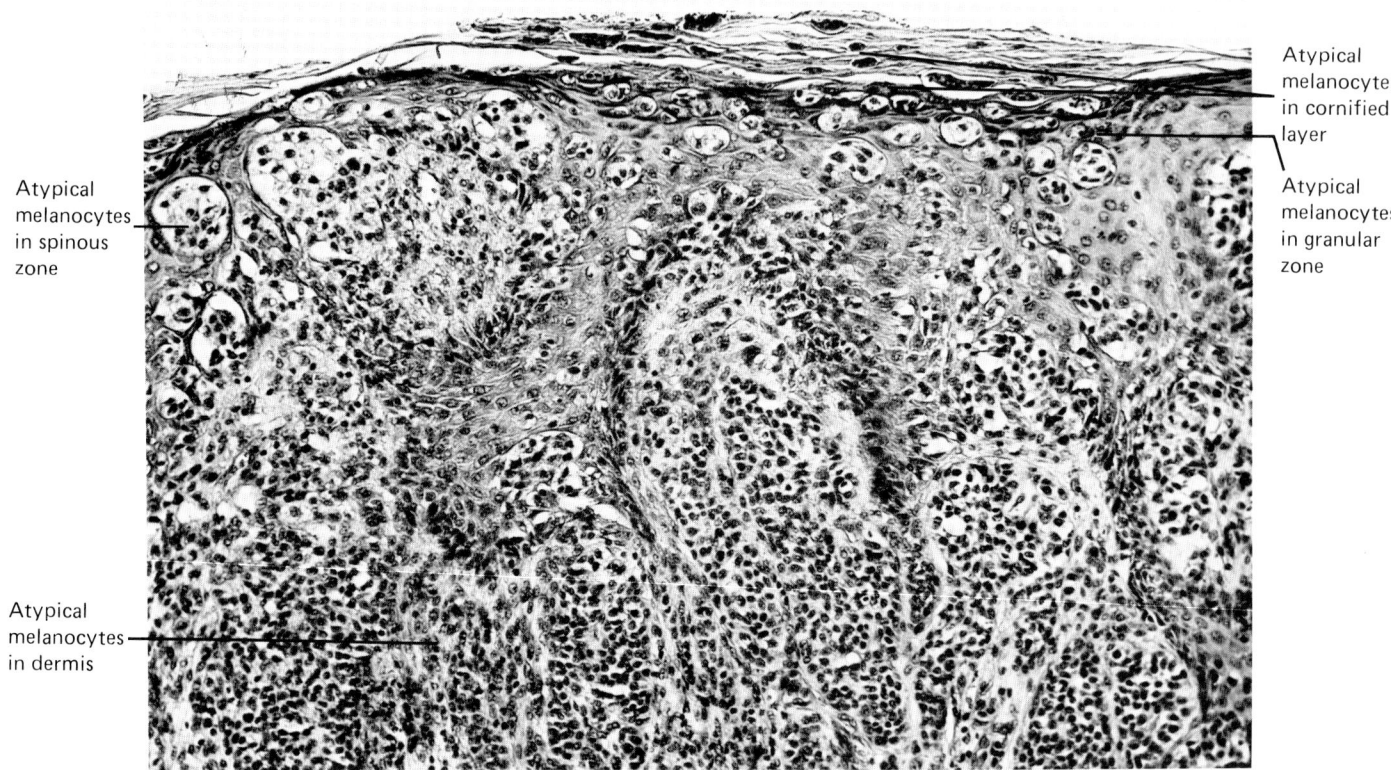

FIGURE 47B. **Malignant melanoma, nodular type.** This higher magnification of the nodular melanoma pictured in Fig. 47A shows changes in the epidermis that are indistinguishable from those of superficial spreading malignant melanoma, namely, atypical melanocytes, both singly and in nests, at all levels of the epidermis including the cornified layer. It is for this reason, among others, that we favor the concept that nodular melanoma, in most instances, is simply a form of superficial spreading malignant melanoma in which the vertical growth component has overtaken the horizontal one. (Reduced from ×173)

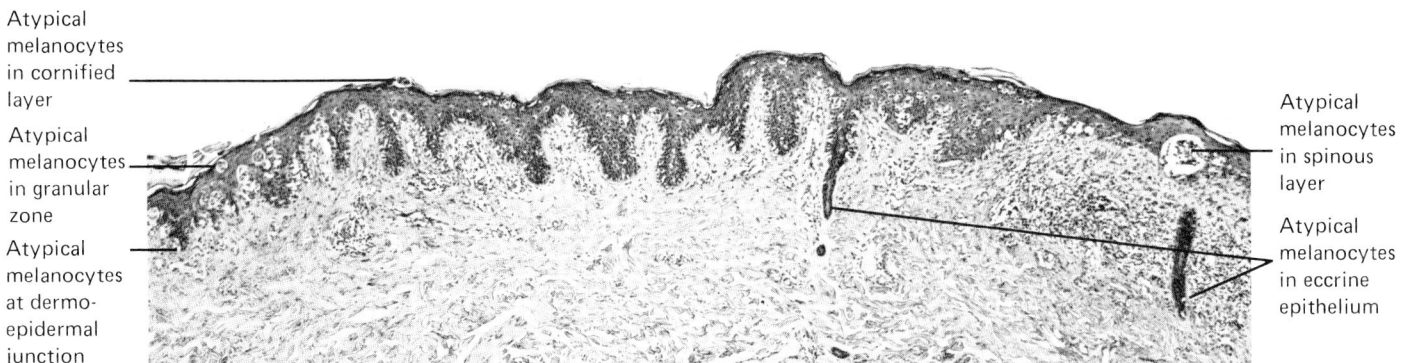

FIGURE 48A. **Malignant melanoma** in situ **with extensive involvement of epidermal and adnexal epithelium.** *The atypical melanocytes in this broad superficial spreading malignant melanoma* in situ *are seen to have lodged in all layers of the epidermis, including the cornified layer, and in the eccrine ducts. (Reduced from ×52)*

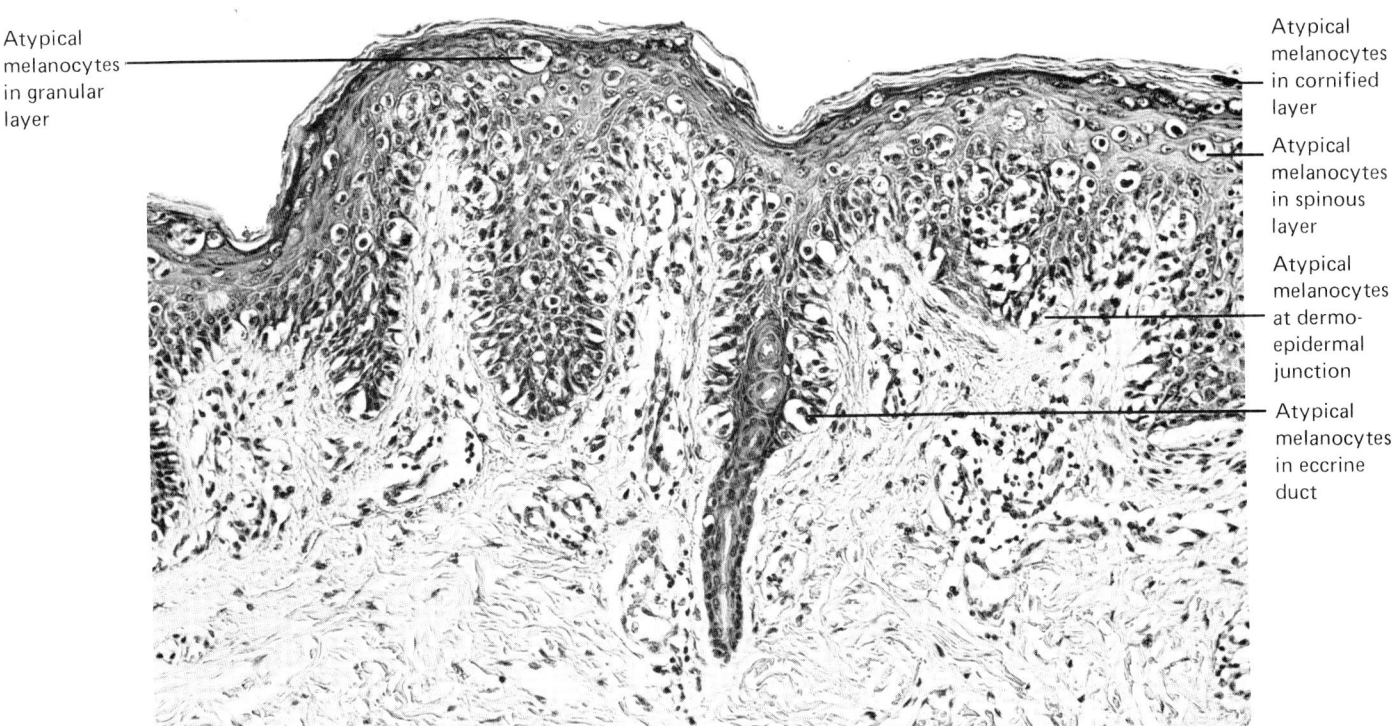

FIGURE 48B. **Malignant melanoma** in situ **with extensive involvement of epidermal and adnexal epithelium.** *A higher-power view of Fig. 48A shows "buckshot" scatter of atypical melanocytes within the epithelium of an eccrine duct of this horizontally extending malignant melanoma. (Reduced from ×198)*

atypical melanocytes appear in the dermis, the lesion is termed lentigo maligna melanoma, but nonetheless, the transition of lentigo maligna to lentigo maligna melanoma is a single pathological process in continuity (Fig. 51). If a nodule eventually develops in a lentigo maligna melanoma, the atypical melanocytes that comprise it are invariably spindle-shaped (Fig. 52). Elastotic material (i.e., solar elastosis), a sign of long-standing exposure to sunlight, is always present in the upper part of the dermis in lesions of both lentigo maligna and lentigo maligna melanoma. Usually, the solar elastosis is plentiful and prominent.

Acral lentiginous malignant melanoma, which we have

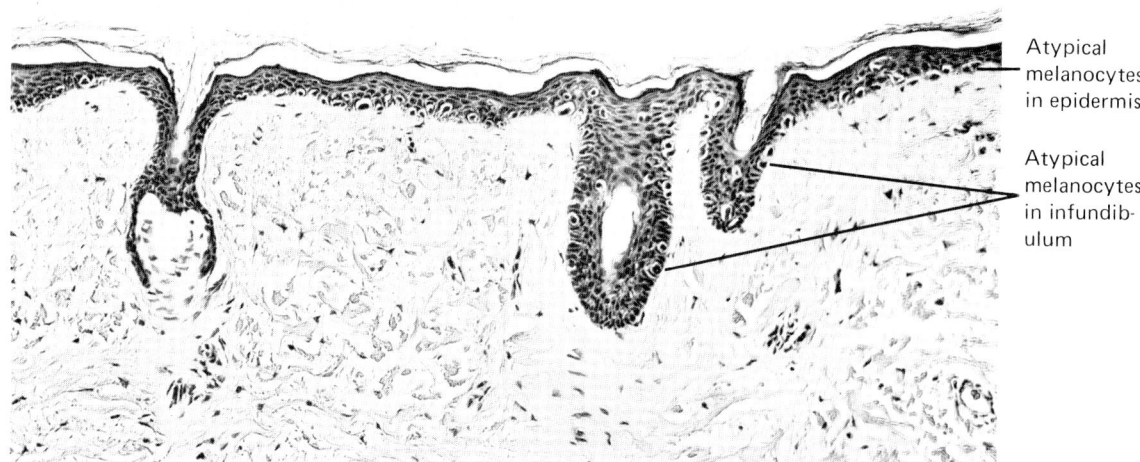

FIGURE 49A. **Lentigo maligna, early stage.** *Among the early changes in lentigo maligna are the appearance of atypical melanocytes disposed singly within the basal layer of the epidermis and within epithelial structures of adnexa, as pictured here. Note the severe solar elastosis and the thinned epidermis that is devoid of rete ridges. (Reduced from ×166)*

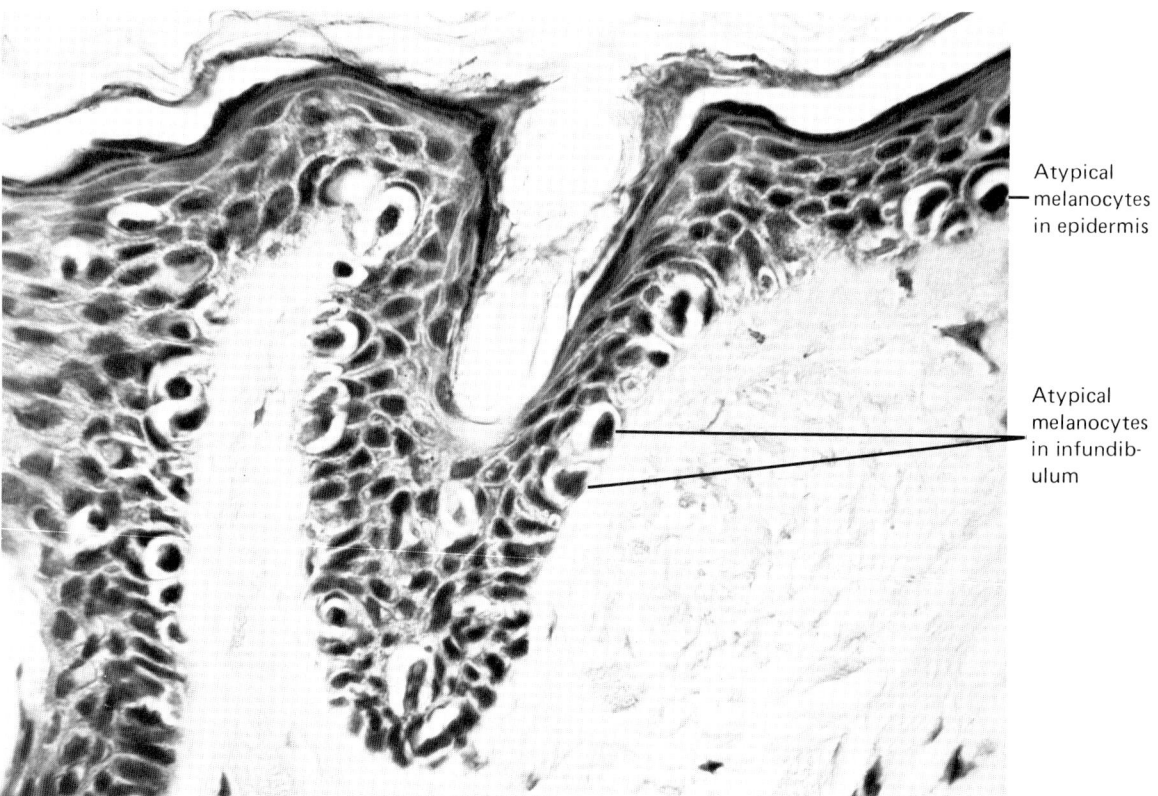

FIGURE 49B. **Lentigo maligna, early stage.** *The atypical melanocytes in lentigo maligna are more apparent in this higher magnification of Fig. 49 A. These melanocytes have nuclei that are large, hyperchromatic, and pleomorphic, and cytoplasms that also vary in volume and staining qualities. (Reduced from ×700)*

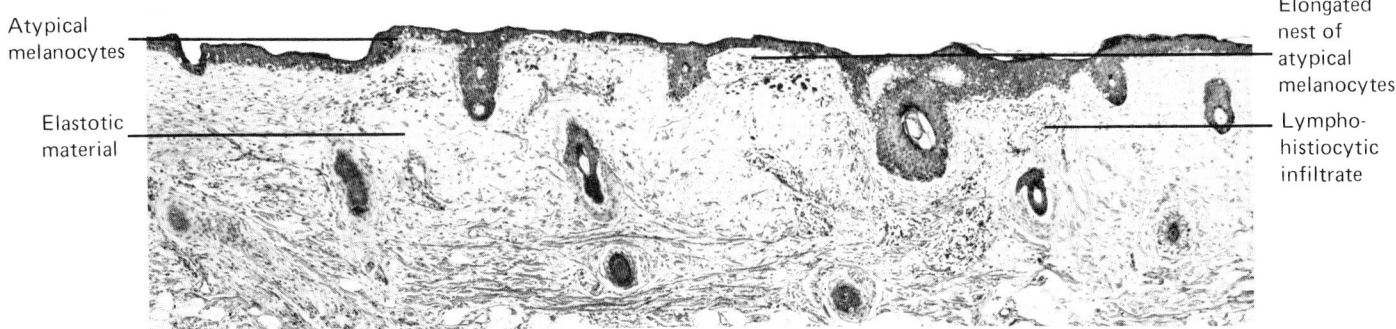

FIGURE 50A. **Lentigo maligna.** *Diagnosis of lentigo maligna can be made with scanning power, as in this photomicrograph, because of the increased number of melanocytes, both singly and in elongated nests, that parallel the skin surface at the dermoepidermal junction. Note the marked solar elastosis and the moderately dense lymphohistiocytic infiltrate with melanophages in the upper part of the dermis. (Reduced from ×49)*

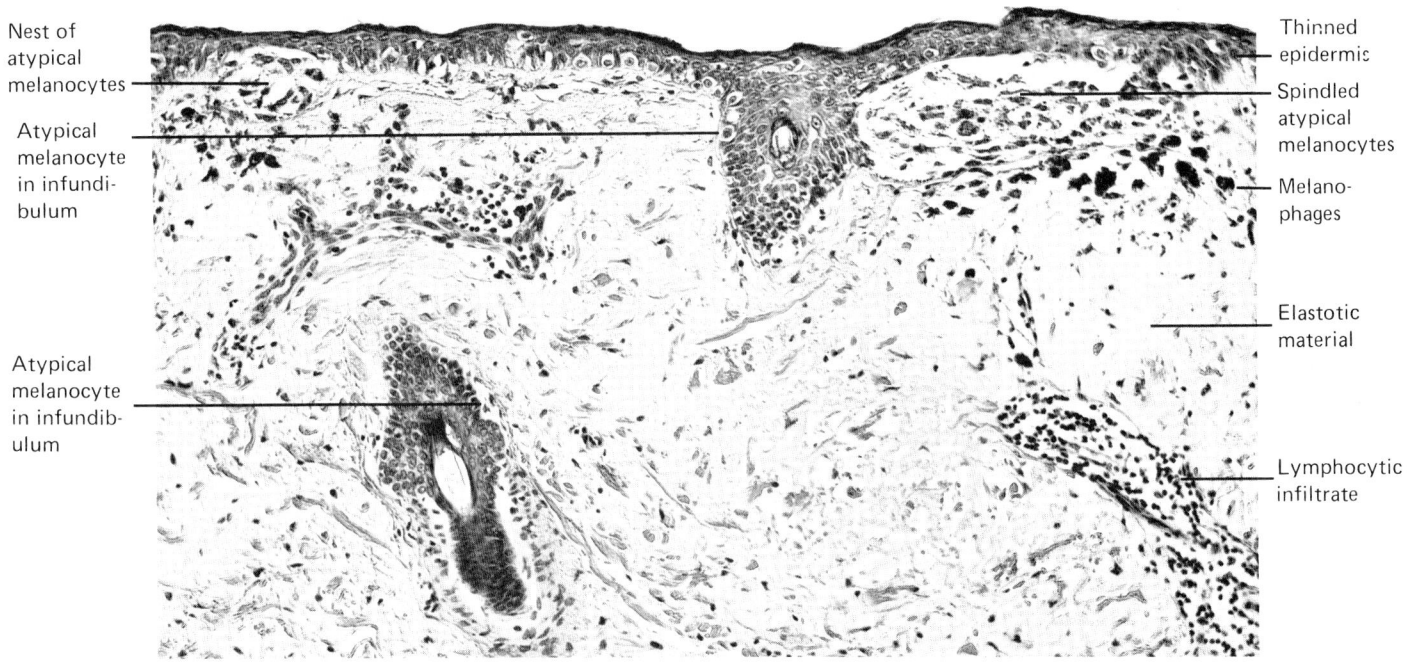

FIGURE 50B. **Lentigo maligna.** *This higher magnification of Fig. 50A shows the increased number of atypical melanocytes, both singly and in nests, within the epidermis. On the right-hand side of the photomicrograph, at the dermoepidermal junction, there is an elongated nest of atypical melanocytes that is oriented parallel to the skin's surface. This orientation is typical of nests of melanocytes within the epidermis of lentigo maligna and lentigo maligna melanoma, in contrast to the perpendicular alignment of elongated nests of melanocytes in the epidermis of the nevus of large spindle and/or epithelioid cells. (Reduced from ×173)*

also dubbed palmar-plantar-periungual malignant melanoma, has many clinical and histologic features like those of lentigo maligna melanoma. Because acral lentiginous malignant melanoma also spreads horizontally within the epidermis of the acral regions for such a long time, it may, like lentigo maligna, attain the size of a large patch, 10 cm or more in diameter. Often, after many years, some of the increased numbers of dendritic, spindle-shaped, or cuboidal melanocytes that were originally confined within the epidermis of acral lentiginous malignant melanoma *in situ*

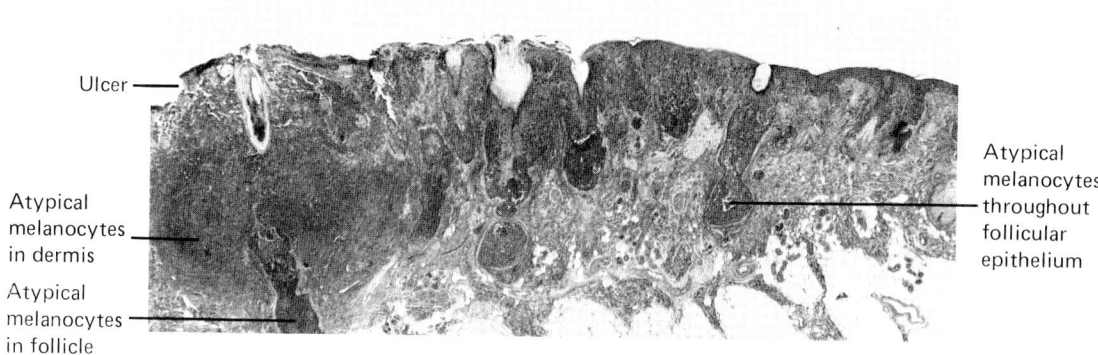

FIGURE 51A. ***Malignant melanoma, lentigo maligna type.*** *Scanning magnification reveals that this is a lentigo maligna type of malignant melanoma because of the extensive involvement of epithelium of adnexa, especially hair follicles, by the spindle-shaped melanocytes. On the right-hand side of the photomicrograph, the malignant melanoma is largely* in situ *(lentigo maligna), whereas on the left-hand side there is extension of atypical melanocytes to the base of the specimen in the deep reticular dermis (lentigo maligna melanoma). (Reduced from ×17)*

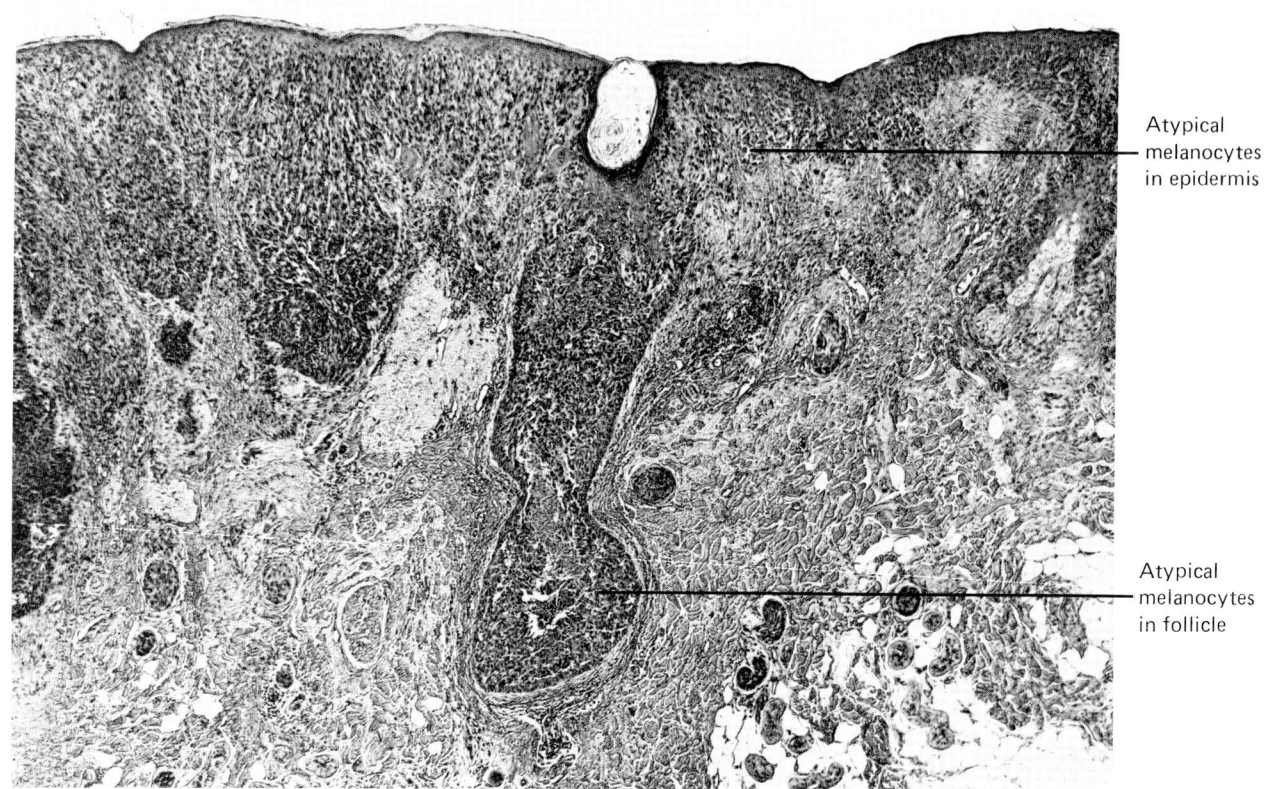

FIGURE 51B. ***Malignant melanoma, lentigo maligna type.*** *The increased number of atypical melanocytes seen in this higher magnification of Fig. 51A are not only present within the epidermis, but largely replace the infundibular portion of the hair follicle pictured. These changes, plus the marked solar elastosis, are typical of lentigo maligna and lentigo maligna melanoma. (Reduced from ×68)*

extend into the dermis where they assume spindle or cuboidal shapes. The earliest histologic change within the epidermis of acral lentiginous malignant melanomas is proliferation of melanocytes as individual units whose nuclei are not atypical, but whose cellular shapes are often remarkably dendritic (Fig. 53). Dendrites may extend as far up as the granular layer. If one is not alert to these subtle cytologic changes in early lesions of acral lentiginous malignant melanoma *in situ,* the lesion may be easily misinterpreted as a benign simple lentigo or simply as melanocytic hyperplasia. In time, the dendritic melanocytes congregate into nests of different sizes and shapes (Fig. 54). The epidermis of these lesions at this *in situ* stage is usually heavily pigmented. The eventual clinical consequences of these histologic changes are formation of papules and/or nodules surrounded by an irregularly shaped and colored pigmented patch.

Superficial spreading malignant melanoma also begins as a pigmented macule that evolves into a patch in which atypical, usually pagetoid, melanocytes are confined to the epidermis (Fig. 55). Unlike the situation in lentigo maligna and acral lentiginous malignant melanoma *in situ* where there is proliferation of *individual* melanocytes within the epidermis for years, in superficial spreading malignant melanoma *in situ, nests* of atypical melanocytes form relatively early in the course. However, for reasons still inexplicable, some atypical melanocytes within the epidermis of superficial spreading malignant melanoma migrate into the dermis after months, or at most a few years, rather than decades as is often the case in lentigo maligna and acral lentiginous types of malignant melanoma (Fig. 56). With the development of vertical growth of atypical melanocytes, a papular and subsequently nodular lesion often forms within the pigmented patch or plaque of the original process. The sites of predilection for superficial spreading malignant melanoma, the back in men and the legs in women, are clearly different from those of lentigo maligna melanoma and acral lentiginous malignant melanoma. The different distribution of superficial spreading malignant melanoma in the two sexes may result, in part, from differences in sun exposure.

The term superficial spreading malignant melanoma is unfortunate because the word "superficial" implies to some physicians and surgeons that these neoplasms are superficial in location when, in fact, they may penetrate deep into the dermis and into the subcutaneous fat. In addition, superficial spreading malignant melanoma usually spreads superficially for a much shorter distance than either lentigo maligna melanoma or acral lentiginous malignant melanoma.

Nodular malignant melanoma, just as the other variants of malignant melanoma, must also begin as a pigmented macule that in a relatively short time, probably less than 1 year, evolves so that atypical, usually cuboidal, neoplastic melanocytes come to form a papule and then a nodule in the dermis. This phenomenon of papulation to nodulation occurs along the entire front of the epidermis that contains atypical melanocytes. Therefore, unlike lentigo maligna, acral lentiginous malignant melanoma *in situ,* and superficial spreading malignant melanoma *in situ* in which melanocytes in only a relatively limited focus of the epidermis descend into the dermis to produce a papule or nodule that is surrounded by a pigmented patch or plaque, the atypical melanocytes along the entire small front of nodular malignant melanoma *in situ* appear en masse in the dermis (Fig. 47). The resultant nodule in nodular malignant melanoma is not surrounded by a broad patch or plaque of pigmentation. However, we do not agree with Clark and his associates (1975) that "nodular melanomas are comprised exclusively of a vertical-growth phase." In our opinion, nodular malignant melanomas, like all malignant melanomas, first have a horizontal growth phase within the epidermis and quickly thereafter assume a vertical growth phase within the dermis. The unique feature of nodular malignant melanomas is the relative suddenness with which the vertical growth phase supervenes. Clark and co-workers seem to acknowledge the superficially spreading phase of nodular malignant melanoma when they write of the criterion for differentiating nodular malignant melanoma from superficial spreading malignant melanoma in which a nodule has developed. The distinction, according to them, is that the atypical melanocytes within the epidermis of nodular malignant melanoma extend for no more than three rete ridges beyond the nodule, whereas in superficial spreading malignant melanoma more than three rete ridges are traversed (Fig. 57). In our opinion, even three rete ridges represent horizontal spread. Careful scrutiny of clinical lesions of nodular malignant melanoma will also sometimes reveal evidence of horizontal spread of melanocytes, namely, a rim of pigmentation to one side of the nodule or around it. In long-standing lesions of nodular malignant melanoma there may only be a few atypical melanocytes within the epidermis and those disposed only as single cells in the basal layer rather than in nests at all levels of the epidermis. In other lesions of nodular malignant melanoma, the features in the epidermis are indistinguishable from those of superficial spreading malignant melanoma.

An unequivocal judgment about whether a malignant melanoma is of lentigo maligna, acral lentiginous, superficial spreading, or nodular types cannot always be made

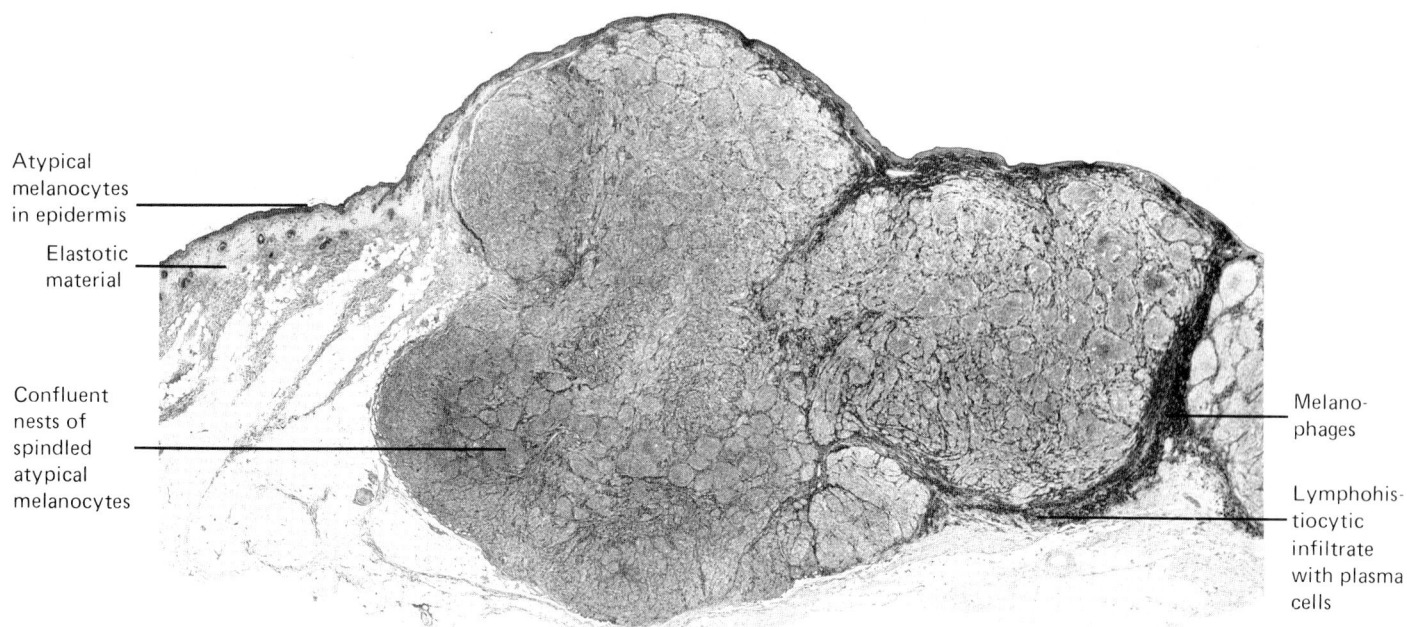

FIGURE 52A. **Malignant melanoma, lentigo maligna type.** *This large nodule within a lentigo maligna melanoma extends deep into the subcutaneous fat. Note that there is very little inflammatory-cell infiltrate around the neoplasm. The patient from whom this melanoma was excised lived with the disease for many years and, despite the depth of penetration (thickness) by the malignant neoplasm, had no evidence of metastases. (Reduced from ×12)*

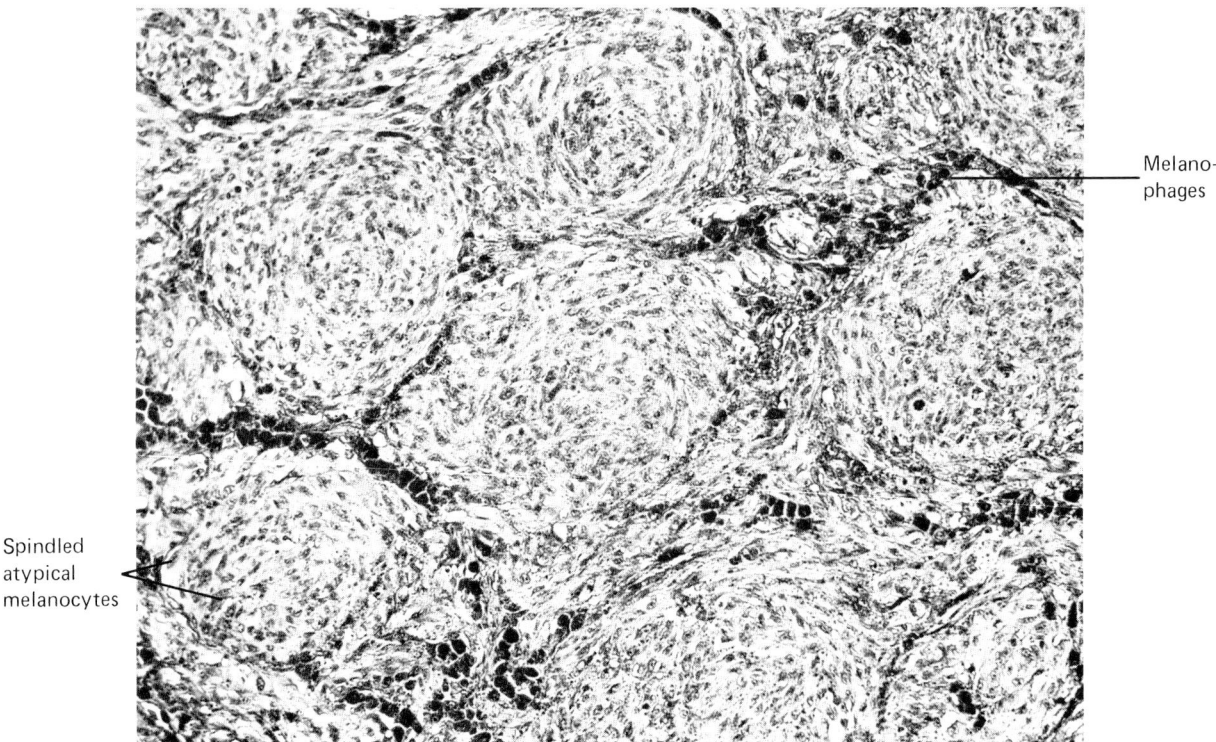

FIGURE 52B. **Malignant melanoma, lentigo maligna type.** *This higher-power view of Fig. 52B reveals the spindle shape of the neoplastic cells that are arranged in variously sized nests. (Reduced from ×158)*

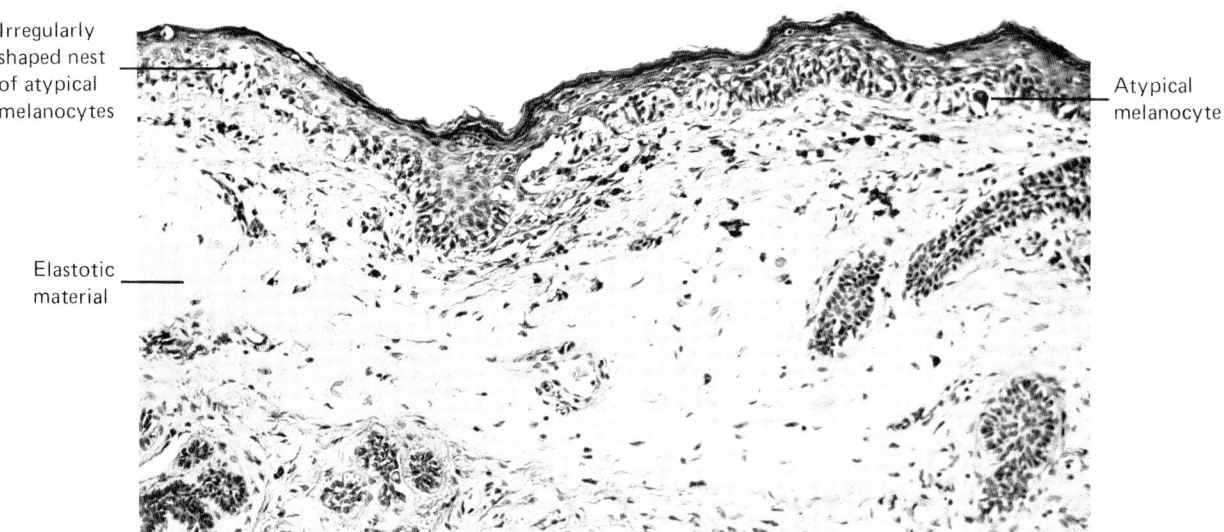

FIGURE 52C. **Malignant melanoma, lentigo maligna type.** *In the epidermis to the left of the nodule of malignant melanoma pictured in Fig. 52A there are diagnostic changes of lentigo maligna, namely, atypical melanocytes singly and in variously sized and irregularly shaped nests in a thinned epidermis devoid of rete ridges. Note the extensive elastotic material (solar elastosis), a* sine qua non *for the diagnosis of lentigo maligna and lentigo maligna melanoma. (Reduced from ×158)*

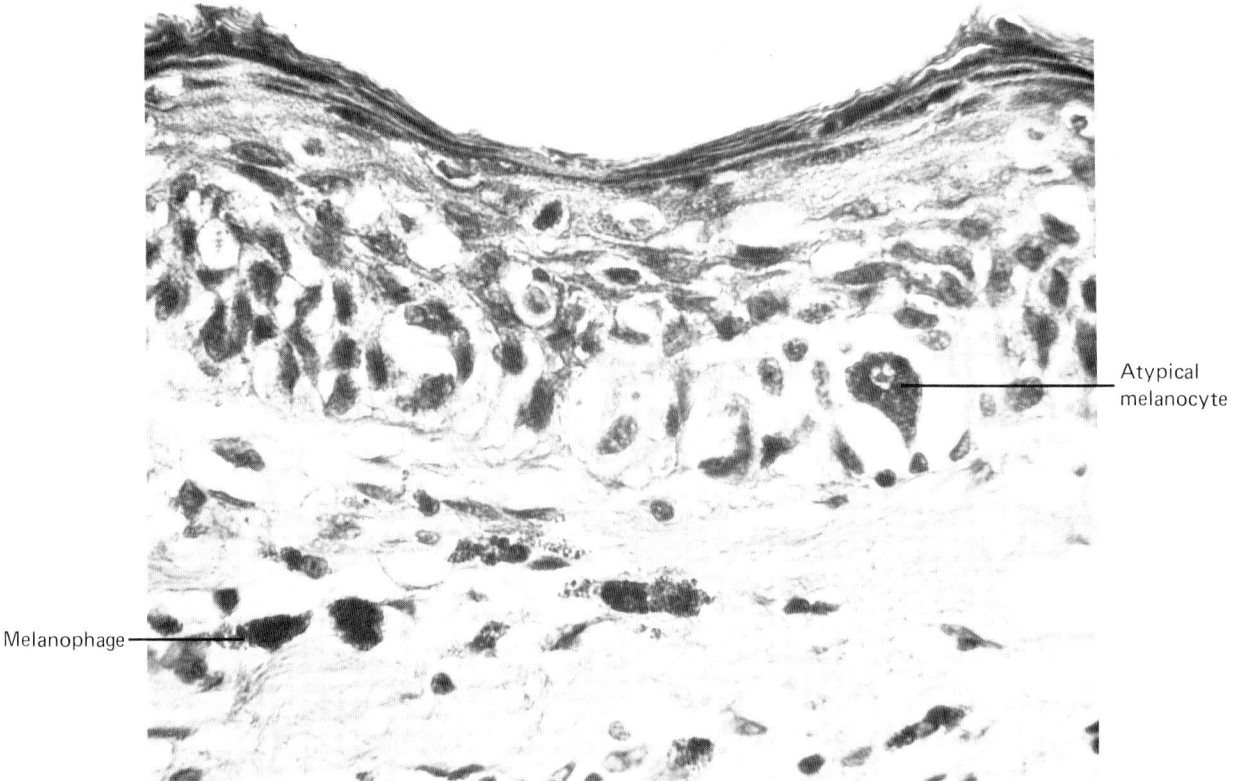

FIGURE 52D. **Malignant melanoma, lentigo maligna type.** *Still higher magnification of Fig. 52C to show more distinctly the atypical melanocytes within the epidermis and melanophages within the dermis of this focus of lentigo maligna. (Reduced from ×760)*

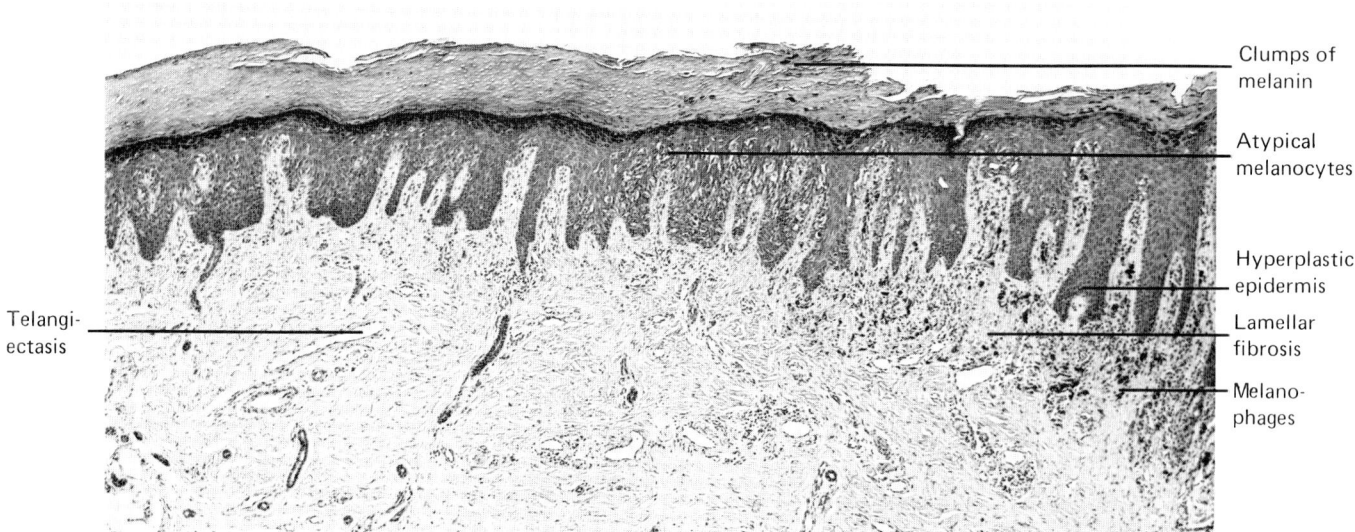

FIGURE 53A. **Malignant melanoma, acral lentiginous type, in situ.** *This specimen comes from volar skin as is evidenced by the compact cornified layer, the prominent granular zone, and the relatively thick epidermis. Within the epidermis there are an increased number of single melanocytes, not only in the basal zone, but at all levels of the epidermis. The papillary dermis on the right side is thickened by fibrosis and contains a sparse lymphohistiocytic infiltrate with numerous melanophages. (Reduced from ×55)*

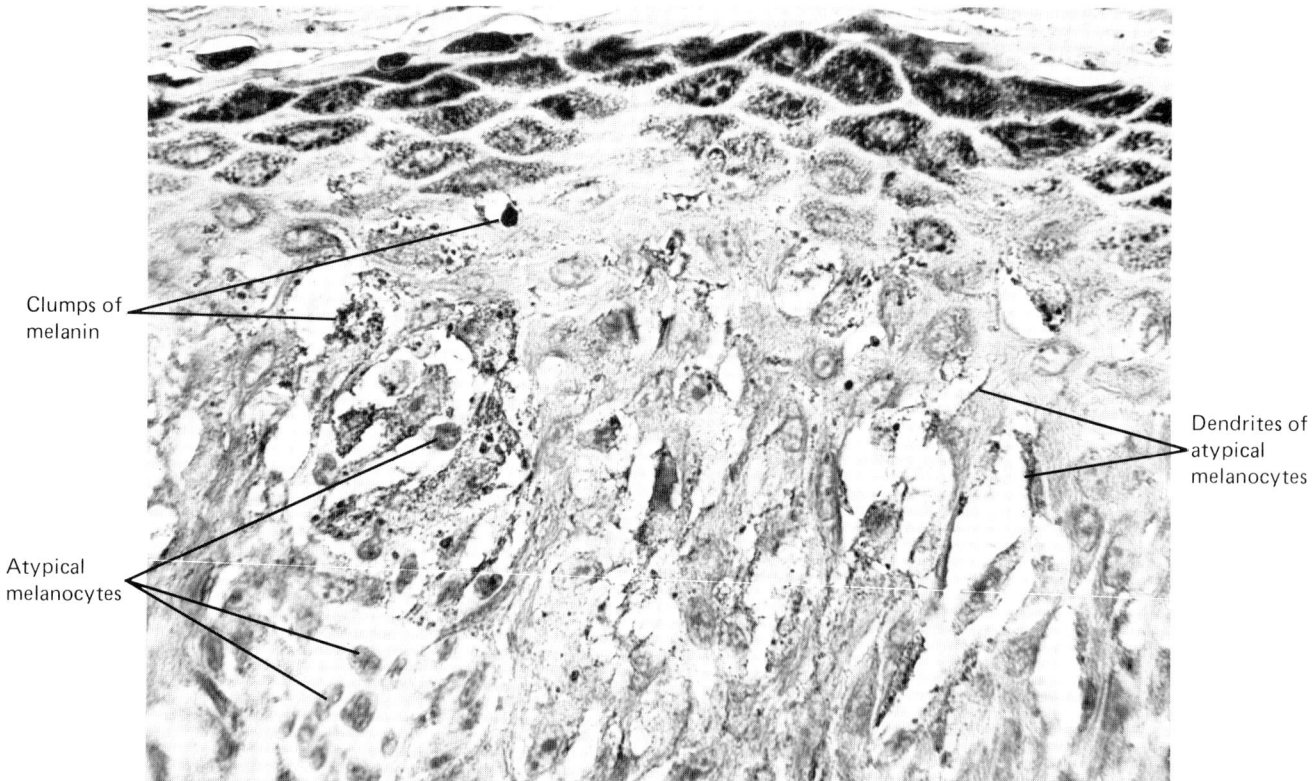

FIGURE 53B. **Malignant melanoma, acral lentiginous type, in situ.** *This higher magnification of Fig. 53A shows the diagnostic features of early acral lentiginous malignant melanoma* in situ, *namely, an increased number of melanocytes having prominent dendrites, some of which extend from the basal to the granular zone. If one is not alert to these changes, such a lesion could easily be misinterpreted as simply melanocytic hyperplasia and not a malignant melanoma* in situ. *(Reduced from ×714)*

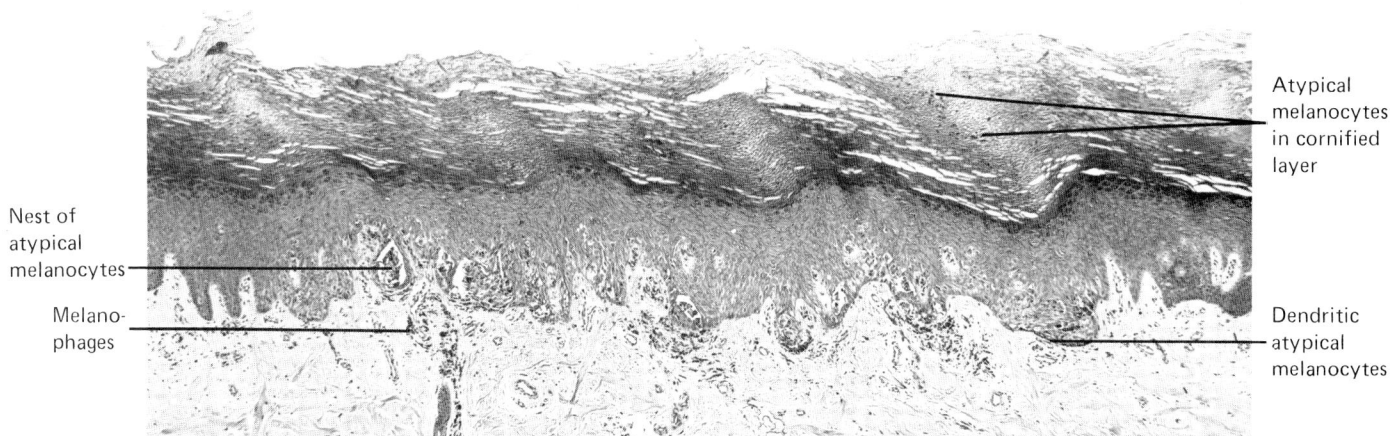

FIGURE 54A. **Malignant melanoma, acral lentiginous type, in situ.** *This is a slightly later stage of the process pictured in Fig. 53. In this specimen there are not only an increased number of dendritic melanocytes, but atypical melanocytes congregated in irregularly shaped nests. There is also a lymphohistiocytic infiltrate with melanophages in the papillary dermis. (Reduced from ×58)*

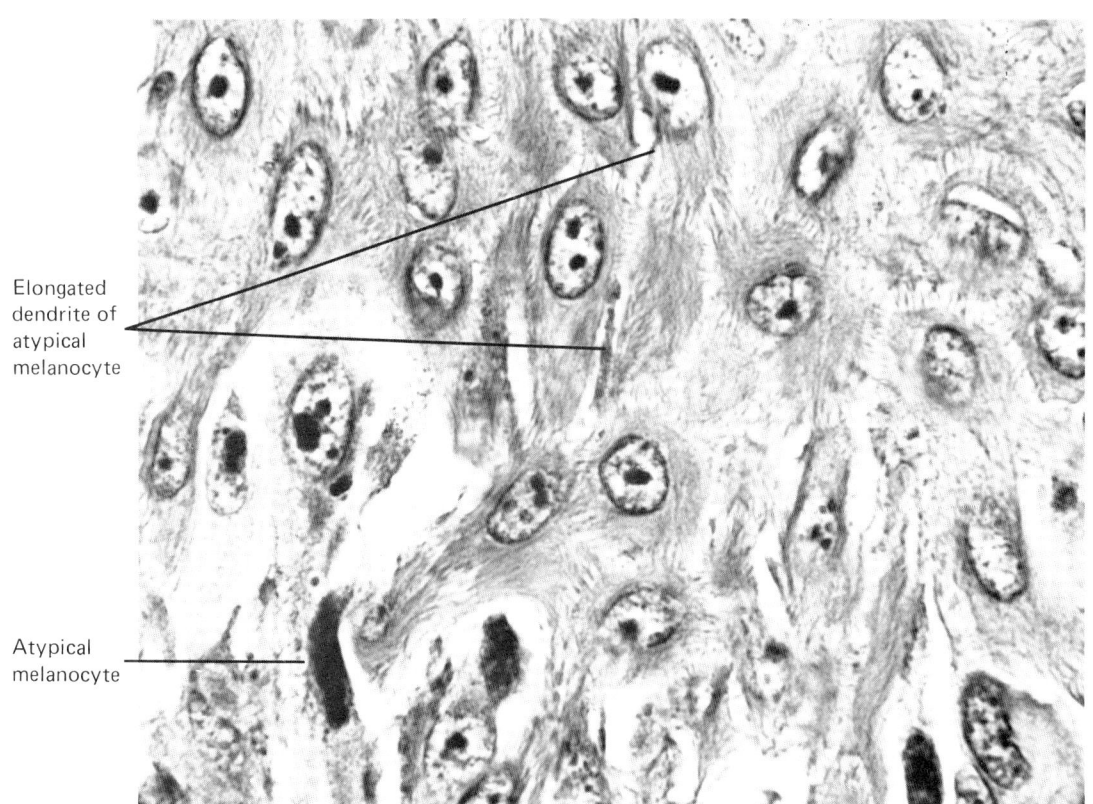

FIGURE 54B. **Malignant melanoma, acral lentiginous type, in situ.** *Higher-power magnification of Fig. 54B shows atypical melanocytes in the lower left-hand portion of the photomicrograph and elongated dendrites that extend between keratinocytes in the middle, signs of acral lentiginous malignant melanoma* in situ. *(Reduced from ×1476)*

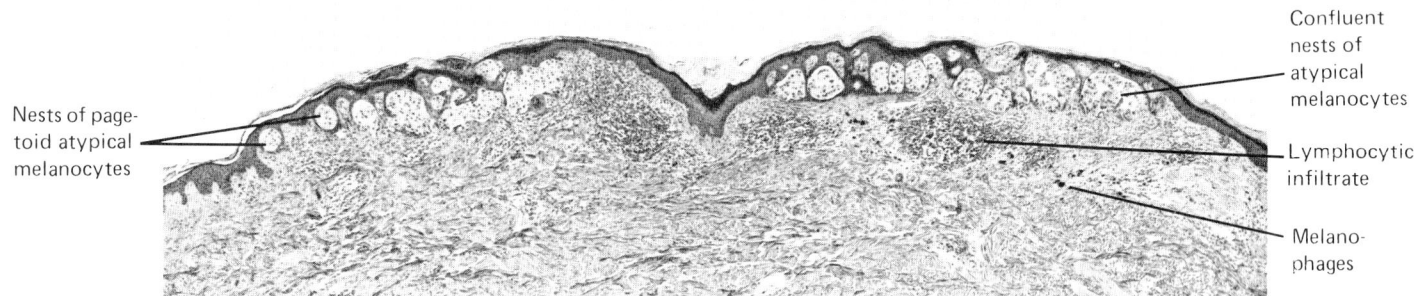

FIGURE 55A. **Malignant melanoma, superficial spreading type, in situ.** *With scanning magnification one can see that there are irregularly shaped aggregates of pagetoid cells, presumably melanocytes, within the epidermis. Note the moderately dense lymphohistiocytic infiltrate in the upper part of the dermis. If under high power some atypical melanocytes are found in the papillary dermis, this would be a malignant melanoma without question. If, however, the atypical melanocytes are confined to the epidermis, the lesion is a malignant melanoma* in situ, *comparable to squamous-cell carcinoma* in situ. *(Reduced from ×35)*

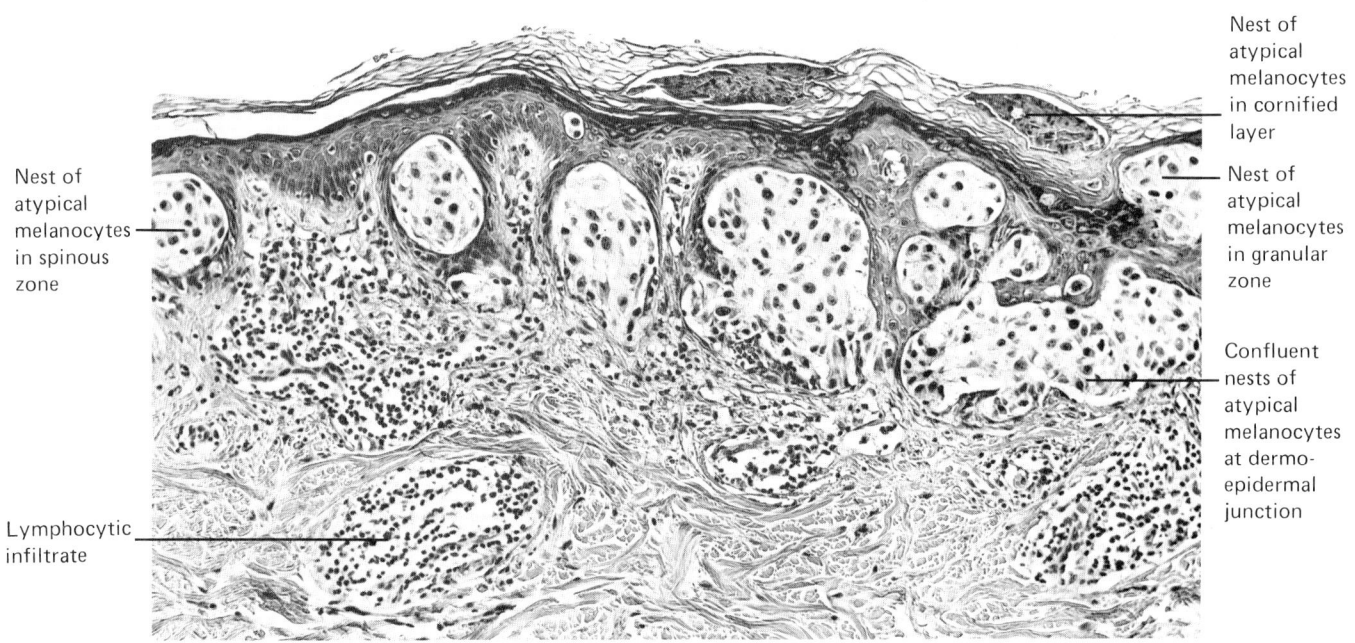

FIGURE 55B. **Malignant melanoma, superficial spreading type, in situ.** *Higher magnification of Fig. 55A shows irregularly shaped nests of atypical melanocytes throughout all levels of the epidermis including the cornified layer. Some of the nests have become confluent. The correct histologic diagnosis in lesions such as this is not simply atypical melanocytic hyperplasia, but malignant melanoma, superficial spreading type,* in situ. *(Reduced from ×164)*

because of overlapping features in a particular lesion. Some malignant melanomas do not seem to conform precisely to any of these four types and such lesions are termed "malignant melanoma, unclassified" by us (Figs. 58 and 59).

Clark's classification of malignant melanoma is a significant contribution in several respects, but perhaps mostly because it enables early recognition of malignant melanomas, clinically and histologically, and by so doing permits surgery to be performed earlier and thus increases the likelihood of cure.

The clinical similarities and differences among the four principal types of primary cutaneous malignant melanoma may be understood and explained within the context of their respective evolutions. Just as the different types of malignant melanoma have clinical, and eventually biological, features in common, so, too, do they have many histologic features in common. In time, each type of malignant melanoma is characterized by an increased number of atypical melanocytes both singly and in nests within the epidermis, within epithelial structures of adnexa, within the dermis to varying depths, and if undisturbed, even within the subcutaneous fat. The presence of atypical melanocytes as single cells or in strands between collagen bundles in the reticular dermis presages a poor prognosis for the patient. Cytologically, any of these types of malignant melanoma may show little or much nuclear atypia. Their cytoplasms may be replete with melanin or almost devoid of it. The cells may be very large (balloon cells) or quite small (small cells). Some cytologic differences may be found among the various types of malignant melanoma, namely, the melanocytes in lentigo maligna and in lentigo maligna melanoma tend to be dendritic and/or spindle-shaped; those of acral lentiginous malignant melanoma are often dendritic and later cuboidal in the *in situ* stage and spindled or cuboidal during the papular or nodular melanomatous phase; those of superficial spreading malignant melanoma are often pagetoid; and those of nodular malignant melanoma are more likely to be large and cuboidal (epithelioid). Nevertheless, any of these cytologic variants may be found in variable numbers in any of the types of malignant melanoma. For example, pagetoid cells may be found in lentigo maligna melanoma and spindle-shaped melanocytes in superficial spreading malignant melanoma.

Another histologic finding that may sometimes be shared by each of the various types of malignant melanomas is more than one population of atypical melanocytes within the dermis. For example, in one part of the neoplasm, atypical melanocytes may have small nuclei with little cytoplasm, whereas in another zone of the same malignant melanoma atypical melanocytes may be pagetoid. The development of more than one population of atypical melanocytes within the dermis of malignant melanoma presages rapid vertical growth of the neoplasm and the likelihood of imminent metastases. In sum, two or more populations of atypical melanocytes in a malignant melanoma implies a more serious prognosis for the patient.

The epidermis in all kinds of malignant melanoma is altered by the pathological process and may respond by becoming thinned, hyperplastic, papillated, verrucous, eroded, ulcerated, or necrotic.

A predominantly lymphocytic infiltrate, in which histiocytes and rarely plasma cells are admixed, is present beneath almost every malignant melanoma *in situ,* irrespective of type (Fig. 60). The density of the inflammatory-cell infiltrate varies from lesion to lesion, but is usually most dense below thin malignant melanomas and less dense as the neoplasms thicken as they descend progressively into the dermis. This may partially explain the observation that the denser the inflammatory-cell infiltrate, the better in most instances is the prognosis. Plasma cells predominate in the sparse infiltrate found within and beneath thick malignant melanomas.

The blood vessels of the superficial vascular plexus dilate in association with thin malignant melanomas, i.e., those that are confined to the papillary dermis. Sometimes, the dilation of the venules of this subpapillary plexus is dramatic.

Desmoplastic malignant melanoma with its intense fibroplasia around atypical spindle-shaped melanocytes is a reactive process of the stroma to the atypical melanocytes of what is usually a lentigo maligna melanoma and less commonly an acral lentiginous malignant melanoma (Fig. 61). The spindle-shaped melanocytes may contain little or no melanin and may penetrate to the deep reticular dermis or subcutaneous fat (Frolow et al., 1975). The fibrosis may be interpreted as an attempt by the host to contain the neoplasm. The histochemical and electron-microscopic findings of Labrecque et al. (1976) confirm the fibroblastic nature of the stromal response. Some bizarre, pleomorphic neoplastic cells are sometimes found among the fibroblasts and collagen (Conley et al., 1971). Desmoplastic malignant melanoma must be differentiated histologically from squamous-cell carcinoma whose cells are spindle-shaped, atypical fibroxanthoma, and malignant fibrous histiocytoma. The clue to the diagnosis of desmoplastic malignant melanoma is the finding of some atypical melanocytes within the epidermis. Desmoplasia in malignant melanoma is uncommon but dramatic when it occurs. It must be differentiated from the more common and subtle lamellar fibrosis that involves the papillary dermis only (Fig. 62).

The tendency to form an epidermal collarette (elongated, inwardly bowed, embracing peripheral rete ridges) and/or fibroplasia at the base of nodular (Fig. 63) and pedunculated (Fig. 64) malignant melanomas may also be interpreted as an attempt by the host to "wall off" the expanding population of atypical melanocytes in the upper part of the dermis. The attempt fails and patients with nodular and pedunculated malignant melanomas often succumb to metastatic disease. The prognosis for pedunculated malignant melanomas is seemingly among the most grave of all cutaneous malignant melanomas.

Verrucous malignant melanoma, with its crusted, verrucoid, hyperplastic epidermis, is an exuberant expression of the epidermis and papillary dermis to influences upon them by the neoplastic melanocytes and the inflammatory-cell infiltrates (Fig. 65). Ulceration and crusting are

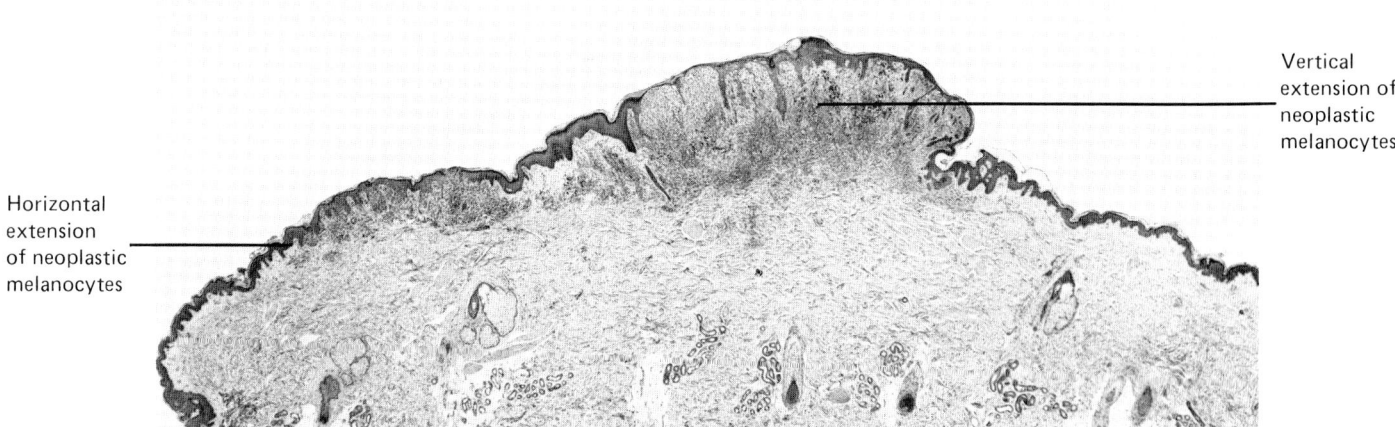

FIGURE 56A. **Malignant melanoma, superficial spreading type.** *This scanning power view shows a nodule of malignant melanoma on the right-hand portion of the photomicrograph and nests of atypical melanocytes that extend considerably beyond the nodule within the epidermis on the left. These are the features of a superficial spreading malignant melanoma in which a nodule has formed. (Reduced from ×18)*

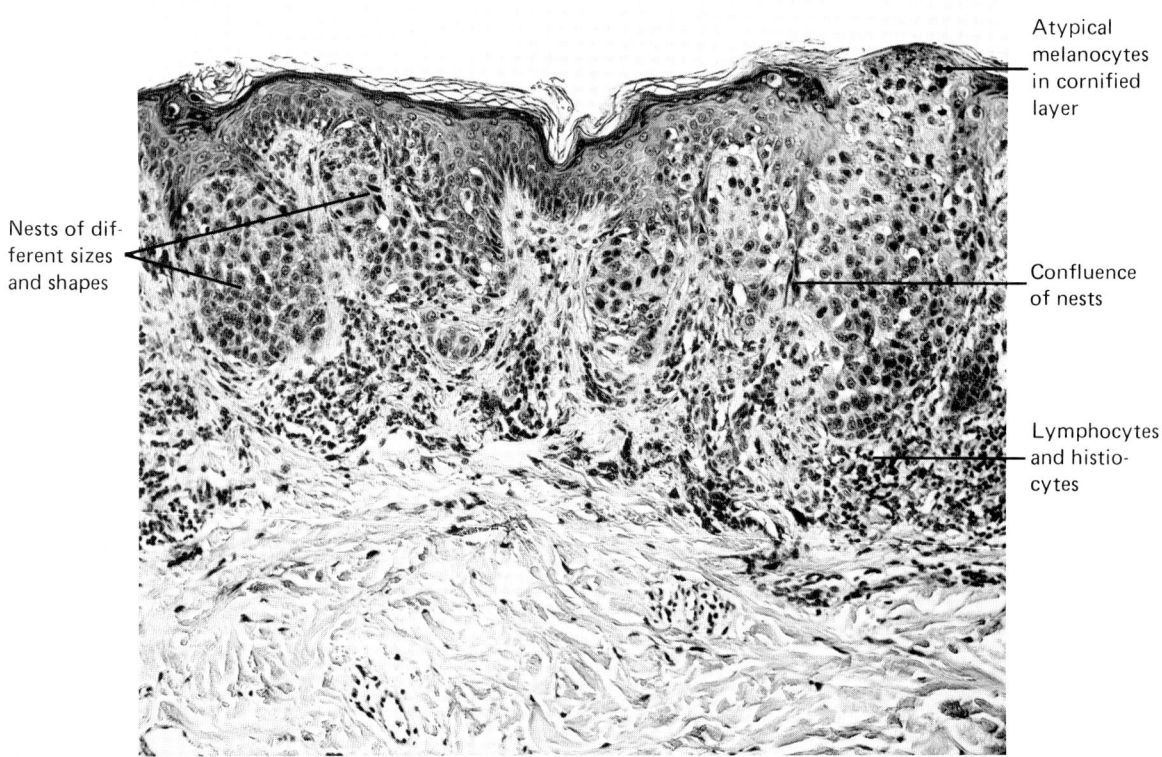

FIGURE 56B. **Malignant melanoma, superficial spreading type.** *This higher magnification of Fig. 56A shows marked variation in the size and shape of the nests of atypical melanocytes within the epidermis, their tendency to confluence, and their presence far above the basal layer. (Reduced from ×152).*

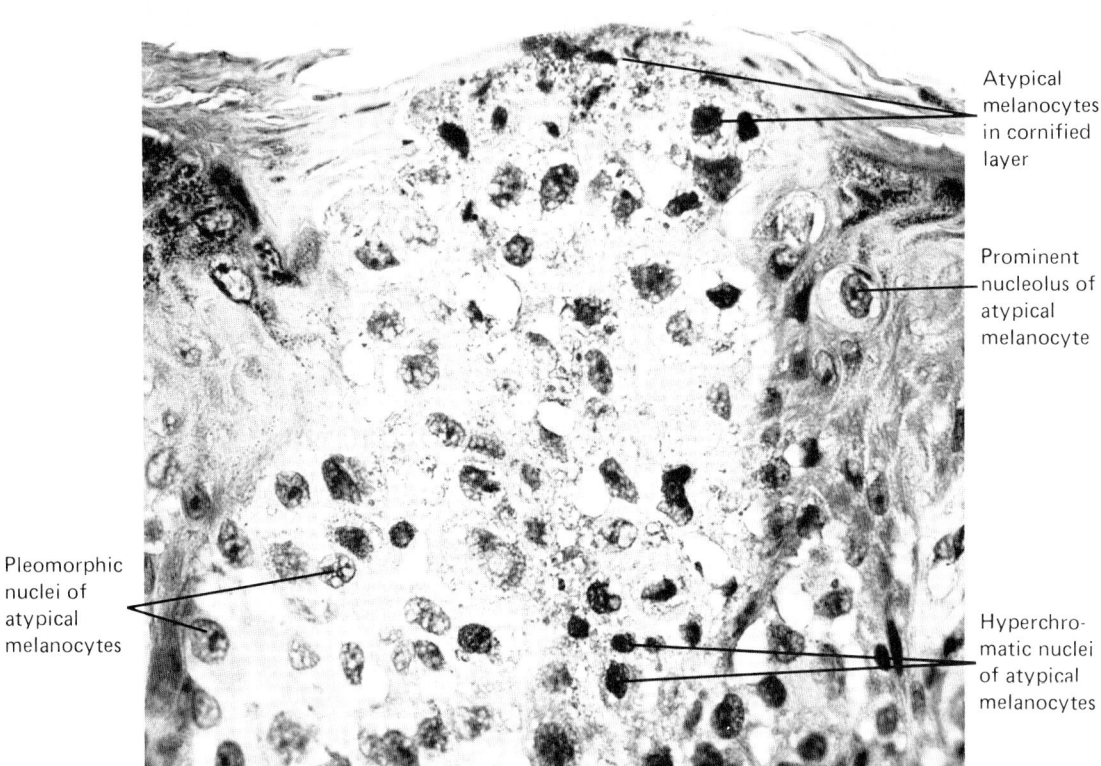

FIGURE 56C. **Malignant melanoma, superficial spreading type.** *Higher magnification of Fig. 56B showing marked cytologic atypia of the melanocytes in the spinous, granular, and cornified layers. (Reduced from ×604)*

common in verrucous malignant melanoma and those changes may also be secondary to direct effects of the neoplastic cells or to trauma.

The granulation tissue beneath the ulcer of a malignant melanoma may be so exuberant as to resemble a pyogenic granuloma (Fig. 66). Lesions that at first glance with scanning magnification are thought to be pyogenic granulomas should be studied more carefully at higher magnification to ensure that there are no atypical melanocytes within the granulation tissue.

In our experience, malignant melanoma of all types may arise in association with preexisting acquired melanocytic nevi, especially those that are wholly intradermal (Figs. 67–70). Since we have been doing step sections through all specimens of malignant melanoma, we have found that about 50% of our cases of superficial spreading malignant melanoma show some nevus cells, ranging from very few to as many as those comprising an entire melanocytic nevus (Fig. 69), contiguous with the atypical melanocytes in the dermis. The percentage of associated nevus cells is considerably less in the other types of malignant melanoma. Unfortunately, there are still no certain clinical or histological markers for predicting in which acquired melanocytic nevus a malignant melanoma will develop.

Recently, Reimer et al. (1978) and Clark et al. (1978) have described a type of familial malignant melanoma that develops within large acquired melanocytic nevi, so-called B-K moles. The B-K moles, according to these authors, may be recognized histologically by the presence of nevus cells along a broad front confined to the papillary dermis, the constellation of atypical melanocytes within the epidermis, dense lymphocytic infiltrates, angioneogenesis, and fibroplasia in the papillary dermis. What these authors understand to be a feature of the B-K mole itself, namely, atypical melanocytic hyperplasia within the epidermis, we interpret to be malignant melanoma *in situ* arising in association with a large acquired intradermal melanocytic nevus (Fig. 71).

All types of malignant melanoma in skin have the capability to metastasize, including those that arise in prepubescent children and those in the aged. Malignant melanoma rarely develops in youngsters and then must be dif-

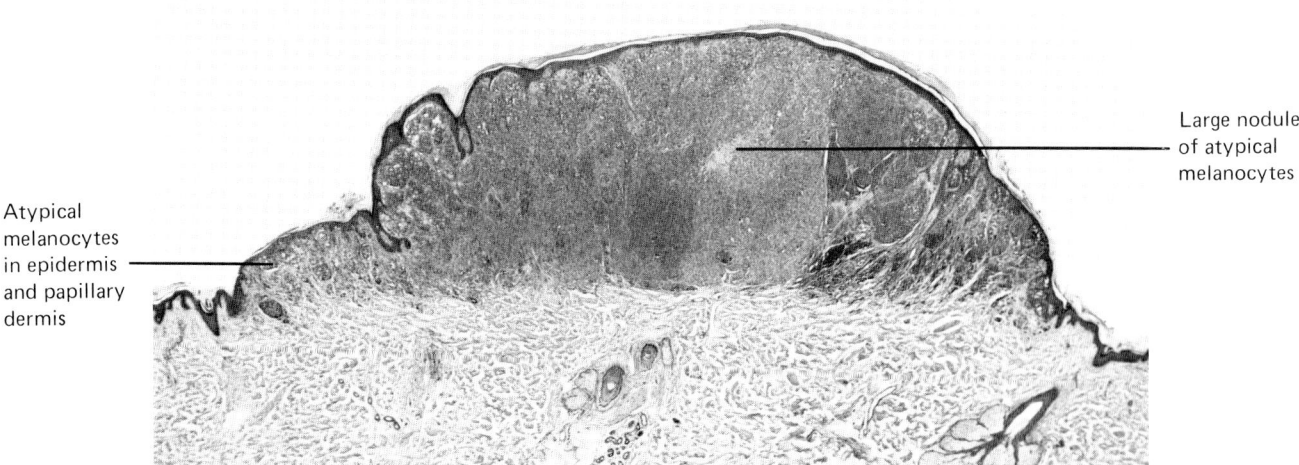

FIGURE 57A. **Malignant melanoma with features of superficial spreading and nodular types.** *To the left of this large nodule of malignant melanoma there are atypical melanocytes within the epidermis and within the papillary dermis. According to Clark, this must be interpreted as a superficial spreading malignant melanoma, rather than a nodular malignant melanoma, because the atypical melanocytes extend for a distance greater than three rete ridges beyond the nodule. (Reduced from ×18)*

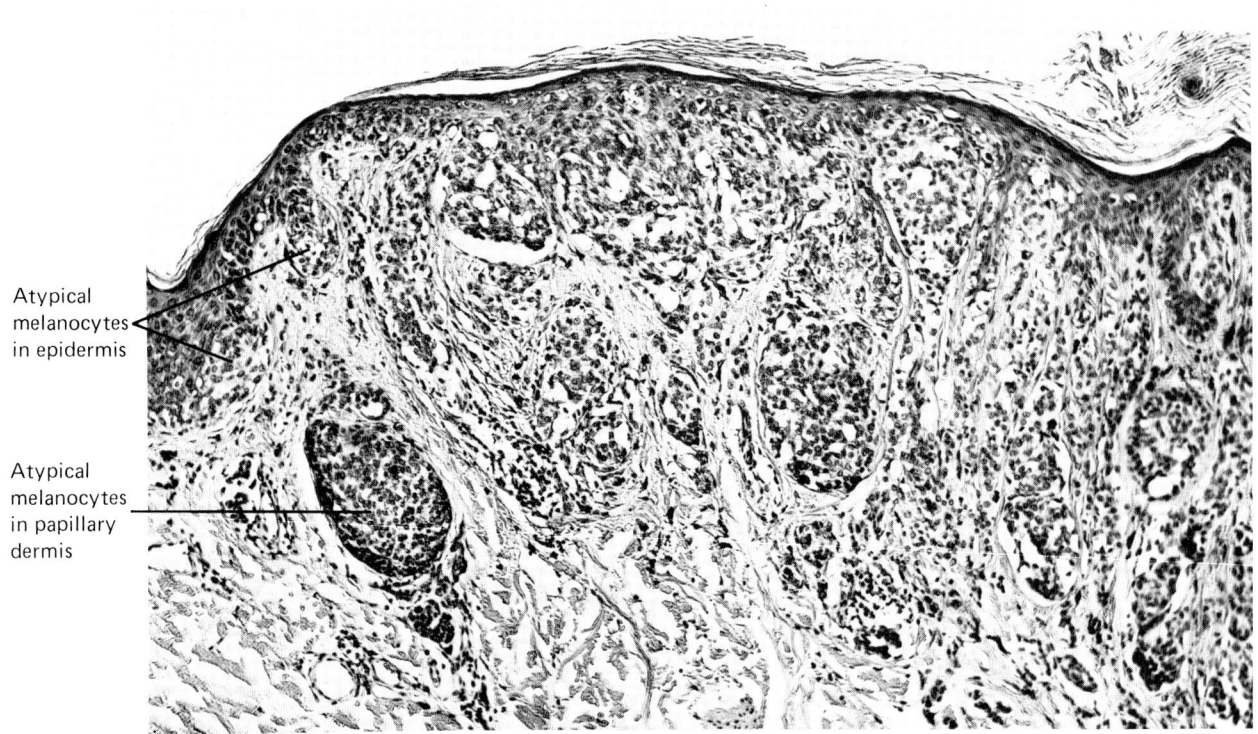

FIGURE 57B. **Malignant melanoma with features of superficial spreading and nodular types.** *This higher-power magnification of Fig. 57A shows the superficial spreading component of the lesion. Note the atypical melanocytes in irregularly shaped nests within the epidermis and the dermis. If these atypical melanocytes had only extended the breadth of two rete ridges, this lesion would be termed nodular malignant melanoma by Clark. (Reduced from ×128)*

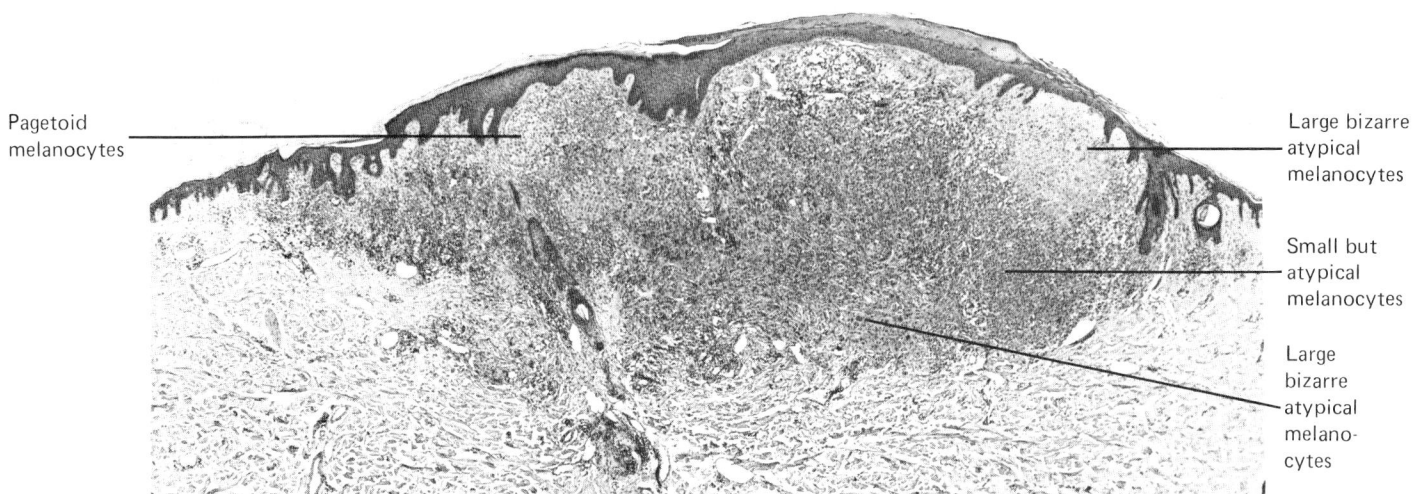

FIGURE 58A. **Malignant melanoma, probably superficial spreading type, with a nodule.** *This specimen illustrates the difficulty in assigning a type to all specimens of malignant melanoma. This lesion is broader than it is tall, which favors a superficial spreading type of malignant melanoma. However, very few atypical melanocytes are present within the epidermis and there is little horizontal extension of atypical melanocytes beyond the nodule, features of nodular melanoma. These details are of less importance than the diagnosis, which is surely primary malignant melanoma. The atypical melanocytes extend into the reticular dermis, beneath which there is a scant inflammatory-cell infiltrate containing melanophages. (Reduced from ×24)*

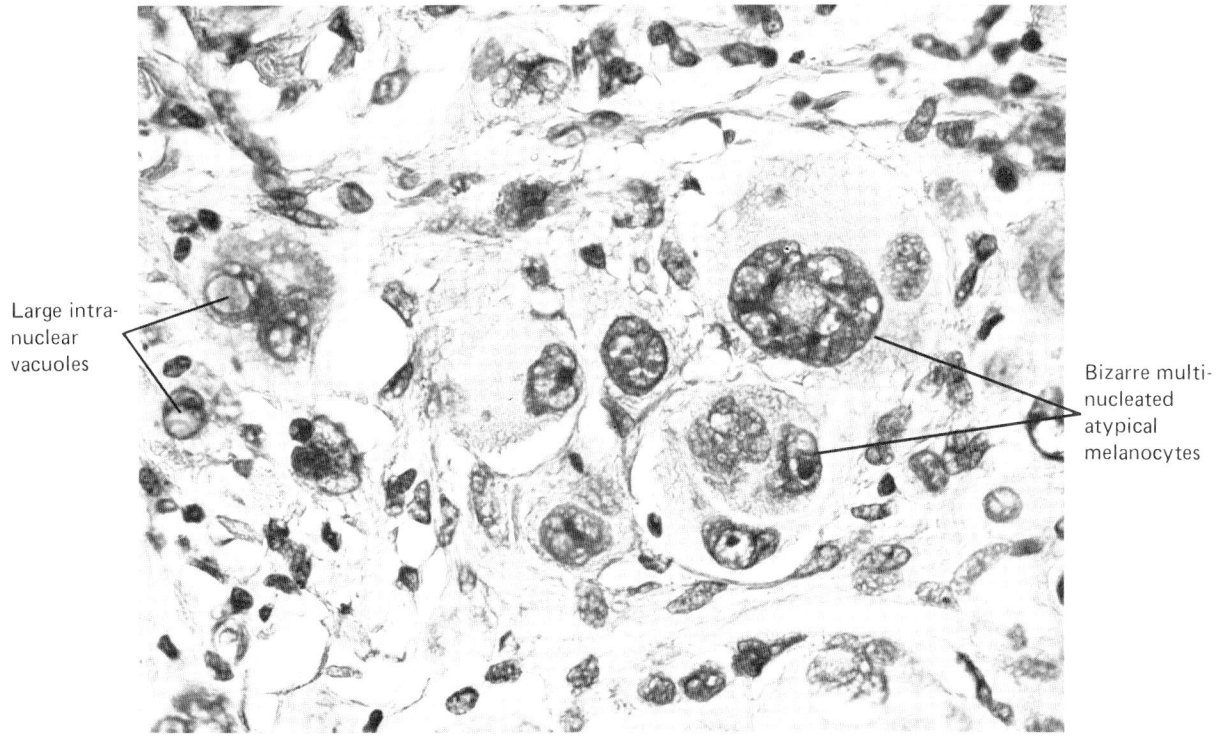

FIGURE 58B. **Malignant melanoma, probably superficial spreading type, with a nodule.** *At the base of the neoplasm pictured in Fig. 58A there are very large atypical melanocytes, many of which are multinucleated, with abundant pale-staining cytoplasm, within which is dusty melanin. Intranuclear vacuoles are common in the atypical melanocytes of malignant melanoma. (Reduced from ×639)*

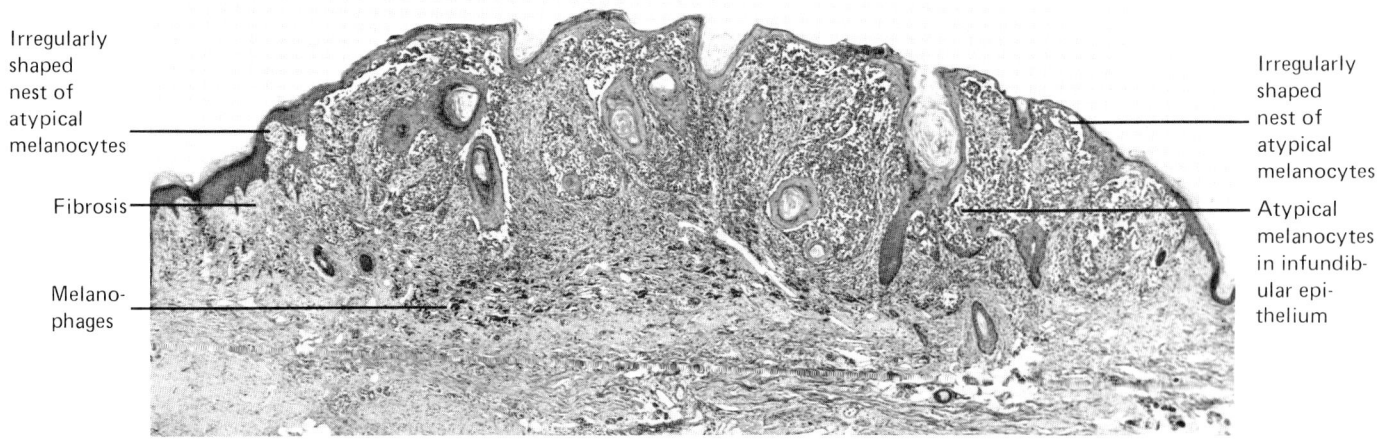

FIGURE 59A. **Malignant melanoma, unclassified.** *This large nodule is characterized by atypical melanocytes within the epidermis and within the epithelium of adnexal structures. Few if any atypical melanocytes are present within the thickened papillary dermis, although there is an inflammatory-cell infiltrate and fibrosis there. (Reduced from ×26)*

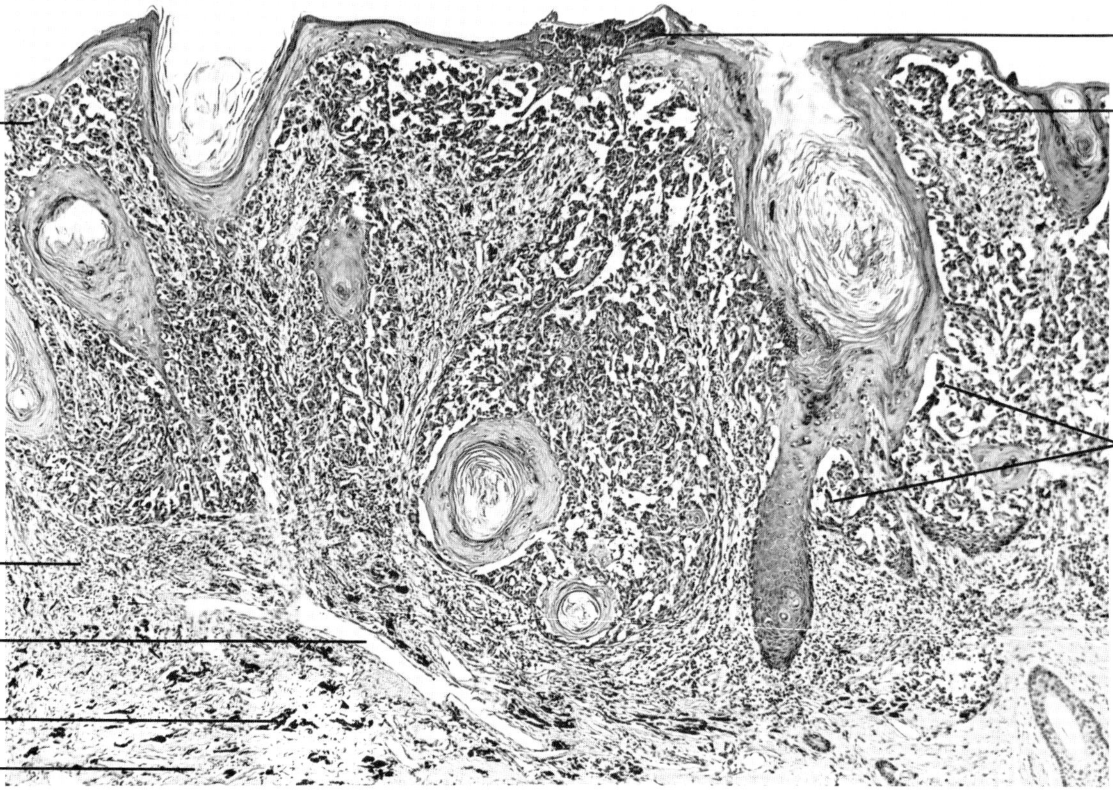

FIGURE 59B. **Malignant melanoma, unclassified.** *Higher magnification of Fig. 59A shows that the numerous atypical melanocytes are confined largely to the markedly hyperplastic epidermis and to adnexal epithelium. This lesion demonstrates how a nodule of malignant melanoma may result from changes in both the epidermis and papillary dermis, yet the atypical melanocytes may be mostly in situ. This particular malignant melanoma cannot be considered the nodular type because atypical melanocytes do not fill the papillary dermis. (Reduced from ×71)*

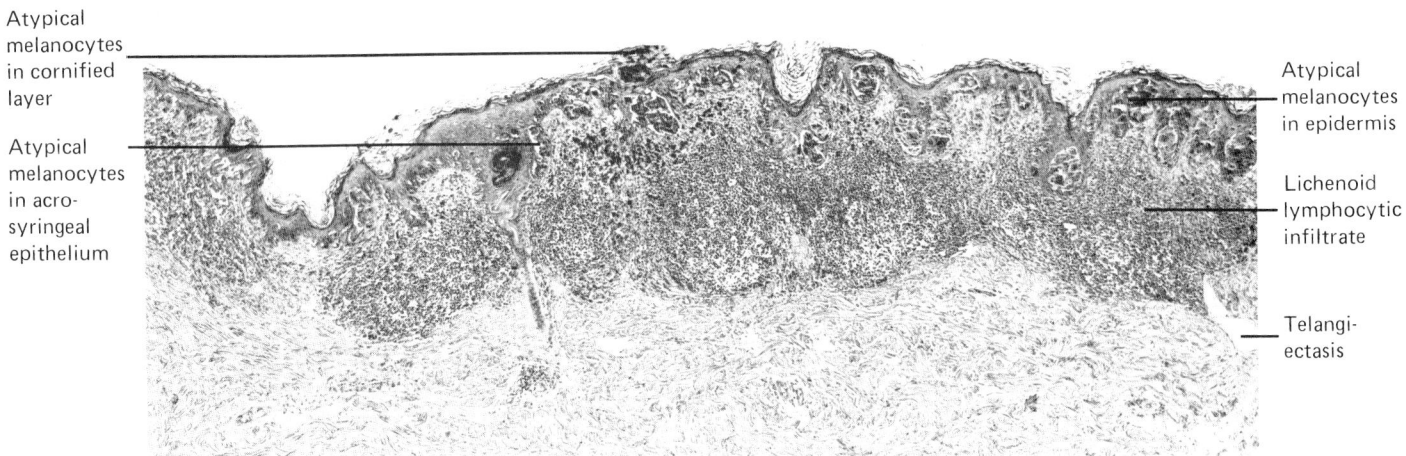

FIGURE 60A. *Dense lichenoid infiltrate of inflammatory cells beneath a superficial spreading malignant melanoma in situ.* A dense band-like (lichenoid) lymphohistiocytic infiltrate may be present beneath malignant melanomas in situ of all types, but especially the superficial spreading type as pictured here. Note also the heavily pigmented irregularly shaped nests of atypical melanocytes at all levels of the epidermis and within the adnexal epithelial structure, namely, an eccrine sweat duct. (Reduced from ×56)

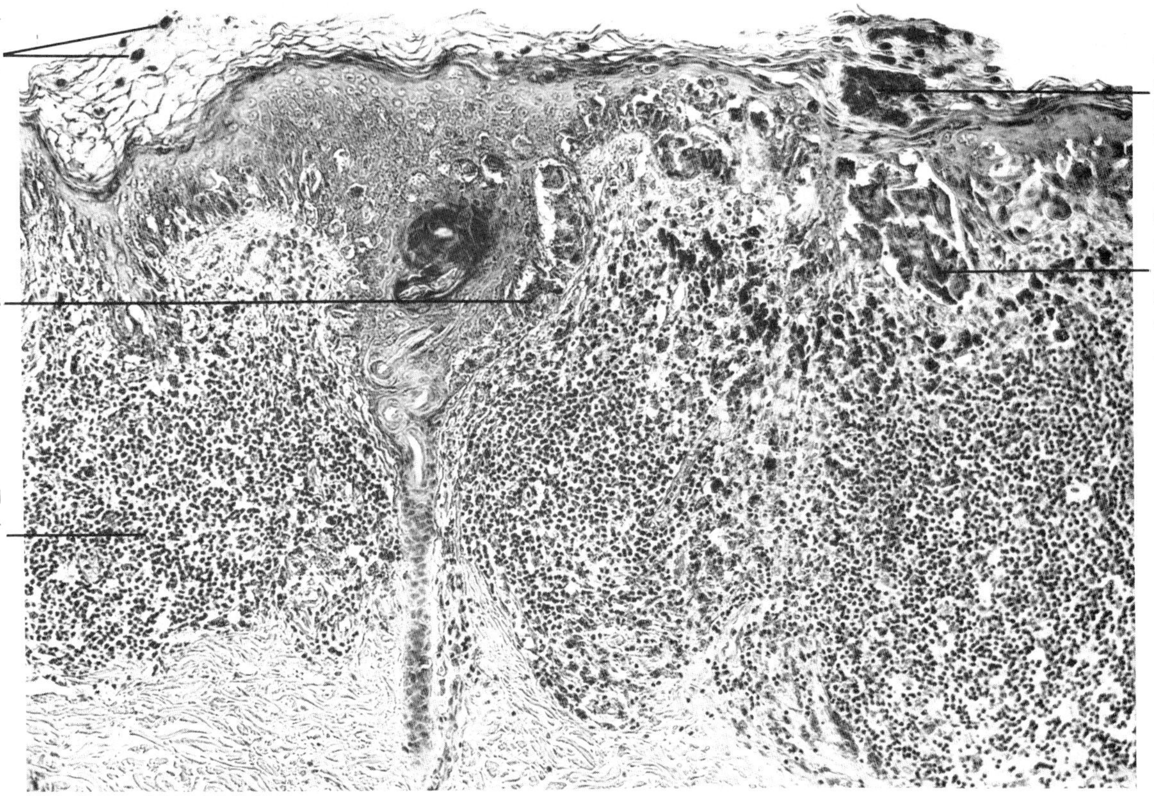

FIGURE 60B. *Dense lichenoid infiltrate of inflammatory cells beneath a superficial spreading malignant melanoma in situ.* Higher magnification of Fig. 60A shows the involvement of the acrosyringium by atypical melanocytes, the presence of atypical melanocytes at all levels of the epidermis including the cornified layer, and a dense lichenoid infiltrate of lymphocytes and histiocytes, which causes the papillary dermis to thicken. (Reduced from ×173)

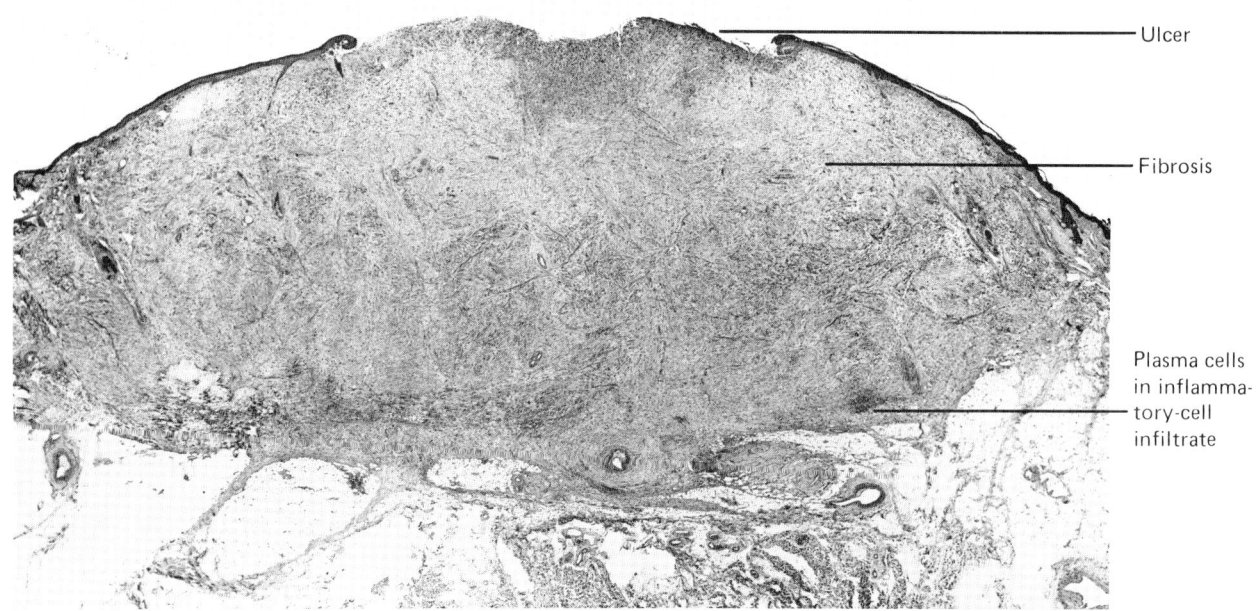

FIGURE 61A. **Malignant melanoma, desmoplastic type.** *In this scanning-power photomicrograph the pathologic process appears to be a form of fibroplasia. Higher magnification will confirm this preliminary impression, and will also reveal atypical spindle-shaped melanocytes within the fibrotic stroma, evidences of desmoplastic (highly and densely fibrotic) malignant melanoma. (Reduced from ×13)*

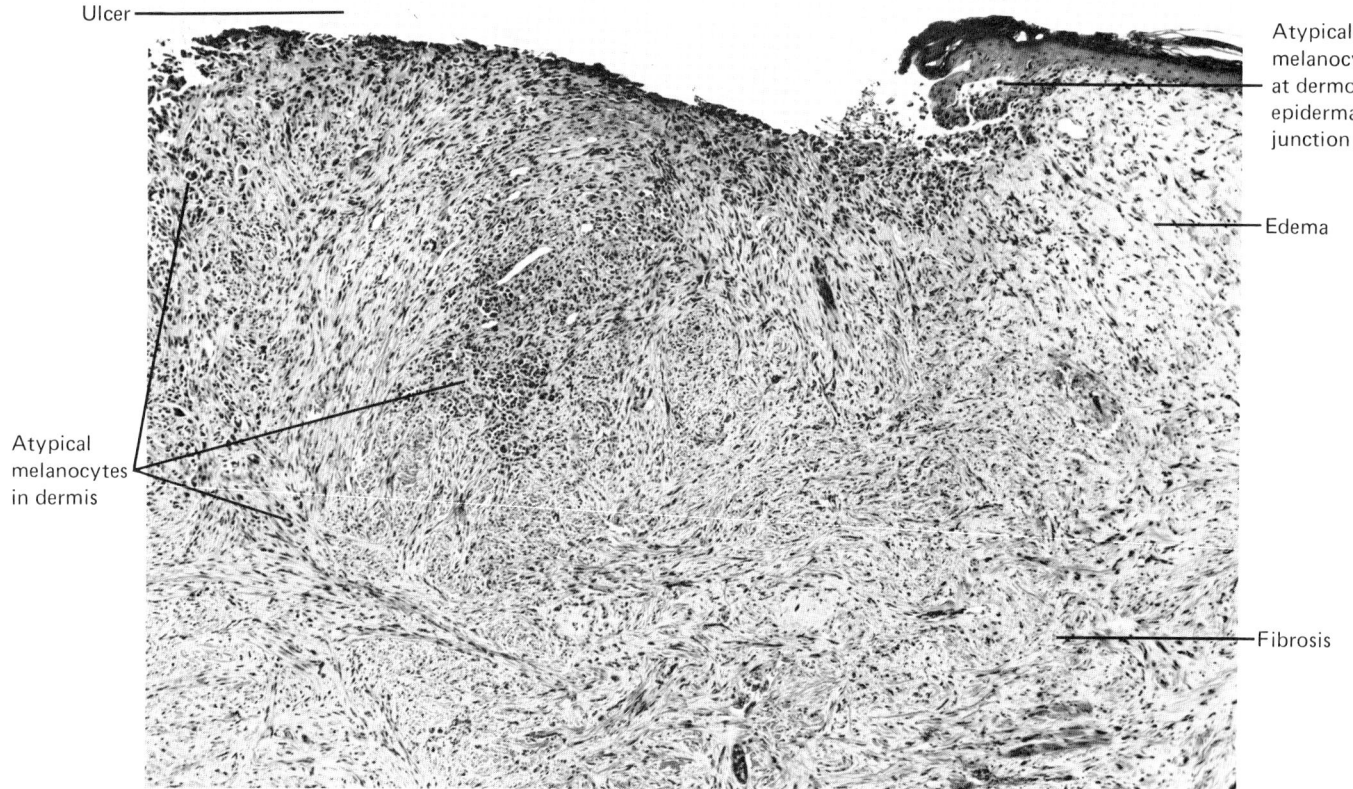

FIGURE 61B. **Malignant melanoma, desmoplastic type.** *This higher-power photomicrograph of Fig. 61A shows atypical melanocytes, singly and in nests, within the epidermis at the side of an ulcer and in the fibrotic dermis. Without the presence of atypical melanocytes within the epidermis, a diagnosis of primary cutaneous malignant melanoma could not be made with certainty. (Reduced from ×75)*

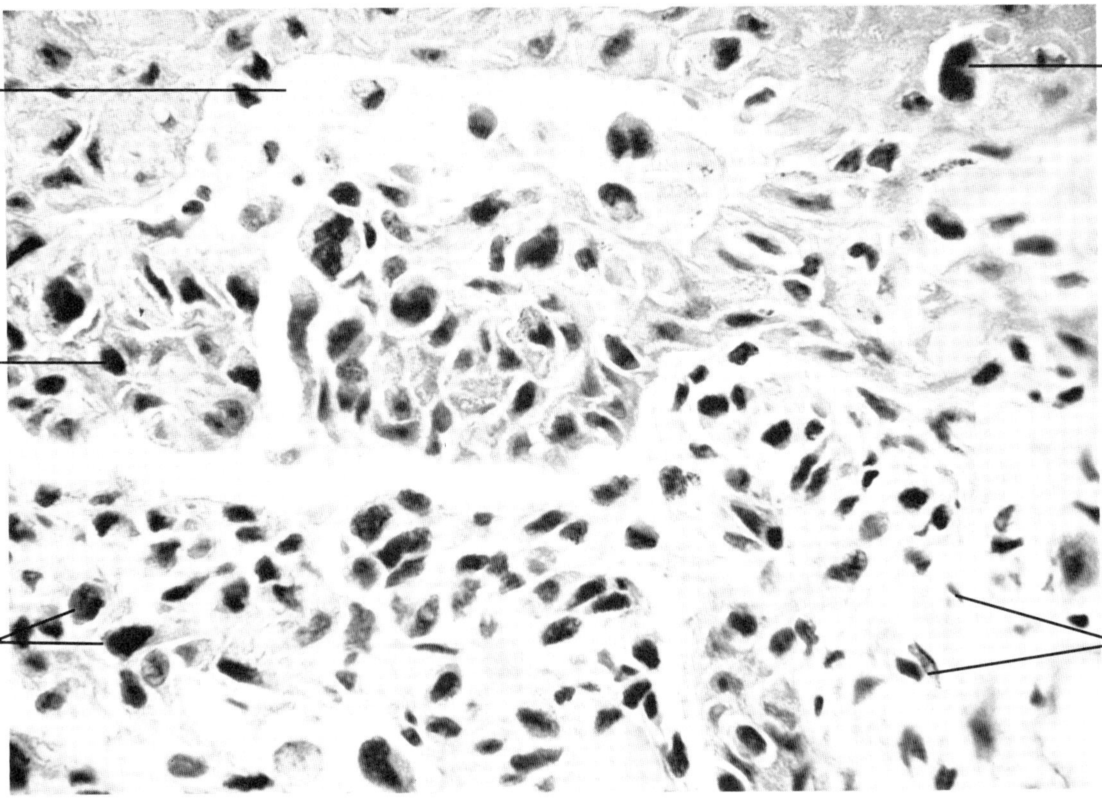

FIGURE 61C. **Malignant melanoma, desmoplastic type.** *Still higher magnification of Figure 61A showing the changes at the side of the ulcer that reveal indubitable features of primary cutaneous malignant melanoma, namely, atypical melanocytes at the dermoepidermal junction and within the epidermis. (Reduced from ×740)*

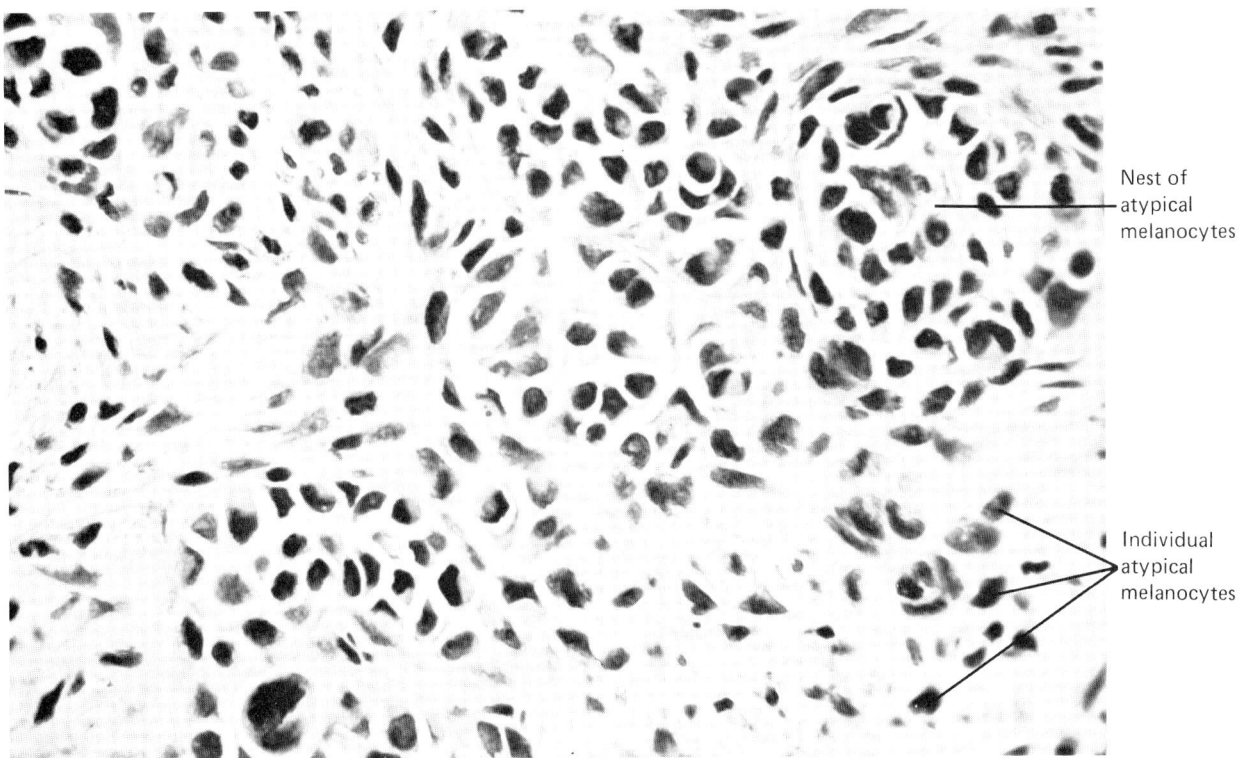

FIGURE 61D. **Malignant melanoma, desmoplastic type.** *Higher-power view of Fig. 61A showing the changes beneath the ulcer, namely, nests of markedly atypical melanocytes within the dermis. Note also the atypical melanocytes distributed singly within the dermis. In the desmoplastic malignant melanoma the atypical melanocytes are best recognized in the epidermis and in the upper part of the dermis. They are largely obscured by fibrosis in the mid and lower portions of the dermis. (Reduced from ×740)*

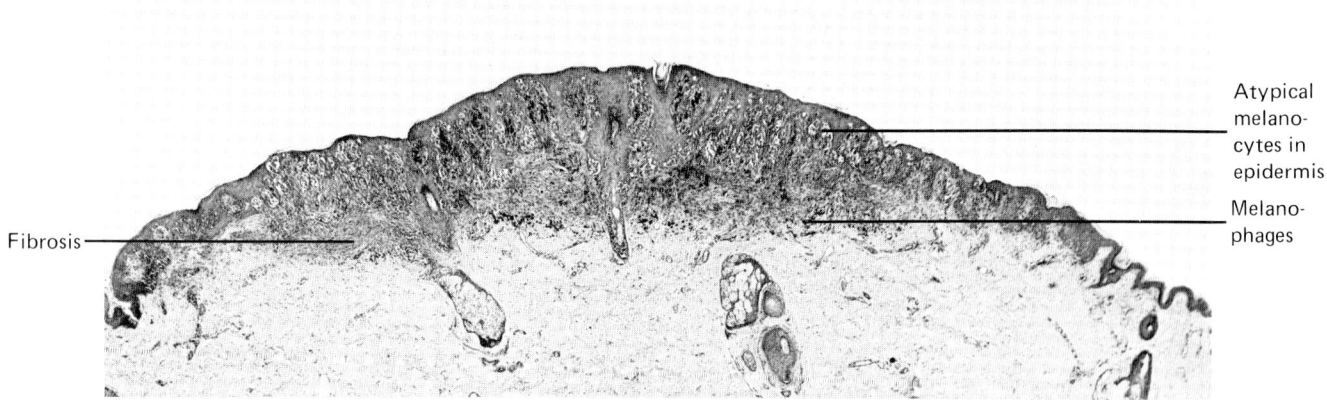

FIGURE 62A. **Lamellar fibrosis associated with a superficial spreading malignant melanoma.** *This is a superficial spreading malignant melanoma because of the horizontal extension of melanocytes within the epidermis considerably beyond the bulk of the intradermal portion of the neoplasm, the irregularity in size and shape of melanocytes within the epidermal and follicular epithelium, and the "buckshot" scatter of melanocytes throughout the epidermis. Early signs of lamellar fibrosis are seen beneath and surrounding atypical melanocytes in the upper part of the dermis. (Reduced from ×24)*

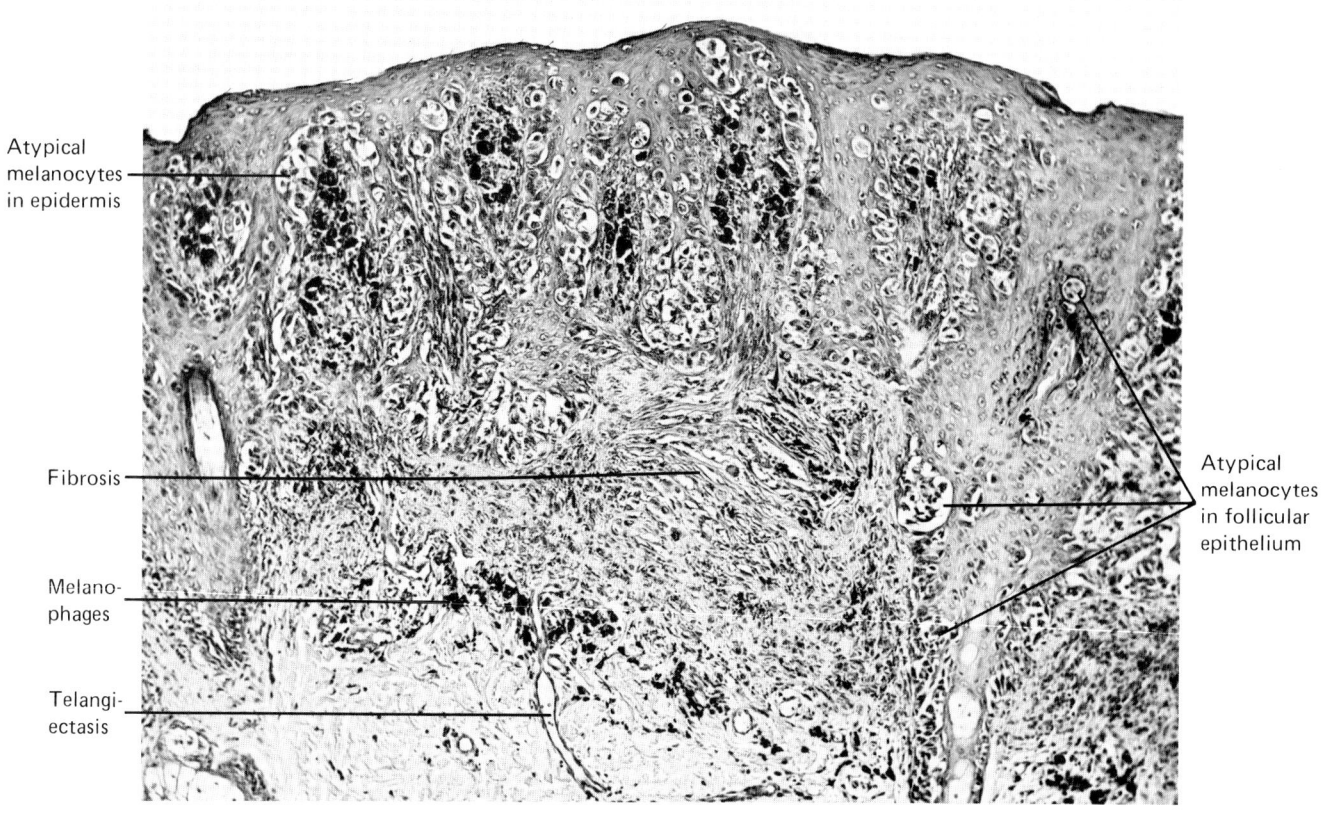

FIGURE 62B. **Lamellar fibrosis associated with a superficial spreading malignant melanoma.** *This higher magnification of Fig. 62A illustrates all of the intraepithelial features of superficial spreading malignant melanoma and the lamellar fibrosis to better advantage. Note that there are a few atypical melanocytes intermingled with fibrocytes and melanophages in the zone of fibrosis. (Reduced from ×113)*

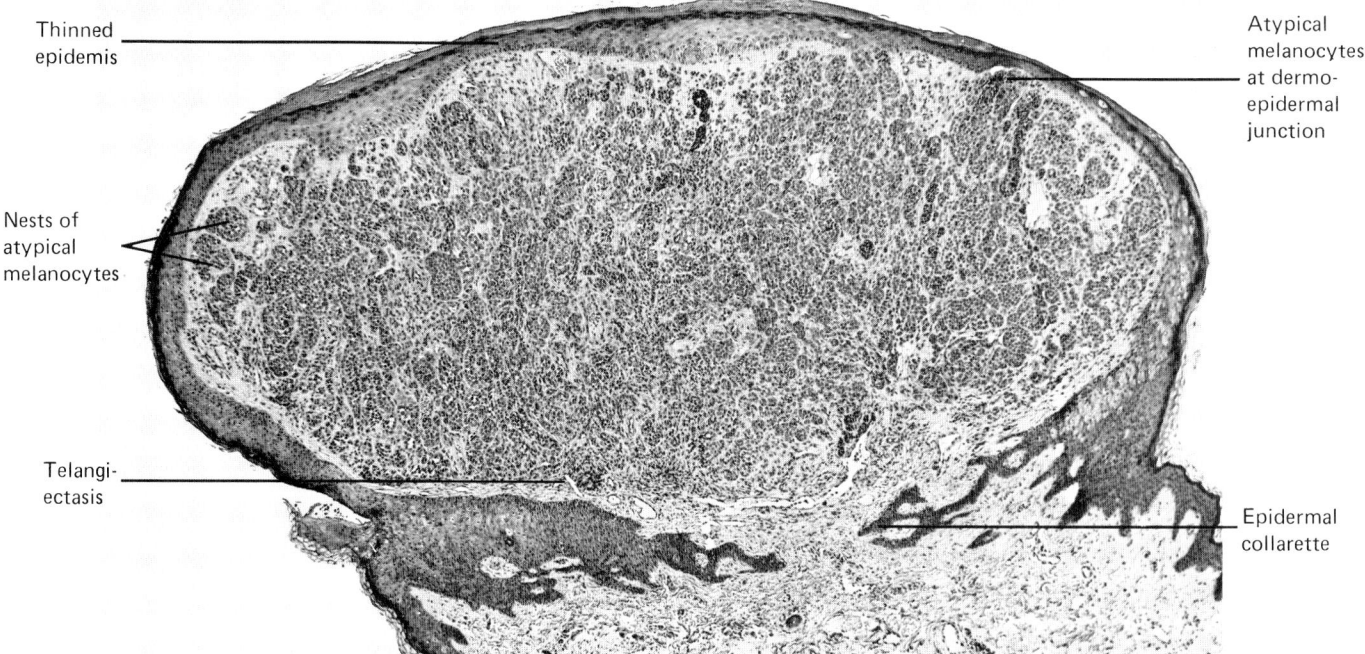

FIGURE 63A. **Malignant melanoma, nodular type, with epidermal collarette.** *Some nodular melanomas, such as the one pictured here, may be misinterpreted as metastatic malignant melanoma to skin or even, at first glance, as a pyogenic granuloma. The relatively large size of this neoplasm, the presence of a few atypical melanocytes at the dermoepidermal junction, and the prominent collarette of epidermal epithelium indicate that this is a primary cutaneous malignant melanoma of the nodular type. Note the near absence of an inflammatory-cell infiltrate beneath this thick neoplasm. (Reduced from ×51)*

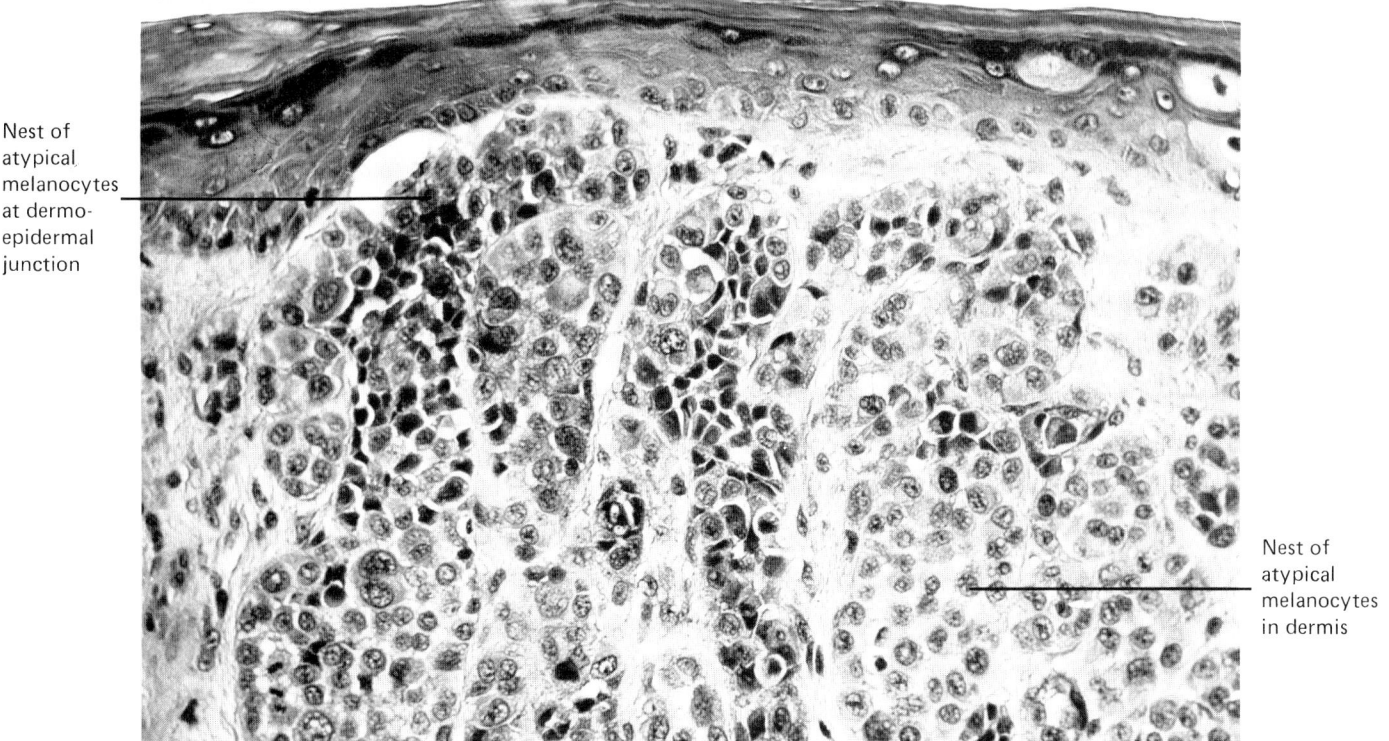

FIGURE 63B. **Malignant melanoma, nodular type, with epidermal collarette.** *Higher magnification of Fig. 63B shows one aggregate of atypical melanocytes at the dermoepidermal junction, an indication of primary malignant melanoma. However, similar changes may be found in some instances of metastatic malignant melanoma to skin. (Reduced from ×381)*

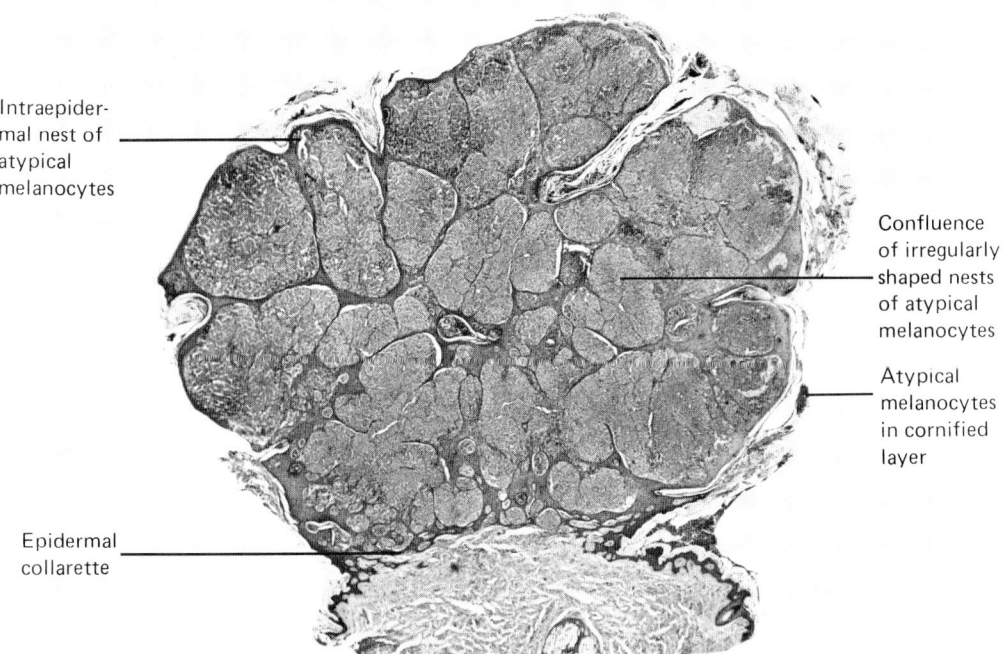

FIGURE 64. *Malignant melanoma, pedunculated type, with epidermal collarette.* *This exophytic papillomatous malignant melanoma with its embracing collarette of epidermis can be differentiated histologically from a papillomatous melanocytic nevus by architectural features easily noted with this scanning-power magnification, namely, the nests of melanocytes are large, irregular in size and shape, and fill the dermis so completely because of confluence that practically no connective tissue is visible. Changes such as these do not occur in melanocytic nevi. (Reduced from ×14)*

ferentiated histologically from the much more common nevus of large spindle and/or epithelioid cells of Spitz (benign juvenile melanoma), which is wholly benign and never metastasizes. Any lesion thought to be metastasizing benign juvenile melanoma was almost certainly a malignant melanoma from the outset. We do not agree with Helwig who implies that these nevi in children occasionally metastasize (Helwig, 1975).

In sum, the terms lentigo maligna melanoma, acral lentiginous malignant melanoma, superficial spreading malignant melanoma, and nodular malignant melanoma are clinical and histologic descriptions of different types of malignant melanoma. Spindle, dendritic, pagetoid, and cuboidal are the usual cytologic features of these types of malignant melanoma. Measurement of depth of extension (maximal thickness) of a malignant melanoma into the skin is an attempt to gauge prognosis and to guide therapy.

IV. CLINICOPATHOLOGICAL CORRELATIONS IN MALIGNANT MELANOMA

The three morphologic features most helpful to the clinical diagnosis of primary malignant melanoma in skin (except for the wholly nodular type) are irregularity in color, irregularity in shape, and irregularity in the surface of the lesions.

Variegation in color is perhaps the most important hallmark of primary cutaneous malignant melanoma because it is the change that occurs first, before irregularity in shape or surface contour. The usual colors present in malignant melanoma are hues of brown, ranging from light tan to deep chocolate. In addition, there may be mottling by dark blue and black and other areas may even be hypopigmented to utter whiteness. A less frequent finding is shades of redness within the clinical lesion of malignant melanoma. All of these colors may be accounted for histologically. The variations of brown result from an increased number of melanin-producing melanocytes at all levels of the epidermis as well as melanocytes and melanophages within the dermis (Fig. 72). The amount of melanin within epidermal keratinocytes is also markedly increased. Black is a reflection of abundant melanin within the cornified layer of the epidermis and blue is the consequence of abundant melanin in the mid and lower portions of the dermis (the Tyndall effect). Whitening is a sign of spon-

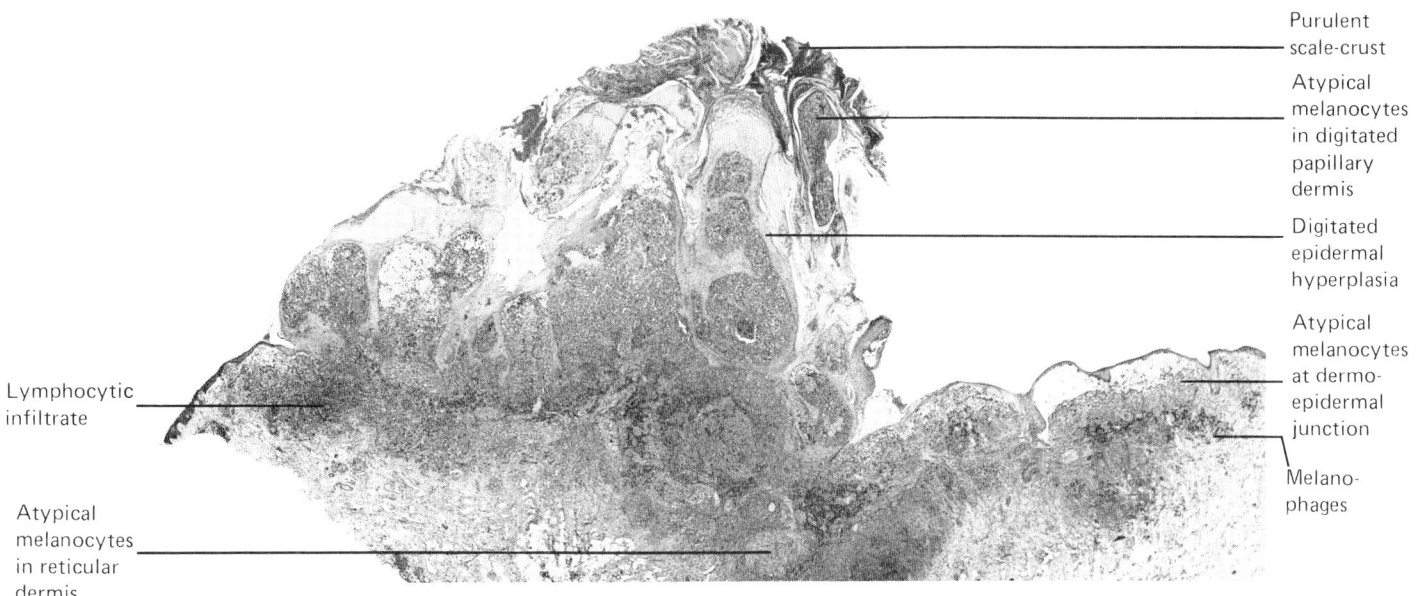

FIGURE 65A. **Malignant melanoma, verrucous type.** *This digitated variant of malignant melanoma is a kind of superficial spreading malignant melanoma with a verrucous surfaced nodule. The epidermis in this lesion has become papillated and covered by huge scale-crusts. (Reduced from ×8.5)*

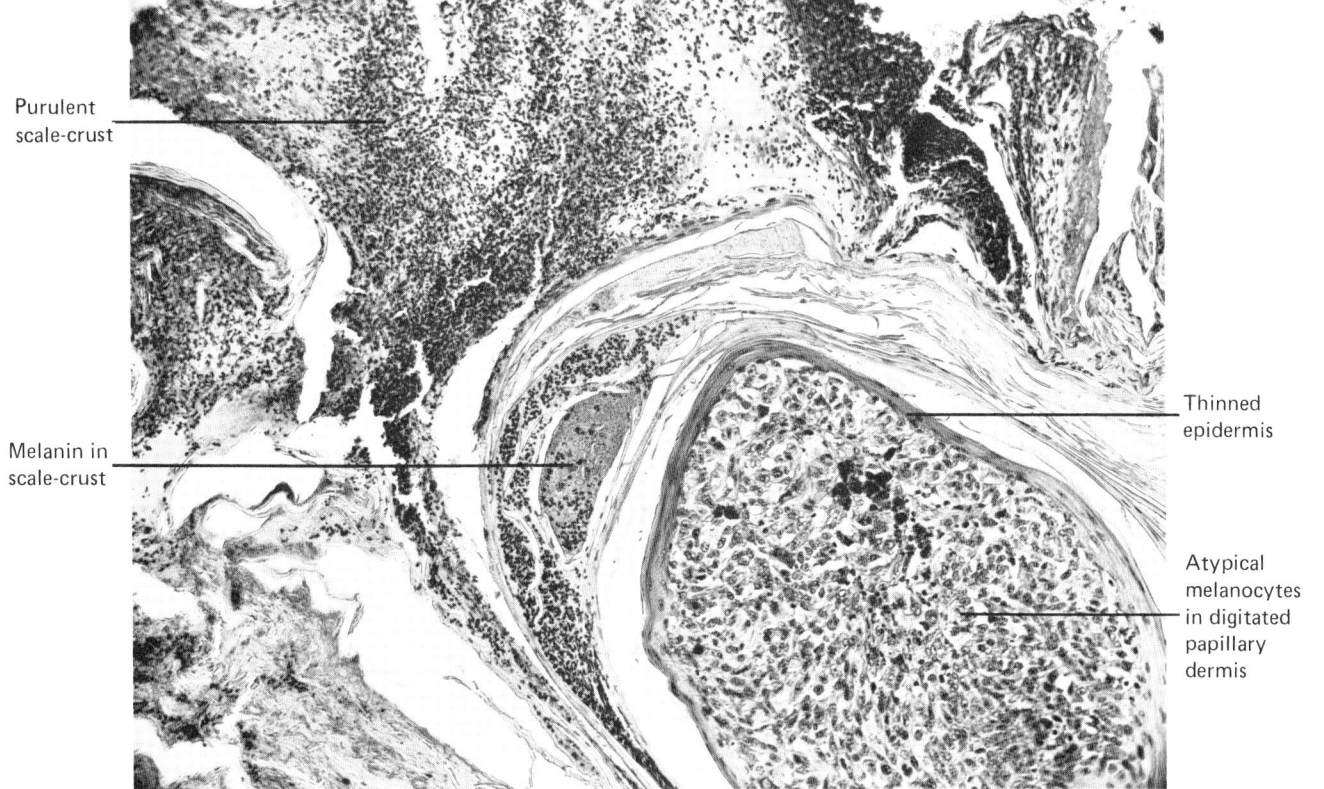

FIGURE 65B. **Malignant melanoma, verrucous type.** *Higher magnification of Fig. 65A shows atypical melanocytes within the digitated papillary dermis, the thinned epidermis, and the covering of purulent scale-crusts. (Reduced from ×164)*

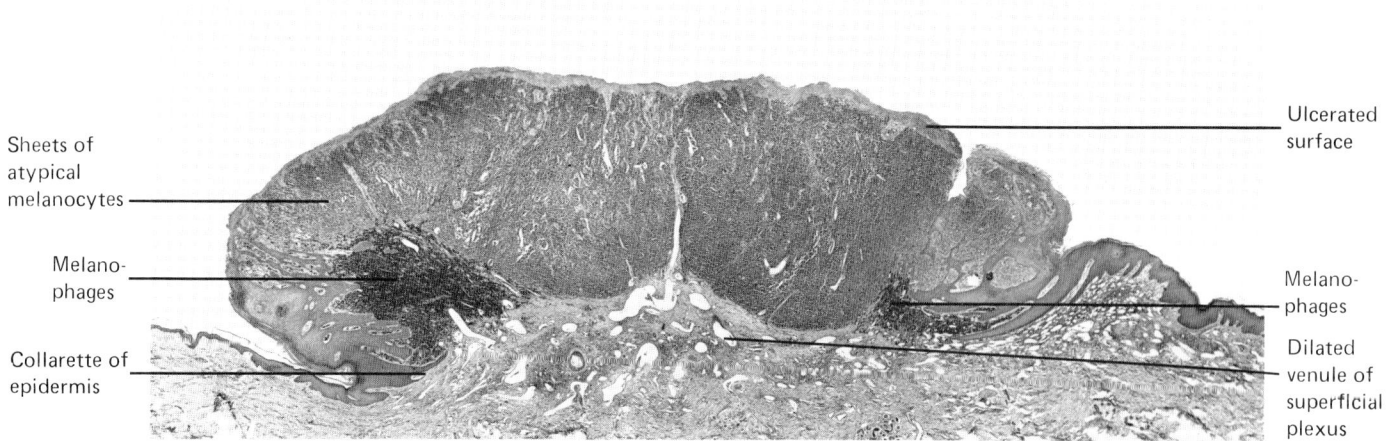

FIGURE 66A. **Malignant melanoma, nodular type, with ulceration.** *The architectural pattern of this nodular malignant melanoma bears some resemblance to a pyogenic granuloma. Both lesions are predominantly exophytic, highly vascular, embraced by a collarette of epidermis, and tend to ulceration. The dense cellular infiltrate of atypical melanocytes in this section makes this lesion a malignant melanoma. Note also the zones of melanosis immediately beneath the neoplasm. (Reduced from ×11)*

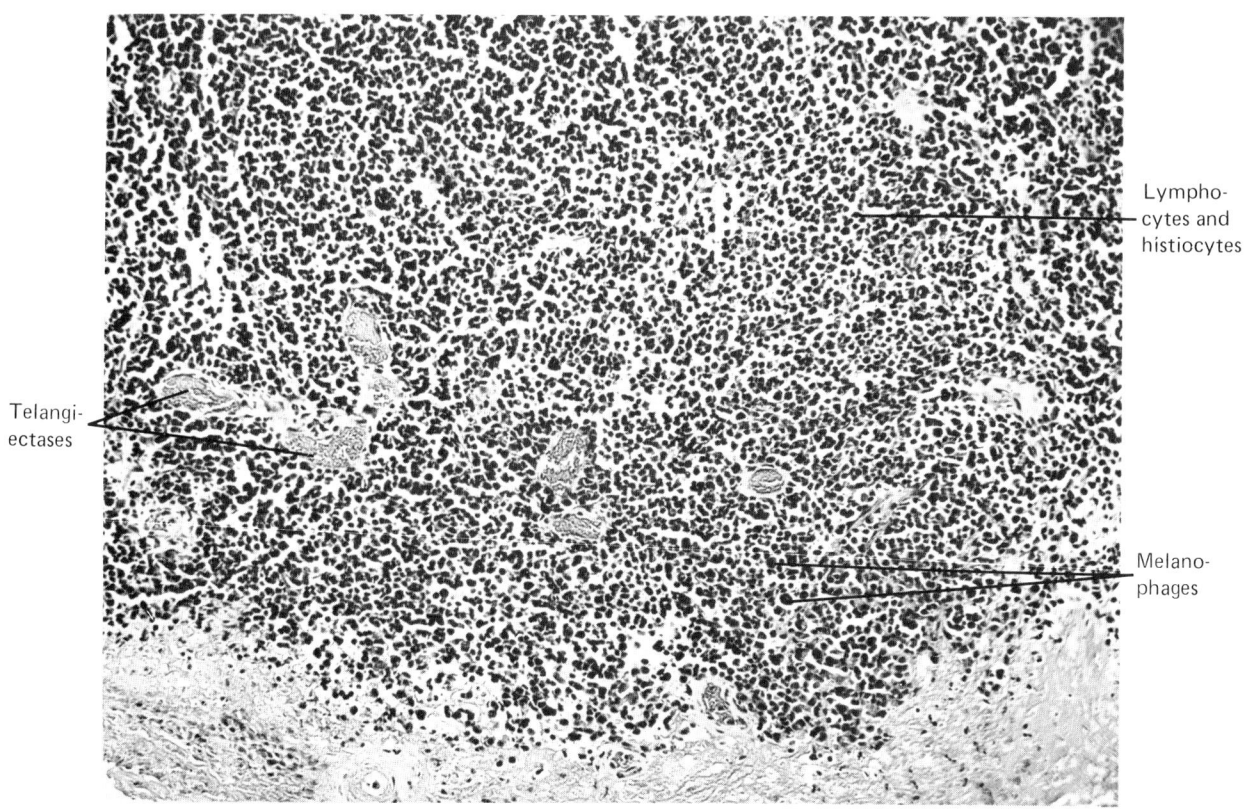

FIGURE 66B. **Malignant melanoma, nodular type, with ulceration.** *Beneath the sheets of atypical melanocytes shown in Fig. 66A there are sheets of melanophages, i.e., macrophages that have engulfed melanin produced by the neoplastic cells. (Reduced from ×164)*

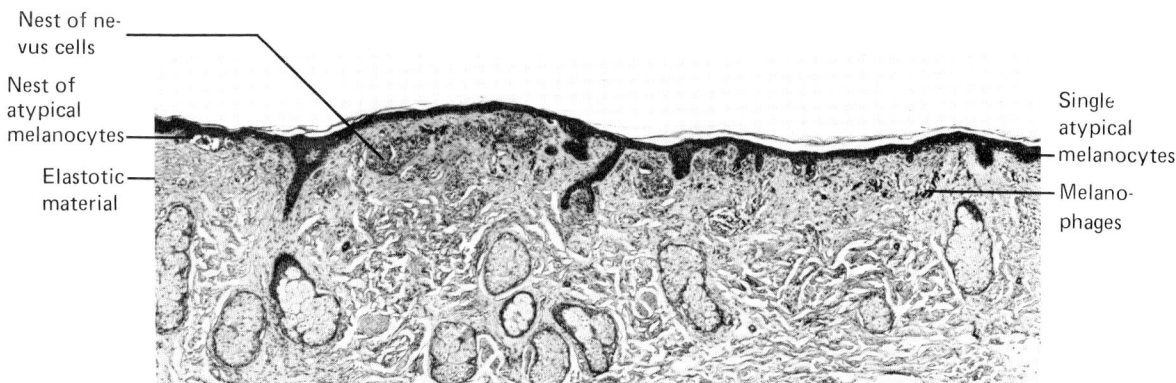

FIGURE 67A. **Lentigo maligna overlying an intradermal melanocytic nevus.** *With scanning power one can see that there are atypical melanocytes, singly and in nests, within the epidermis and orderly nests of nevus cells in the upper portion of the dermis. Even with scanning magnification this lesion can be identified as a lentigo maligna above an intradermal melanocytic nevus and not simply a compound melanocytic nevus, because the nests of melanocytes within the epidermis are irregular in size and shape and the lesion is very broad, extending to both lateral margins. (Reduced from ×34)*

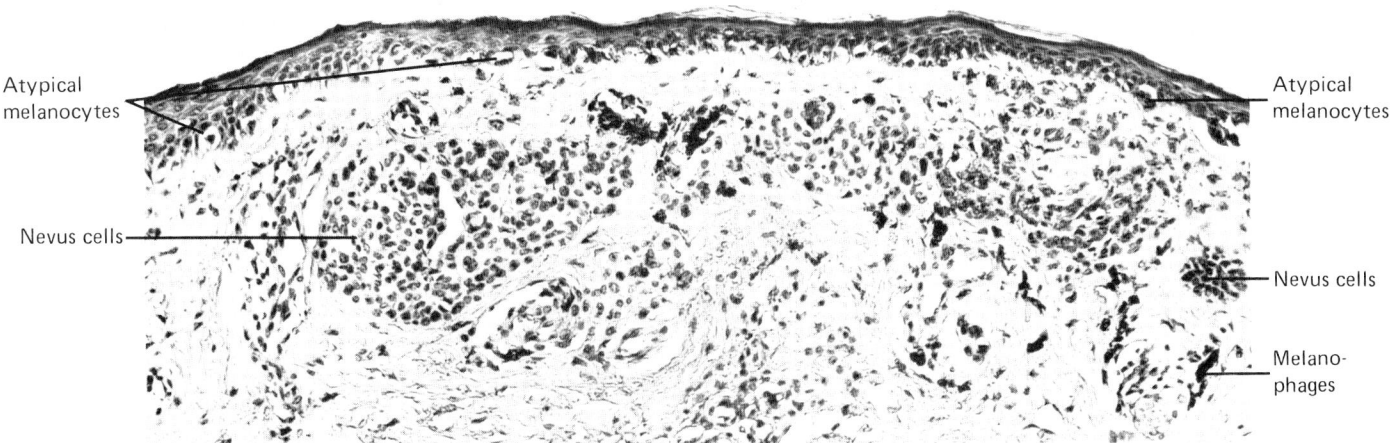

FIGURE 67B. **Lentigo maligna overlying an intradermal melanocytic nevus.** *There are an increased number of atypical melanocytes arranged singly in the thinned epidermis and nests of nevus cells within the upper part of the dermis of this higher power view of Fig. 67A. All types of malignant melanoma, including lentigo maligna, may arise in association with a preexisting melanocytic nevus. (Reduced from ×173)*

taneous regression in malignant melanoma, a process that begins with an extremely dense lichenoid infiltrate of lymphocytes and ends by fibrosis within a thickened papillary dermis (Figs. 73–76). Signs of partial regression are seen commonly in superficial spreading malignant melanoma, but practically never in nodular malignant melanoma. The dense infiltrates of lymphocytes and histiocytes permeate the thin malignant melanomas (those confined to the papillary dermis) and destroy the atypical melanocytes there and in the epidermis. As a result of the action of lymphocytes, there usually are few or no melanocytes within the epidermis above these fibrotic foci, but there are often numerous melanophages immediately below them (Fig. 77). How white, off-white, or blue-white the lesion appears is usually a reflection of the number and depth of melanophages and the extent to which the papillary dermis is thickened by fibrosis. Partial regression of a thin superficial spreading malignant melanoma is common (Figs. 78–80). An uncommon phenomenon is the complete regression of a primary malignant melanoma that leaves only a residual whitish patch (Fig. 76). Paradoxically, this phenomenon of total regression of a seemingly thin malignant melanoma may be accompanied by the development of metastases of the neoplastic cells from the skin to internal

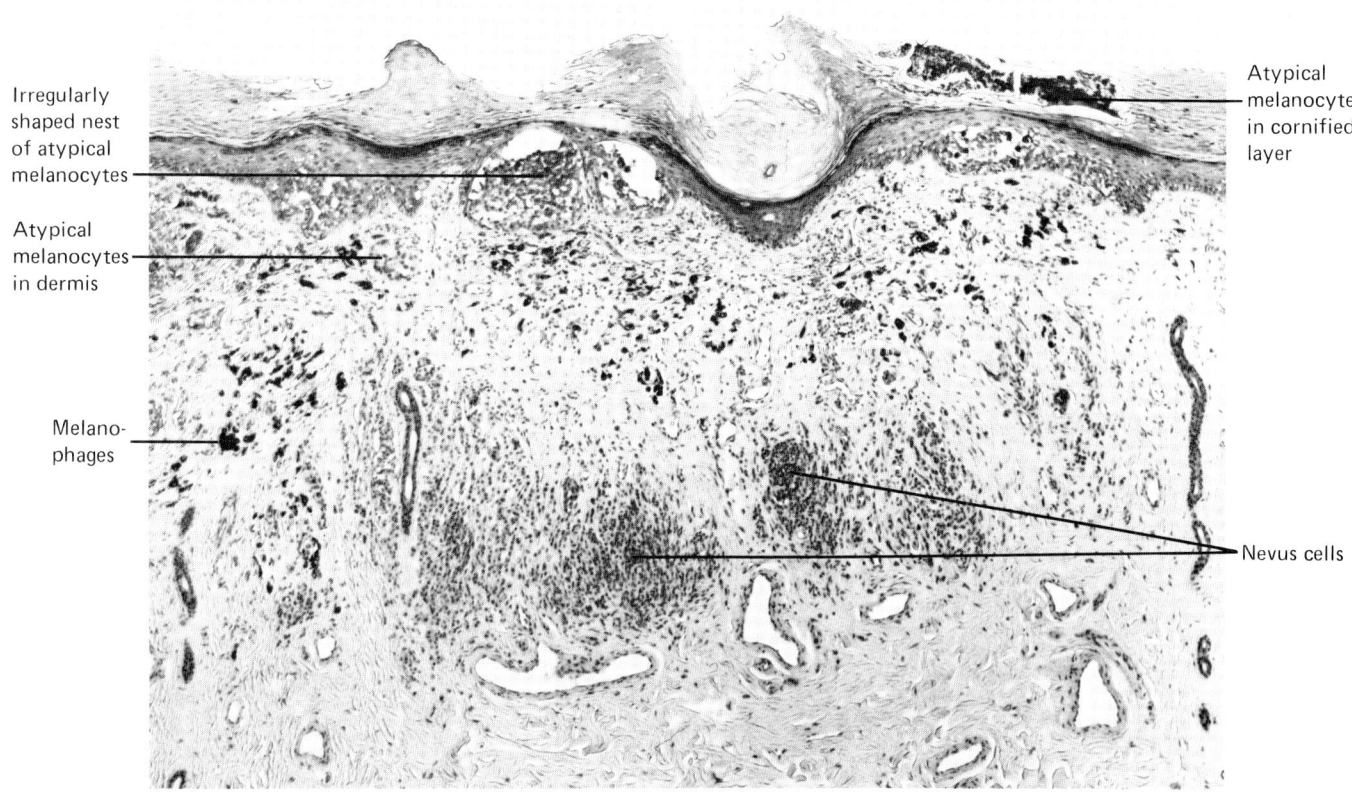

FIGURE 68. ***Malignant melanoma, acral lentiginous type, above an intradermal melanocytic nevus.*** *The acral lentiginous malignant melanoma shown here arose in association with a preexisting intradermal melanocytic nevus. This association seems to be most common in superficial spreading malignant melanoma and least common in nodular malignant melanoma. (Reduced from ×70)*

organs (Gromet et al., 1978). The subtle shades of red are a reflection of widely dilated blood-filled vessels of the superficial vascular plexus.

Concurrent with, or shortly after, the appearance of mottled pigmentation within a malignant melanoma is the development of a scalloped or crenulated periphery. This is explained histologically by the varying rates of centrifugal spread of melanin-producing melanocytes within the epidermis (Fig. 46). This uncontrolled horizontal extension of melanocytes within the epidermis, so characteristic of malignant melanoma and so uncharacteristic of melanocytic nevi, is the major factor responsible for the irregular outline of the lesion. Naturally, melanocytes within the epidermis of a benign melanocytic nevus also proliferate for a time and extend horizontally. However, most acquired melanocytic nevi are usually much smaller than malignant melanomas and their horizontal growth ceases in time, unlike the horizontal and eventually vertical growth of malignant melanomas, which, undisturbed, is unceasing unto death. If an acquired pigmented lesion repeatedly measures less than 10 mm in diameter in follow up, it is almost certain to be a melanocytic nevus rather than a malignant melanoma (Mihm and Fitzpatrick, 1977).

The last important clinical feature to emerge in the evolution of malignant melanoma is the altered surface configuration of the lesion. That contour in high relief may grossly take the form of papules and nodules, some of which may become ulcerated or crusted (Fig. 66). Those that are not ulcerated or crusted often show obliteration of the normal skin-surface markings. These clinical changes in topography may be explained histologically by migration of atypical melanocytes upward in the epidermis and downward into the dermis and even the subcutaneous fat (Fig. 47). It is this vertical growth, both upward and downward, that is largely responsible for the changes on the surface of malignant melanoma. The loss of skin markings

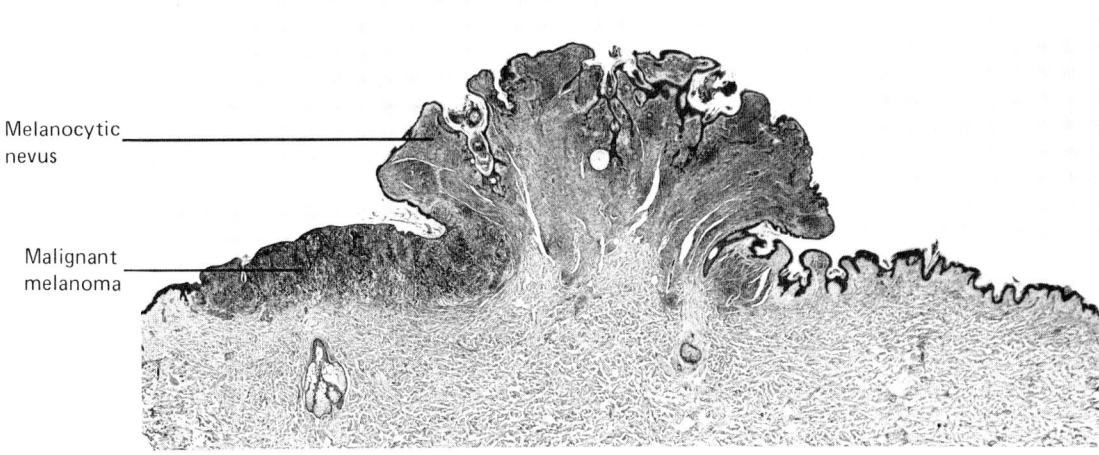

FIGURE 69A. ***Malignant melanoma, superficial spreading type, contiguous to a papillated melanocytic nevus.*** *The number of cells of a melanocytic nevus found in association with a malignant melanoma, especially of the superficial spreading type, varies from few to many as pictured here. (Reduced from ×12)*

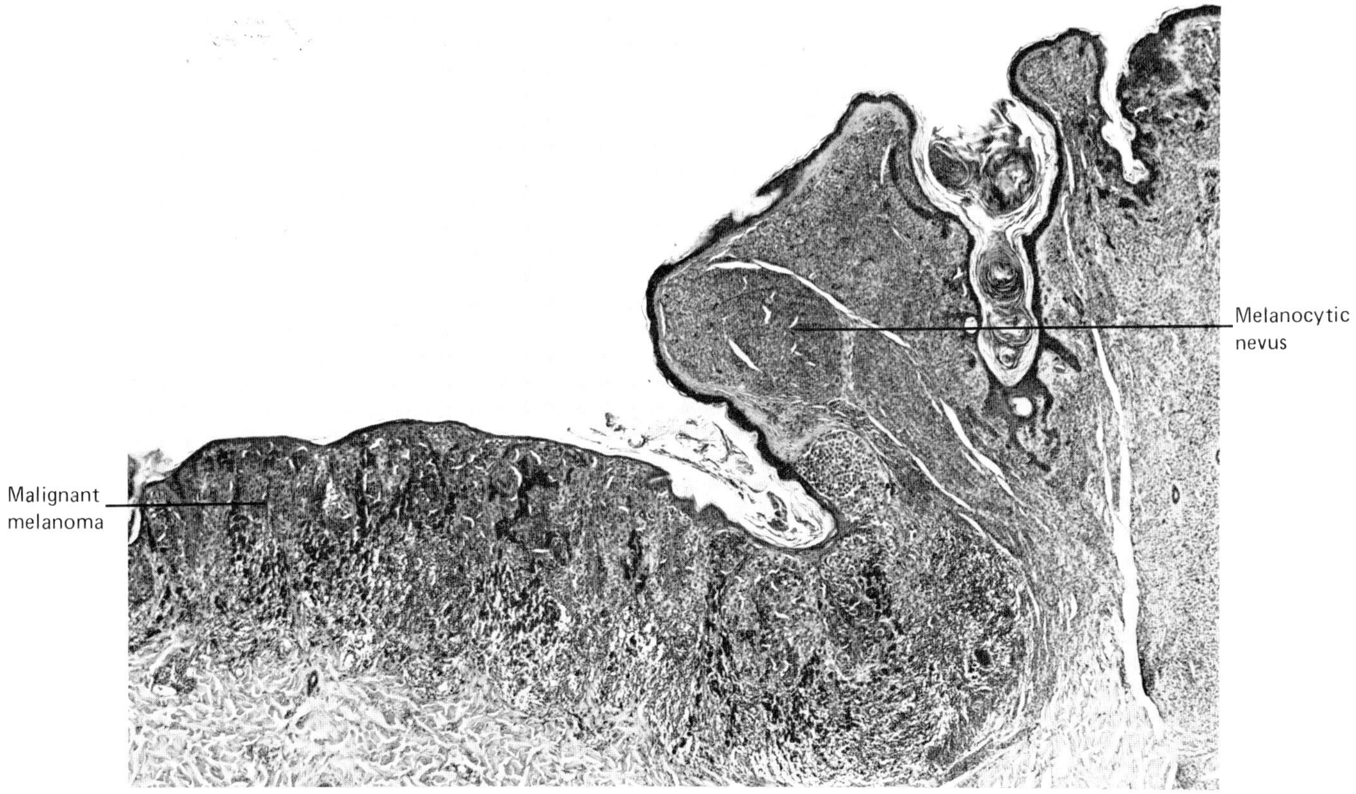

FIGURE 69B. ***Malignant melanoma, superficial spreading type, contiguous to a papillated melanocytic nevus.*** *In this higher magnification of Fig. 69A the superficial spreading malignant melanoma on the left seems to merge with the melanocytic nevus on the right. (Reduced from ×180)*

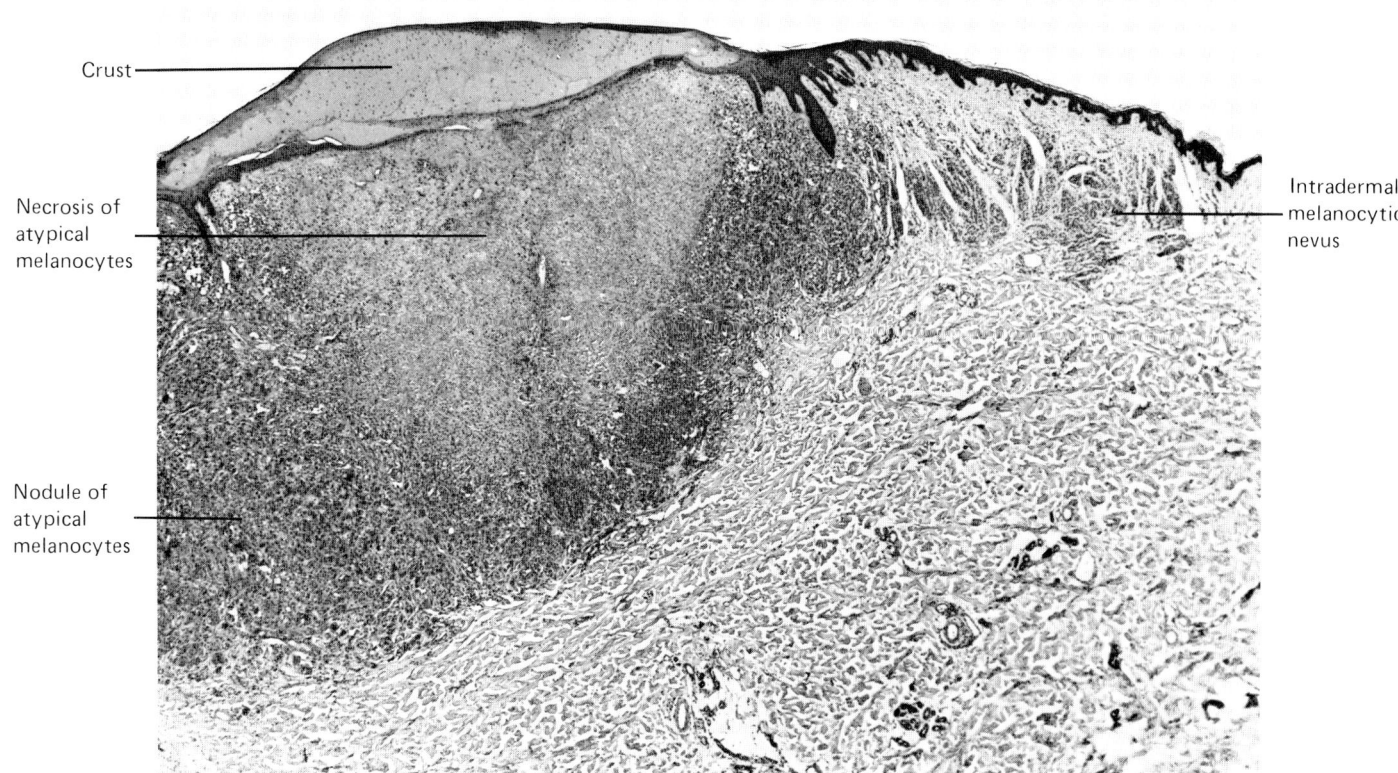

FIGURE 70. **Malignant melanoma, nodular type, in association with an intradermal melanocytic nevus.** *On the left-hand side of this photomicrograph there is a large nodular malignant melanoma that has undergone necrosis and is covered by a huge scale-crust. In the upper part of the dermis on the right side of the photomicrograph contiguous to the malignant melanoma there is a melanocytic nevus, intradermal type. (Reduced from ×24)*

results from effacement, by the neoplastic melanocytes, of the normal pattern that exists between the epidermal rete ridges and the dermal papillae. As the papillary dermis becomes increasingly filled by atypical melanocytes and the overlying epidermis becomes increasingly compressed by them, the skin markings normally visible to the naked eye become obliterated.

What has just been written about clinical–pathological correlation applies to all forms of malignant melanoma, but less so to the nodular type. The prototypic lesion of nodular malignant melanoma has little or no mottling in color (usually uniformly dark brown or black), is devoid of irregular margins (usually sharply circumscribed), and without bumpiness of its surface (usually smooth). However, in many nodular malignant melanomas there are exceptions in each of these characteristic features. For example, there may be some play of color at its periphery, and papillation, ulceration, or crusting of its surface.

V. HISTOLOGIC CRITERIA FOR THE DIAGNOSIS OF MALIGNANT MELANOMA (TABLE 5)

It cannot be emphasized too strongly that a biopsy specimen of adequate size is essential for accurate diagnosis of malignant melanoma. That means that the specimen should, when possible, be taken preferably by scalpel excision, be rimmed by normal appearing skin, and contain subcutaneous fat (Fig. 81). Except for this statement, there are exceptions to almost every rule that has been enunciated about the histologic diagnosis of malignant melanoma. It should be also emphatically underscored that the most important features for the diagnosis of malignant melanoma are architectural rather than cytologic. For this reason, the final diagnosis of malignant melanoma is best made with scanning, rather than with high-power, magnification.

For us, the critical zone to be examined microscopically

in an attempt to differentiate malignant melanoma from unusual melanocytic nevi, such as the nevus of large spindle and/or epithelioid cells, halo nevi, irritated junction or compound melanocytic nevi, and recurrent melanocytic nevi following shave biopsy (Kornberg and Ackerman, 1975) is the circumference of these melanocytic processes. The peripheral regions of importance are the most lateral aspects of the intraepidermal portion of the melanocytic lesion, the upper half of the epidermis, and the base of the lesion whether in the dermis or in the subcutaneous fat (Fig. 82). At the lateral margins of melanocytic nevi of all types there is sharp demarcation of the melanocytic component within the epidermis (Fig. 83), whereas in malignant melanoma of all types, except less commonly in nodular melanoma, there tends to be horizontal extension of individual melanocytes beyond the bulk of melanocytes both within the epidermis and the dermis (Fig. 54). Within the upper half of the epidermis one should look for melanocytes, either singly or in small collections. In melanocytic nevi, the melanocytes tend to be grouped into nests that are present either at the dermoepidermal junction or in the lower portion of the epidermis (Fig. 83). In contrast, in malignant melanoma irrespective of type, melanocytes are commonly scattered like buck-shot in the upper half of the epidermis, even unto the cornified layer (Fig. 47). At the base of a melanocytic lesion in the dermis, one should determine if the nuclei of the melanocytes are smaller, the same size, or even larger than the nuclei of melanocytes within the upper portion of the dermis and within the epidermis. In melanocytic nevi, the nuclei of melanocytes (or nevocytes) tend to become smaller (an aspect of maturation) as they descend progressively into the dermis (Fig. 84), whereas in malignant melanoma of all types there tends to be little or no maturation of melanocytes (Fig. 85).

Having examined the circumference of the melanocytic lesion, where the most telling signs for differentiation of benignancy from malignancy are to be found, it is then useful to search for other architectural features while still using scanning magnification. A helpful clue to recognition of a melanocytic nevus or a malignant melanoma is the size and shape of the nests of melanocytes within the epidermis and the dermis. In melanocytic nevi, the nests of melanocytes tend to be relatively uniform in size and shape, whereas in malignant melanoma they are usually variable in size and irregular in shape (Fig. 86). Furthermore, the nests of melanocytes in the epidermis of melanocytic nevi are very well circumscribed and discrete, whereas those in malignant melanoma are poorly circumscribed and often confluent like run-on sentences (Fig. 86). Nests, cords, strands, and individual nevocytes are found in the dermis

TABLE 5

Histologic Criteria for the Diagnosis of Malignant Melanoma

Architectural Pattern

Increased number of atypical melanocytes, singly and/or in nests within the epidermis.

Horizontal extension of atypical melanocytes, singly and/or in nests, within the epidermis beyond the bulk of the intraepidermal and intradermal components of the neoplasm.

Failure of nuclei of the atypical melanocytes to become smaller with progressive descent into the dermis.

Atypical melanocytes present singly and/or in nests at all levels of the epidermis, even including the cornified layer.

Variation in size and shape of intraepidermal and intradermal nests of atypical melanocytes.

Confluence of the nests of atypical melanocytes within the epidermis and the dermis.

Extension of atypical melanocytes, singly and/or in nests, down epithelial structures of adnexa, namely, hair follicles and eccrine sweat ducts.

Cytologic Features

Atypical melanocytes with large, hyperchromatic, pleomorphic nuclei and prominent nucleoli.

Melanocytes in mitosis within the epidermis and the dermis.

Necrotic melanocytes.

of compound and intradermal melanocytic nevi, whereas sheets and irregularly shaped aggregates of atypical melanocytes are common findings in the dermis of malignant melanomas (Fig. 58).

The differences that obtain within the epidermis of melanocytic nevi and malignant melanomas occur also within the epithelial structures of the adnexa. When melanocytes of melanocytic nevi are present within the epithelium of hair follicles and eccrine sweat ducts, as is often the situation in congenital and in Spitz's nevi, they are arranged as in the epidermis, i.e., uniform in size and shape and discrete. When melanocytes of malignant melanomas are present within the epithelial structures of adnexa, as they often are, especially in lentigo maligna melanoma, they are often scattered like buck-shot, and when nested, the nests are variable in size and irregular in shape and tend to

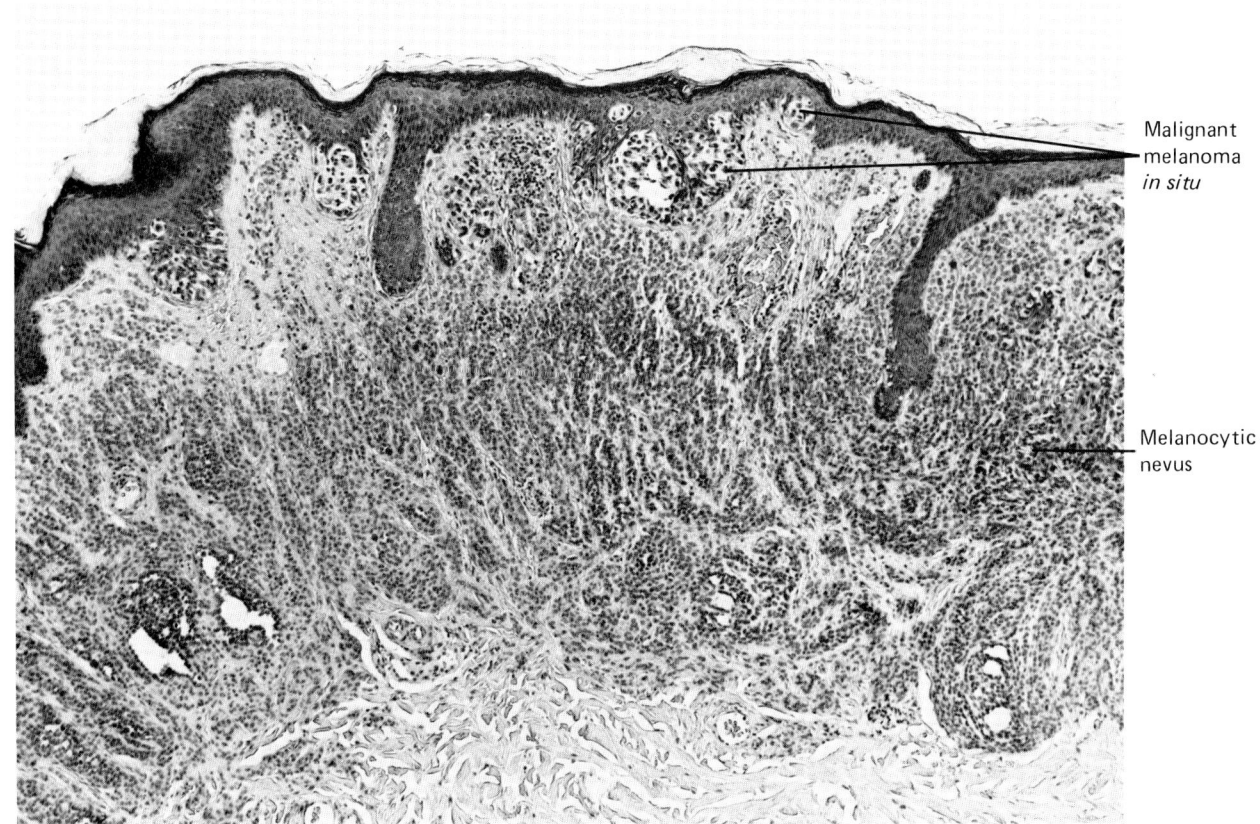

FIGURE 71A. *Malignant melanoma* **in situ** *overlying a large acquired intradermal melanocytic nevus (so-called B-K mole)*. The patient from whom this biopsy was obtained had many acquired melanocytic nevi on the trunk that measured between 2 and 3 cm in diameter. The histologic features illustrated here are those of a broad melanocytic nevus confined to thickened papillary dermis and atypical melanocytes scattered singly and in nests of various sizes and shapes within the epidermis. (Reduced from ×84)

confluence (Fig. 87). Adnexal epithelial structures are sometimes destroyed completely by the advance of cells of malignant melanoma within the dermis, but adnexal structures are not affected in a destructive way by nevocytes of melanocytic nevi. In the dermis, there is usually considerable connective tissue around nevus cells of melanocytic nevi, whereas little or no connective tissue is found in and about the conglomerations or sheets of atypical melanocytes in malignant melanomas.

A predominantly lymphocytic infiltrate is often present in a malignant melanoma as may be the case in a halo nevus and in a Spitz's nevus. One helpful differentiating feature is that in malignant melanoma the inflammatory-cell infiltrate is usually situated at or immediately beneath the advancing margin of atypical melanocytes in the dermis (Fig. 73), whereas in a halo nevus it is diffusely distributed throughout the nevus (Fig. 88) and in a Spitz's nevus it is present just around blood vessels throughout the nevus (Fig. 84). The lymphocytes at the base of a malignant melanoma may intermingle with the atypical melanocytes in the lowermost portion of the neoplasm. The finding of an inflammatory-cell infiltrate per se is not a helpful feature for differentiating a malignant melanoma from a melanocytic nevus; only the position of the infiltrate in relation to the melanocytes or nevus cells aids in diagnosis. As a rule, the deeper the atypical melanocytes in a malignant melanoma reach into the dermis, the less dense the inflammatory-cell infiltrate tends to become.

In our view, cytologic considerations are much less helpful than architectural ones for the differentiation of melanocytic nevi from malignant melanomas. However, care should be taken to examine melanocytes for evidence of nuclear atypia (Fig. 89), necrosis, (Fig. 90), and mitotic figures (Fig. 91). Large darkly staining nucleoli are also common features of malignant melanomas, but practically never of melanocytic nevi (Fig. 92). Large pink or pale gray

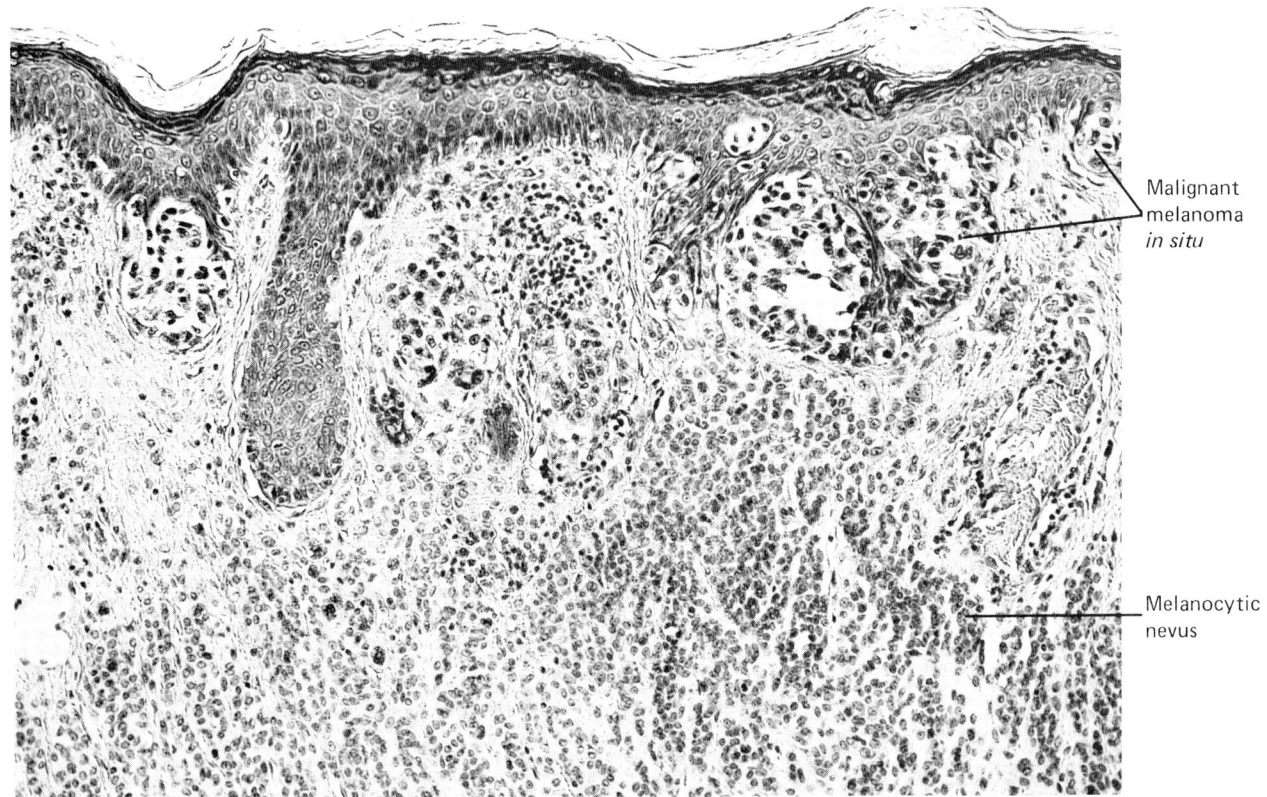

FIGURE 71B. ***Malignant melanoma* in situ *overlying a large acquired intradermal melanocytic nevus (so-called B-K mole).*** *In this higher magnification of Fig. 71A the features of malignant melanoma* in situ *above an intradermal melanocytic nevus may be seen to better advantage. Note also the sparse inflammatory-cell infiltrate and the lamellar collagen. In sum, this is a large melanocytic nevus upon which a malignant melanoma is evolving. (Reduced from ×190)*

intranuclear vacuoles are commonly found in malignant melanomas, especially of the superficial spreading and nodular types (Fig. 93). Except in the nevus of large spindle and/or epithelioid cells, and some stages of halo nevi, the nuclei of melanocytic nevi are not usually atypical. However, some Spitz's nevi may show greater nuclear atypia than do most malignant melanomas. Neither do nevocytes tend to undergo necrosis or to exhibit mitoses (except for Spitz's nevus and for large congenital melanocytic nevi that have been biopsied shortly after birth). In contrast, the nuclei of all types of malignant melanoma tend to be atypical to variable degrees, though sometimes slightly so in early stages of lentigo maligna and in malignant melanomas composed of small cells. The finding of mitotic figures in the deeper portion of the neoplasm supports a diagnosis of malignant melanoma. In some malignant melanomas, especially the nodular types, there may be as many as 10 to 15 mitotic figures per high-power field. This is never the case in melanocytic nevi, not even Spitz's nevi, where some mitotic figures may be found. The presence of many mitotic figures per high-power field or of atypical mitotic figures in a melanocytic lesion favors the diagnosis of malignant melanoma and, in our experience, the more mitotic figures per high-power field, the worse the prognosis tends to be. Pagetoid cells, i.e., cells with abundant pale staining cytoplasms and dusty melanin within them, are a feature of malignant melanomas (especially the superficially spreading type) and practically never of melanocytic nevi.

The finding of multinucleated melanocytic giant cells, thought by Spitz to be the single most important histologic feature for differentiation of benign juvenile melanoma from malignant melanoma, is of dubious importance in our view. Many types of multinucleated melanocytes may be

72 The Histology of Cutaneous Malignant Melanoma

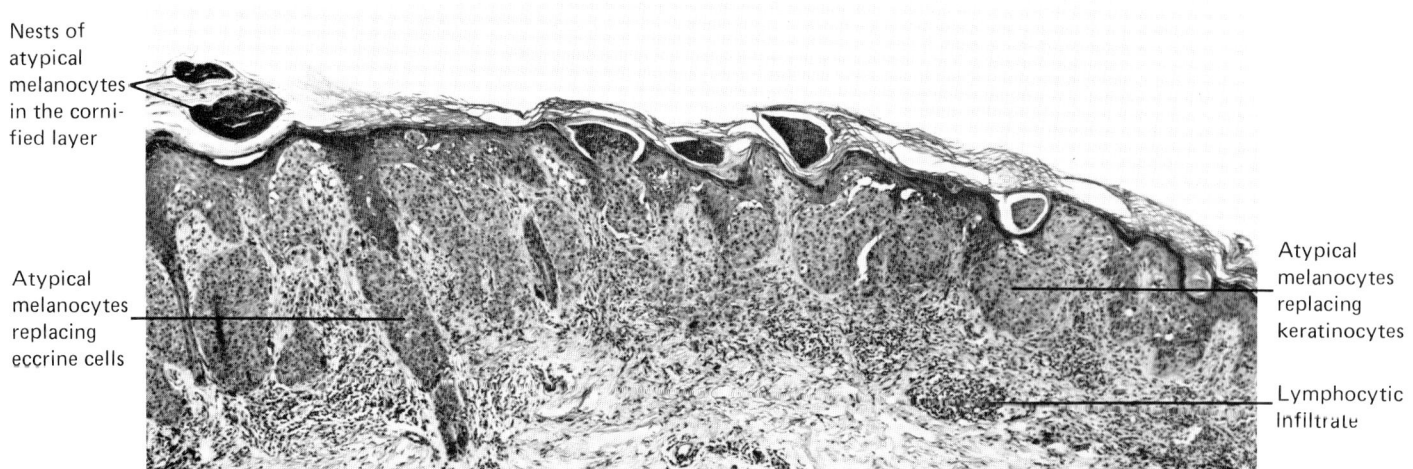

FIGURE 72A. **Malignant melanoma, superficial spreading type.** *This lesion illustrates how atypical melanocytes within the epidermis of malignant melanoma are not rooted to the basal-cell zone, but ascend through all levels into the cornified layer. The pigmented masses within the epidermis are not parakeratotic cells, but nests of necrotic melanocytes. (Reduced from ×61)*

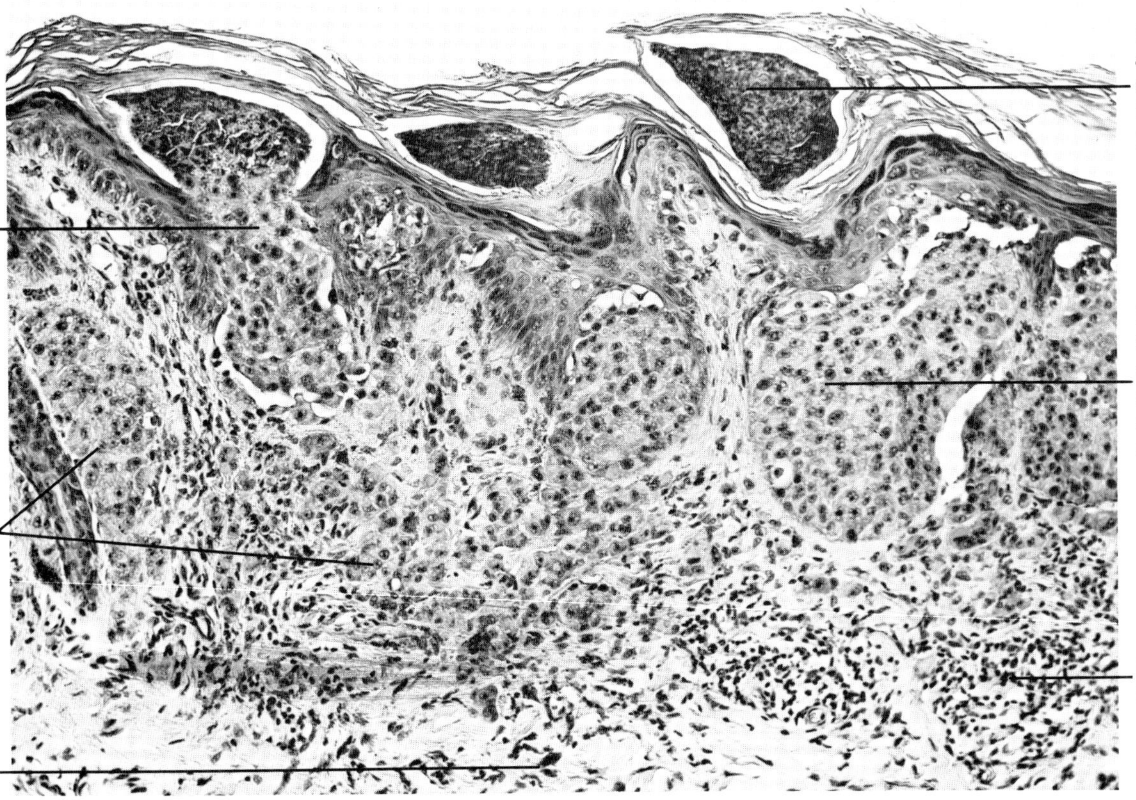

FIGURE 72B. **Malignant melanoma, superficial spreading type.** *This higher magnification of Fig. 72A shows to better advantage the irregular nests of necrotic melanocytes within the epidermis of a superficial spreading malignant melanoma. On the left-hand portion of the photomicrograph one can see the extension of the atypical melanocytes through the epidermis into the cornified layer. Note the irregularity in size and shape of the nests of atypical melanocytes in both the epidermis and the dermis. (Reduced from ×173)*

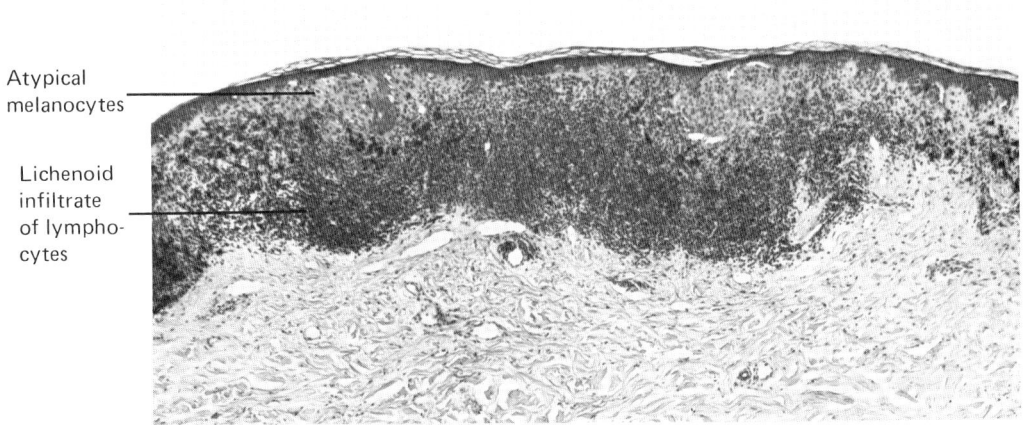

FIGURE 73A. **Dense lichenoid inflammatory-cell infiltrate prior to regression of a malignant melanoma.** *A prelude to regression of malignant melanoma illustrated here is a dense lymphocytic infiltrate that permeates the front of atypical melanocytes within the papillary dermis. Without such an infiltrate of inflammatory cells there can be no involution of the malignant neoplasm. (Reduced from ×54)*

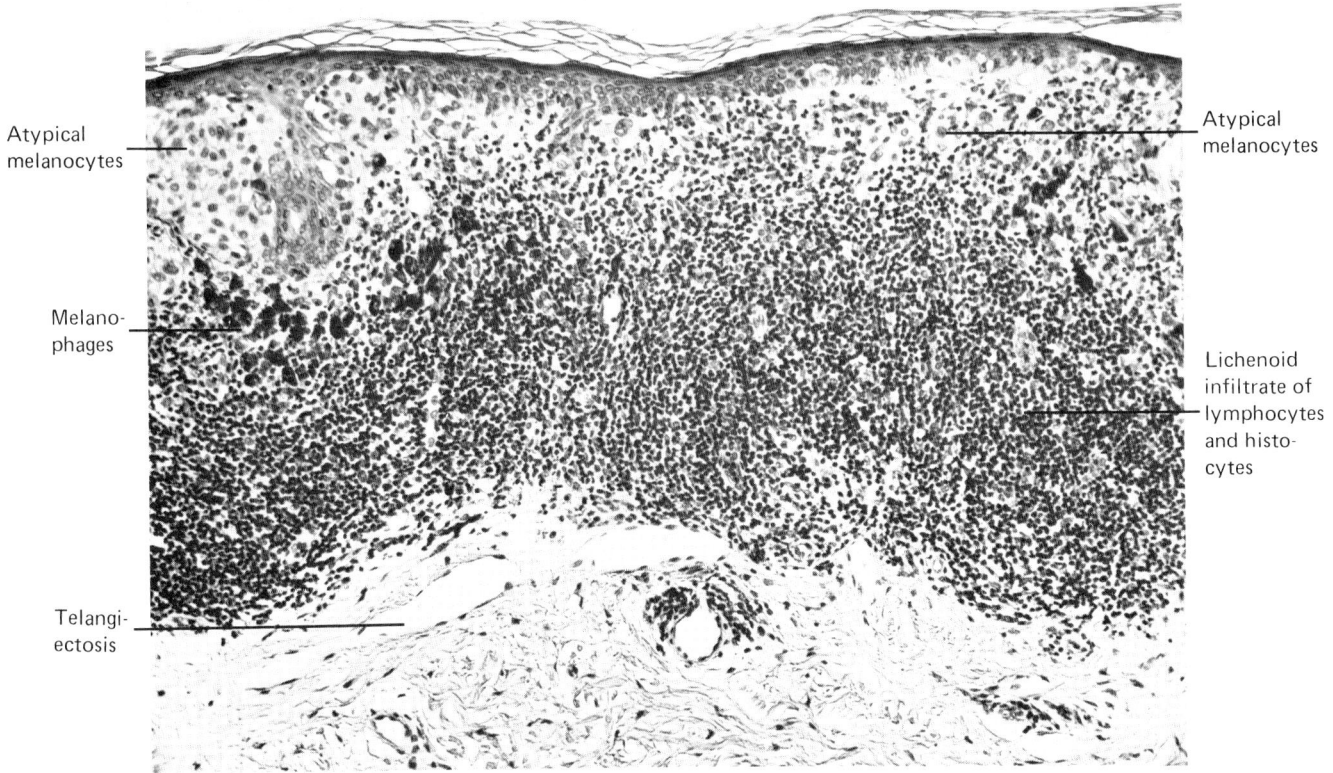

FIGURE 73B. **Dense lichenoid inflammatory-cell infiltrate prior to regression of a malignant melanoma.** *Within the epidermis there is an increased number of atypical melanocytes, singly and in nests, and in the markedly thickened papillary dermis there is a dense band-like lymphohistiocytic infiltrate with numerous melanophages. Some atypical melanocytes may have penetrated the papillary dermis but are totally obscured by the dense lichenoid inflammatory-cell infiltrate requisite for subsequent regression of the malignant melanoma. (Reduced from ×164)*

74   The Histology of Cutaneous Malignant Melanoma

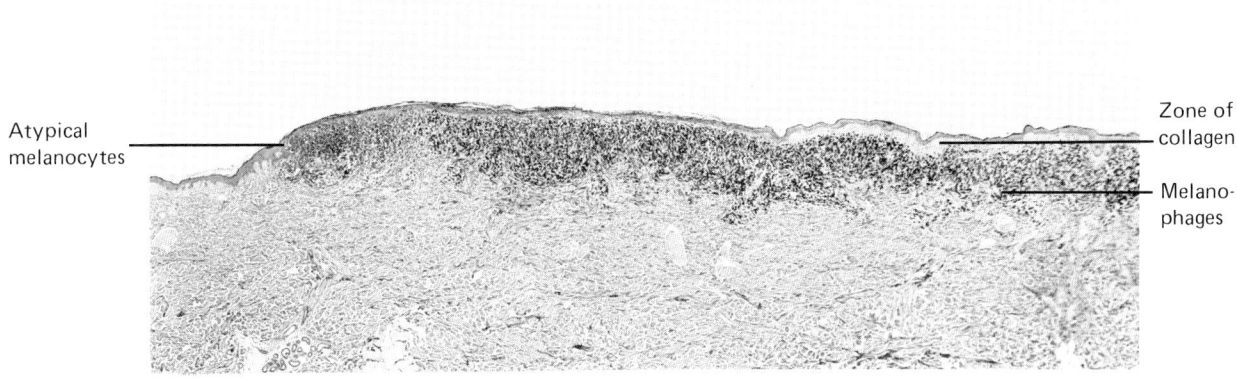

FIGURE 74A. **Progression of stages in spontaneous regression of superficial spreading malignant melanoma.** *On the left side of this photomicrograph the lichenoid infiltrate that fills the thickened papillary dermis is seen to obscure the dermoepidermal junction, whereas on the right side there is a thin zone of collagen between the infiltrate and the epidermis. The sequence, from left to right, bespeaks eradication in part by a lymphocytic infiltrate of a malignant melanoma situated at the dermoepidermal junction and in the papillary dermis. Residual melanophages confined to the papillary dermis and thinning of the epidermis are other features. (Reduced from ×17)*

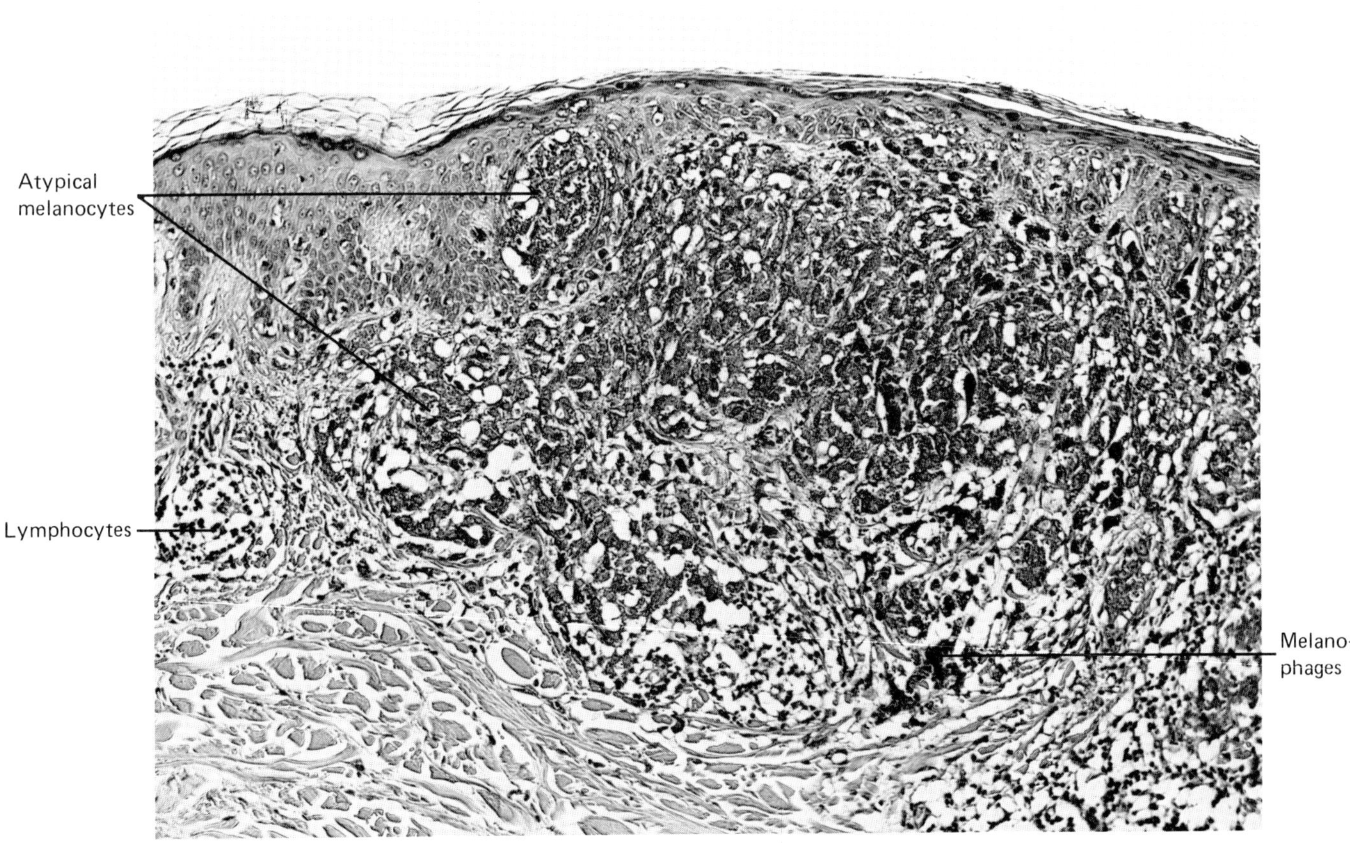

FIGURE 74B. **Progression of stages in spontaneous regression of superficial spreading malignant melanoma.** *In this higher magnification of the left-hand portion of Fig. 74A the malignant melanoma, lymphocytic infiltrate, and melanophages are seen better. (Reduced from ×175)*

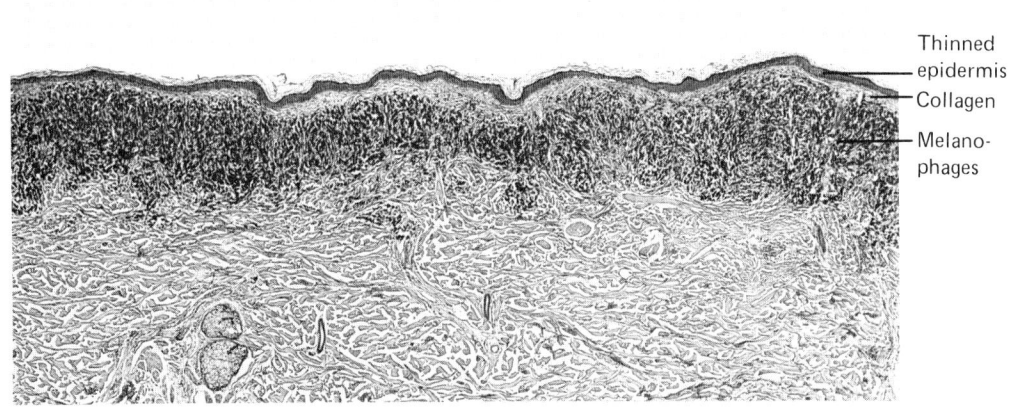

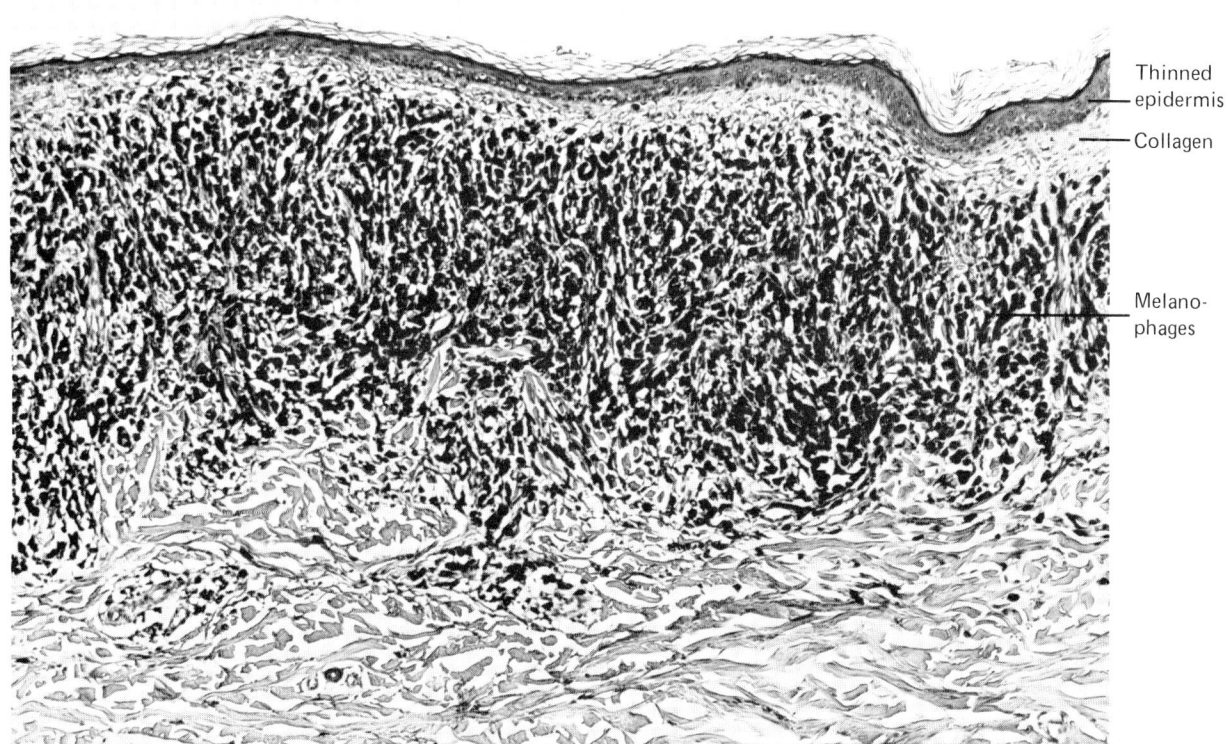

FIGURES 75A & B. ***Lichenoid infiltrate of melanophages as residua of malignant melanoma that underwent complete local regression.*** *These changes mark the site of a previous superficial spreading malignant melanoma that reached into the papillary dermis where it was obliterated by a dense predominantly lymphocytic infiltrate. A thin zone of fibrotic collagen separates the band of melanophages from the thinned epidermis. (Reduced from ×26 and ×100)*

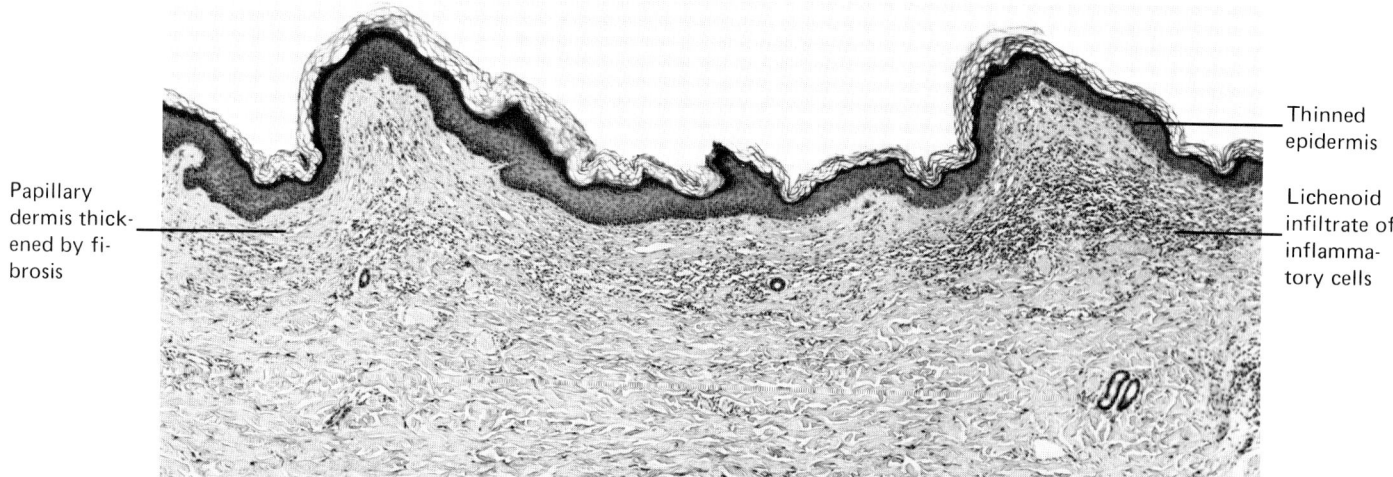

FIGURE 76A. **Residual changes following complete local regression of malignant melanoma.** *There is a normal compliment of normal appearing melanocytes within the epidermis, a flat epidermis devoid of rete ridges, and marked fibrosis of the thickened papillary dermis, beneath which is a lymphohistiocytic infiltrate. All are signs of a malignant melanoma that has been eliminated at this site. This portion of the lesion would be whitish clinically because of the fibrosis in the thickened papillary dermis. (Reduced from ×54)*

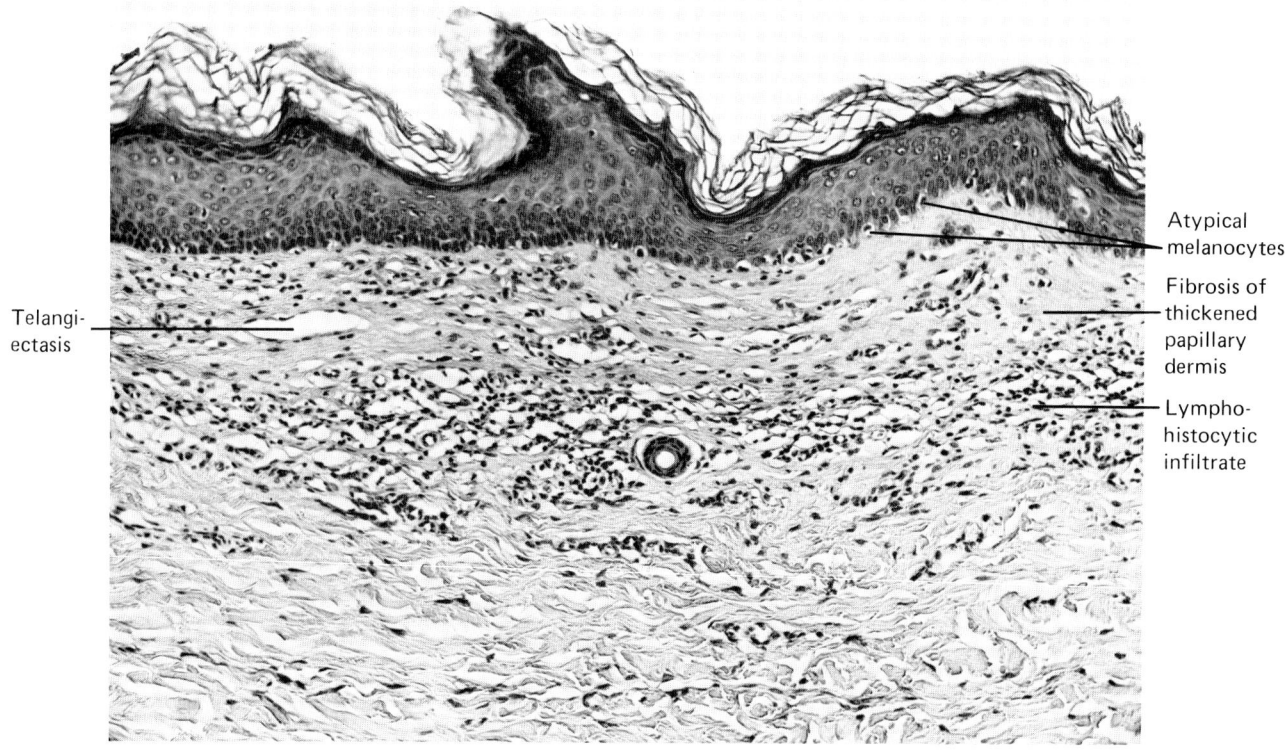

FIGURE 76B. **Residual changes following complete local regression of malignant melanoma.** *This closer view of Fig. 76A illustrates the flattened undersurface of the epidermis, the zone of fibrosis beneath it, and a sparse band of mononuclear inflammatory cells. These are evidences of a previously long-standing inflammatory-cell infiltrate in the upper part of the dermis that did battle with a thin malignant melanoma and defeated it. The only melanocytes that remain of what once was a malignant melanoma at this site are the few normal appearing "clear cells" in the basal layer of the epidermis. (Reduced from ×164)*

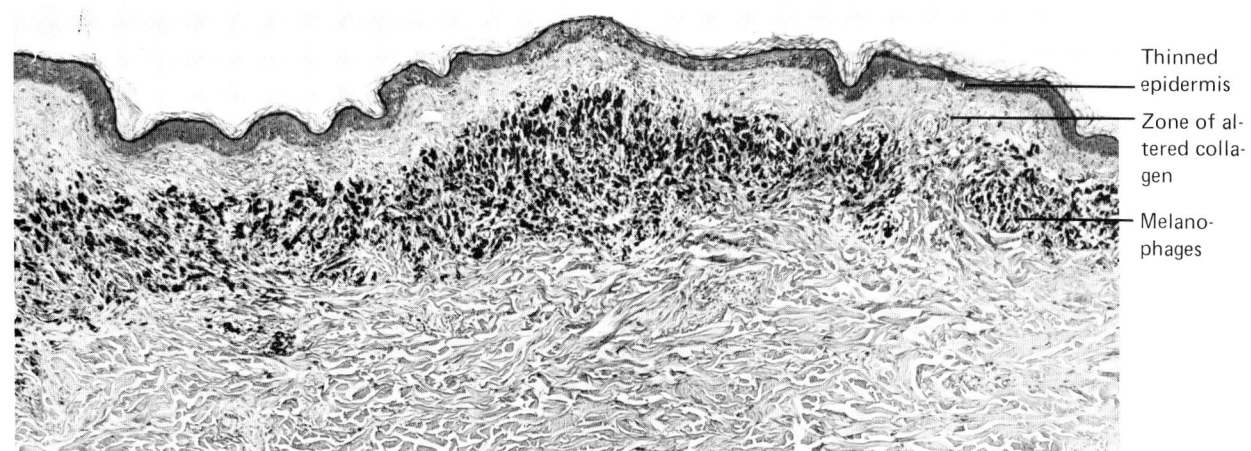

FIGURE 77A. **Lichenoid infiltrate of melanophages beneath a zone of fibrosis in a malignant melanoma that has regressed spontaneously and entirely.** *After a dense lymphocytic infiltrate has wiped out a superficial spreading malignant melanoma, the only residua may be a broad zone of melanophages separated from a thinned epidermis by a narrow band of collagen, as shown here. The interaction between the lymphocytes and atypical melanocytes takes place in the papillary dermis which thickens markedly as a result of the litter of the battle. (Reduced from ×54)*

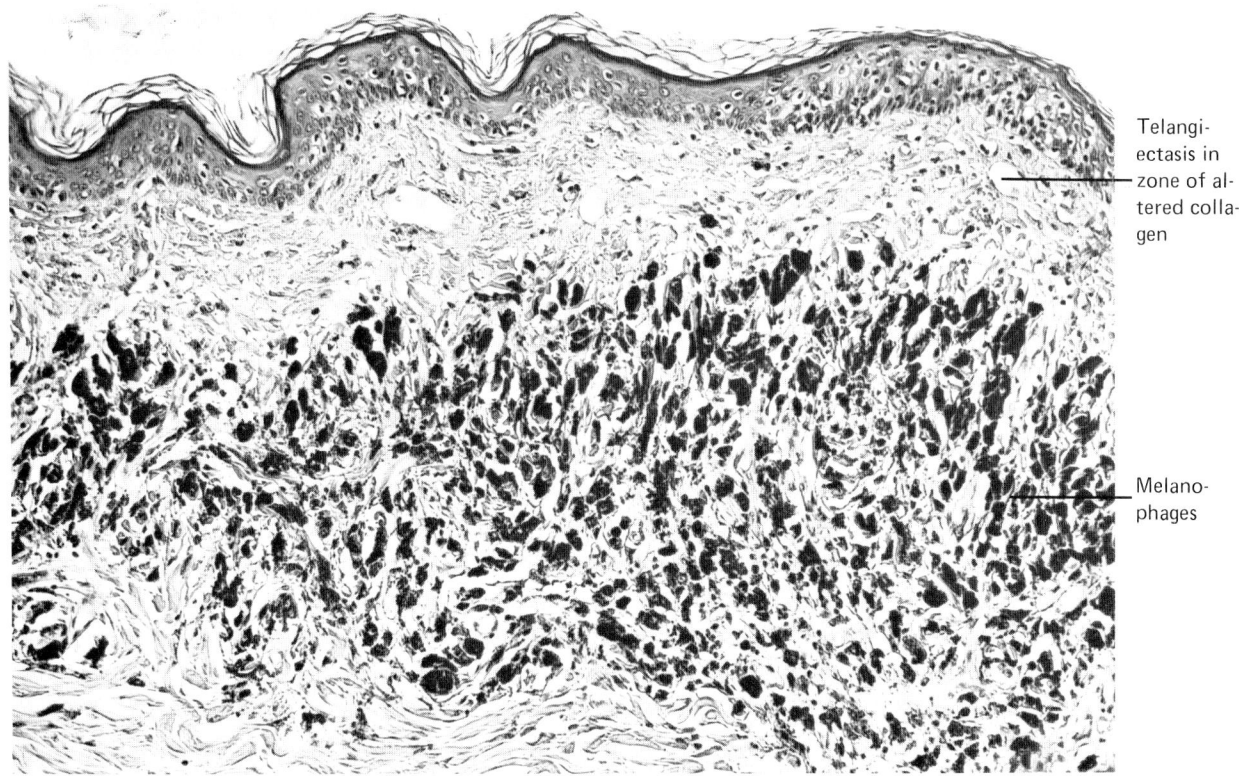

FIGURE 77B. **Lichenoid infiltrate of melanophages beneath zone of fibrosis in malignant melanoma that has regressed spontaneously and entirely.** *A thinned epidermis devoid of atypical melanocytes, a zone of coarse collagen, and a broad band of melanophages are telltale signs of a site where a superficial spreading malignant melanoma has undergone spontaneous regression. Such changes do not mean or presage cure. Changes such as those pictured here may be found concurrent with evidences of metastatic extension from the primary lesion at this very site. (Reduced from ×180)*

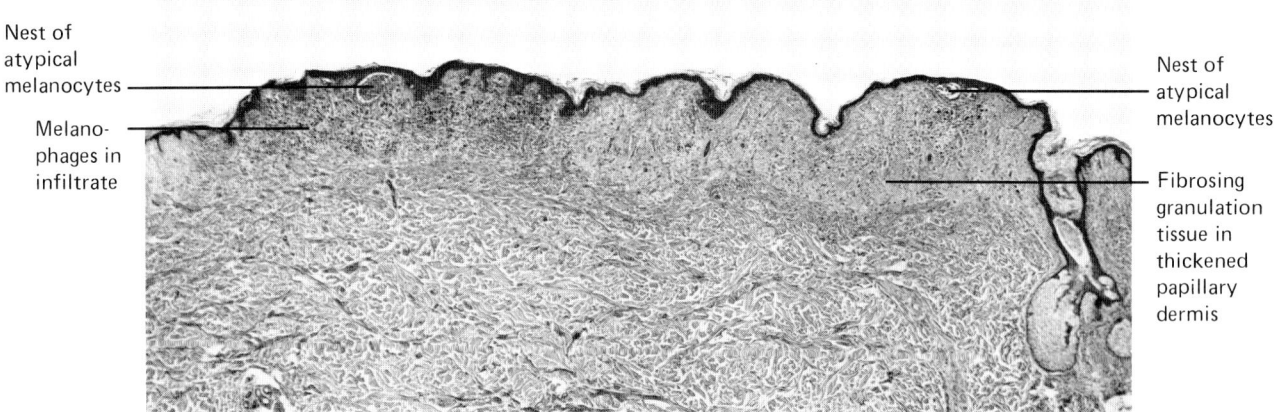

FIGURE 78A. ***Malignant melanoma with evidences of partial regression.*** *On the left of this photomicrograph there is a typical superficial spreading malignant melanoma and on the right there is a markedly widened and fibrotic papillary dermis, indication of regression of the malignant melanoma in that zone. (Reduced from ×23)*

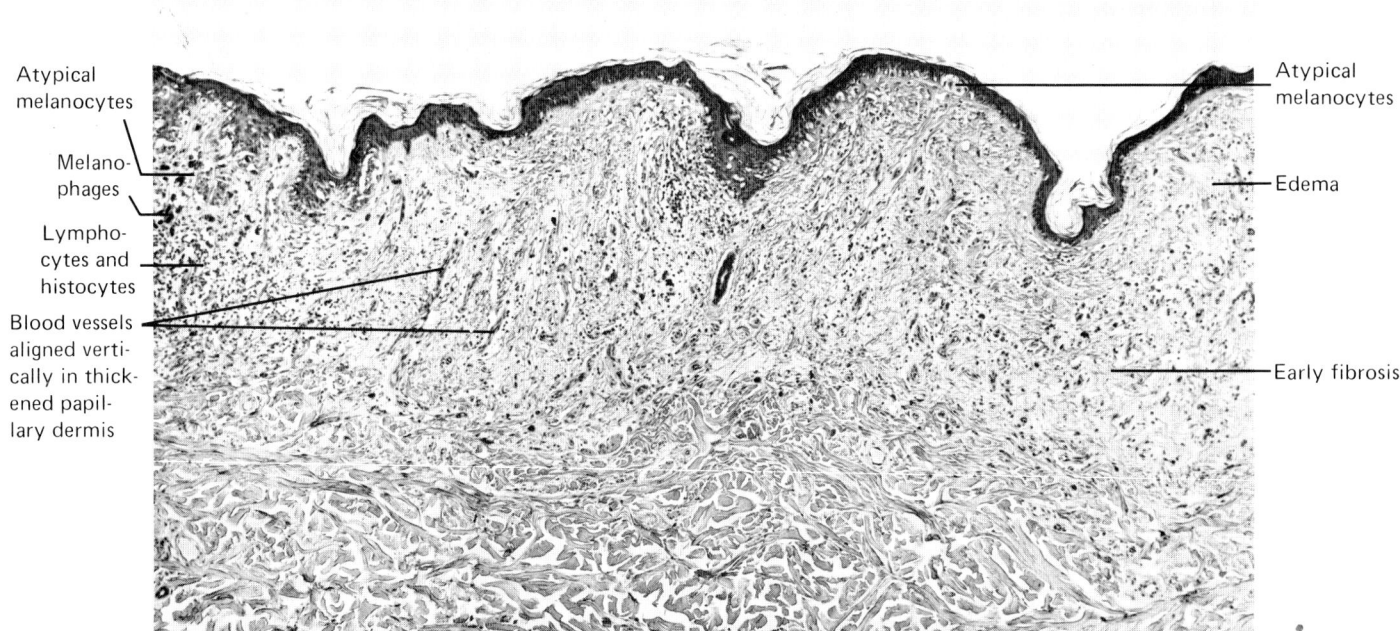

FIGURE 78B. ***Malignant melanoma with evidences of partial regression.*** *In this higher power view of Fig. 78A the widened papillary dermis and its sharp demarcation from the reticular dermis may be seen to better advantage. The dominant feature in the altered papillary dermis is fibrosing granulation tissue. Atypical melanocytes within the epidermis are the only residue of the malignant melanoma that was formerly at this site before it was eliminated by a dense lichenoid infiltrate of lymphocytes. The melanophages bear testimony to the earlier presence of atypical pigmented-producing melanocytes in the dermis. (Reduced from ×78)*

seen in malignant melanomas (Fig. 94) ranging from these that resemble Langhan's histiocytic cells to gigantic cells with bizarre nuclei and pale granular cytoplasms. In some instances, admittedly rare, the multinucleated cells of malignant melanomas may be indistinguishable cytologically from those of Spitz's nevus. Lastly, melanocytic giant cells are found in fewer than 50% of Spitz's nevi. Therefore, we do not emphasize the significance of giant cells in the diagnosis of melanocytic lesions.

The diagnosis of malignant melanoma primary in the skin, irrespective of type, cannot be made with certainty in the absence of atypical melanocytes within the epidermis. This is equally applicable to both ordinary melanotic and amelanotic malignant melanomas. If atypical melanocytes are present only within the dermis and the epidermis is absolutely free of them, the diagnosis is more likely to be metastatic, rather than primary, malignant melanoma or recurrent malignant melanoma following partial surgical excision. Because virtually all primary cutaneous malignant melanomas begin within the epidermis, it is to the surface epithelium that one must first look for atypical melanocytes. There is to be found the most important bits of evidence of malignant melanomas that originate in the skin.

In conclusion, without several clear-cut criteria for the histologic diagnosis of cutaneous malignant melanoma, accurate microscopic diagnosis of pigmented skin lesions in general becomes impossible. Histologic diagnosis of malignant melanoma cannot be made on the basis of any single criterion, but rather by using a combination of them. Exceptions may be found to each of the architectural and cytologic features of malignant melanoma listed in Table 5. Not every one of these features is present in every malignant melanoma and, conversely, some features usually associated with malignant melanoma may be seen in banal melanocytic nevi. If any one criterion is uniformly diagnostic of malignant melanoma, it is the finding of numerous mitotic figures per high-power field, especially in the lower portion of the neoplasm. This is practically never the case in benign neoplasms or hamartomas of melanocytes.

VI. HISTOLOGIC DIFFERENTIAL DIAGNOSIS OF MALIGNANT MELANOMA

The major simulators of primary cutaneous malignant melanomas are melanocytic nevi, namely, congenital nevi biopsied shortly after birth, unusual junction nevi, traumatized junction or compound nevi (Figs. 95 and 96), nevi of large spindle and/or epithelioid cells (benign juvenile melanomas) (Fig. 97), halo nevi (Fig. 98), and recurrent melanocytic nevi following partial removal, usually by shave excision and light electrodesiccation (Figs. 99 and 100) (Table 6). Pagetoid Bowen's disease (Fig. 101) and both mammary (Figs. 102 and 103) and extramammary Paget's disease may be mistaken for pagetoid (superficial spreading) malignant melanomas (Table 7). Another simulator of primary malignant melanoma is epidermotropically metastatic malignant melanoma (Kornberg et al., 1978). Each of these conditions may be differentiated from primary malignant melanomas, especially on the basis of architectural features. It is not surprising that architectural pattern is more helpful for the diagnosis of melanocytic nevi, pagetoid carcinomas, and malignant melanomas than are cytologic details when one reflects that in almost every difficult histologic problem involving a melanocytic lesion, reference to even still lower power, the macroscopic or gross morphology, i.e., the clinical appearance of the lesion, tends to be decisive. It is usually easy for a skilled clinician to decide whether a lesion is a melanocytic nevus (Spitz, halo, recurrent, etc.), Paget's disease, Bowen's disease, or a malignant melanoma.

Two exceedingly difficult melanocytic lesions to interpret histologically are a nevus of large spindle and/or epithelioid cells developing within an ordinary melanocytic nevus (Fig. 104) and a second nodular clutch of epithelioid cells arising in a spindle-cell type of Spitz's nevus (Fig. 105). In both circumstances one must differentiate epithelioid nevocytes of a Spitz's nevus from epithelioid melanocytes of a malignant melanoma that has arisen within a preexisting melanocytic nevus. At times, the difficult decision for or against malignancy cannot be made with certainty, and in these instances complete excision of the melanocytic lesion or the biopsy site should be performed.

Lentigo maligna is one form of malignant melanoma *in situ* that may often be misinterpreted as a simple junction nevus (Fig. 106). When one sees nests of melanocytes within the epidermis above severely solar-damaged dermis, the more likely diagnosis is lentigo maligna rather than junction nevus, a rarity in older individuals. A clue to the diagnosis of lentigo maligna is the finding of spindle-shaped melanocytes in elongated nests oriented parallel to the surface of the specimen.

Heavily pigmented desmoplastic malignant melanomas may sometimes be misinterpreted histologically as blue nevi (Fig. 107). Both show spindle-shaped melanocytes, melanophages, and fibrosis in the dermis. However, desmoplastic forms of malignant melanoma, like virtually all primary cutaneous malignant melanomas, have atypical melanocytes within the epidermis. Such is not the case in blue nevi.

Some examples of primary nodular malignant melanomas may be confused histologically with large nodules of

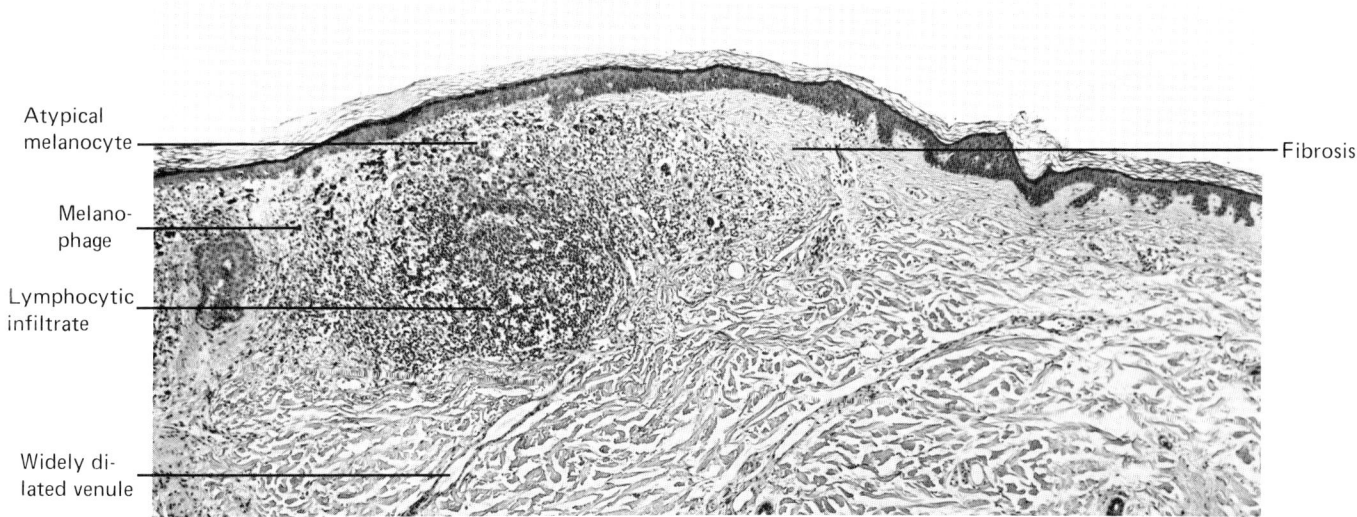

FIGURE 79A. **Malignant melanoma with evidences of partial regression.** *On the left side of this photomicrograph there is a dense lichenoid infiltrate of lymphocytes and melanophages that largely obscures atypical melanocytes of a superficial spreading malignant melanoma. On the right side there are fibrotic changes in the widened papillary dermis, signs of resolution of a similar process to that on the left. (Reduced from ×62)*

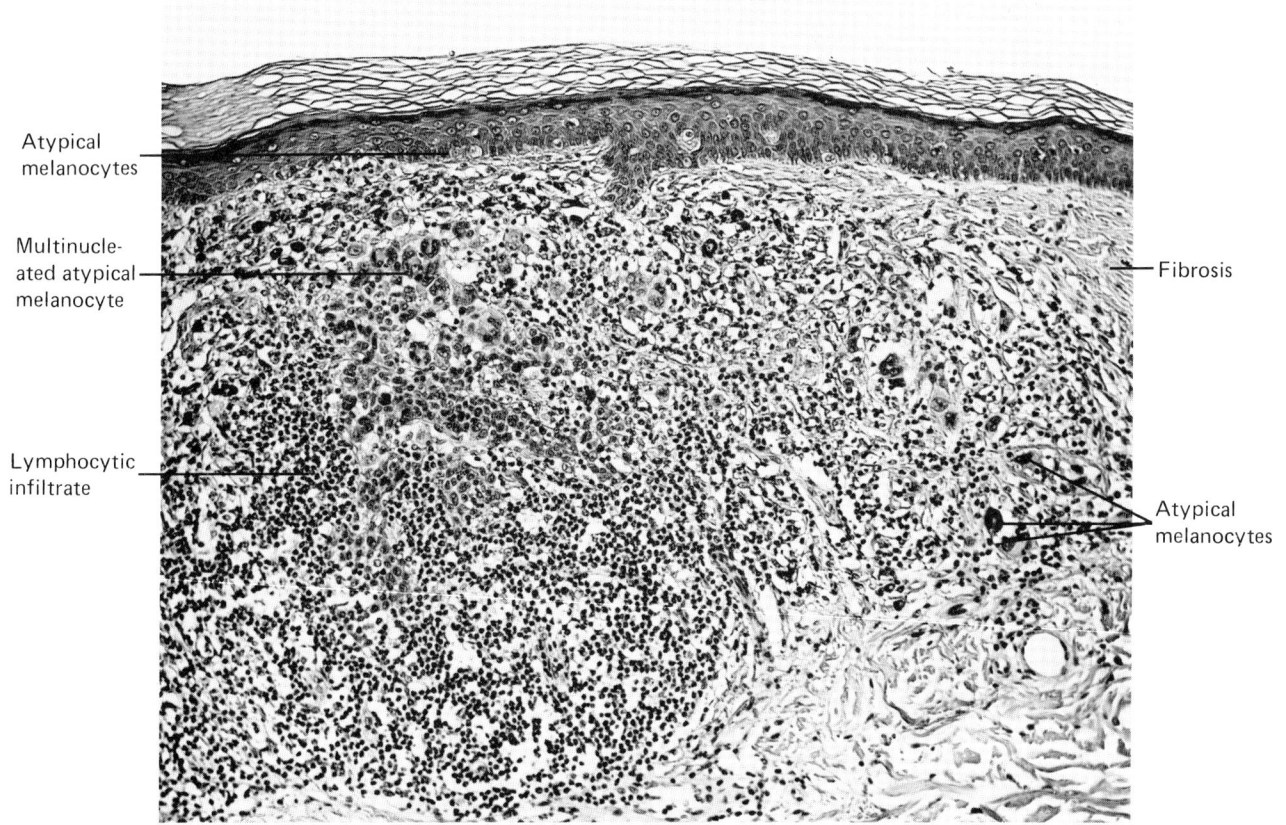

FIGURE 79B. **Malignant melanoma with evidences of partial regression.** *Higher magnification of Fig. 79A to show atypical melanocytes in the epidermis and in the dermis, in the latter surrounded by a dense predominantly lymphocytic infiltrate, a prelude to eradication of the neoplastic cells. (Reduced from ×158)*

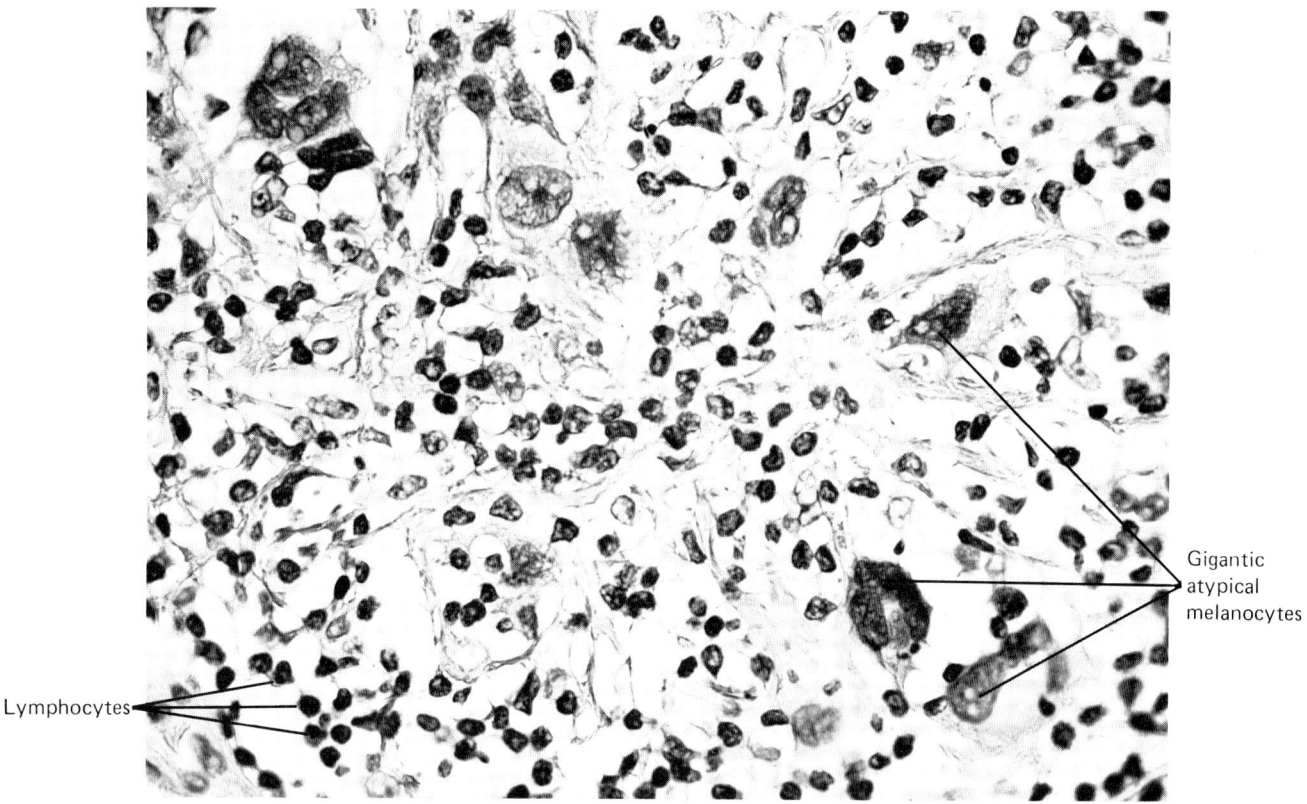

FIGURE 79C. **Malignant melanoma with evidences of partial regression.** *Still higher magnification of Fig. 79A to reveal the strikingly atypical melanocytes enmeshed in a dense infiltrate of lymphocytes. (Reduced from ×572)*

metastatic malignant melanomas that are seated just beneath the epidermis. If many sections are cut through the block of a specimen of nodular malignant melanoma, some of them will almost always reveal, at the very least, a few atypical melanocytes disposed singly within the epidermis. This is the critical feature for differentiation of primary from metastatic malignant melanomas.

Nests of atypical mononuclear cells within the epidermis in cases of mycosis fungoides (so-called Pautrier's microabscesses) sometimes may be confused with nests of atypical melanocytes when the specimen is examined with scanning magnification (Fig. 108). More careful inspection of a lesion of mycosis fungoides with higher magnification will reveal no increased number of solitary melanocytes between the intraepidermal nests of mononuclear cells, no predilection of the nests for the dermoepidermal junction, and no irregular hyperpigmentation of the epidermis by melanin. Furthermore, the atypical lymphocytes in nests of mycosis fungoides often have characteristic convoluted, cerebriform, or raisin-like nuclei.

VII. MALIGNANT MELANOMA METASTATIC TO THE SKIN

Very rarely, atypical melanocytes may be found within the epidermis of lesions of malignant melanomas that are metastatic to the skin (epidermotropically metastic malignant melanoma) (Fig. 109). This exceptional form of a metastatic malignant melanoma may usually be differentiated histologically from a primary cutaneous malignant melanoma despite the fact that atypical melanocytes are present within the epidermis of both conditions. The microscopic clues to the recognition of epidermotropically metastatic malignant melanoma are the occasional presence of atypical melanocytes within lymphatics, the small size and sharp circumscription of the neoplasm, and the fact that the melanocytic process is almost always confined to the upper part of the dermis. Unlike most types of primary malignant melanoma in skin, there is usually no horizontal extension of individual atypical melanocytes within the epidermis beyond the bulk of the small, compact neoplasm of epidermotropically metastatic malignant melanoma. An

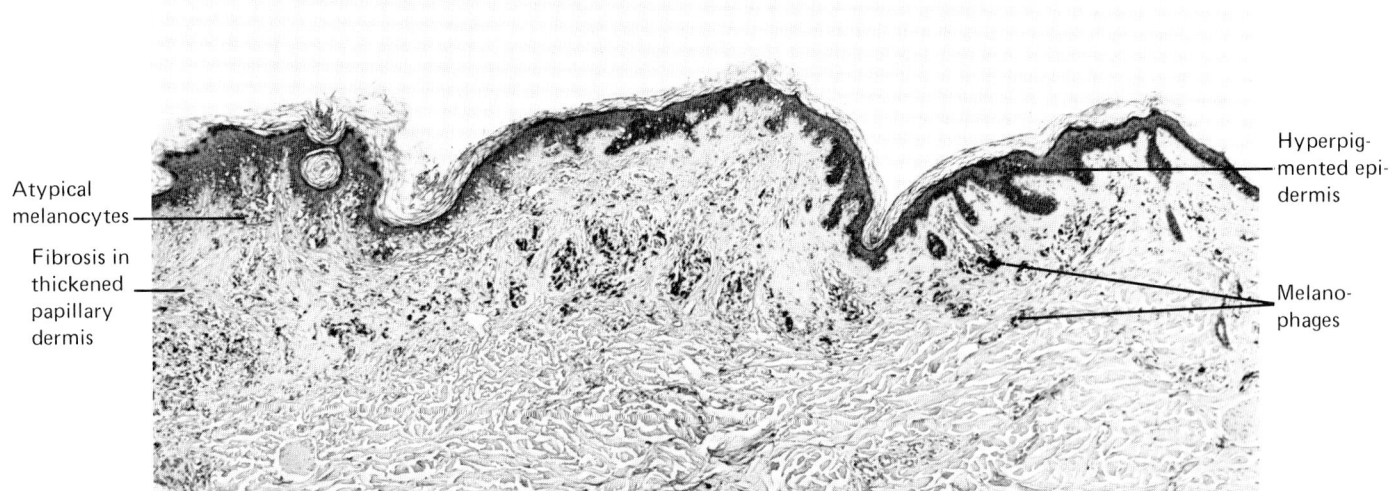

FIGURE 80A. **Residual changes of malignant melanoma that underwent partial regression.** *Contiguous to the changes seen in Fig. 76A are these: atypical melanocytes mostly disposed singly, but also in small nests, within the epidermis and marked thickening of papillary dermis by fibrosis. Numerous melanophages are seated beneath the fibrosis and around the vessels of the superficial plexus. This is an earlier stage in regression of malignant melanoma, because the dense lichenoid infiltrate has waned, melanophages are present, but atypical melanocytes still remain within the epidermis. (Reduced from ×54)*

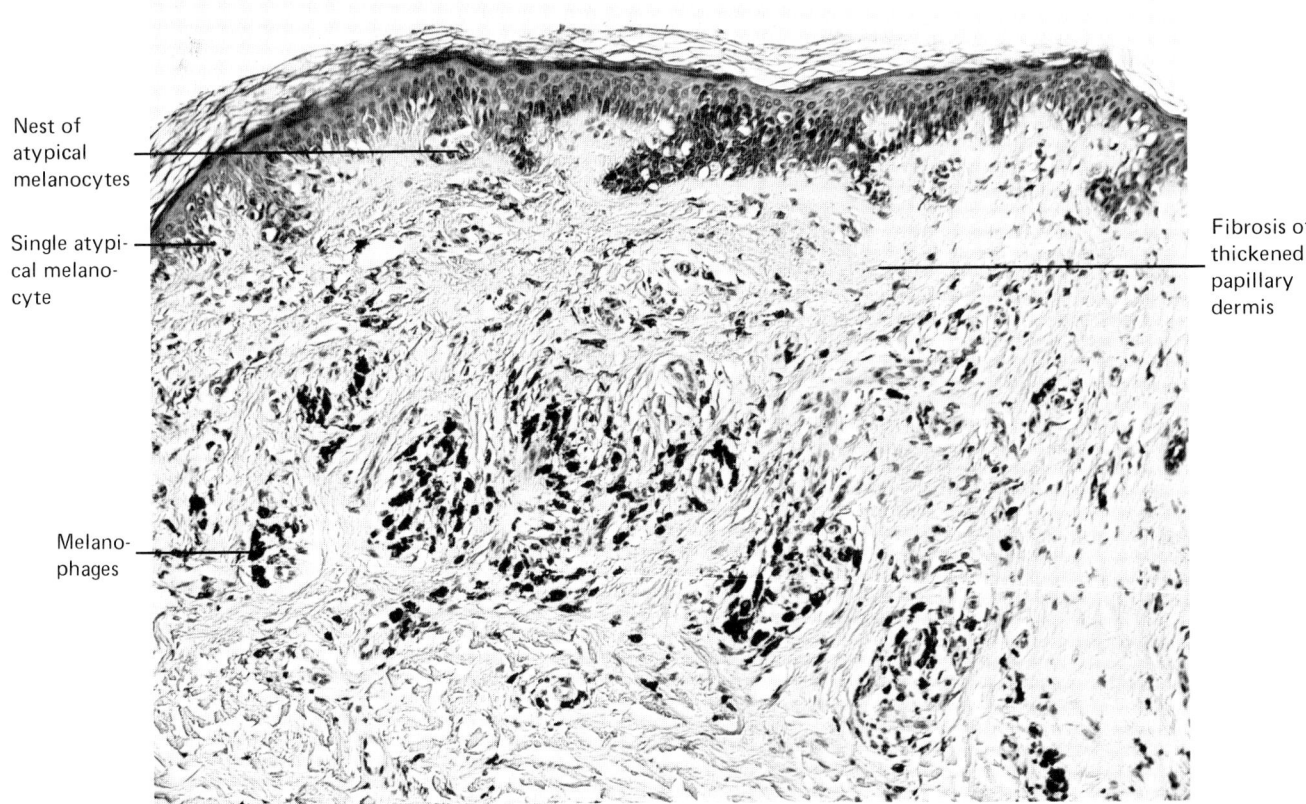

FIGURE 80B. **Residual changes of malignant melanoma that underwent partial regression.** *In this higher magnification of Fig. 80A the fibrosis and subjacent melanophages are better seen. They are testimony to a previous intense and prolonged inflammatory reaction in the superficial dermis involving a band-like lymphocytic infiltrate and a very superficial malignant melanoma. All that now remains of the neoplasm are a few atypical melanocytes within the epidermis. (Reduced from ×164)*

TABLE 6*
Histologic Differential Diagnosis of Superficial Spreading Malignant Melanoma

Superficial spreading malignant melanoma (pagetoid melanoma)	Benign juvenile melanoma (nevus of large spindle and/or epithelioid cells, Spitz's nevus)	Pseudomelanoma (recurrent melanocytic nevus following partial surgical excision)	Halo nevus (leukoderma acquisitum centrifugum, Sutton's nevus)
1. Poor circumscription of the intraepidermal melanocytic component with horizontal extension of individual atypical melanocytes within the epidermis.	1. Sharp lateral demarcation of the intraepidermal melanocytic component (no horizontal spread of individual atypical melanocytes).	1. Sharp circumscription of the intraepidermal melanocytic component (no horizontal spread of individual melanocytes within the epidermis).	1. Sharp circumscription of the intraepidermal melanocytic component (if the lesion is a junction or compound nevus).
2. Epidermal hyperplasia unusual.	2. Epidermal hyperplasia usual.	2. Epidermal hyperplasia unusual.	2. Epidermal hyperplasia unusual.
3. Increased number of melanocytes, both singly and in nests, in the upper half of the epidermis.	3. Few single or nested melanocytes in the mid or upper half of the epidermis.	3. Increased number of melanocytes, singly and in nests, in the upper half of the epidermis.	3. No significant increase in the number of melanocytes in the upper half of the epidermis.
4. Marked variation in size and shape of nests of melanocytes within the epidermis.	4. Nests of melanocytes, when present, relatively uniform in size and shape within the epidermis.	4. Nests of melanocytes within the epidermis vary in size and shape.	4. Nests of intraepidermal melanocytes, when present, are relatively uniform in size and shape.
5. Nests of melanocytes within the epidermis are irregular in size, but not particularly elongated.	5. Nests of melanocytes within epidermis tend to be elongated, and arranged perpendicularly to the surface.	5. Nests of melanocytes within the epidermis tend to be elongated and arranged parallel to the surface of the specimen.	5. Nests of melanocytes within the epidermis not elongated.
6. Nests of epidermal melanocytes tend to confluence.	6. Sharp circumscription of intraepidermal nests of melanocytes from surrounding keratinocytes.	6. Nests of melanocytes within the epidermis are both discrete and confluent.	6. Nests of melanocytes within the epidermis are relatively discrete if present there.
7. No clefts between nests of melanocytes and keratinocytes, usually.	7. Clefts between nests of melanocytes and keratinocytes often.	7. No clefts between nests of melanocytes and surrounding keratinocytes, usually.	7. No clefts between nests of melanocytes and surrounding keratinocytes.
8. Nests of melanocytes in the dermis tend to confluence with formation of sheets of cells.	8. Nests of nevus cells in the dermis tend to be discrete.	8. Remnants of the original melanocytic nevus may be present in discrete nests in the dermis.	8. Nests of nevus cells in the dermis are discrete when discernible; often partially or totally obscured by the lymphocytic infiltrate.
9. No maturation of melanocytes (decrease in nuclear size) with descent into the dermis.	9. Maturation of melanocytes with descent into the dermis.	9. Remnants of the original nevus, when present, show nuclear maturation.	9. Maturation of nevus cells with progressive descent into the dermis.
10. Pagetoid melanocytes often.	10. Spindle or epithelioid melanocytes, some large	10. No pagetoid cells.	10. No pagetoid cells.
11. Melanocytes, side by side, usually pleomorphic.	11. Melanocytes and nevus cells, side by side, usually similar in appearance, although there may be pleomorphism between noncontiguous melanocytes and nevocytes.	11. Melanocytic nuclei slightly, but not strikingly, atypical.	11. Melanocytes and nevus cells may be slightly atypical.
12. Inflammatory-cell infiltrate when present, band-like beneath and at the sides of the melanocytic component in the dermis.	12. Inflammatory-cell infiltrate patchy around blood vessels throughout the lesion.	12. Inflammatory-cell infiltrate only around the blood vessels of the superficial plexus; beneath the epidermis occasionally.	12. Inflammatory-cell infiltrate may be band-like in the upper part of the dermis or dense and diffuse throughout the lesion.

TABLE 6 (Continued)

Superficial spreading malignant melanoma (pagetoid melanoma)	Benign juvenile melanoma (nevus of large spindle and/or epithelioid cells, Spitz's nevus)	Pseudomelanoma (recurrent melanocytic nevus following partial surgical excision)	Halo nevus (leukoderma acquisitum centrifugum, Sutton's nevus)
13. Stroma not edematous, but may be fibrotic in the thickened papillary dermis, a sign of spontaneous resolution.	13. Stroma often edematous (especially in children); may be fibrotic (especially in adults).	13. Stroma fibrotic in at least the upper part of the dermis.	13. Stroma not edematous, but slightly fibrotic in lesions that have resolved completely.
14. Neoangiogenesis, when present, beneath the zone of neoplastic cells.	14. Neoangiogenesis prominent in the upper portion of the dermis (especially in young children).	14. Neoangiogenesis in the scarred area only.	14. Blood vessels throughout the lesion are dilated and have thickened walls lined by plump endothelial cells.
15. Extension into subcutaneous fat may occur when nodules form.	15. Extension into subcutaneous fat rare.	15. No involvement of the subcutaneous fat.	15. No extension into subcutaneous fat.

* From Ackerman, A. B. and Niven, J. Differential Diagnosis in Dermatopathology. Philadelphia, Lea and Febiger Co., to be published.

additionally confusing feature of epidermotropically metastatic malignant melanoma is the presence of an inflammatory-cell infiltrate beneath the neoplasm, just as in primary malignant melanoma. Also perplexing is the occasional finding of dendritic melanocytes within the epidermal and dermal portions of epidermotropically metastatic malignant melanomas, a feature that further complicates differentiation from primary malignant melanoma. Some patients reputed to have had several primary malignant melanomas almost certainly had but one primary malignant melanoma and several epidermotropic metastases.

The more common expression of malignant melanoma metastatic to the skin is one or more nodules of atypical melanocytes containing various amounts of melanin within the dermis and/or the subcutaneous fat with little or no surrounding inflammatory-cell infiltrate (Fig. 110). The nodules are usually well circumscribed, but there is a tendency for some of the atypical melanocytes at the periphery of the aggregations to interpose themselves between collagen bundles or among lipocytes. The nuclei of these metastatic cells are usually strikingly atypical, many are in mitosis, and there is often marked necrosis of the neoplastic cells. However, there usually is only one population of atypical melanocytes in the infiltrates of metastatic malignant melanomas in contrast to those of primary malignant melanomas where there may be two or more populations of atypical melanocytes. A rather common manifestation of metastatic melanoma to the skin is the finding of the conglomeration of atypical melanocytes within a large blood vessel, usually a vein (Fig. 111).

A metastatic malignant melanoma that presents itself as a small nodule in the upper half of the dermis and is replete with melanin within melanocytes and macrophages must be differentiated from a cellular blue nevus. The crucial distinguishing features of these two forms of heavily pigmented melanocytic lesions are the atypical nuclei and mitotic figures of malignant melanoma.

Sometimes a metastasis of a malignant melanoma to skin is amelanotic in histologic appearance. In these instances, electron microscopy may reveal atypical melanosomes within the cytoplasms of the atypical cells and therefore confirm the judgment of malignant melanoma. Metastatic malignant melanoma may even mimic angiosarcoma (Fig. 112).

One special clinical variety of metastatic malignant melanoma to skin is termed "satellitosis" and refers to metastatic lesion(s) in the immediate vicinity of the primary malignant melanoma (Fig. 113). In a large surgical specimen it is sometimes possible to see both the primary malignant melanoma and one or more satellites in the dermis or the subcutis (Fig. 114). There are no atypical melanocytes in the epidermis above satellite nodules in contrast to their presence above the dermal component of the primary malignant melanoma. Furthermore, there is usually little or no inflammatory-cell infiltrate surrounding satellites. Another histologic clue to satellitosis is the tendency of atypical melanocytes at the periphery of the nodules to extend outward between collagen bundles giving the impression of a "star-burst" (Fig. 115). In most of our cases, when satellitosis of malignant melanoma was found in the

TABLE 7*
Histologic Differential Diagnosis of Superficial Spreading Malignant Melanoma

Pagetoid malignant melanoma in situ (superficial spreading malignant melanoma in situ)	Paget's disease of the breast	Extramammary Paget's disease	Pagetoid Bowen's disease
1. Cornified cells of stratum corneum usually normal.	1. Orthokeratotic hyperkeratosis.	1. Orthokeratotic hyperkeratosis usually.	1. Parakeratotic hyperkeratosis usually.
2. Atypical melanocytes sometimes scattered within the stratum corneum.	2. Atypical epithelial pale cells within the stratum corneum often.	2. Atypical epithelial pale cells within the stratum corneum often.	2. No atypical cells within the stratum corneum.
3. Atypical melanocytes with abundant pale cytoplasm singly, but more usually in nests, along the dermoepidermal junction and scattered throughout the epidermis.	3. Atypical epithelial cells with abundant pale cytoplasm, singly and in nests, at and above the dermoepidermal junction, and scattered throughout the epidermis, but predominantly in its lower part.	3. Atypical epithelial cells with abundant pale cytoplasm, singly and in nests, above the dermoepidermal junction throughout the epidermis, predominantly in its lower part.	3. Atypical epidermal cells with abundant pale cytoplasm, singly but more usually in nests, above the dermoepidermal junction and at all levels of the epidermis.
4. Nests of atypical melanocytes tend to confluence.	4. Nests of atypical epithelial cells are sharply demarcated from the surrounding keratinocytes; little tendency to confluence.	4. Nests of atypical epithelial cells are sharply demarcated from the surrounding keratinocytes; little tendency to confluence.	4. Nests of atypical melanocytes tend to confluence.
5. No intercellular bridges between the atypical melanocytes within the nests.	5. No intercellular bridges between pale epithelial cells in nests.	5. No intercellular bridges between pale epithelial cells in nests.	5. Intercellular bridges are often visible between pale cells in nests.
6. Keratinocytes surrounding the atypical melanocytes have normal nuclei.	6. Keratinocytes surrounding the nests of pale epithelial cells have normal nuclei.	6. Keratinocytes surrounding the nests of pale epithelial cells have normal nuclei.	6. Keratinocytes surrounding the nests of pale cells usually have atypical nuclei.
7. Multinucleated atypical melanocytes occasionally.	7. No multinucleated epithelial cells.	7. No multinucleated epithelial cells.	7. Atypical keratinocytes multinucleated often.
8. No dyskeratotic cells.	8. No dyskeratotic cells.	8. No dyskeratotic cells.	8. Dyskeratotic cells usual.
9. No acinar structures within the epidermis.	9. Acinar structures within the epidermis occasionally.	9. Acinar structures with the epidermis occasionally.	9. No acinar structures within the epidermis.
10. Basal keratinocytes not flattened by nests of atypical melanocytes.	10. Basal keratinocytes flattened by nests of atypical epithelial cells often.	10. Basal keratinocytes are often flattened by nests of atypical epithelial cells.	10. Basal keratinocytes are not flattened by nests of atypical epidermal cells.
11. Atypical melanocytes, singly and in nests, within epithelium of adnexal structures (i.e., hair follicles and eccrine ducts) often.	11. Atypical epithelial cells, singly and in nests, within lactiferous ducts.	11. Atypical epithelial cells within adnexal epithelial structures occasionally.	11. No atypical keratinocytes within epithelium of adnexal structures usually.

* From Ackerman, A. B. and Niven, J. Differential Diagnosis in Dermatopathology. Philadelphia, Lea and Febiger Co., to be published.

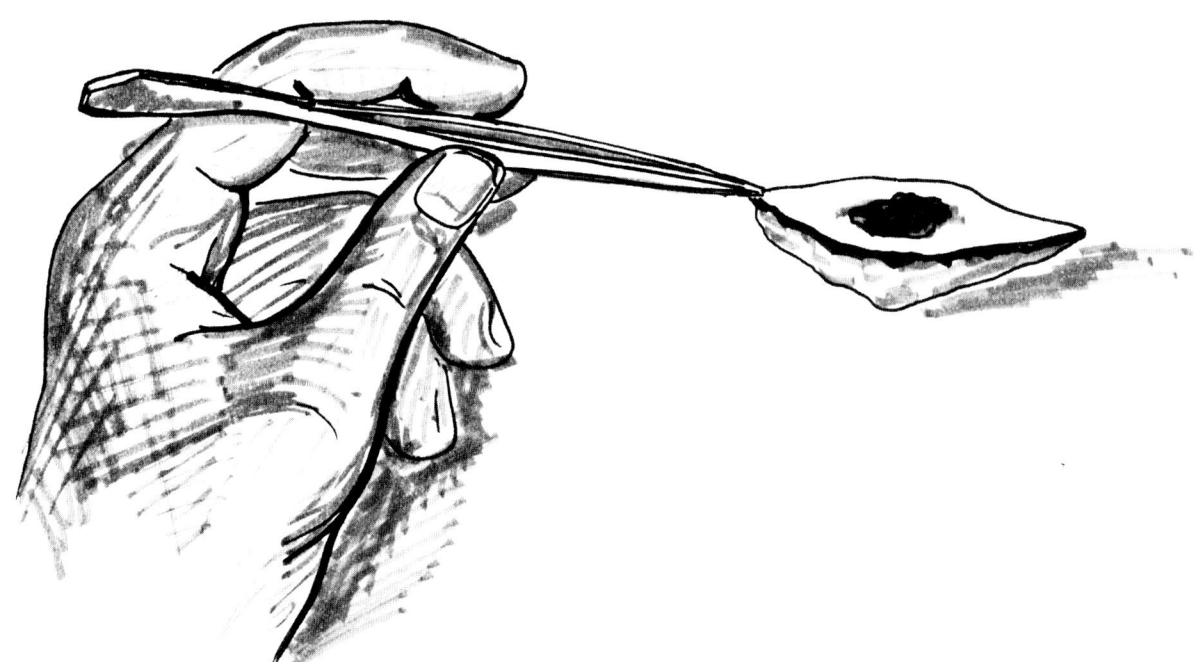

FIGURE 81. *Total excisional biopsy of a lesion suspected of being malignant melanoma.* This is the recommended procedure for removal of a lesion thought clinically to be a malignant melanoma. Note the narrow margin of normal skin around the excised specimen, the presence of subcutaneous fat, and the delicate handling of the tissue.

skin there was concomitant metastasis to the regional lymph nodes. Some small satellite nodules may be misinterpreted histologically as unusual intradermal melanocytic nevi.

Patients with disseminated metastases of malignant melanoma develop, rarely, a diffuse slate-blue or metallic gray pigmentation of the skin. Histologic sections studied by conventional microscopy of biopsy specimens from such generalized melanosis reveals free melanin and melanophages within the dermis, but no atypical melanocytes there. However, individual atypical melanocytes throughout the dermis of these lesions have been identified by electron microscopy (Konrad and Wolff, 1974).

VIII. MELANOSIS

A distinction must be made between melanin-containing macrophages (melanophages) and melanin-containing melanocytes. Sheets of melanophages (melanosis) may be found in association with atypical melanocytes in primary cutaneous malignant melanomas (Fig. 116) and in malignant melanomas metastatic to the skin. Melanophages alone, in the absence of atypical melanocytes, may be seen in malignant melanomas of the skin that have undergone spontaneous regression (Fig. 77) and in lymph nodes draining a primary malignant melanoma. These melanophages should not be misinterpreted as atypical melanocytes of metastatic lesions of malignant melanomas. When the pathologist is uncertain as to whether the heavily pigmented cells are melanophages or atypical melanocytes, bleaching the specimen with potassium permanganate will enable histologic judgments about whether the nuclei are normal as in histiocytes (macrophages) or abnormal as in melanoma cells. Numerous melanophages may also occur in benign melanocytic processes such as blue nevi. Therefore the presence of sheets of melanophages implies nothing about benignancy or malignancy. However, when one sees melanosis in the skin, one should always consider the possibility of malignant melanoma, either primary or secondary.

As has been mentioned previously, diffuse slate-blue or gray pigmentation may develop over the entire skin in some patients with disseminated metastases of malignant melanoma. Biopsy of the slate gray pigmentation reveals epidermal hyperpigmentation (Silberberg et al., 1968) and granules of free melanin scattered within the dermis and within melanophages, but no atypical melanocytes appear to be there in sections viewed by conventional microscopy. However, many scattered atypical melanocytes, a phenomenon termed "single-cell metastasization," have been found in studies by electron microscopy and DOPA reactions (Konrad and Wolff, 1974).

If the pathologist is unsure whether the brown granular pigment in a specimen is melanin or hemosiderin, he may do a Fontana-Masson stain for melanin and/or a Perl stain for iron. As a rule these two pigments may be differentiated from one another in sections stained by hematoxylin and eosin, hemosiderin being more golden yellow and more refractile than melanin. This quality of hemosiderin may be better appreciated by decreasing the intensity of transmitted light in the microscope by lowering the condenser.

IX. CRITIQUE OF METHODS FOR ASSESSING PROGNOSIS OF MALIGNANT MELANOMA BASED ON HISTOLOGIC FINDINGS

A. LEVELS OF INVASION AS PROGNOSTIC GUIDES

Clark (1970), like several other authors before him, recognized that, as a rule, the deeper the atypical melanocytes of malignant melanoma are situated in the dermis, the worse the patient's prognosis. In an attempt to devise a consistent method for gauging depth of invasion, Clark quantified malignant melanoma *in situ* (i.e., atypical melanocytes confined to the epidermis) as level I, malignant melanoma that extended into the papillary dermis as level II, malignant melanoma that filled the entire papillary dermis and abutted upon the reticular dermis along a broad front as level III, malignant melanoma that extended into the reticular dermis as level IV, and malignant melanoma that reached into the subcutaneous fat as level V. On the basis of these five levels, Clark and his co-workers came to regard depth of invasion of malignant melanoma as the major criterion for predicting the biologic behavior of malignant melanoma.

There is no question that the levels of invasion proposed by Clark correlate in large measure with the biologic behavior of malignant melanomas. However, in time, some limitations to the concept of levels of invasion became evident. For example, those malignant melanomas with the worse prognoses are the most exophytic ones, namely, the pedunculated, sessile, and nodular types. In these instances of malignant melanomas with exceedingly poor prognoses, the level of invasion according to the criteria of Clark may be no more than level II because the growth is almost wholly upward, away from the reticular dermis rather than downward into it. Therefore, a pedunculated or sessile malignant melanoma may be only level II morphologically, but equivalent to level V biologically (Fig. 117).

A second criticism of the levels of invasion pertains to the thickening of the papillary dermis that usually accompanies extension of atypical melanocytes from the epidermis into the dermis. As a result of marked widening of the papillary dermis by neoplastic cells, angioneogenesis, and concurrent fibrosis, the neoplasm within the papillary dermis may be quite thick, yet be only level II because of the considerable expansion of the papillary dermis (Fig. 79).

A third difficulty with the level method as predictive of prognosis of malignant melanoma concerns the extension of atypical melanocytes into the epithelial structures of adenexa, especially hair follicles, but also eccrine ducts (Fig. 59). This is especially important in lentigo maligna, in which atypical melanocytes are not only present within the epidermis, but within adnexal structures often to the level of the sebaceous duct and sometimes even as far as the coils of eccrine sweat glands. If the atypical melanocytes are wholly within the epithelium, the lesion is considered by Clark to be a level I malignant melanoma. However, should the atypical melanocytes that are lodged some distance down epithelial structures of adnexa emerge and traverse the slender periadnexal dermis there and then enter into the contiguous reticular dermis, what was a level I malignant melanoma almost instantly becomes a level IV malignant melanoma by convention. Should one consider lentigo maligna that extends to the level of the coils of sweat glands level I or level IV?

The level method proposed by Clark does not take into account differences in depth of extension of malignant melanoma within the reticular dermis itself. The reticular dermis is the broadest zone in the sequence of levels I to V and yet it is considered to be only a single level, namely, level IV. No distinction is made between malignant melanoma that extends just into the reticular dermis, i.e., the uppermost part of the reticular dermis, and malignant melanoma that extends to the deep reticular dermis just above the subcutaneous fat. It is likely that there are prognostic differences between malignant melanomas that have progressed to only the upper part, to the middle, and to the deepest portion of the reticular dermis.

Another difficult judgment using the level method is whether a neoplasm should be called deep level II, level III, or superficial level IV. These are very subjective judgments and competent pathologists often come to different conclusions about them in reviewing the same specimen (Suffin et al., 1975, Roses et al., 1979). The descriptive definition of level IV by Clark et al. (1969) is somewhat imprecise, i.e., "isolated intrusion of cells between collagen bundles of the upper reticular dermis at the base of level III tumors is not considered sufficient for classification as a level IV lesion.

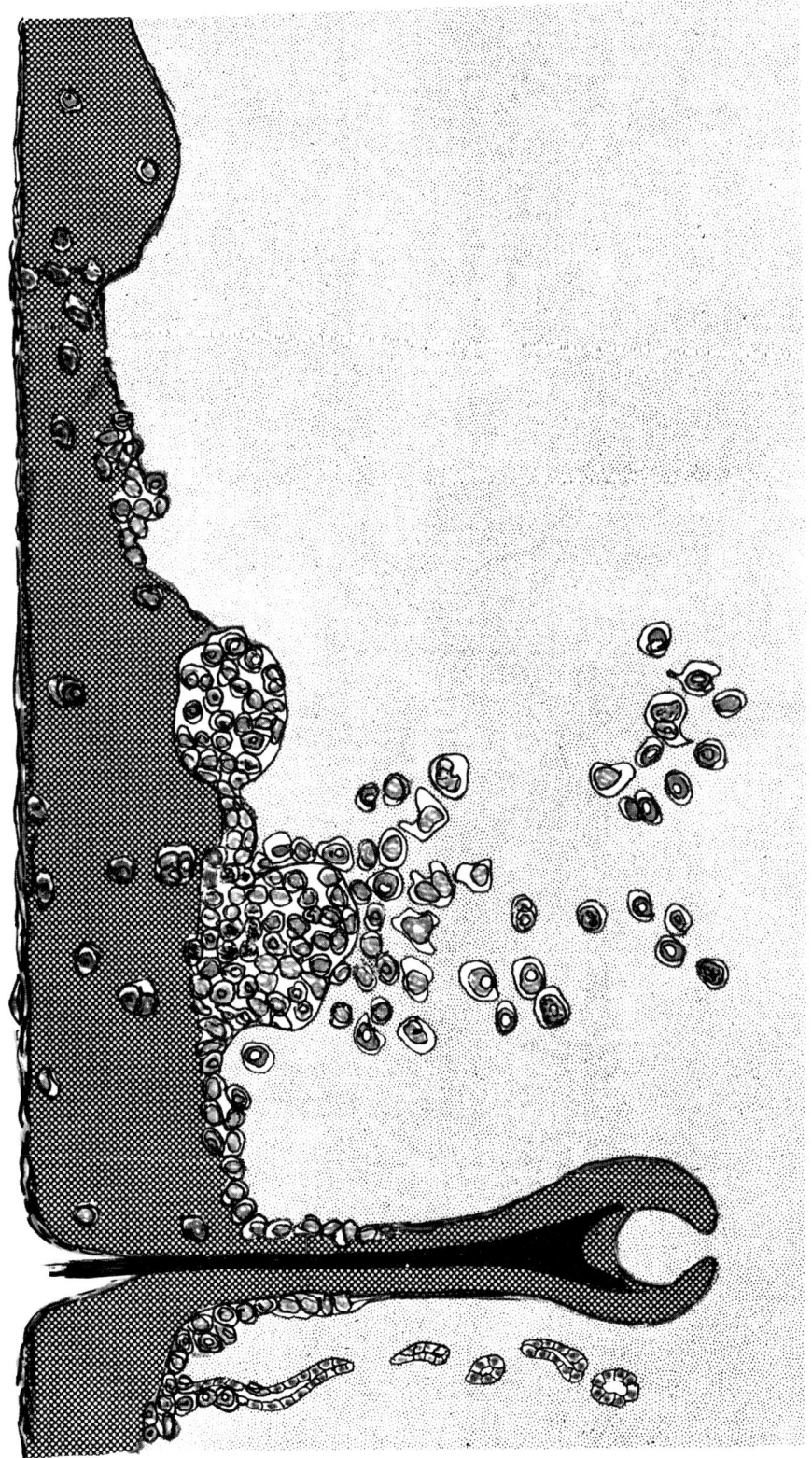

FIGURE 82. **Crucial zone for histologic diagnosis of malignant melanoma: the periphery of the lesion.** *The histologic diagnosis of malignant melanoma is best made by studying architectural features with the scanning objective of the microscope and especially those at the periphery of the neoplasm, namely, "buckshot" scatter of melanocytes throughout the epidermis, horizontal extension of melanocytes within the epidermis at the peripheries beyond the bulk of the neoplasm within the dermis, and failure of maturation of melanocytes at the base of the neoplasm in the dermis or the subcutis.*

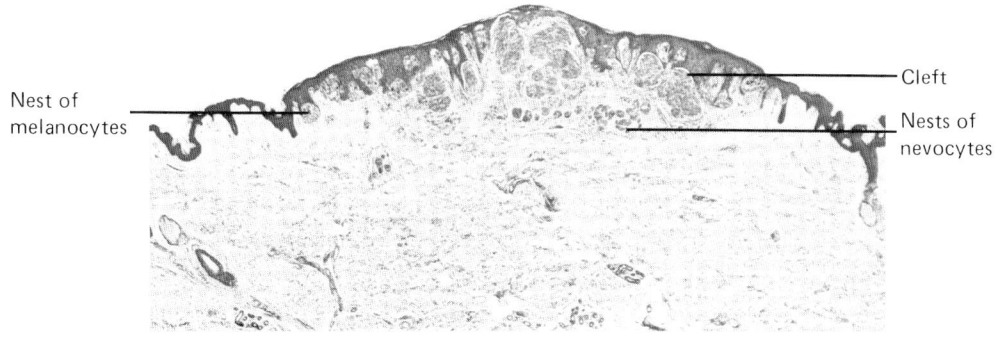

FIGURE 83A. **Nevus of large spindle and/or epithelioid cells (Spitz's nevus).** *This scanning-power view illustrates the sharp circumscription of this melanocytic process and the maturation of the cells as they descended progressively into the dermis: two important signs of a benign melanocytic nevus that are usually absent in a malignant melanoma. (Reduced from ×19)*

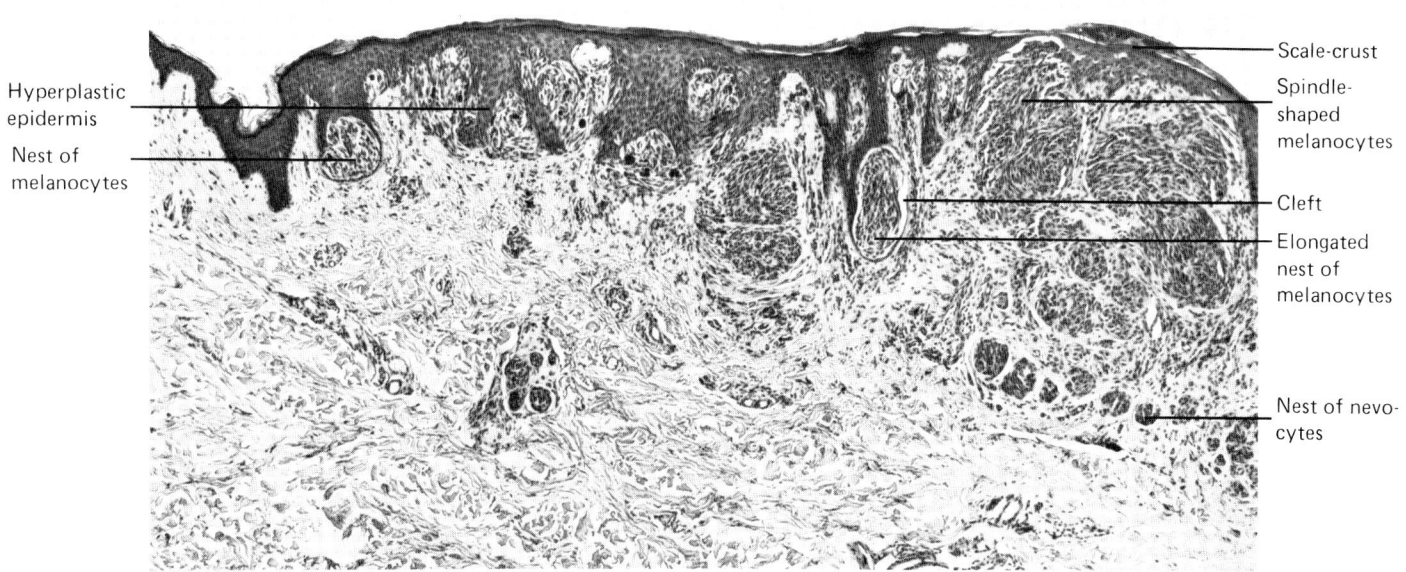

FIGURE 83B. **Nevus of large spindle and/or epithelioid cells (Spitz's nevus).** *Higher magnification of Fig. 83A shows the absence of horizontal extension of melanocytes to the side of the farthest nest of melanocytes on the left side of this photomicrograph. Such sharp lateral demarcation is one sign of a melanocytic nevus in contrast to malignant melanoma. Note that the nuclei of the nevus cells at the base of this lesion are smaller (more mature) than those of the melanocytes within the epidermis. This is a Spitz's nevus because the nuclei are spindle shaped, some of them are large, the intraepidermal nests are elongated and oriented perpendicular to the surface of the specimen, and clefts separate the nests of melanocytes from keratinocytes. (Reduced from ×66)*

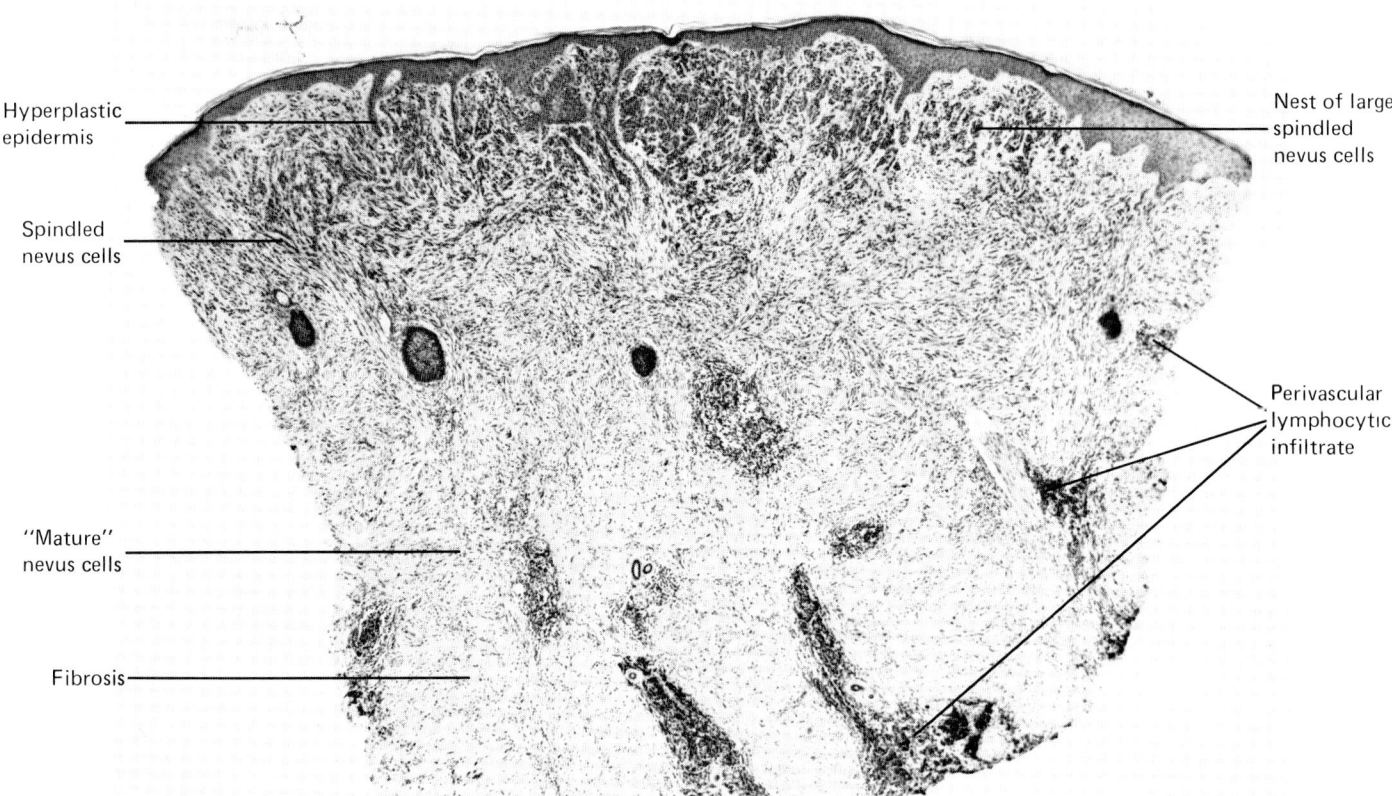

FIGURE 84A. *Nevus of large spindle and/or epithelioid cells (Spitz's nevus) exhibiting maturation of nevus cells. This lesion can be diagnosed as Spitz's nevus, rather than a malignant melanoma, because of the absence of atypical melanocytes from the epidermis, the maturation of nevus cells with progressive descent into the fibrotic dermis, and the presence of inflammatory-cell infiltrates around blood vessels throughout the lesion. Nevertheless, a preferred biopsy specimen would have included the lateral and deep margins of the specimen where the crucial clues to benignancy or malignancy of melanocytic lesions reside, rather than the partial punch excision that was done here.*

There should be distinct invasion well into the reticular dermis." Because levels II, III, and IV have very different implications for surgery, accuracy and unanimity in reading are desirable. Furthermore, wide variations in the thickness of a malignant melanoma (see below) occur within each of these three levels.

B. Thickness as Prognostic Guide

Another method for assessing prognosis in malignant melanoma was devised by Breslow (1970) and utilizes measurement of the thickness of the malignant melanoma from the uppermost portion of the granular zone of the epidermis to the cells at the base of the neoplasm. He found that the thicker the malignant melanoma, the worse the prognosis. Very thin malignant melanomas rarely, if ever, metastasize. Although this method of measurement, by a micrometer in the eyepiece of the microscope, has proved to be an excellent prognosticator of the biological course of malignant melanoma and is more objective than is the judging of levels of invasion, it, too, has some limitations. For example, because the neoplasm is measured from the top of the granular zone to the base of the neoplasm, variations in the normal thickness of the epidermis will inevitably affect the reading of total thickness of the neoplasm. Therefore, the total thickness of malignant melanoma on an eyelid will appear to be thinner than the same sized malignant melanoma on palms or soles by virtue of the marked difference in the normal thickness of the epidermis in those different anatomic sites. If the epidermis is hyperplastic, even greater differences will result. Perhaps these problems could be avoided if the bottom of the epidermis in the suprapapillary plate were used as the uppermost limit rather than the top of the granular layer. Secondly, if a

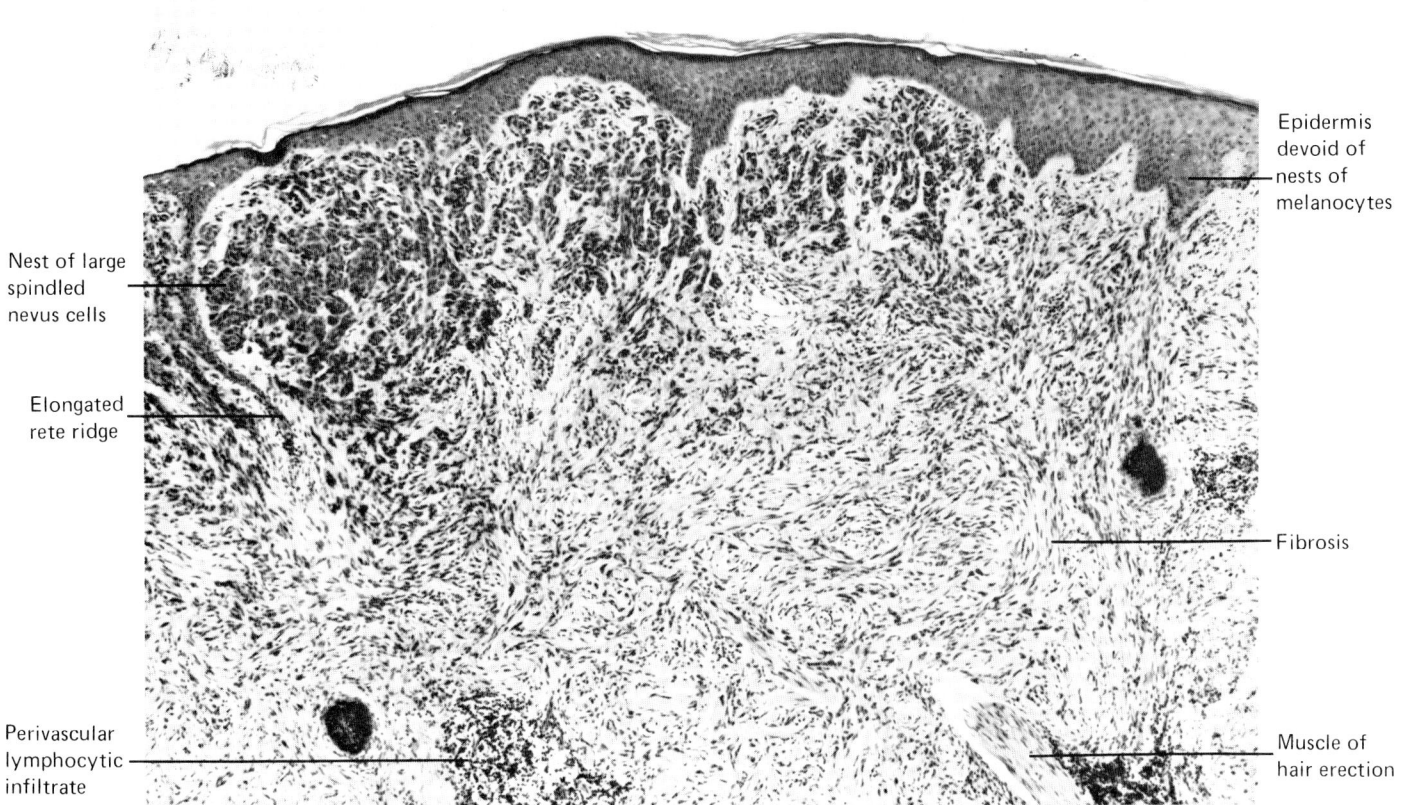

FIGURE 84B. *Nevus of large spindle and/or epithelioid cells (Spitz's nevus) exhibiting maturation of nevus cells.* This higher magnification of Fig. 84A shows an epidermis devoid of atypical melanocytes and a dermis replete with nevus cells. Those in the upper part of the dermis are large and cuboidal, whereas those in the lower portion are small and spindled. Note the fibrosis and the perivascular inflammatory-cell infiltrate. These are typical features of Spitz's nevus. (Reduced from ×82)

specimen is ulcerated, the pathologist can only guess the site of the granular zone as the upper boundary for measurement or he has to use the base of the ulcer as the upper limit. Neither compromise is precise. Thirdly, a problem sometimes arises when a malignant melanoma develops in association with a preexisting melanocytic nevus and the atypical melanocytes of the malignant melanoma are interspersed among or are contiguous with the nevus cells. In such circumstances it is often difficult to discern precisely where at the base of the neoplasm to measure, that is, what is malignant melanoma and what is still benign nevus (Fig. 118). Fourthly, if the specimen containing the malignant melanoma is embedded improperly or is sectioned tangentially, the neoplasm when measured may seem to be much thicker than it truly is. Fifthly, Breslow's method does not attempt to deal with the question of extension of atypical melanocytes down adnexal epithelial structures and the significance thereof to prognosis. Lastly, if thin sections (e.g., of 3 micra) are cut, the tissue stretches when it is placed on the slide and leads to a reading of more thickness than is actual. Breslow concedes (personal communication, 1978) that

> Tumor thickness also has its problems. If blocks are not prepared at right angles to the surface of the tumor or are not embedded and cut properly, the tangential section which results will increase apparent thickness. Fortunately a deviation of as much as 22°, 50′ will only result in an 8% error. Though there are many uncontrolled variables in histologic technique which might alter thickness, the method works and its extreme precision indicates that these variables are not important.

Despite these limitations, at the moment the measurement of malignant melanoma by use of an ocular micrometer as proposed by Breslow is the best method for pre-

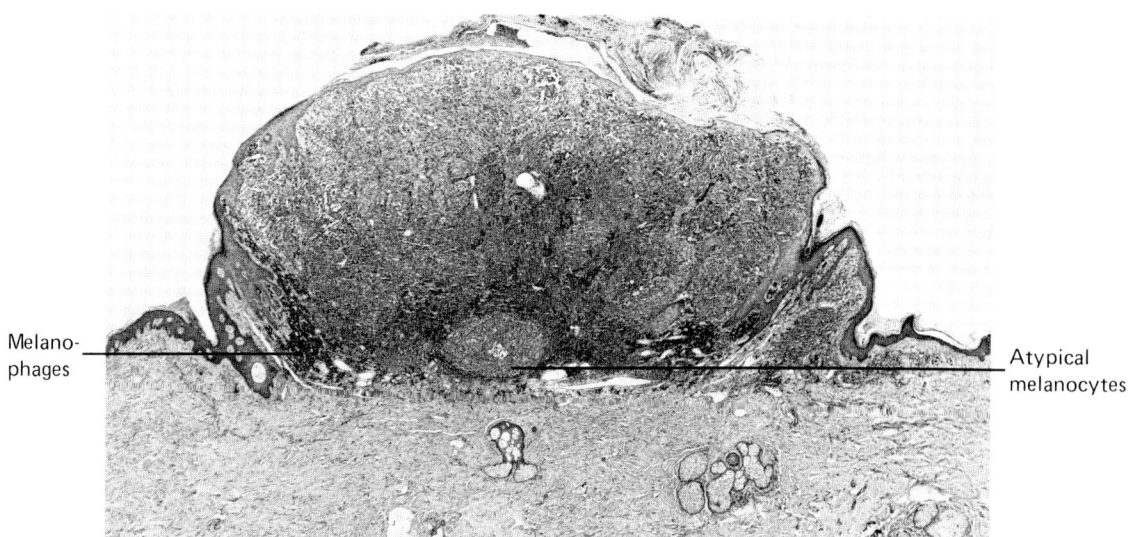

FIGURE 85A. **Failure of maturation of melanocytes in nodular malignant melanoma.** *A common finding in malignant melanoma, in contrast to a melanocytic nevus, is the failure of the nuclei of atypical melanocytes in the dermis to become smaller as they descend, a feature which is best appreciated with higher magnification. Note also signs of regression in the papillary dermis to the right of the nodule and a second well-circumscribed population of atypical melanocytes near the base of the nodule, a poor prognostic sign. (Reduced from ×18)*

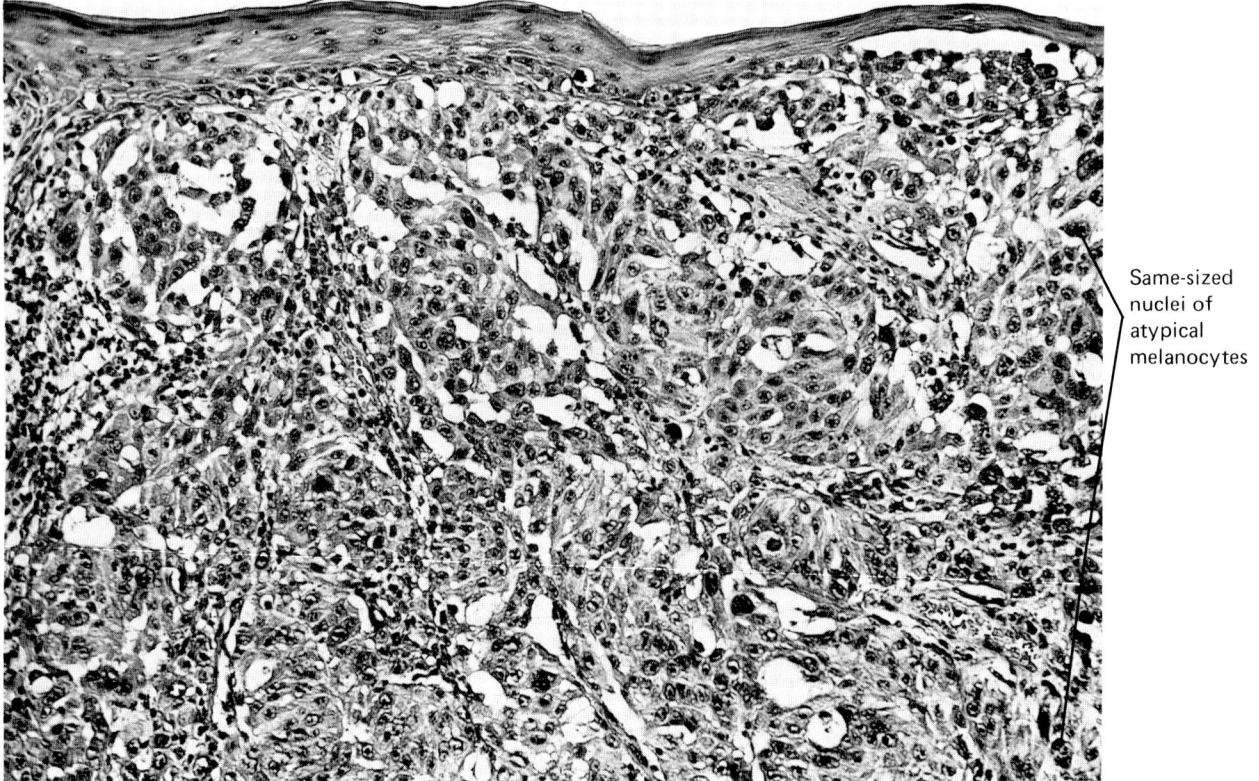

FIGURE 85B. **Failure of maturation of melanocytes in nodular malignant melanoma.** *A higher-power view of Fig. 85A illustrates that the atypical nuclei of cells at the base of this photomicrograph are about as large as those near the epidermis, a feature characteristic of malignant melanoma. (Reduced from ×200)*

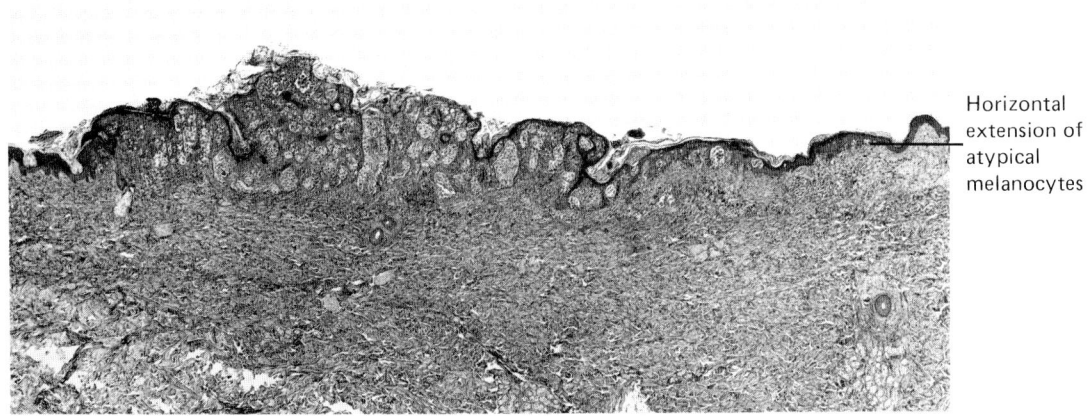

FIGURE 86A. *Malignant melanoma, superficial spreading type, with marked variation in size and shape of nests of atypical melanocytes.* Not only are no two nests of atypical melanocytes shown here the same size or shape, but the nests tend to confluence. Note also the wide, lateral extension of the atypical melanocytes within the epidermis to the right of the bulk of the neoplasm. (Reduced from ×17)

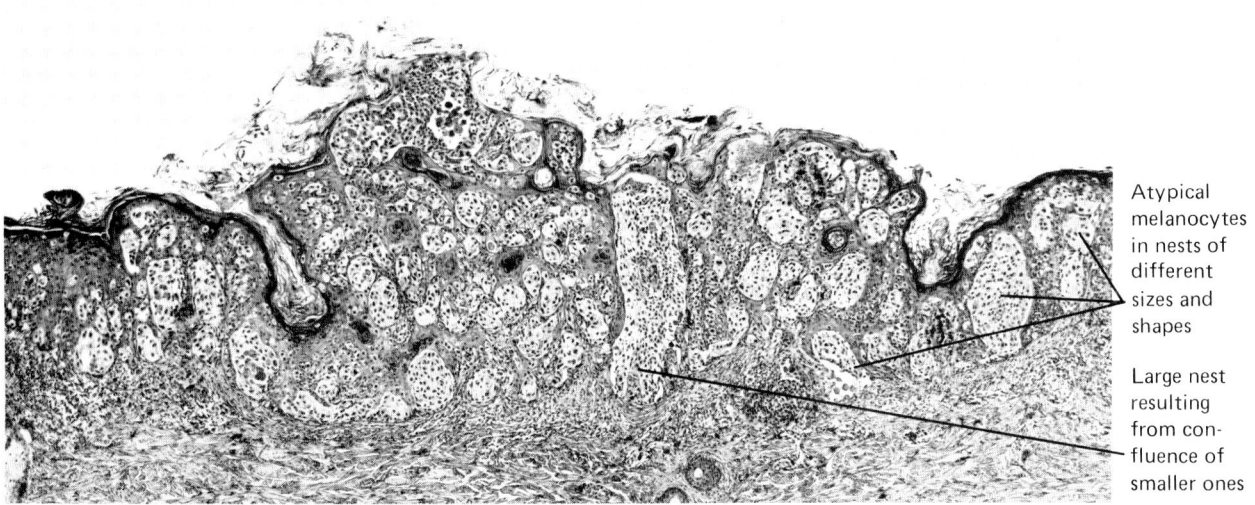

FIGURE 86B. *Malignant melanoma, superficial spreading type, with marked variation in size and shape of nests of atypical melanocytes.* Higher magnification of Fig. 86A shows better the aggregates of atypical melanocytes in their marked variation of size and shape and tendency to confluence, important features of malignant melanoma. The atypical melanocytes are also scattered singly at all levels of the epidermis, to and including the cornified layer. (Reduced from ×48)

dicting biologic behavior of malignant melanoma (Hansen and McCarten, 1974; Wanebo et al., 1975; Balch et al., 1978; Breslow et al., 1978). However, an even more accurate gauge of prognosis might be calculation of the total volume of the malignant melanoma. This could be done by measuring the breadth and varying depths of the neoplasm in step sections through the tissue block. It may be that prognosis turns more upon the volume of the neoplastic cells irrespective of the particular type of malignant melanoma (Breslow, 1970).

> According to Breslow (personal communication)
> The major defect in Clark's system is the wide variation, 10 × or more, in thickness for level III and IV tumors, a consequence of the variation in skin thickness and in differences in the surface contour of the tumors. Since the rate of metastasis has been

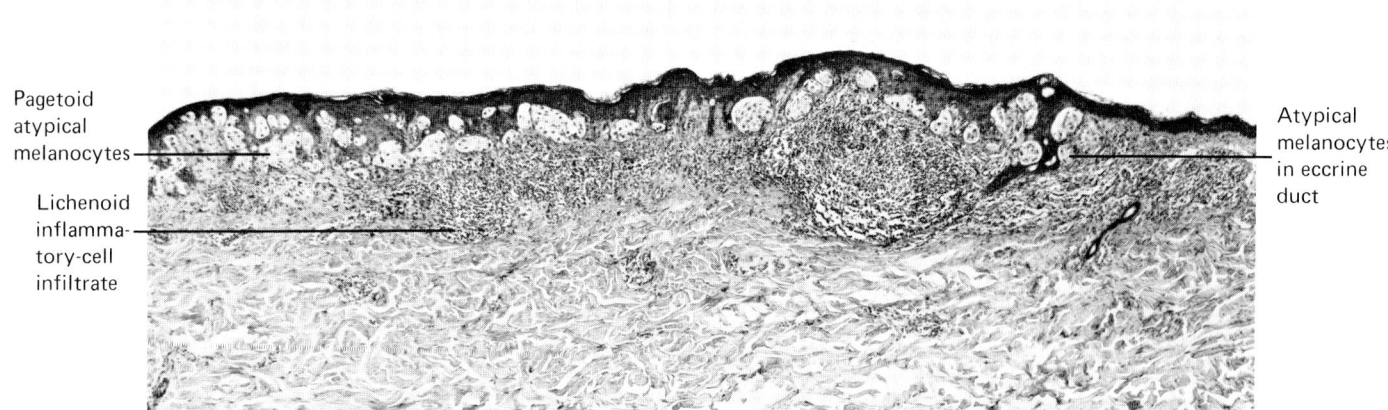

FIGURE 87A. **Malignant melanoma, superficial spreading type, in situ *with involvement of eccrine duct.*** *Atypical pagetoid melanocytes in this thin superficial spreading malignant melanoma are situated within epithelium of the epidermis and the eccrine sweat duct and in the papillary dermis. The dense lichenoid infiltrate of lymphocytes and histiocytes is an expected occurrence beneath thin malignant melanomas of all varieties. (Reduced from ×47)*

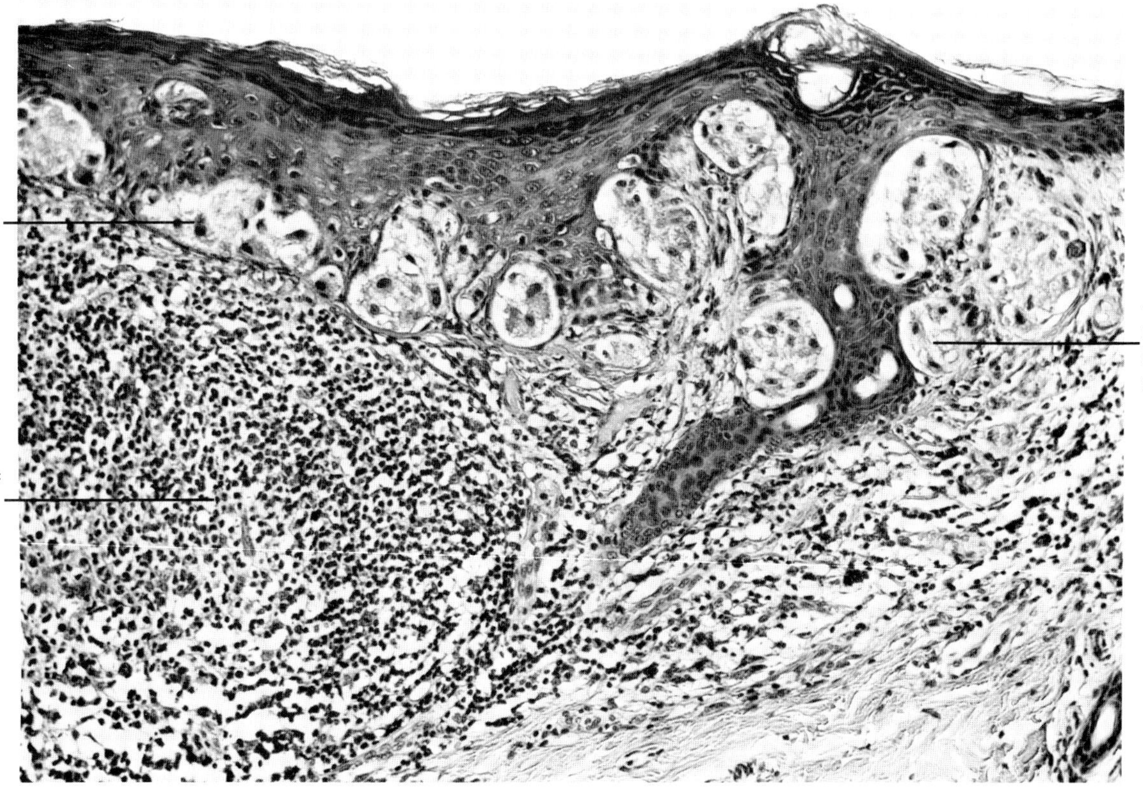

FIGURE 87B. **Malignant melanoma, superficial spreading type, in situ *with involvement of eccrine duct.*** *In this higher magnification of Fig. 87A the atypical pagetoid melanocytes may be seen within both epidermal and eccrine epithelium. Note that the nests in both positions vary considerably in size and shape and tend to confluence. (Reduced from ×198)*

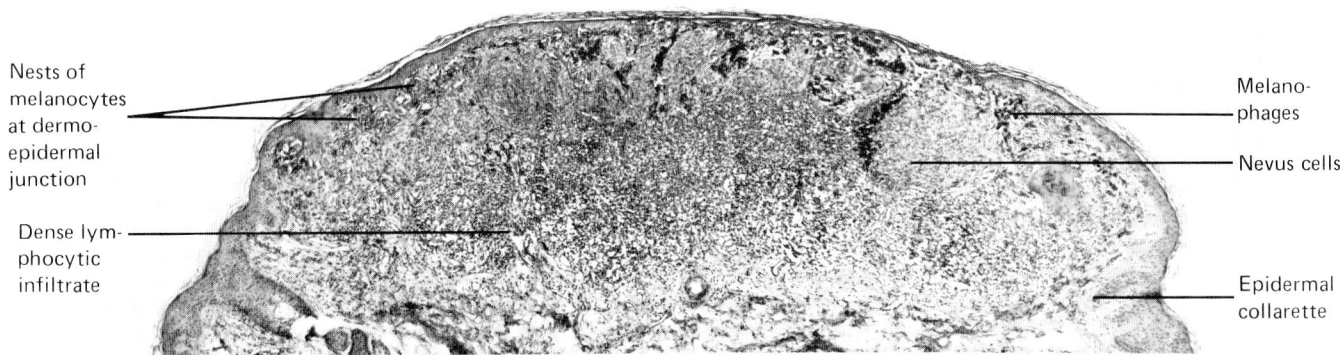

FIGURE 88A. **Halo nevus.** *Because this melanocytic lesion is slightly dome-shaped, well-circumscribed, and partially enclosed by an epidermal collarette, it is a melanocytic nevus. Because the predominantly lymphocytic infiltrate extends throughout the lesion, it is a halo nevus. In a nodular malignant melanoma, in contrast, the inflammatory-cell infiltrate, if present, is at the advancing lower border of the neoplasm, rather than diffusely throughout it. (Reduced from ×48)*

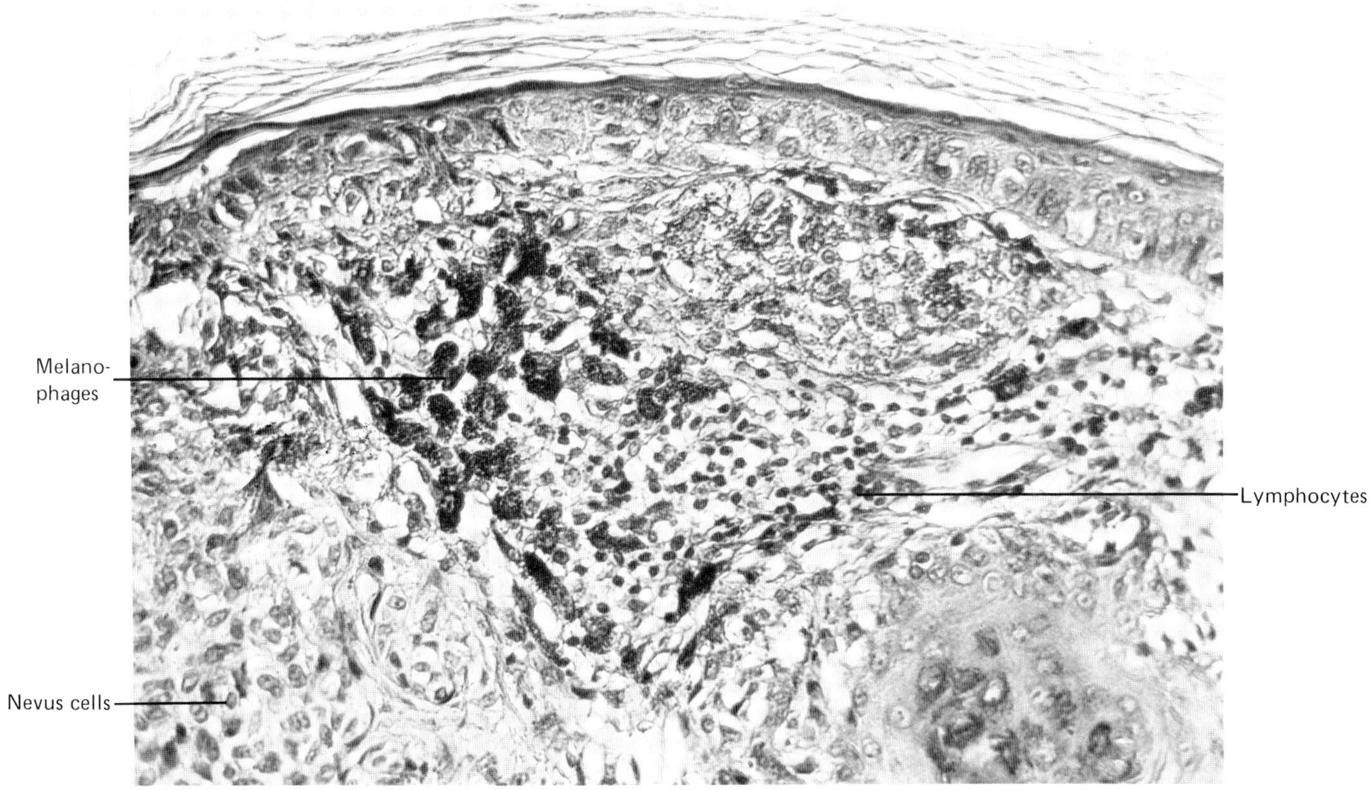

FIGURE 88B. **Halo nevus.** *Some nevocytes are still recognizable in this higher-power view of the halo nevus pictured in Fig. 88A. (Reduced from ×378)*

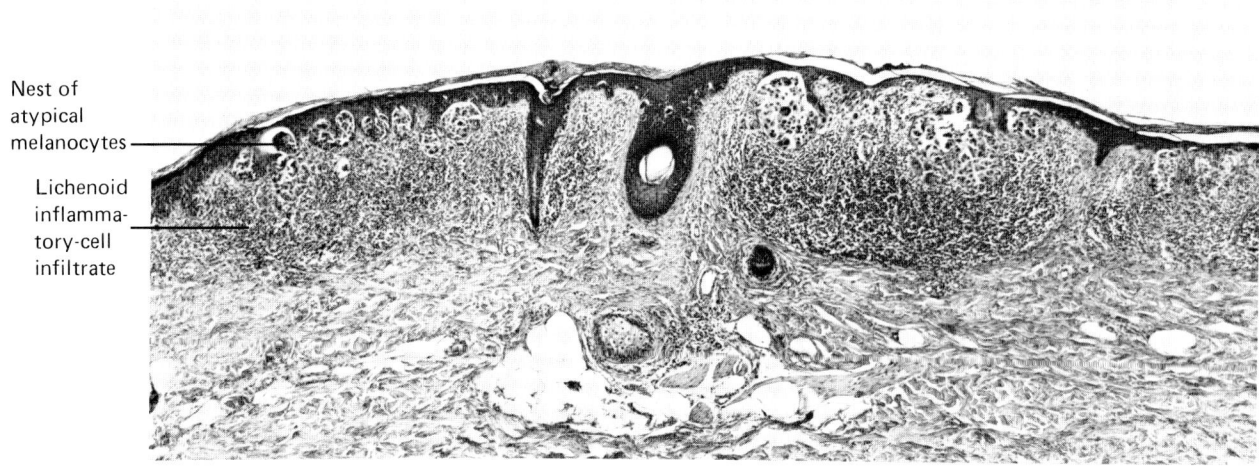

FIGURE 89A. **Malignant melanoma, superficial spreading type, with cytologic atypia.** *The atypical melanocytes in this superficial spreading malignant melanoma are within the epidermis, in the epithelial structures of adnexa (eccrine ducts and hair follicles), and in the papillary dermis, which, moreover, is thickened by a dense lichenoid infiltrate of lymphocytes and histiocytes. (Reduced from ×47)*

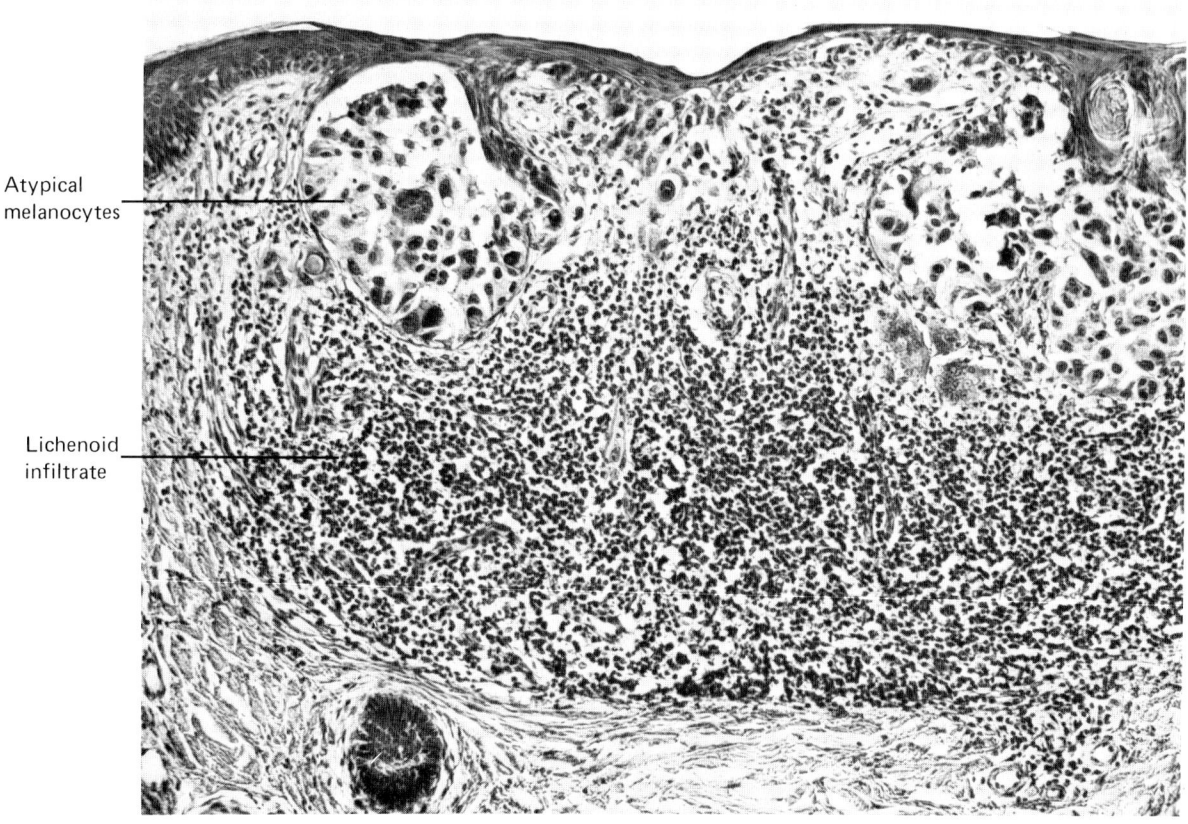

FIGURE 89B. **Malignant melanoma, superficial spreading type, with cytologic atypia.** *Higher magnification of Fig. 89A demonstrates the marked variation in size and shape of the nests of atypical melanocytes in this slender malignant melanoma. Note the dense inflammatory-cell infiltrate. (Reduced from ×175)*

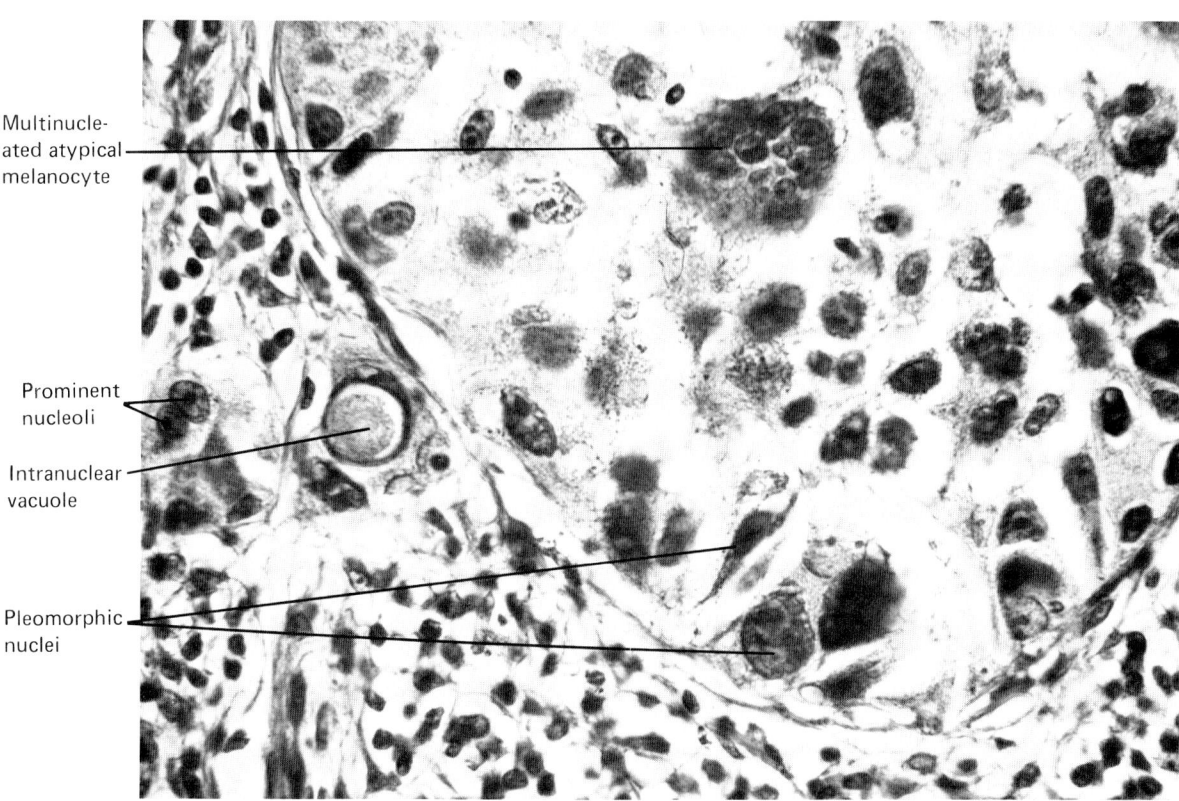

FIGURE 89C. *Malignant melanoma, superficial spreading type, with cytologic atypia.* This still higher-power view of Fig. 89B dramatically reveals the cytologic atypia of the melanocytes, to wit, nuclei that are either large, hyperchromatic, or multiple, and cellular shapes that are pleomorphic or bizarre. (Reduced from ×700)

found to closely correlate with tumor thickness, the level of invasion cannot be as good as thickness in evaluation of prognosis. This was the finding of several independent studies. The final question with regards to the level of invasion is whether it is an indirect measure of tumor thickness or is an independent prognostic variable? If it is the latter, we should continue to evaluate level even if it is less useful than thickness, but if the former is true, the level can be ignored. Two studies of over 400 tumors, by means of multifactorial analysis have found that once thickness has been measured there is little or no additional prognostic information to be derived from evaluating the level of invasion. The level appears to be a dependent variable of thickness and to have no independent value of its own.

The notion recently advanced (Gromet et al., 1978) that the assessment of prognosis of malignant melanoma by measuring "tumor thickness" may be invalid in lesions where there are histologic signs of regression, calls into question the validity of the entire concept that measurement is a gauge of prognosis in all lesions of cutaneous malignant melanoma. Focal evidence of regression of the neoplasm (i.e., whitening clinically, fibrosis throughout the thickened papillary dermis histologically) is so common in all forms of superficially spreading malignant melanoma that if its presence renders measurement valueless, then the method itself becomes less meaningful. However, the validity of the data of Gromet et al. can be questioned because they failed to do step sections through every specimen.

C. Thickness Plus Number of Mitotic Figures as a Prognostic Guide

Recently, it has been proposed by Schmoeckel and Braun-Falco (1978) that prognosis in patients with malignant melanoma may be predicted with greatest accuracy by a prognostic index, defined as "the product of tumor thickness (mm) and the number of mitoses/mm^2." On the basis of their calculations these authors also concluded that

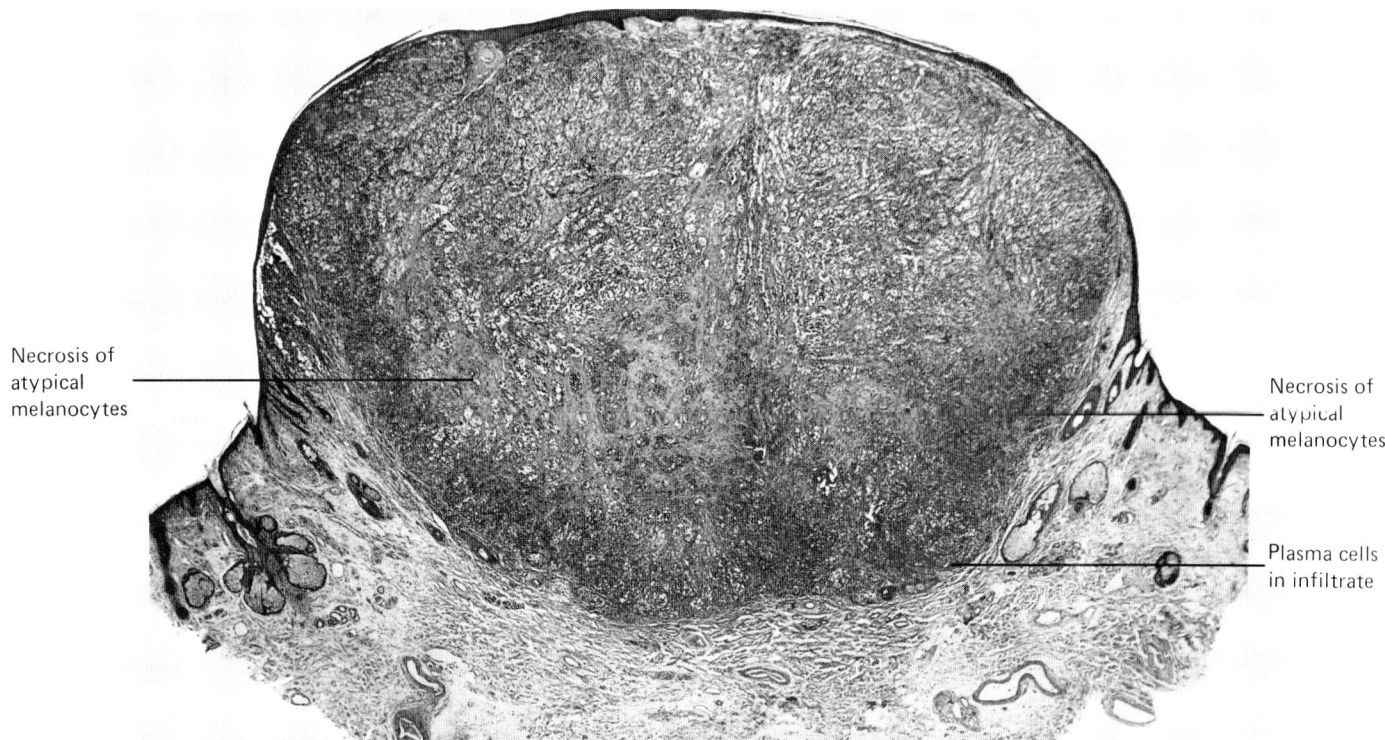

FIGURE 90A. **Necrosis within a nodular malignant melanoma.** *The large irregularly shaped zones of necrosis in the lower half of this nodular malignant melanoma appear as mingled granular and amorphous eosinophilic material in sections stained by hematoxylin and eosin. Plasma cells are usually found only beneath thick malignant melanomas and are a sign of poor prognosis. (Reduced from ×14)*

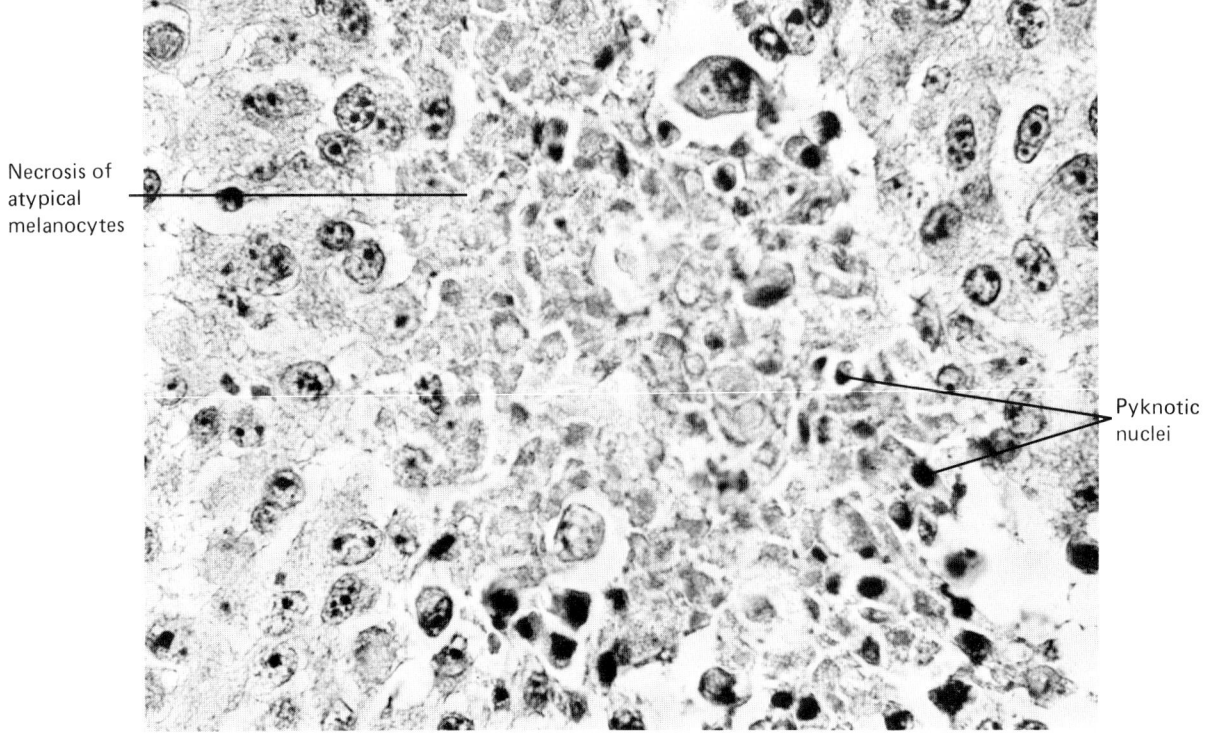

FIGURE 90B. **Necrosis within a nodular malignant melanoma.** *The nuclear signs of necrosis, namely, pyknosis, karyorrhexis, and karyolysis, are all present in this higher magnification of the nodular melanoma pictured in Fig. 90A. Necrotic melanocytes are a feature of malignant melanoma, but not of melanocytic nevi except those that have been traumatized. (Reduced from ×840)*

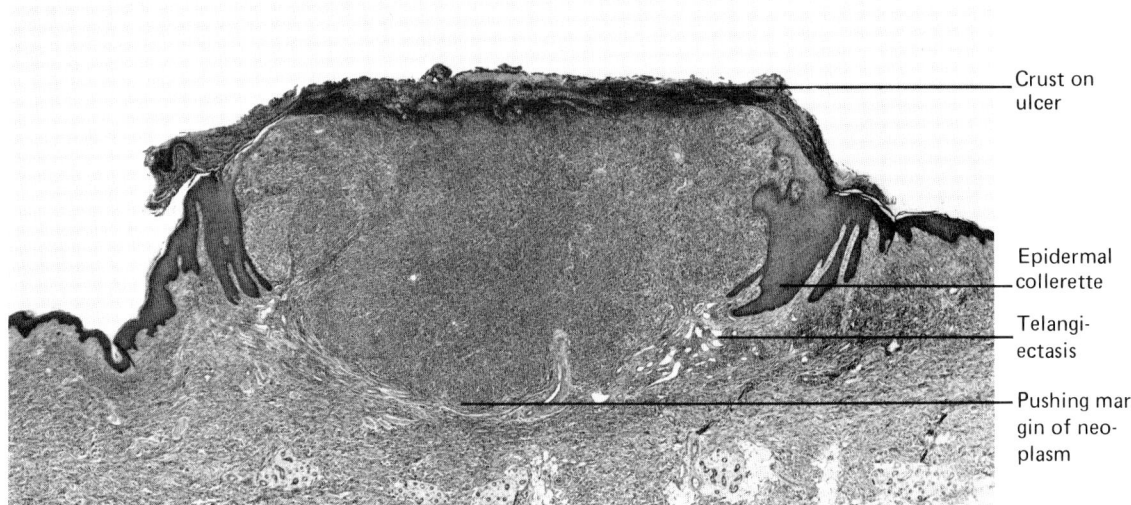

FIGURE 91A. **Nodular malignant melanoma with many mitotic figures.** *Primary cutaneous malignant melanoma tends to expand into the dermis with pushing margins, as illustrated in this large, ulcerated, nodular lesion, unlike metastases from a primary malignant melanoma, which tend to infiltrate between the collagen bundles. Both the primary malignant melanoma and its metastases may have numerous mitotic figures as will be seen in Fig. 91B which is a higher magnification of this primary lesion.*

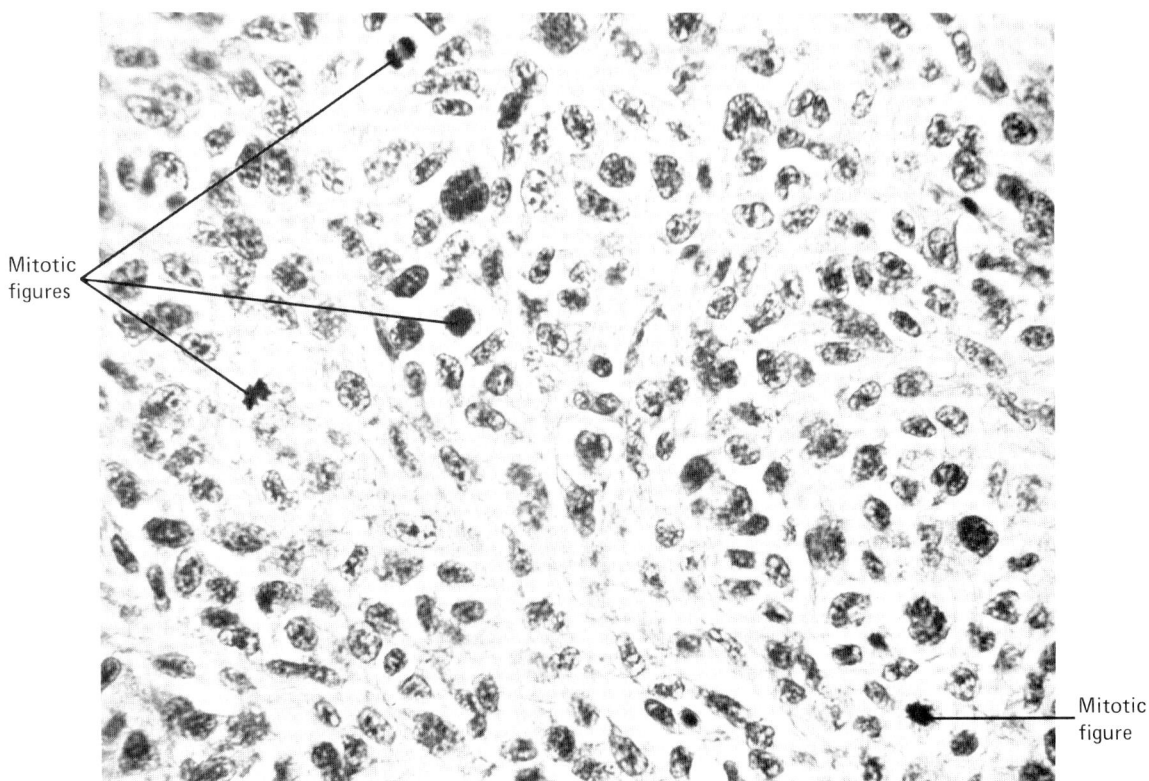

FIGURE 91B. **Nodular malignant melanoma with many mitotic figures.** *A melanocytic neoplasm with this number of mitotic figures in any high-power field is almost certain to be a malignant melanoma and not a banal melanocytic nevus.*

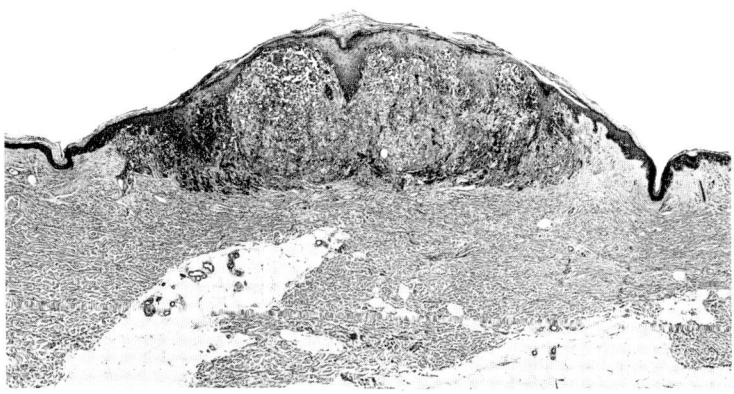

FIGURE 92A. ***Malignant melanoma, nodular type, with prominent nucleoli.*** *In this scanning-power view of a small nodular malignant melanoma, note that the atypical melanocytes completely fill the upper part of the dermis in sheets of cells and wholly obscure the collagen there. (Reduced from ×20)*

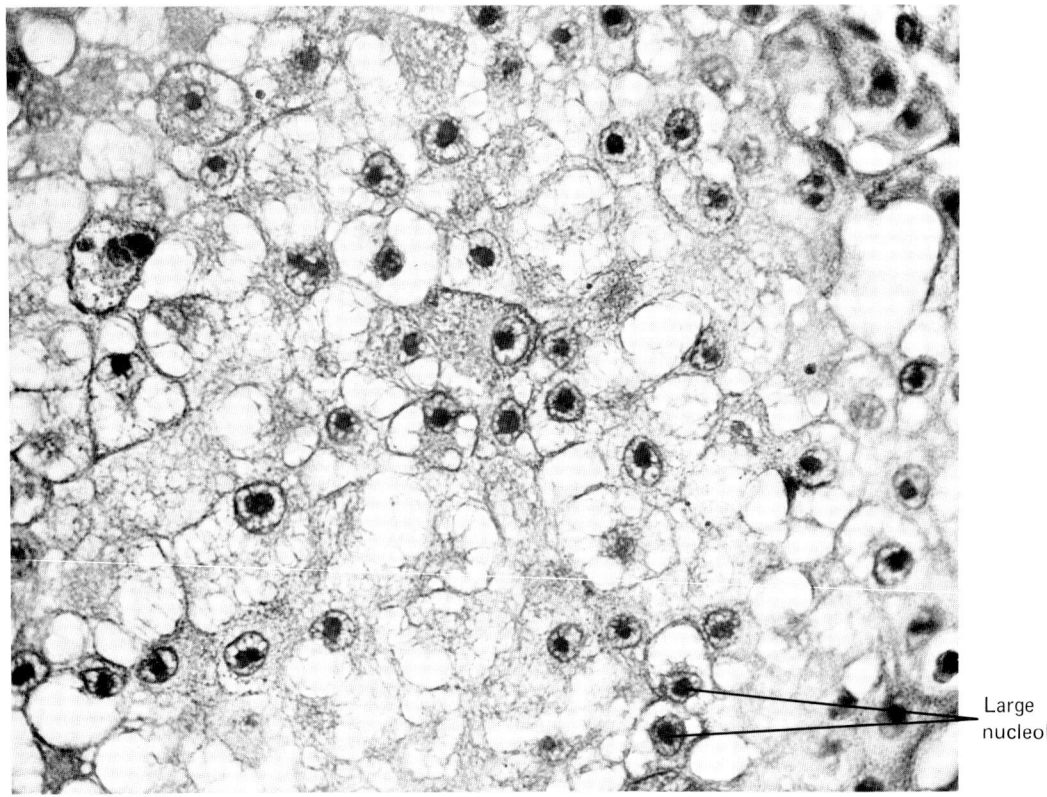

FIGURE 92B. ***Malignant melanoma, nodular type, with prominent nucleoli.*** *An important sign of the atypicality of the melanocytes shown here is presence of large, hyperchromatic, pleomorphic nucleoli. Such nucleoli are features of cells of malignant melanomas and not those of melanocytic nevi of any type, although slightly enlarged nucleoli may be seen in Spitz's nevi.*

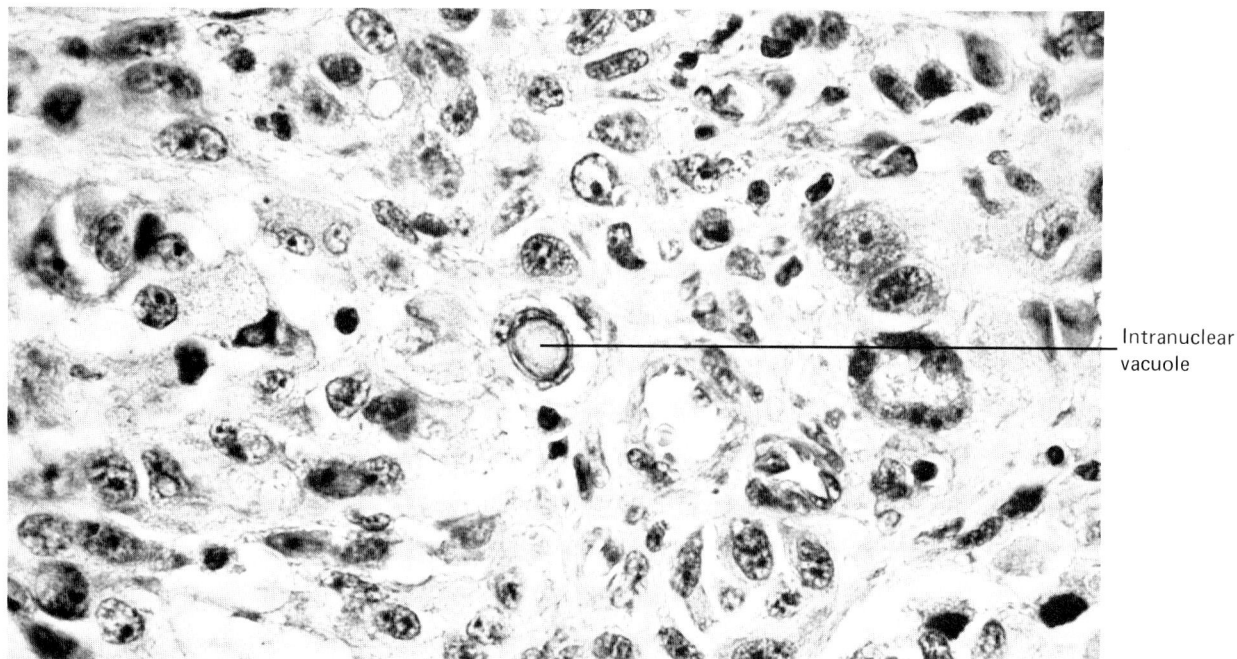

FIGURE 93A. ***Intranuclear vacuole in a cell of a malignant melanoma.*** *A common and characteristic finding in some nuclei of atypical melanocytes of malignant melanomas are vacuoles such as the one pictured here. In sections stained by hematoxylin and eosin they are colored pink-purple, like raspberries. (Reduced from ×800)*

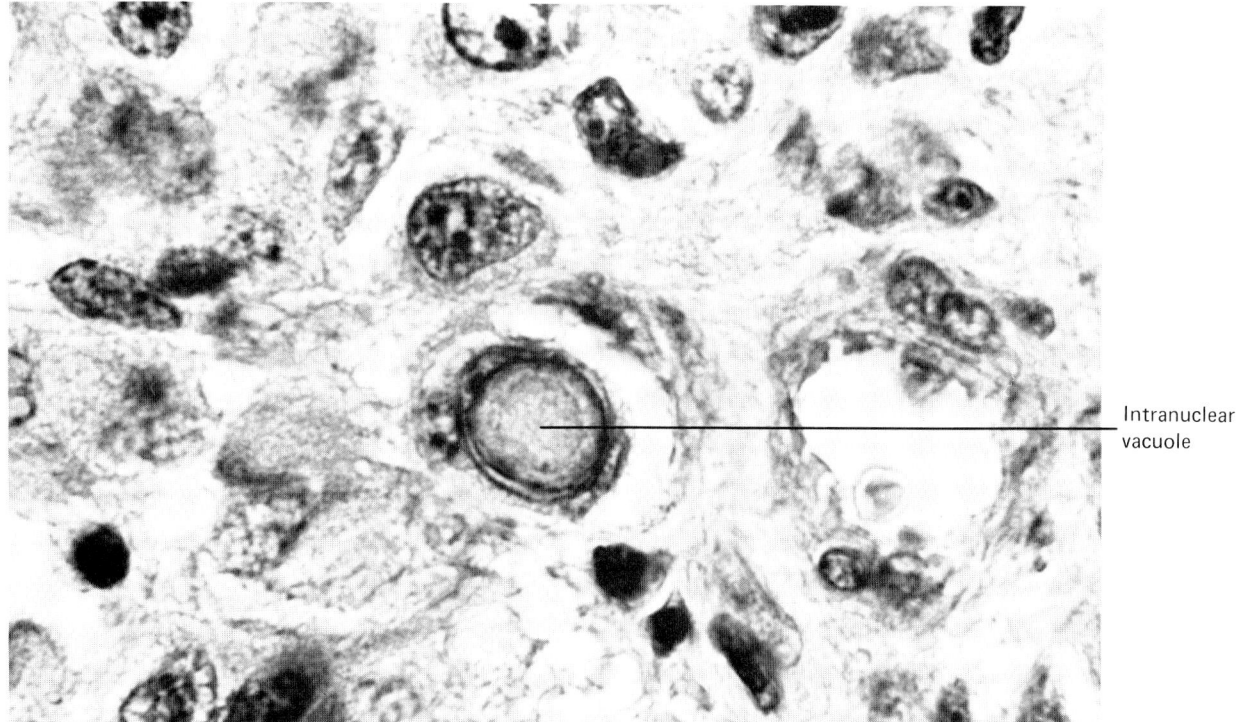

FIGURE 93B. ***Intranuclear vacuole in a cell of malignant melanoma.*** *Higher magnification of Fig. 93A shows a large intranuclear vacuole within an atypical melanocyte of a malignant melanoma. (Reduced from ×1675)*

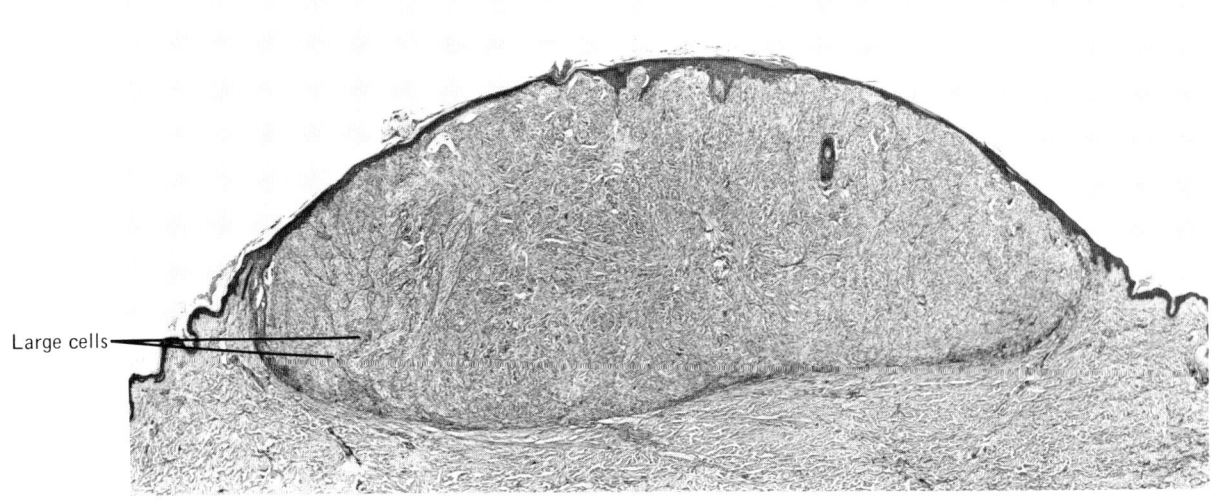

FIGURE 94A. **Malignant melanoma, nodular type, with atypical multinucleated melanocytic giant cells.** *Merely with scanning magnification, some of the cells within this nodular melanoma are seen to be abnormally large. Note also that the atypical melanocytes in this malignant melanoma, in contrast to a melanocytic nevus, completely fill that part of the dermis they occupy and obscure the collagen there. (Reduced from ×14)*

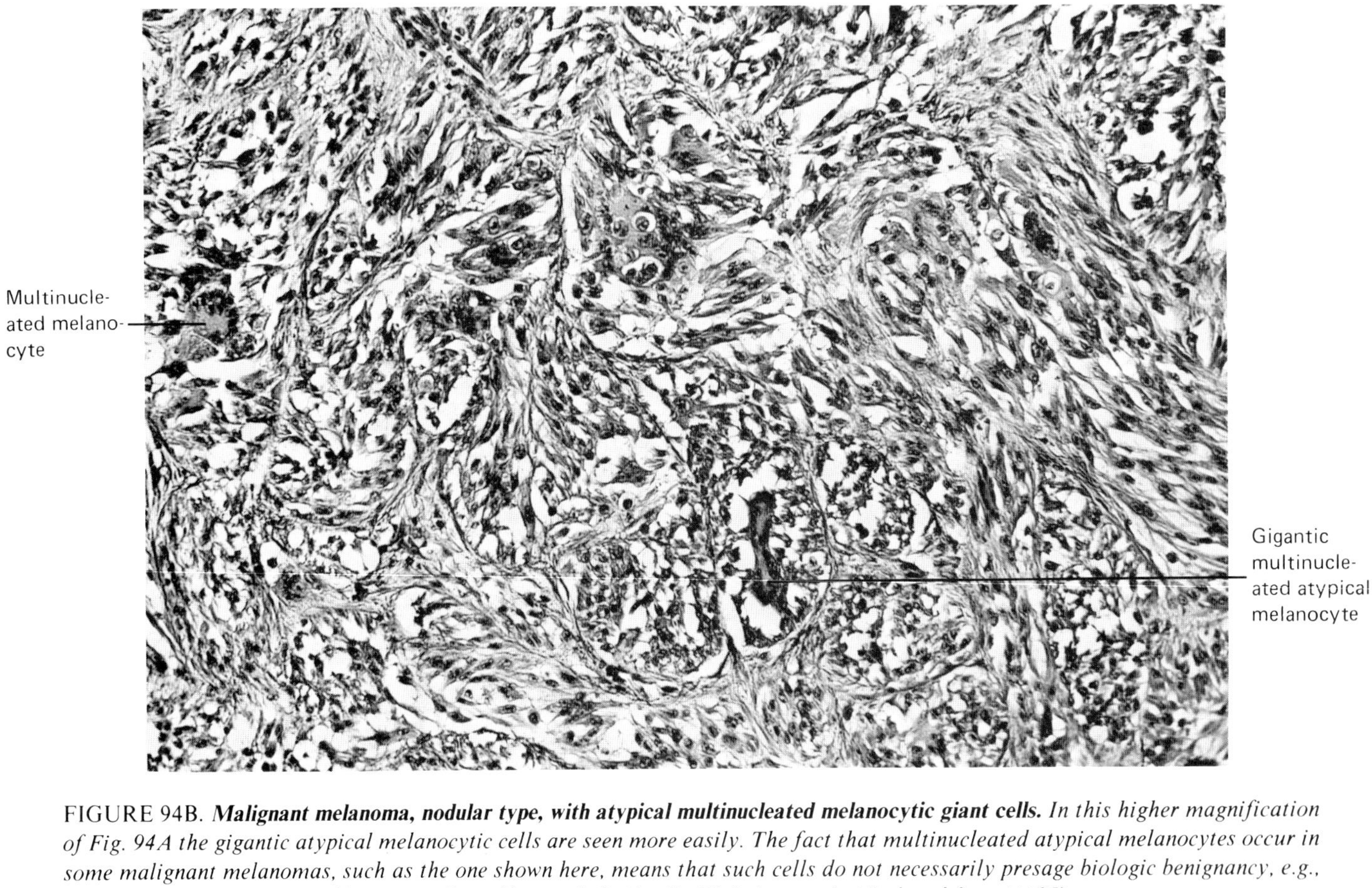

FIGURE 94B. **Malignant melanoma, nodular type, with atypical multinucleated melanocytic giant cells.** *In this higher magnification of Fig. 94A the gigantic atypical melanocytic cells are seen more easily. The fact that multinucleated atypical melanocytes occur in some malignant melanomas, such as the one shown here, means that such cells do not necessarily presage biologic benignancy, e.g., their presence in the nevus of large spindle and/or epithelioid cells (Spitz's nevus). (Reduced from ×185)*

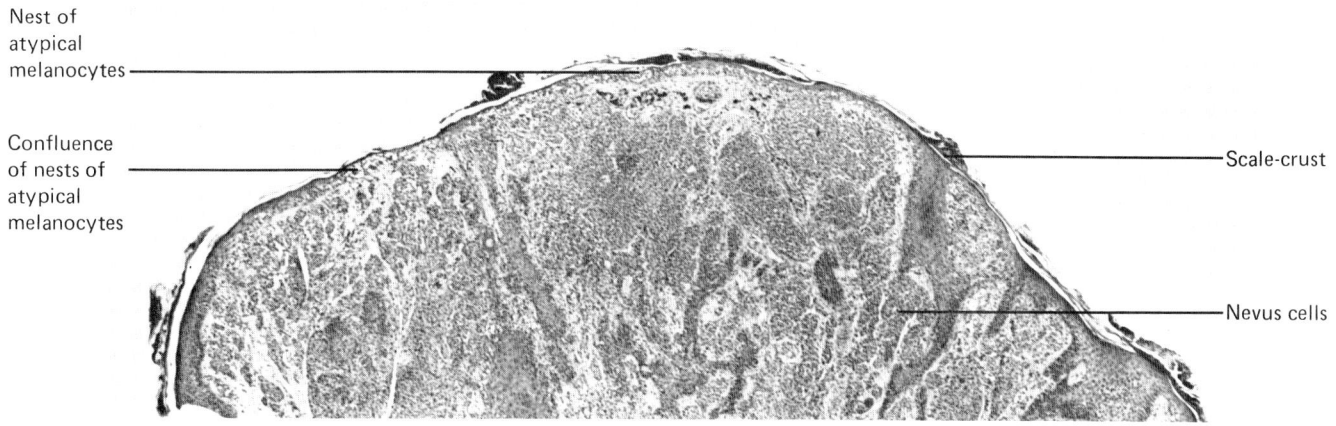

FIGURE 95A. ***Traumatized compound melanocytic nevus.*** *That this compound melanocytic nevus had been traumatized may be inferred from the several mounds of scale-crusts on its surface. The discrete nests, cords, and strands of nevocytes within the dermis mark this lesion as a benign melanocytic nevus. (Reduced from ×37)*

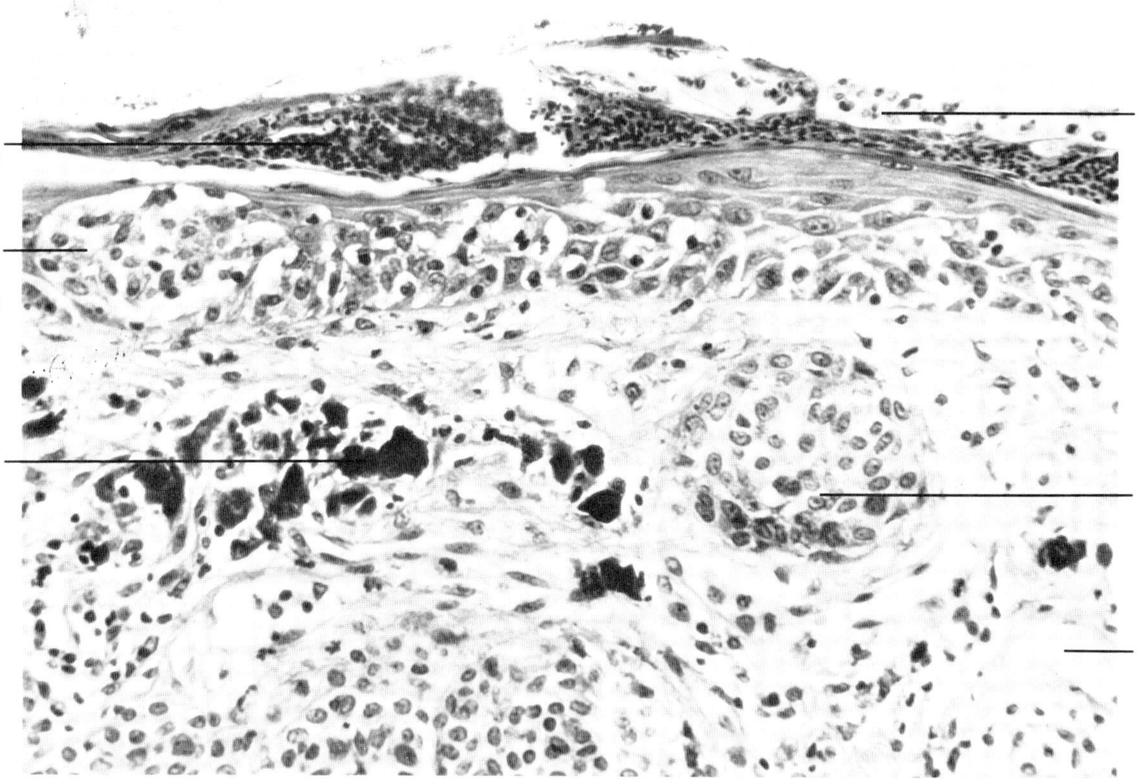

FIGURE 95B. ***Traumatized compound melanocytic nevus.*** *This higher-power view of the surface of the lesion pictured in Fig. 95A shows irregularly shaped nests of melanocytes within an epidermis covered by scale-crusts. In the context of the signs of trauma to the epidermis (i.e., the scale-crusts containing neutrophils) and the nests of typical nevocytes within the dermis, this lesion is surely benign despite the unusual arrangement of the melanocytes within the epidermis. (Reduced from ×378)*

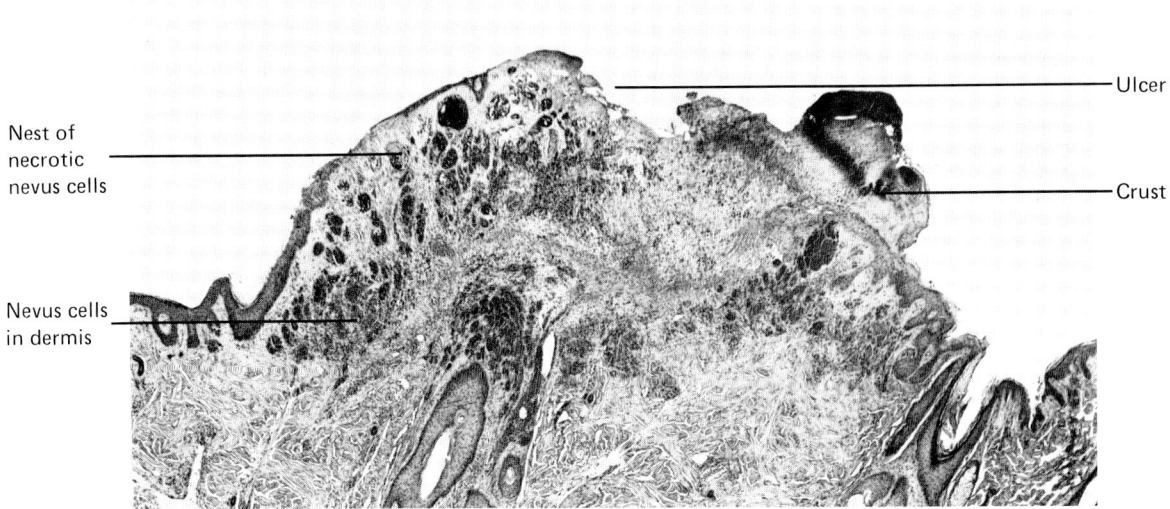

FIGURE 96A. **Ulcerated melanocytic nevus.** This dome-shaped benign melanocytic nevus has been severely traumatized. It is ulcerated and covered by a crust and some of the nevus cells in the upper part of the dermis have undergone necrosis. Lesions such as these should not be misinterpreted as malignant melanoma. (Reduced from ×24)

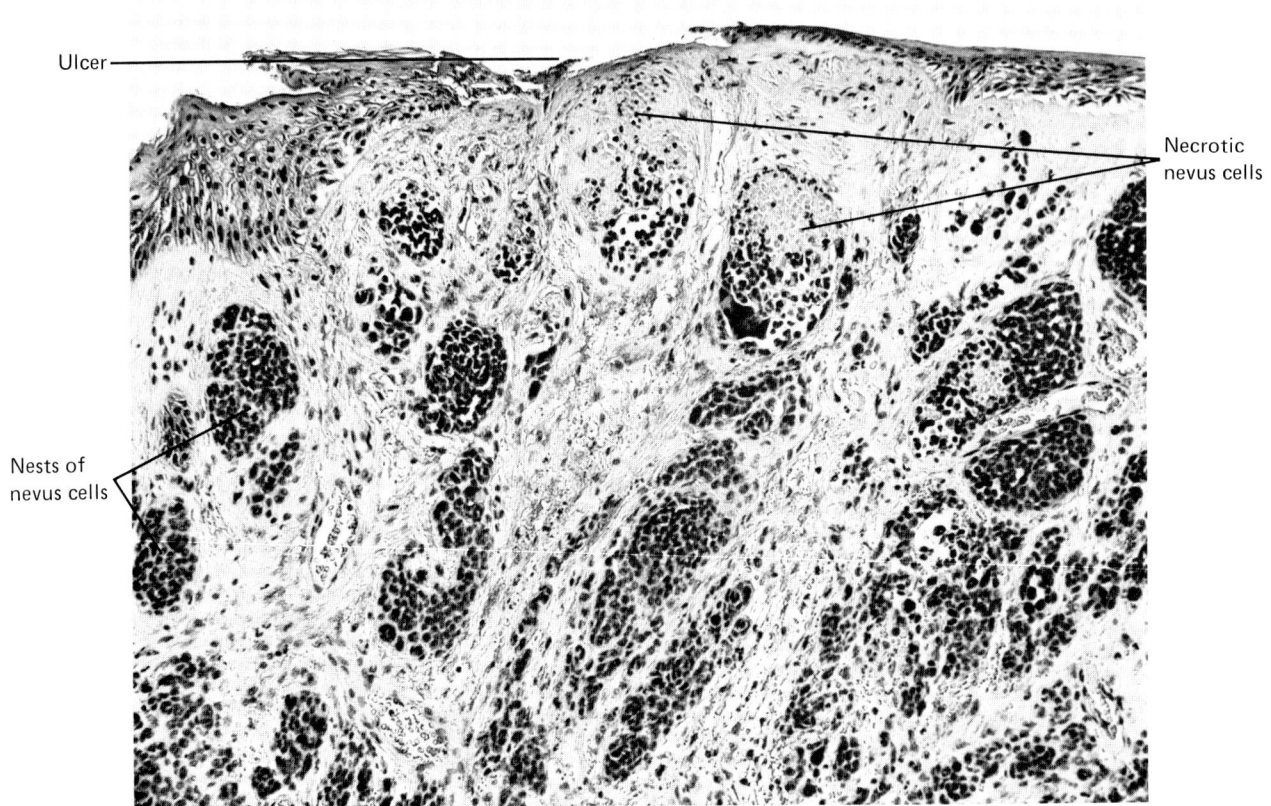

FIGURE 96B. **Ulcerated melanocytic nevus.** This higher magnification of Fig. 96A shows ulceration above nests of nevus cells. Some of the nevocytes in the upper portion of the dermis are necrotic. (Reduced from ×167)

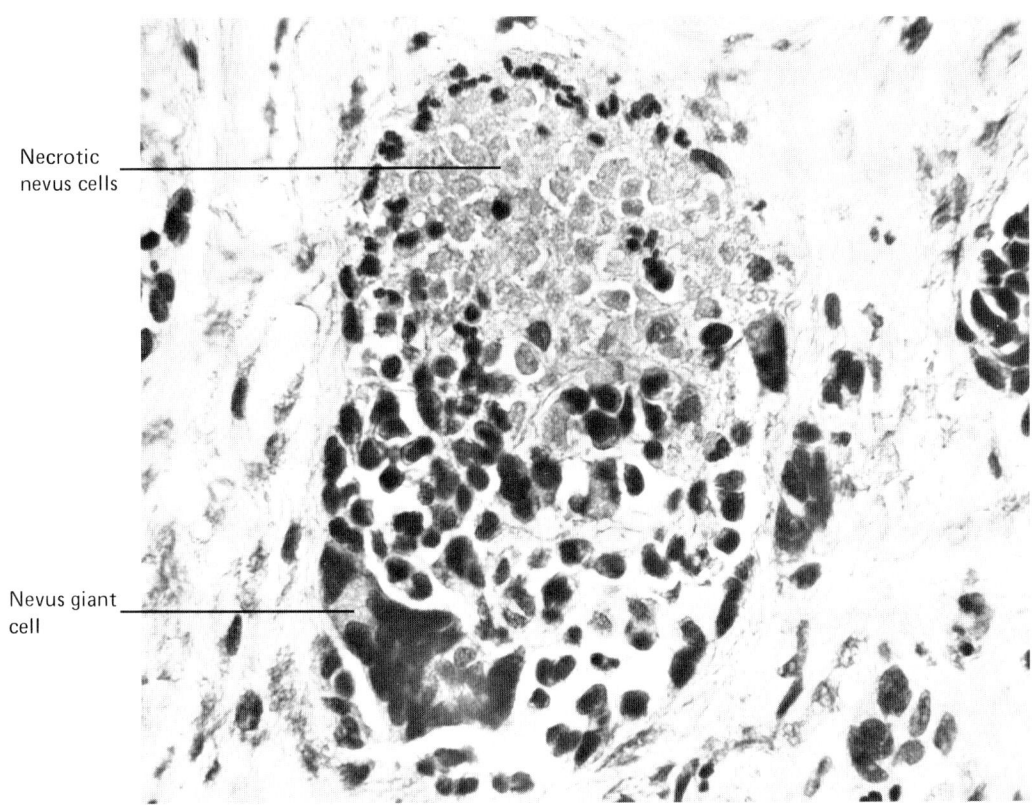

FIGURE 96C. **Ulcerated melanocytic nevus.** *Nest of nevus cells, many of which are necrotic, beneath ulcerated surface of specimen. Although necrosis of melanocytes is a feature of malignant melanoma, nevocytes may undergo necrosis under extraordinary circumstances such as these. (Reduced from ×640)*

"the mitotic rate proved to be as good a parameter as the prognostic index and better than tumor thickness or levels of invasion." At the time of this writing the work of Schmoeckel and Braun-Falco was just published so that no judgment has yet been made by other workers about the efficacy of their method for predicting outcome of malignant melanomas.

Surely there are many other considerations besides the histologic features of depth (levels), thickness, and number of mitotic figures in attempting to assess prognosis of malignant melanoma. Genetic characteristics, immunologic (cellular and humoral) capabilities, and factors inherent in the melanoma cells themselves are but a few that doubtlessly influence the capacity of the host to contain the neoplasm. Methods for accurate quantification of these and other variables must be developed.

X. ANALOGIES BETWEEN CUTANEOUS MALIGNANT MELANOMA AND OTHER NEOPLASMS OF THE SKIN

The common keratinocytic neoplasms in the skin have some features in common with malignant melanomas. For example, both superficial basal-cell carcinomas and intraepidermal squamous-cell carcinomas (squamous-cell carcinomas *in situ*) tend to spread horizontally and to remain within the epidermis or contiguous with it for years before a vertical component of "invasive" basal-cell carcinoma or squamous-cell carcinoma supervenes (Fig. 119). In a sense, a solar keratosis may be likened to a lentigo maligna as relatively innocuous though "precancerous"; Bowen's disease (a type of squamous-cell carcinoma *in situ*) to superficial spreading malignant melanoma *in situ* as

106 The Histology of Cutaneous Malignant Melanoma

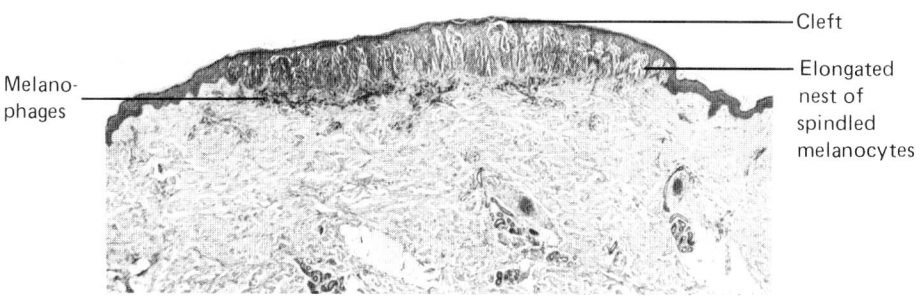

FIGURE 97A. **Nevus of large spindle and/or epithelioid cells (Spitz's nevus).** *This is a melanocytic nevus and not a malignant melanoma because the lesion is small and well circumscribed. A straight line can be drawn vertically at either side of the melanocytic component within the epidermis, because there is no horizontal extension of melanocytes within the epidermis to the sides of this gently domed nodule. (Reduced from ×23)*

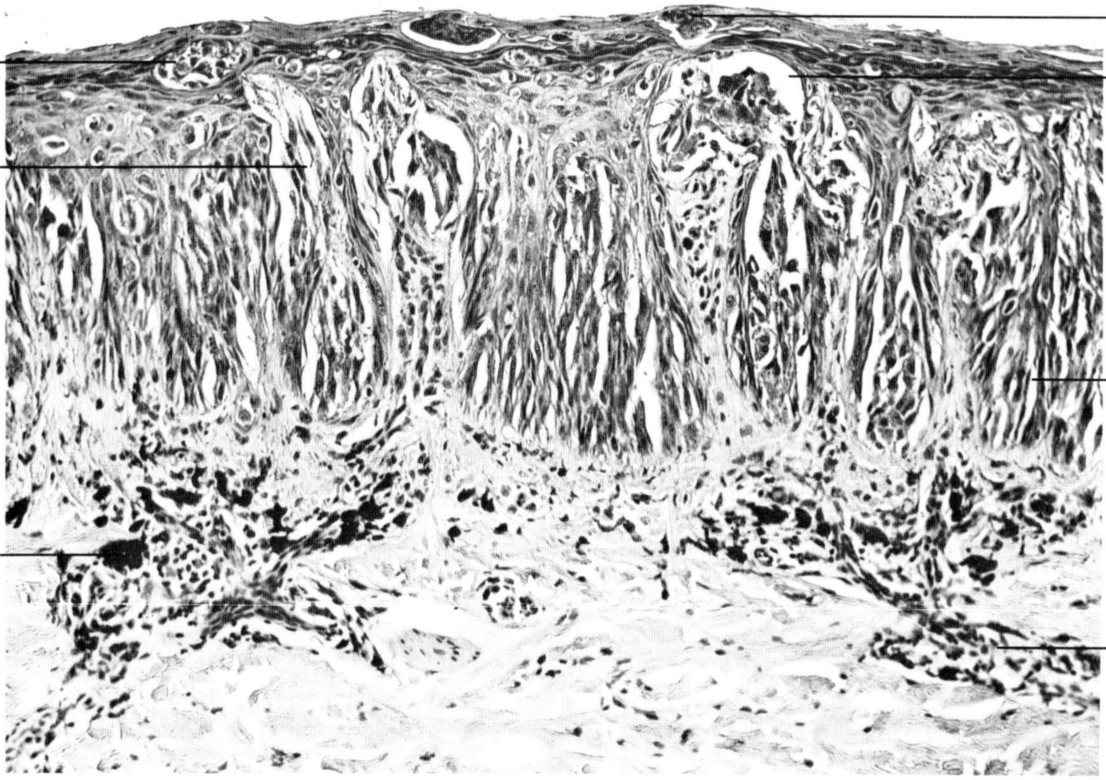

FIGURE 97B. **Nevus of large spindle and/or epithelioid cells (Spitz's nevus).** *This higher power view of Fig. 97A illustrates some features that Spitz's nevus may share with malignant melanoma, namely, an increased number of atypical melanocytes, nests of melanocytes that vary in size and shape, and melanocytes scattered like buckshot throughout the epidermis including the cornified layer. Unlike malignant melanoma, however, the spindle-shaped melanocytes are arranged in elongated nests oriented perpendicular to the surface of the specimen and are surrounded by clefts. (Reduced from ×182)*

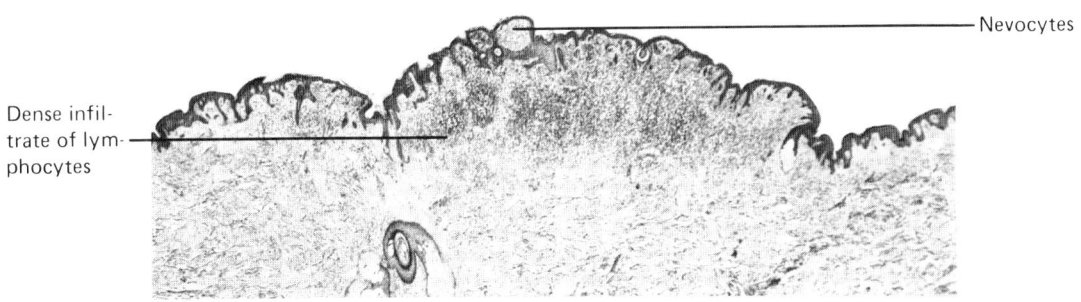

FIGURE 98A. **Halo nevus.** This is a melanocytic nevus because the lesion is sharply demarcated and a halo nevus because the lymphocytic infiltrate permeates the nevocytes and largely obscures them. (Reduced from ×19)

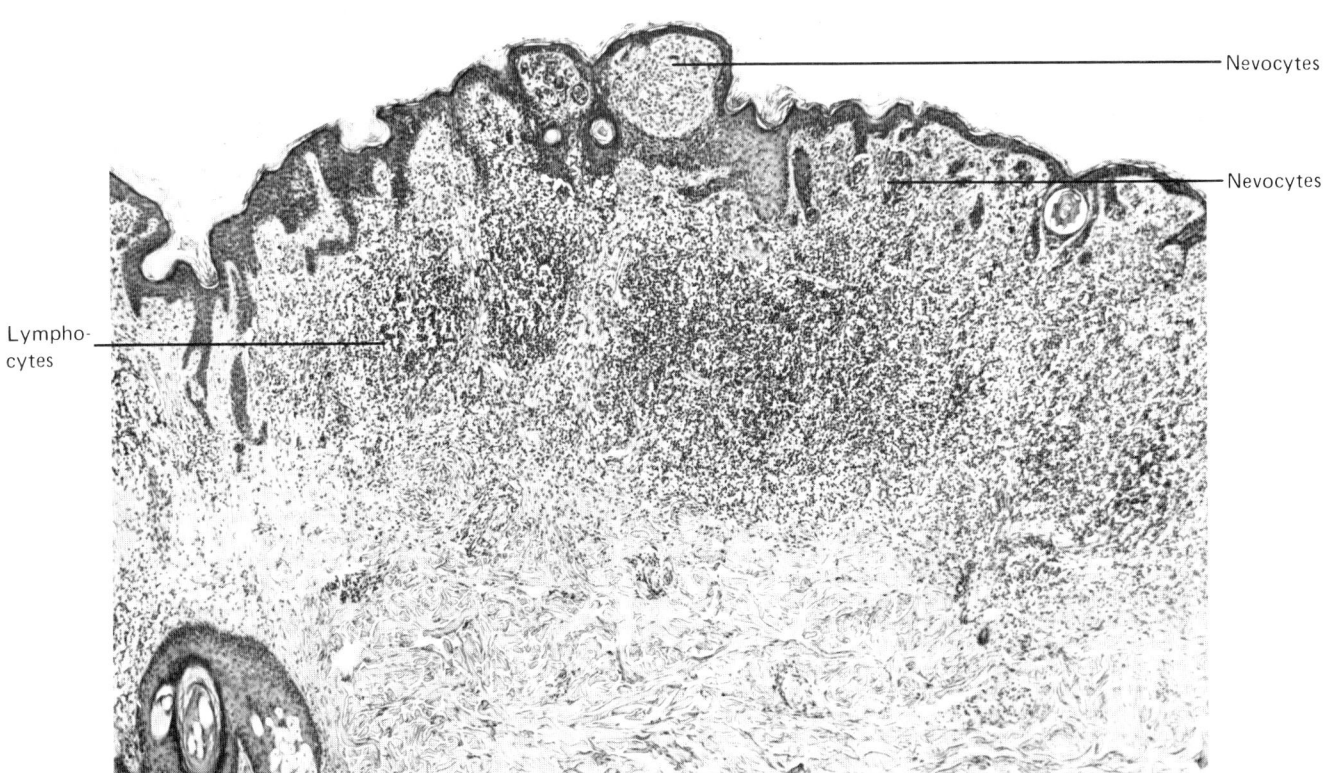

FIGURE 98B. **Halo nevus.** Higher-power view of Fig. 97A to illustrate the nests of nevocytes in the upper part of the dermis and the dense predominantly lymphocytic infiltrate that obscures much of the nevus. The lymphocytes are instrumental in the destruction of the nevocytes, just as they are in those malignant melanomas that undergo partial or total regression. (Reduced from ×66)

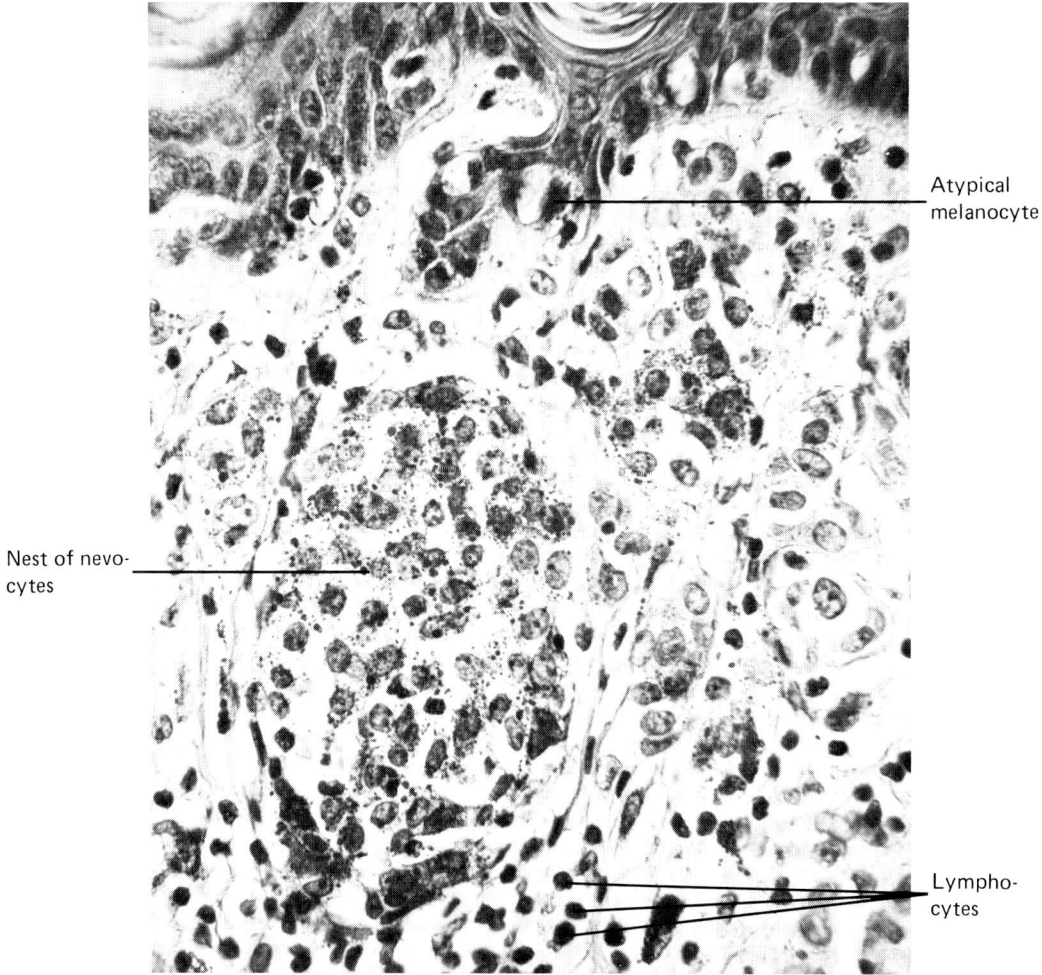

FIGURE 98C. **Halo nevus.** *The nests of melanocytes in the epidermis and of nevus cells in the dermis of this halo nevus pictured in Figs. 98A and 98B will eventually succumb to the lymphocytic infiltrate and disappear completely.*

more consequential but still "precancerous" processes; and squamous-cell carcinoma that arises *de novo* to nodular malignant melanoma as much more serious biologically cancerous conditions. Just as every solar keratosis or Bowen's disease does not necessarily or inevitably eventuate as squamous-cell carcinoma, so too, not every lentigo maligna or superficial spreading malignant melanoma *in situ* progresses relentlessly into "invasive" malignant melanoma. However, of each of these initially "benign" keratinocytic and melanocytic neoplastic processes, most will evolve into frank malignancies if the patient lives long enough.

A predominantly lymphocytic infiltrate of variable density underlies superficial basal-cell carcinomas, solar keratoses, and squamous-cell carcinomas *in situ*, and all types of malignant melanoma *in situ*. As the proliferation of keratinocytes continues and progressively penetrates deeper into the dermis, the density of the inflammatory-cell infiltrate tends to diminish. The same is true for malignant melanomas as they extend further downward into the dermis. Occasionally, presumably on account of the inflammatory-cell infiltrates, superficial basal-cell carcinomas, solar keratoses, and squamous-cell carcinomas *in situ* are contained and undergo some spontaneous regression. The phenomenon of containment and partial regression is more common in superficial spreading malignant melanoma, but total regression of any of these neoplasms is rare.

Basal-cell carcinomas, squamous-cell carcinomas, and malignant melanomas have several different grossly discernible architectural patterns. Verrucous squamous-cell

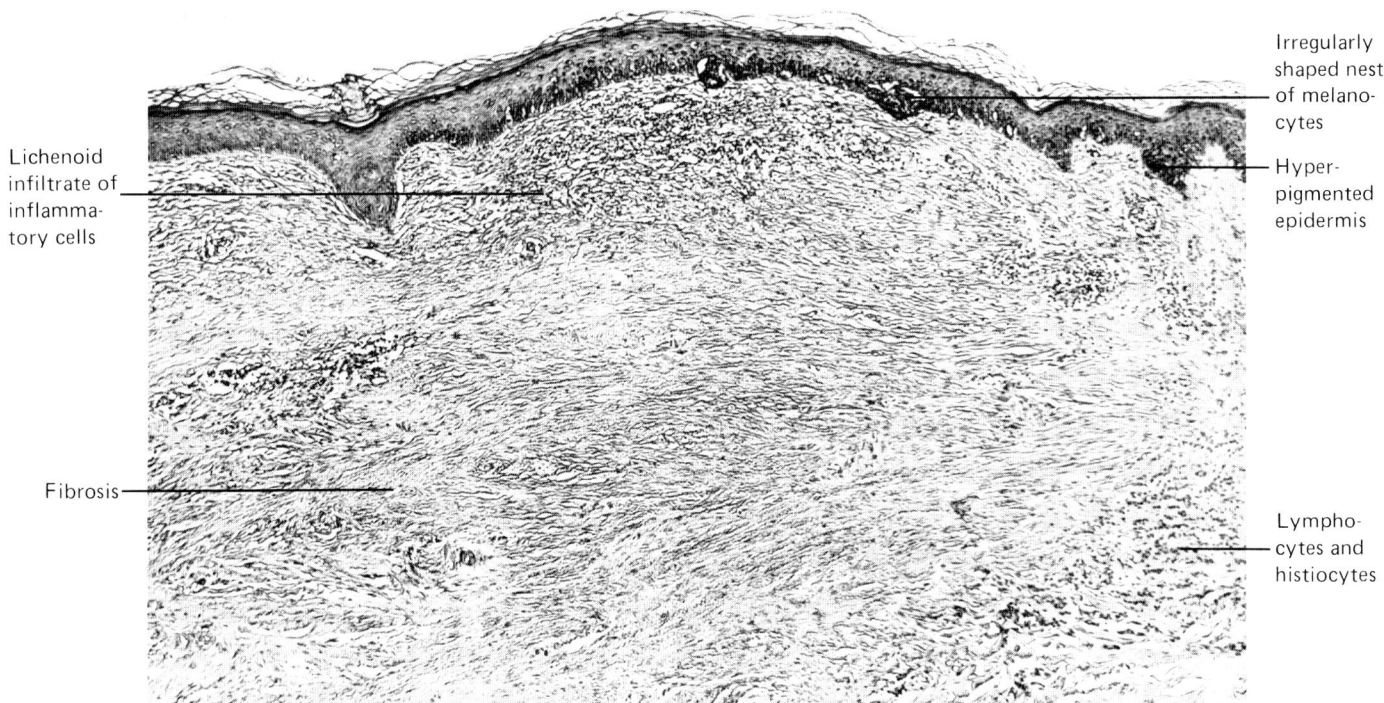

FIGURE 99A. ***Recurrent melanocytic nevus following partial surgical excision (pseudomelanoma).*** *There are no nevocytes beneath the scar within the dermis of this pigmented lesion, so that the pathologist may only infer that the melanocytic hyperplasia and hyperpigmentation within the epidermis represent recurrence of a previous melanocytic nevus, usually intradermal in type. In every instance such as this, the original biopsy specimen should be reviewed to ensure that the initial lesion was truly a melanocytic nevus and not a malignant melanoma. (Reduced from ×79)*

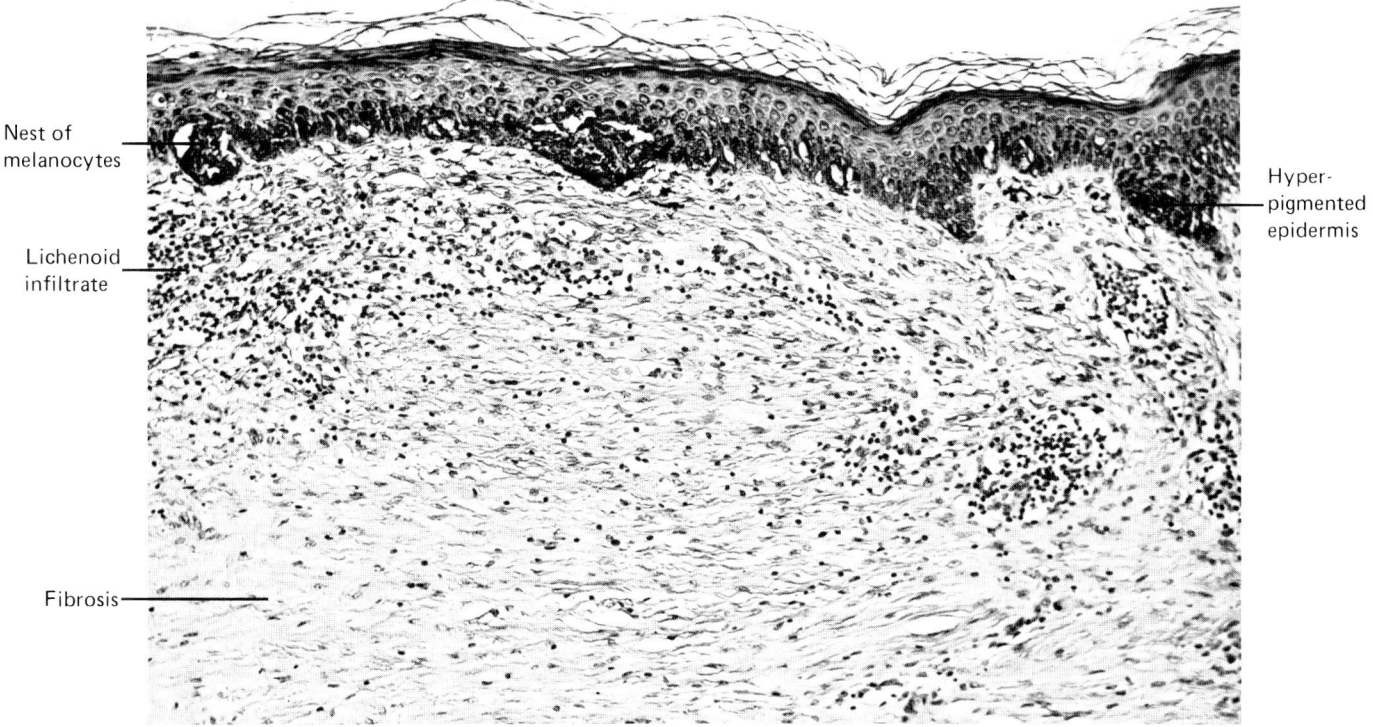

FIGURE 99B. ***Recurrent melanocytic nevus (pseudomelanoma).*** *This closer view of Fig. 99A shows the increased number of melanocytes within the heavily pigmented epidermis, a somewhat lichenoid infiltrate of lymphocytes, and a scar. Note that the nests of melanocytes within the epidermis vary in size and shape. (Reduced from ×170)*

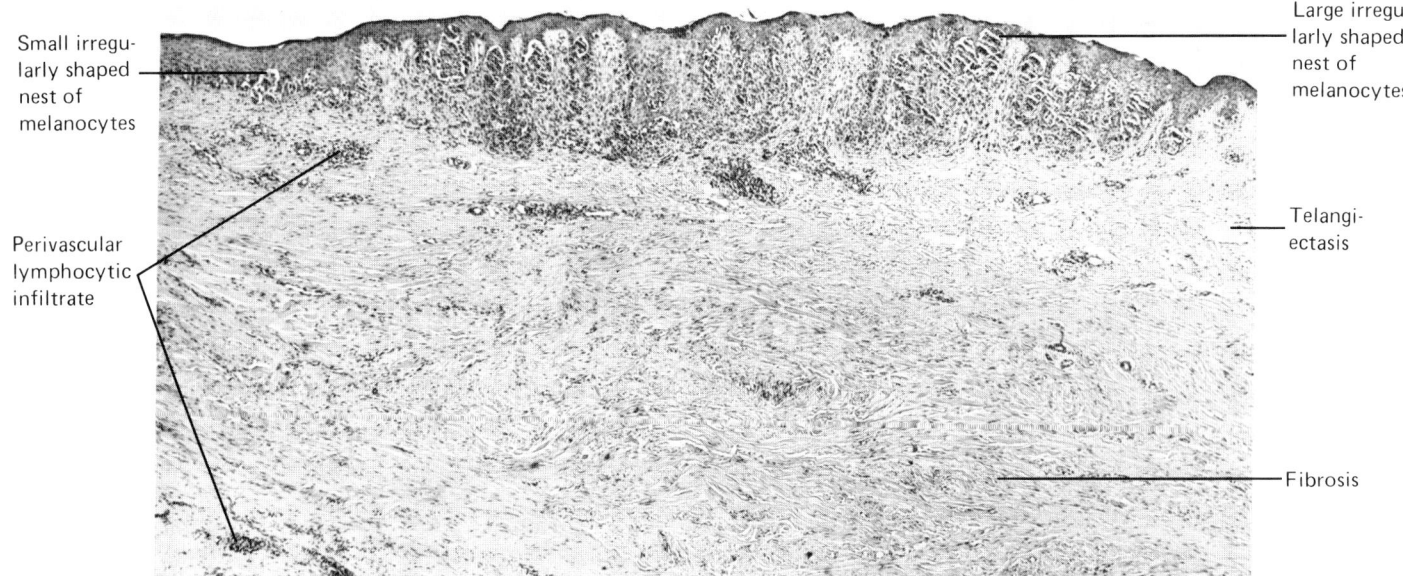

FIGURE 100A. ***Recurrent melanocytic nevus following partial surgical excision (pseudomelanoma).*** *This is a nevus rather than a malignant melanoma because the lesion is well circumscribed and most of the melanocytes are in the lower portion of the epidermis. The sign of a previous surgical procedure is scarring throughout the dermis. Those features suggestive of malignant melanoma are variation in size and shape of the nests of intraepidermal melanocytes and confluence of those nests. There is also an inflammatory-cell infiltrate around the vessels. Were this a recurrent malignant melanoma it would be* in situ. *(Reduced from ×48)*

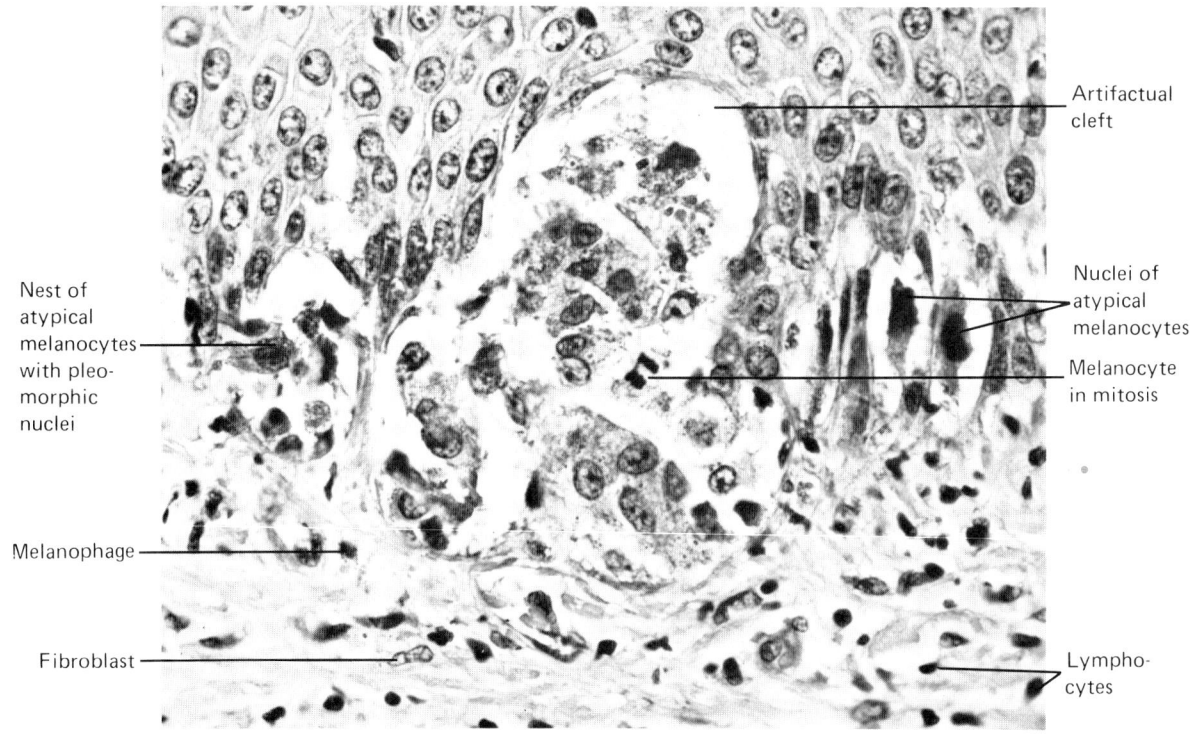

FIGURE 100B. ***Recurrent melanocytic nevus following partial surgical excision (pseudomelanoma).*** *This higher-power view of Fig. 100A shows irregularly shaped and sized nests of atypical melanocytes, some of which are in mitosis. These histologic changes are reminiscent of superficial spreading malignant melanoma and for this reason the recurrent melanocytic nevus following partial surgical excision has been termed "pseudomelanoma." The histologic sections of the original specimen should always be examined. (Reduced from ×640)*

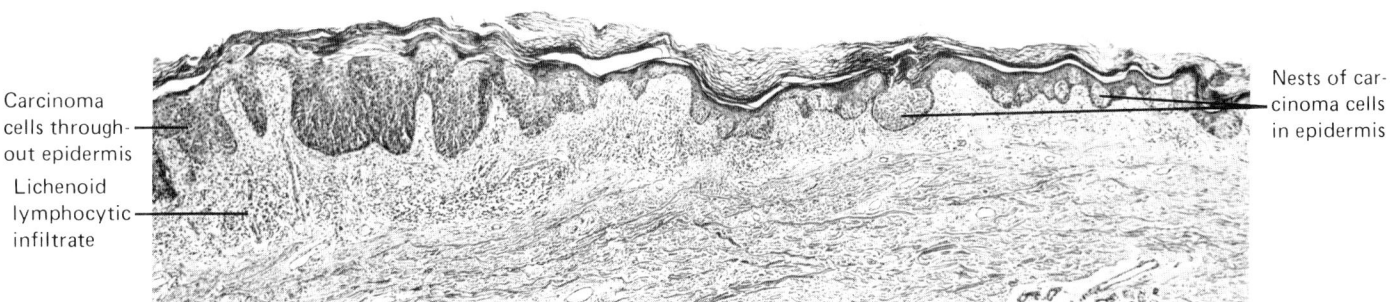

FIGURE 101A. **Pagetoid Bowen's disease.** *Bowen's disease, one form of squamous-cell carcinoma* in situ, *is sometimes characterized by nests of pale-staining keratinocytes that have atypical nuclei (pagetoid cells). The presence of parakeratosis overlying some of these nests indicates that the cells are cornifying, an evidence of squamous differentiation. Note the dense band-like lymphohistiocytic infiltrate in the thickened papillary dermis. (Reduced from ×44)*

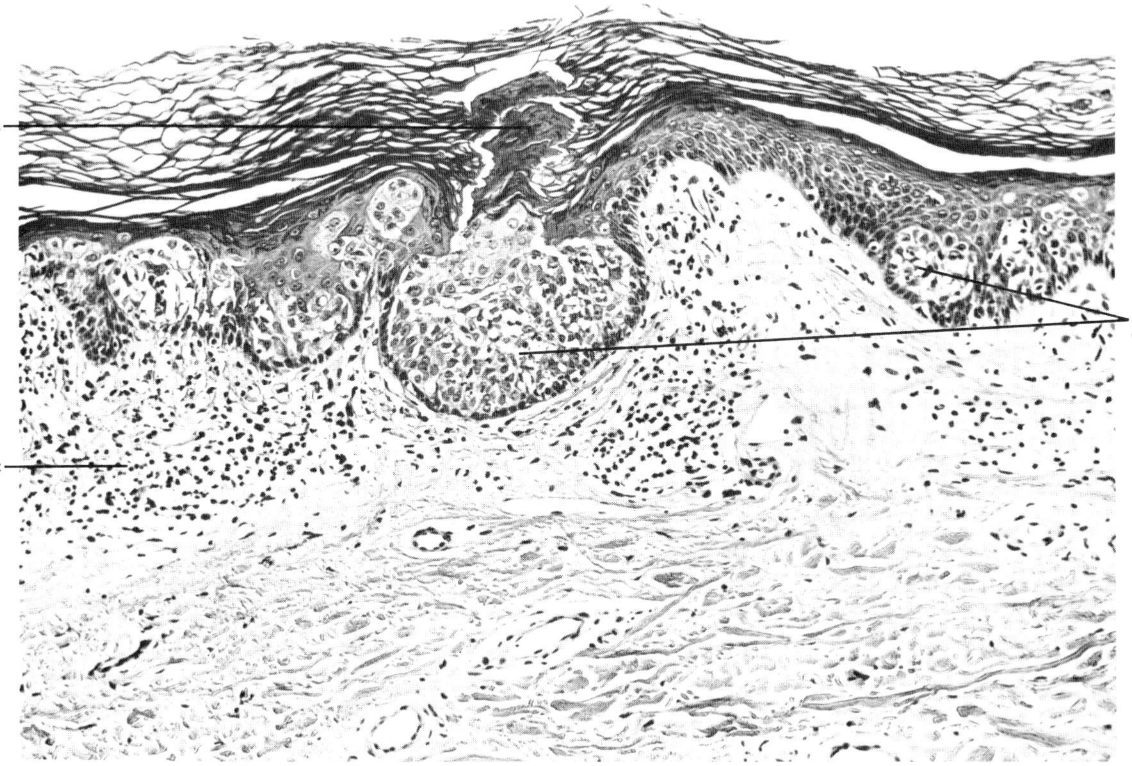

FIGURE 101B. **Pagetoid Bowen's disease.** *This higher magnification of Fig. 101A shows irregularly shaped nests of pale-staining atypical keratinocytes that are situated above the basal layer of the epidermis. Note the focal parakeratosis. (Reduced from ×187)*

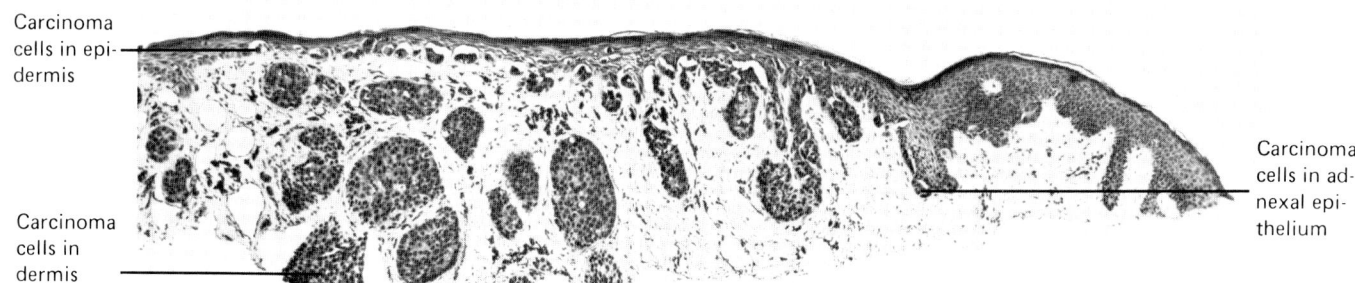

FIGURE 102A. ***Paget's disease of the breast simulating superficial spreading malignant melanoma.*** *In this superficial shaved excision of what clinically was thought to be a malignant melanoma on the breast, the histologic features of mammary Paget's disease pictured here closely resemble those of superficial spreading malignant melanoma. Note the irregularly shaped nests of epithelial cells within the epidermis, at the dermoepidermal junction, within epithelium of adnexal structures, as well as within the dermis. The clefts around the atypical cells within the epidermis are more commonly found in Paget's disease of the breast than in malignant melanoma. (Reduced from ×74)*

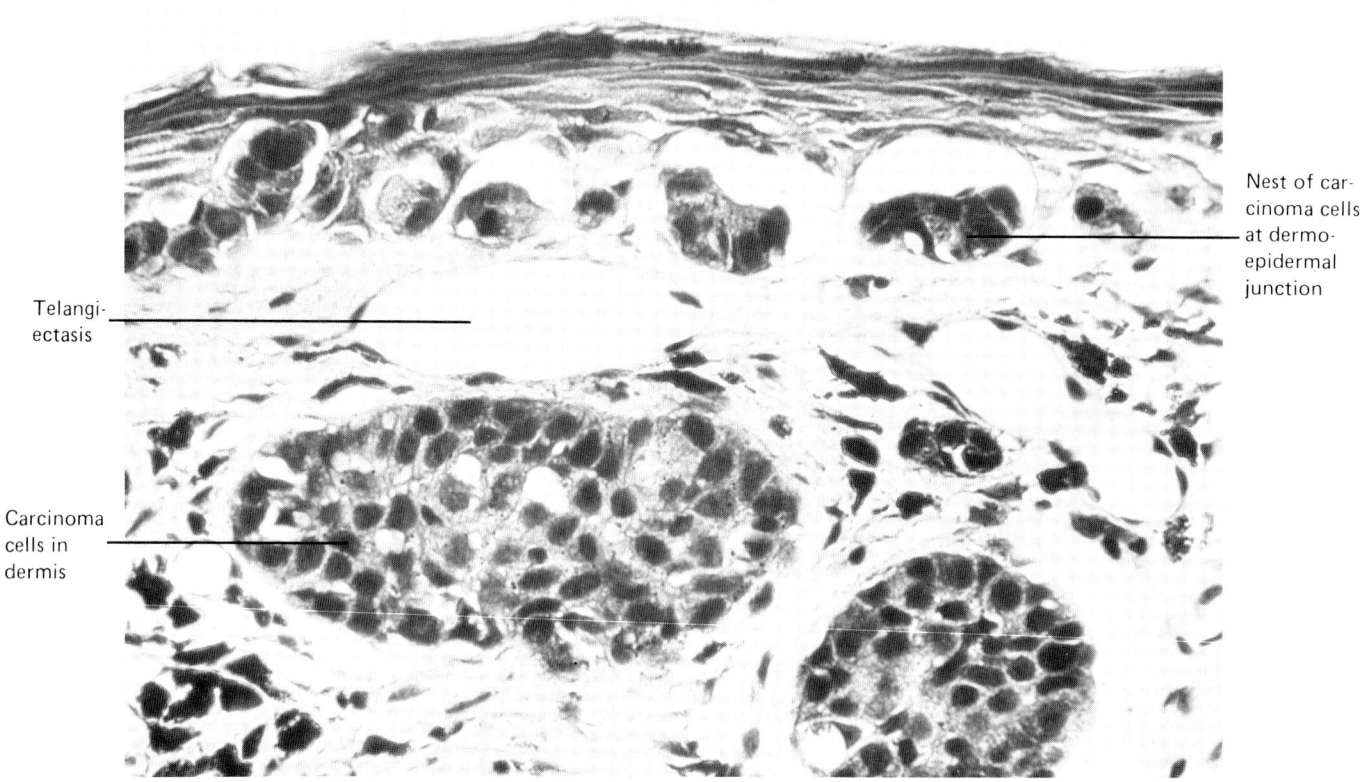

FIGURE 102B. ***Paget's disease of the breast simulating superficial spreading malignant melanoma.*** *Higher magnification of Fig. 102A shows nests of epithelial cells at the dermoepidermal junction and within the dermis. These histologic changes in the epidermis and the dermis must be differentiated from those of superficial spreading malignant melanoma. In only a single field, such as this one pictured, that differentiation may be impossible. These cells were PAS positive–diastase resistant, a feature of Paget's disease. Subsequent surgery revealed an intraductal carcinoma of the breast. (Reduced from ×506)*

carcinoma and verrucous malignant melanoma are examples of one configuration. As cutaneous carcinomas and malignant melanomas become increasingly exophytic, they tend to ulcerate as a consequence of bulky cellularity so near the surface. And, each of these three neoplasms has many fine cytologic variations. Not every basal-cell carcinoma consists only of small basaloid cells; some of their nuclei may be large and pleomorphic, others spindle-shaped, and still other basal-cell carcinomas may even appear squamoid. The atypical cells of squamous-cell carcinoma may be small, cuboidal, spindle-shaped, acantholytic, and dyskeratotic. In malignant melanoma there are many cytologic expressions as already described in this text. Cutaneous carcinomas, like malignant melanomas, may be dark brown or blue-black, e.g., the pigmented basal-cell carcinoma, in which melanin has been transferred to the atypical keratinocytes by apparently normal melanocytes within the neoplasms.

Basal-cell carcinomas and squamous-cell carcinomas that develop in skin that has been severely damaged by sunlight tend to behave in a biologically less aggressive way than those that arise in scars of the sort that result from burns, vaccinations, and radiotherapy. So, too, lentigo maligna melanoma, which always occurs on sun-damaged skin, usually of the face, has a better prognosis as a rule than those malignant melanomas, such as the acral lentiginous, that originate in skin that has not been subjected to the baleful effects of ultraviolet light. Because malignant melanomas often begin in sun-damaged skin, other neoplasms induced by sunlight, such as basal-cell carcinomas, solar keratoses, squamous-cell carcinomas, and keratoacanthomas, may be found together with malignant melanoma in the very same biopsy specimen (Fig. 120).

Although basal-cell carcinomas and squamous-cell carcinomas rarely metastasize, the deeper these neoplasms penetrate into the skin, the greater the local damage and danger of systemic spread. Metastases from malignant melanomas are common compared to those from cutaneous carcinomas, but, in general, the greater the depth of extension of both atypical keratinocytes and melanocytes into the skin and beyond, the worse the prognosis.

Thus, cutaneous malignant melanoma, although a remarkably distinct neoplasm in some respects, is not unique in other respects and has several characteristics in common with cutaneous basal-cell and squamous-cell neoplasms. This is not surprising when one considers that all three are proliferations of atypical cells that tend to arise within the epidermis.

A few words should be said about analogies between extramammary Paget's disease and all of the horizontally spreading types of malignant melanoma. Unlike Paget's disease of the breast, in which atypical pagetoid epithelial cells from an intraductal carcinoma migrate outward along lactiferous ducts into the epidermis, most lesions of extrammary Paget's disease begin as proliferation of atypical pagetoid epithelial cells within the epidermis itself. These cells, whose differentiation is glandular, first spread horizontally within the epidermis for years, as do those of lentigo maligna, acral lentiginous malignant melanoma *in situ,* and superficial spreading melanoma *in situ.* In our opinion, the atypical epithelial cells of extramammary Paget's disease may descend the epithelium of adnexal structures just as do the atypical melanocytes of superficially spreading forms of malignant melanoma. In time, the pagetoid cells of extramammary Paget's disease may move from the confines of epidermal or adnexal epithelium into the dermis and may metastasize, as may all the forms of malignant melanoma. In sum, extramammary Paget's disease in many instances is analogous to all superficially spreading forms of malignant melanoma, i.e., it first spreads horizontally within the epidermis before reaching into the dermis, and usually it is not analogous to Paget's disease of the breast in local behavior.

Finally, pagetoid cells as a cytologic type may be found in several unrelated diseases, namely, Paget's disease of the breast, extramammary Paget's disease, pagetoid Bowen's disease, and pagetoid (superficial spreading) malignant melanoma (Table 7).

XI. SOME OBSERVATIONS AND SPECULATIONS ABOUT MALIGNANT MELANOMA

Among the many enigmatic aspects of malignant melanoma is the fact that when the atypical melanocytes are dispersed, but yet confined, within the richly vascular papillary dermis, the neoplasm rarely metastasizes. However, when the neoplastic melanocytes reach increasingly farther into the relatively less vascular reticular dermis, the chances of hematogenous and lymphatic metastasis greatly increases. One explanation offered by Breslow (personal communication) for this paradoxical phenomenon is the neoangiogenesis that accompanies the aggregations of neoplastic melanocytes. The newly formed capillaries and lymphatics evoked by the neoplastic process are in some way more easily penetrated by the cells of malignant melanoma and these vessels become ready conduits for metastases to skin and other distant parts.

Another startling fact about cutaneous malignant melanomas is that the epidermal melanocytes are the only ones that eventuate into biologic malignancy and not the mela-

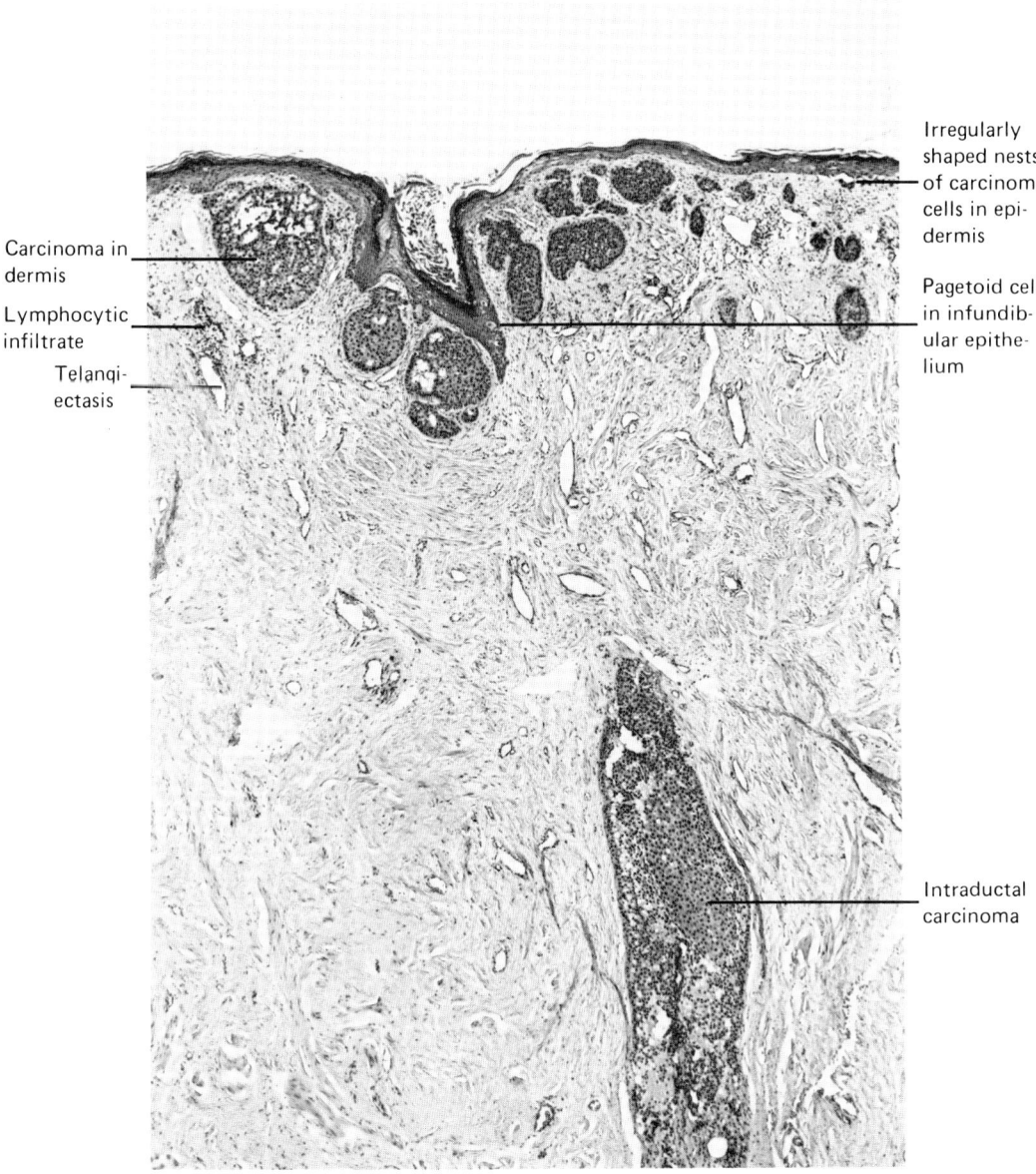

FIGURE 103A. ***Paget's disease of the breast.*** *The changes within the epidermis and in the upper part of the dermis very much resemble the changes of a superficial spreading malignant melanoma. Note, however, that atypical epithelial cells are present also within a lactiferous duct oriented perpendicular to the surface of the specimen. A superficial biopsy of such a specimen could be very confusing to the pathologist. (Reduced from ×45)*

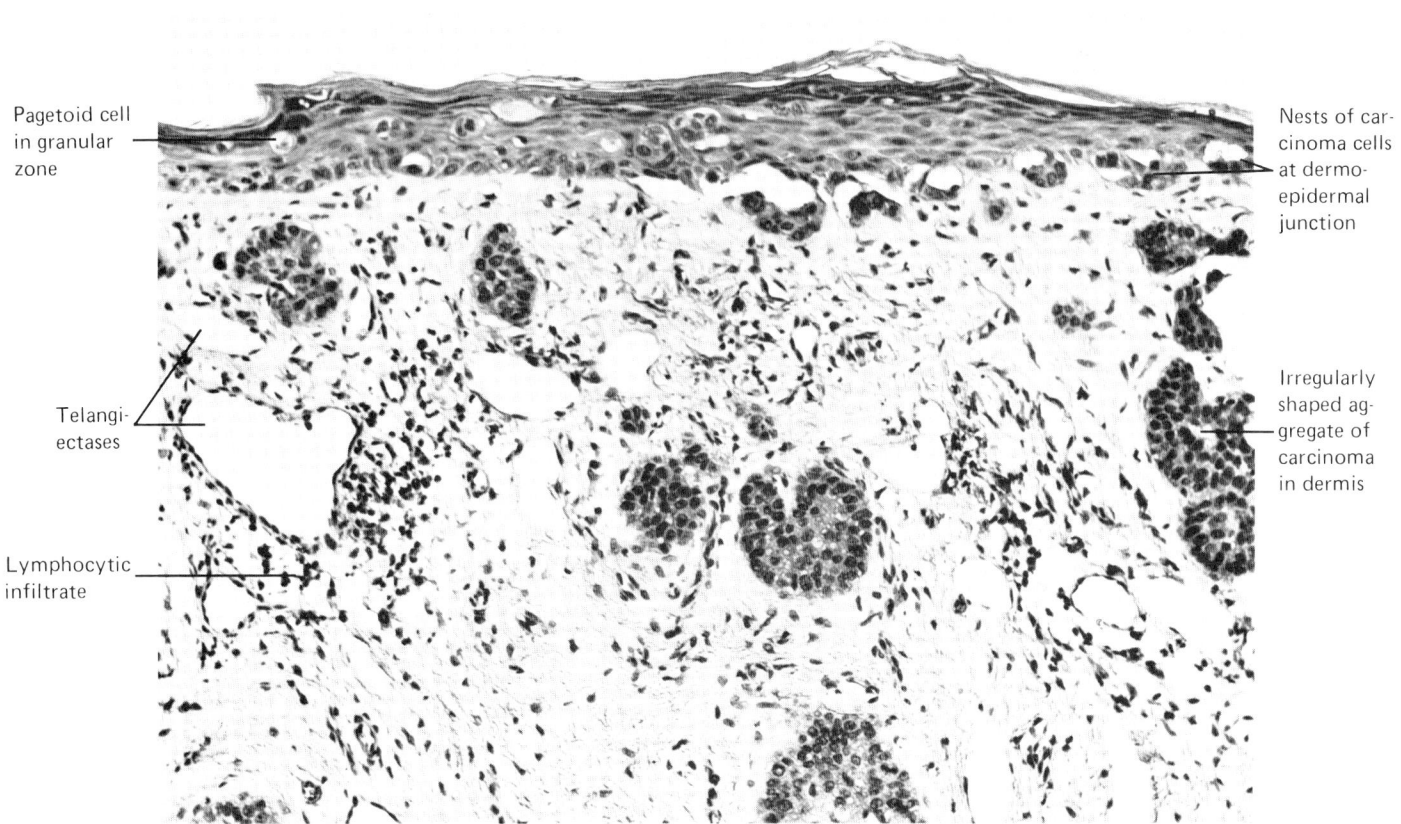

FIGURE 103B. ***Paget's disease of the breast.*** *Higher magnification of Fig. 103A showing histologic changes of Paget's disease that simulate those of superficial spreading malignant melanoma, including "buckshot" scatter of atypical cells at all levels of the epidermis. Special stains such as PAS followed by diastase, aldehyde fuchsin, mucicarmine, and colloidal iron are helpful adjuncts in the differentiation of these two diseases. (Reduced from ×216)*

nocytes in the epithelium of the hair bulb, for example, and practically never the melanocytes in the dermis of blue nevi, Mongolian spots, or the nevi of Ota and Ito. There is something special about epidermal melanocytes and their capacity to become biologically malignant. Could it be due to their exposure in the front line of the skin's defense against electromagnetic energy, especially sunlight? Or could it be owing to influences of the papillary dermis upon them? Or could it be owing to some kind of interaction between them and nevus cells in the dermis because so many malignant melanomas (especially the superficial spreading type) arise in association with preexisting melanocytic nevi?

This brings us to the question of the relationship of malignant melanomas to melanocytic nevi. First, it is important to establish that there is no such thing as junctional "activity" or an "active" junction nevus. Once melanocytes or nevus cells are placed in formalin they should not be described as active. Cytologically, however, melanocytes may be described in sections stained by hematoxylin and eosin as typical or atypical, i.e., having large, hyperchromatic, and pleomorphic nuclei, some with prominent reddish nucleoli, clumped chromatin, or aberrant mitotic figures. A diagnosis of "junctional activity" or "active junction nevus" evades the decision of whether a lesion is a benign or malignant melanocytic process, i.e., a junction melanocytic nevus or malignant melanoma *in situ*. In most instances, this judgment can be made with near certainty if the criteria previously given for the diagnosis of malignant melanoma are taken as guides. In rare instances, it may be impossible to certify that a particular melanocytic lesion is a junction nevus or a malignant melanoma *in situ*. In such cases, a morphologic descriptive diagnosis may be made with an appended note to explain the difficulties in interpretation to the clinician and to advise that the lesion should be excised completely rather than "be watched."

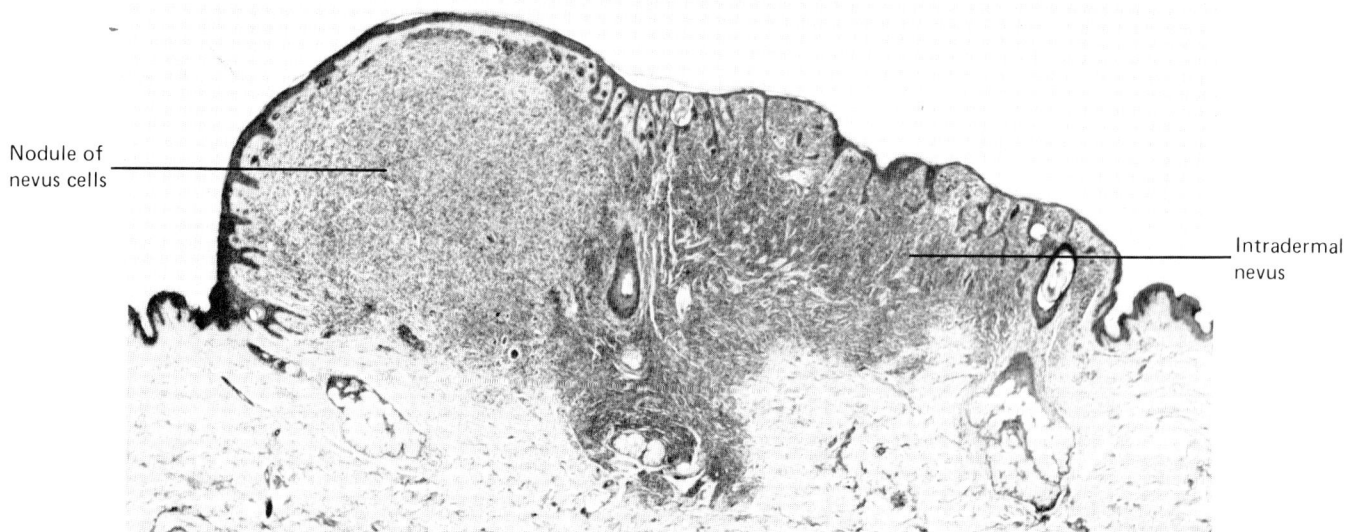

FIGURE 104A. ***Unusual melanocytic nevus with Spitz-like features.*** *On the right side of this photomicrograph there is a conventional intradermal melanocytic nevus. However, in the dome-shaped nodule on the left is a second population of cells having large nuclei and abundant cytoplasm. Under higher power will they be found to have features of a malignant melanoma or a Spitz's nevus? (Reduced from ×28)*

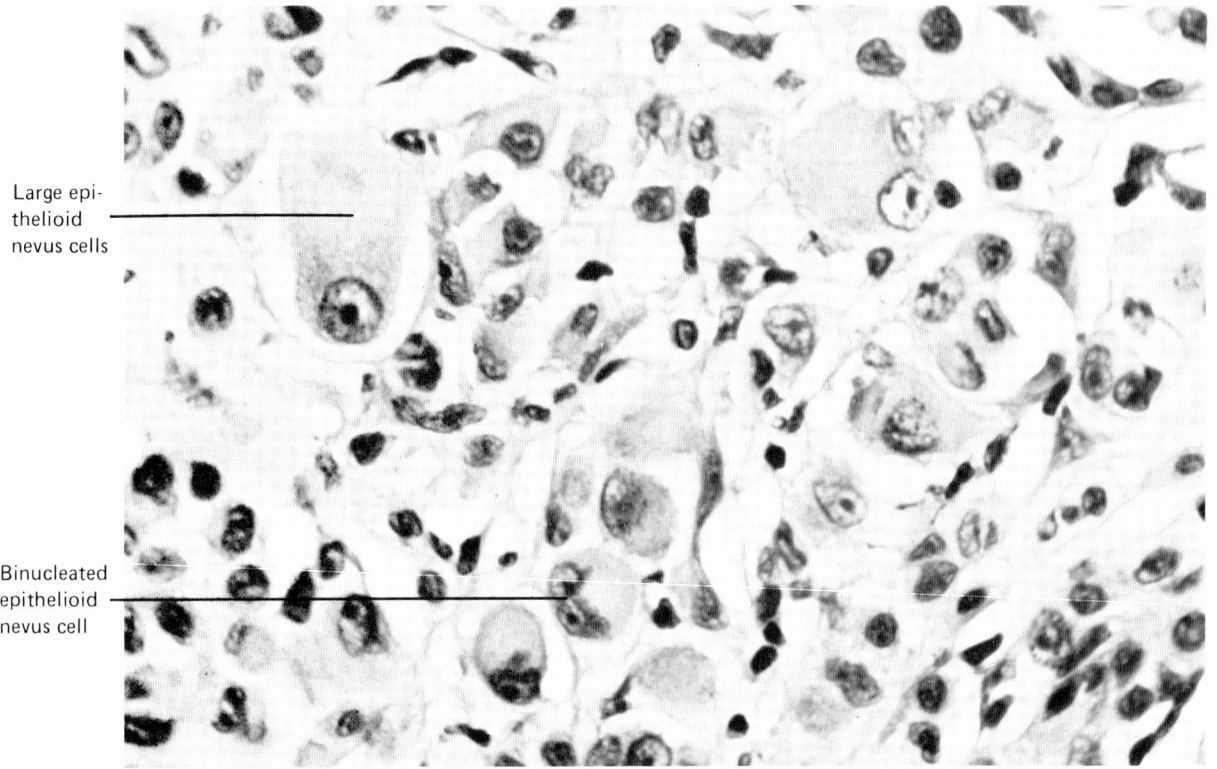

FIGURE 104B. ***Unusual melanocytic nevus with Spitz-like features.*** *This higher magnification of Fig. 104A shows very large cells with pleomorphic nuclei, prominent nucleoli, and abundant pale-staining cytoplasm. Some are binucleated. The absence of atypical melanocytes in the epidermis plus the epithelioid quality of these cells suggests that this is a nevus of large epithelioid cells (Spitz) in association with an ordinary intradermal melanocytic nevus. (Reduced from ×892)*

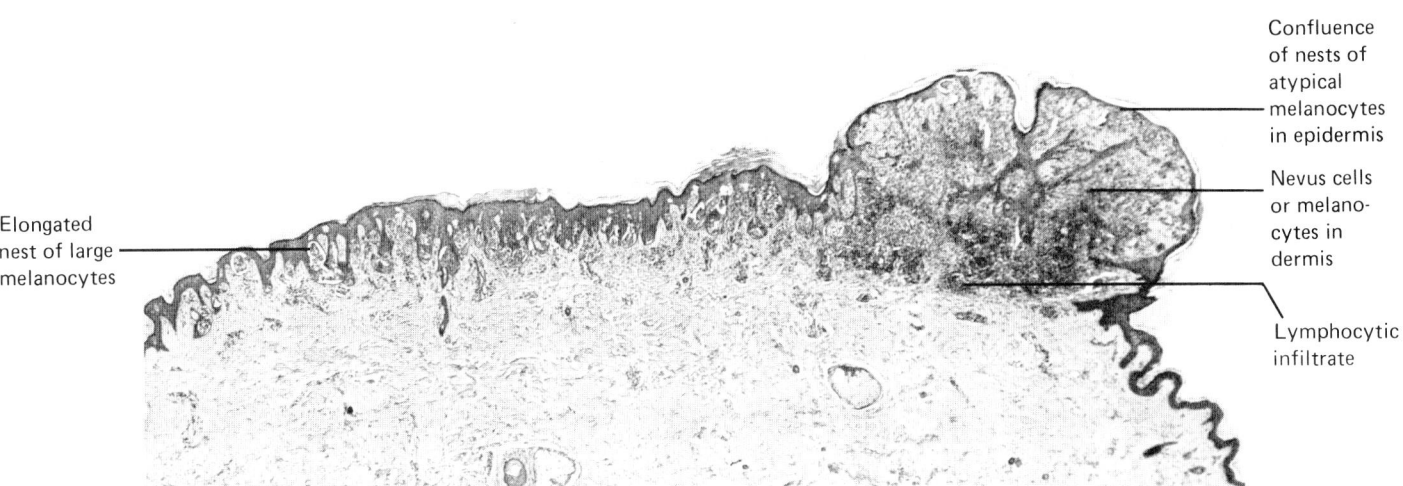

FIGURE 105A. **Nevus of large spindle and/or epithelioid cells with a nodule.** *The changes in the epidermis to the left of the nodule are clearly those of Spitz's nevus as is evidenced by the hyperkeratosis, irregular epidermal hyperplasia, and elongated nests of melanocytes oriented perpendicular to the surface of the specimen and separated from the surrounding keratinocytes by clefts. The melanocytic changes within the nodule on the right are more difficult to interpret. (Reduced from ×24)*

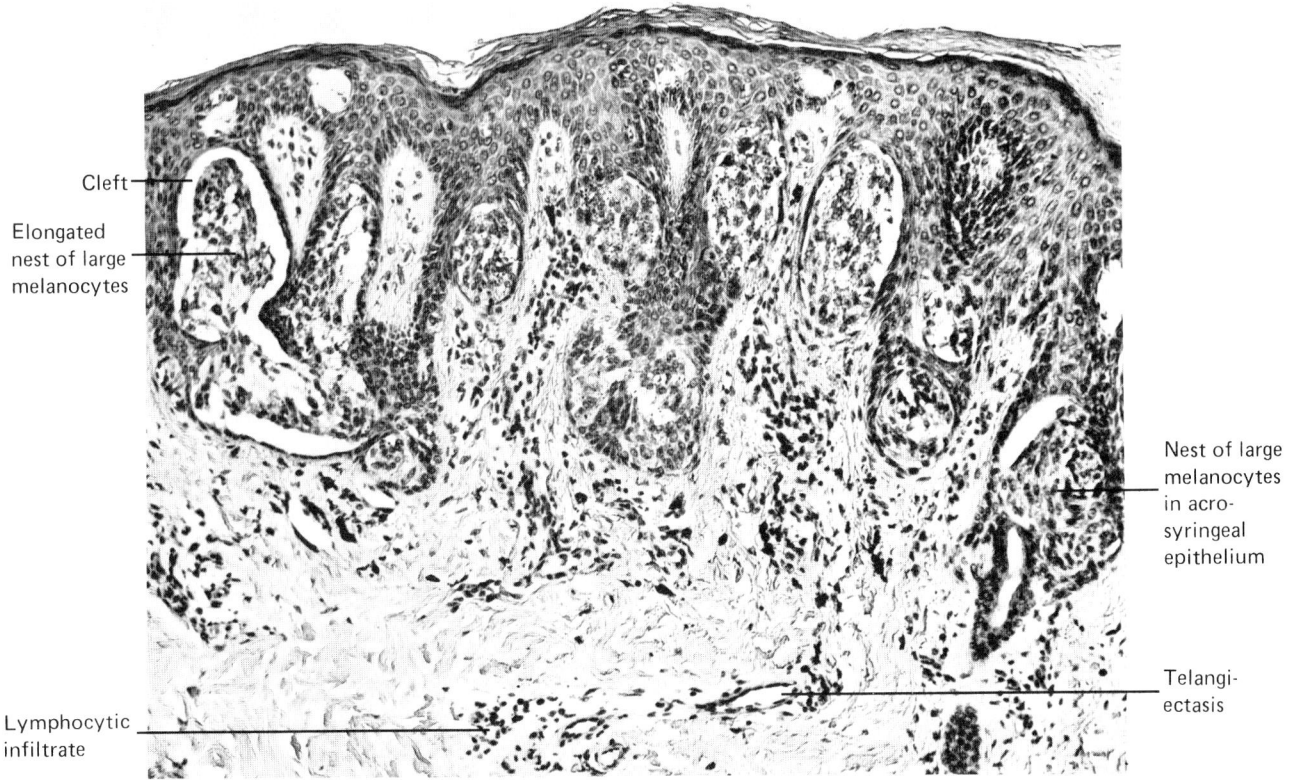

FIGURE 105B. **Nevus of large spindle and/or epithelioid cells with a nodule.** *Higher magnification of the changes in the flat portion of Fig. 105A shows to better advantage the elongated nests of melanocytes, the clefts between nests of melanocytes and surrounding keratinocytes, involvement of the acrosyringium by nests of melanocytes, the hyperplastic epidermis, and the inflammatory-cell infiltrate. (Reduced from ×164)*

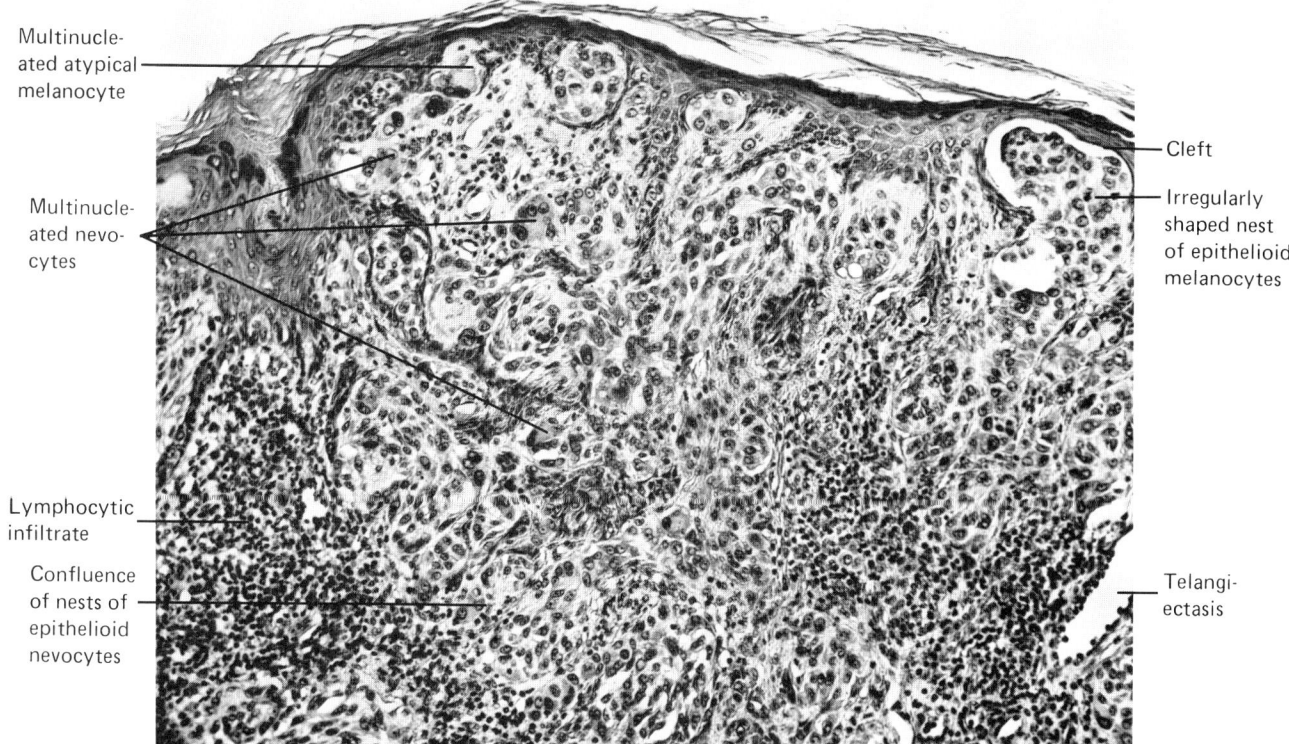

FIGURE 105C. **Nevus of large spindle and/or epithelioid cells with a nodule.** *This higher magnification of the nodule pictured in Fig. 105A shows irregularly shaped nests of atypical melanocytes within the epidermis and irregularly shaped nests of melanocytes or nevus cells within the dermis. Not only are the nuclei large and pleomorphic, but many are multinucleated. (Reduced from ×164)*

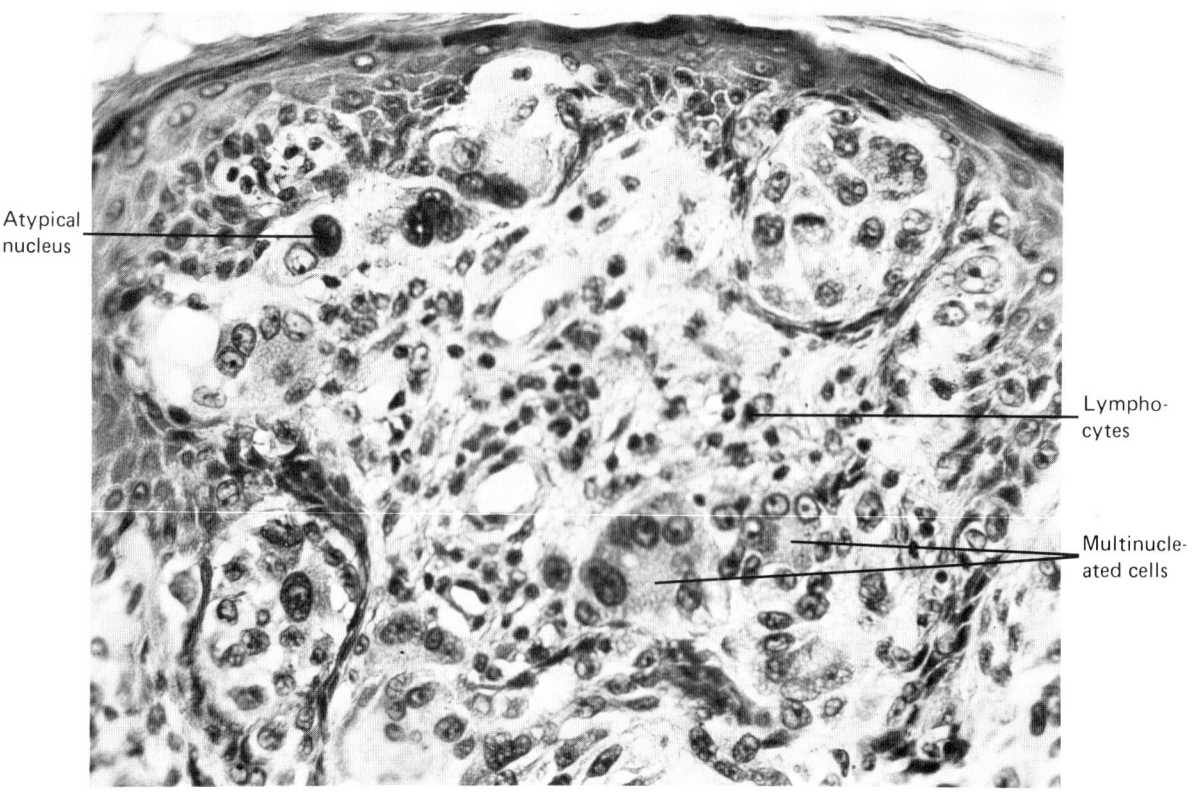

FIGURE 105D. **Nevus of large spindle and/or epithelioid cells with a nodule.** *Still higher magnification of Fig. 105A indicates that the nodule is either directly related to the Spitz's nevus and represents a second clone of nevus cells or is a malignant melanoma arising in association with the Spitz's nevus. We interpreted the entire lesion to be a nevus, especially because the inflammatory-cell infiltrate is throughout rather than beneath the nodule. An unequivocal judgment could not be made about this lesion and that uncertainty was conveyed to the clinician. (Reduced from ×164)*

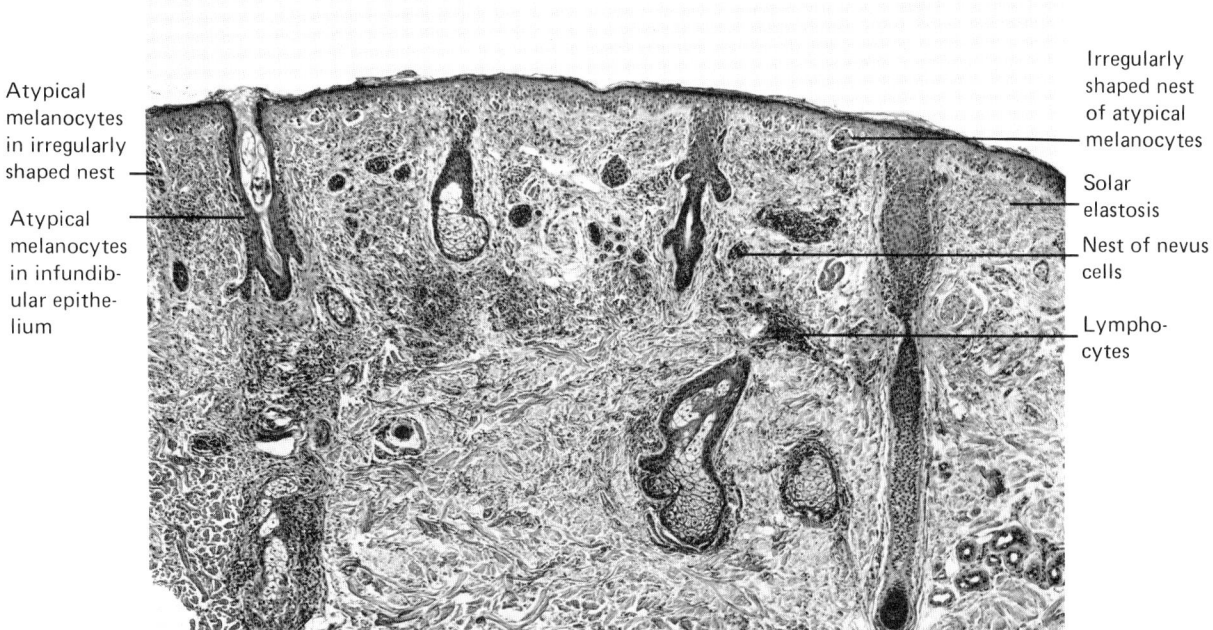

FIGURE 106A. **Lentigo maligna in association with an intradermal melanocytic nevus.** *The increased number of melanocytes, some irregular in size and shape, in a thinned epidermis overlying solar elastosis makes this lesion a lentigo maligna. Note the difference in pattern between the atypical melanocytes in the intraepidermal nests and the typical nevocytes in the intradermal nests. This lesion could be misinterpreted as a compound type of melanocytic nevus if strict criteria for diagnosis are not invoked. An intradermal nevus is uncommon beneath lentigo maligna so that the intraepidermal alterations taken alone may be confused for a junction nevus. (Reduced from ×28)*

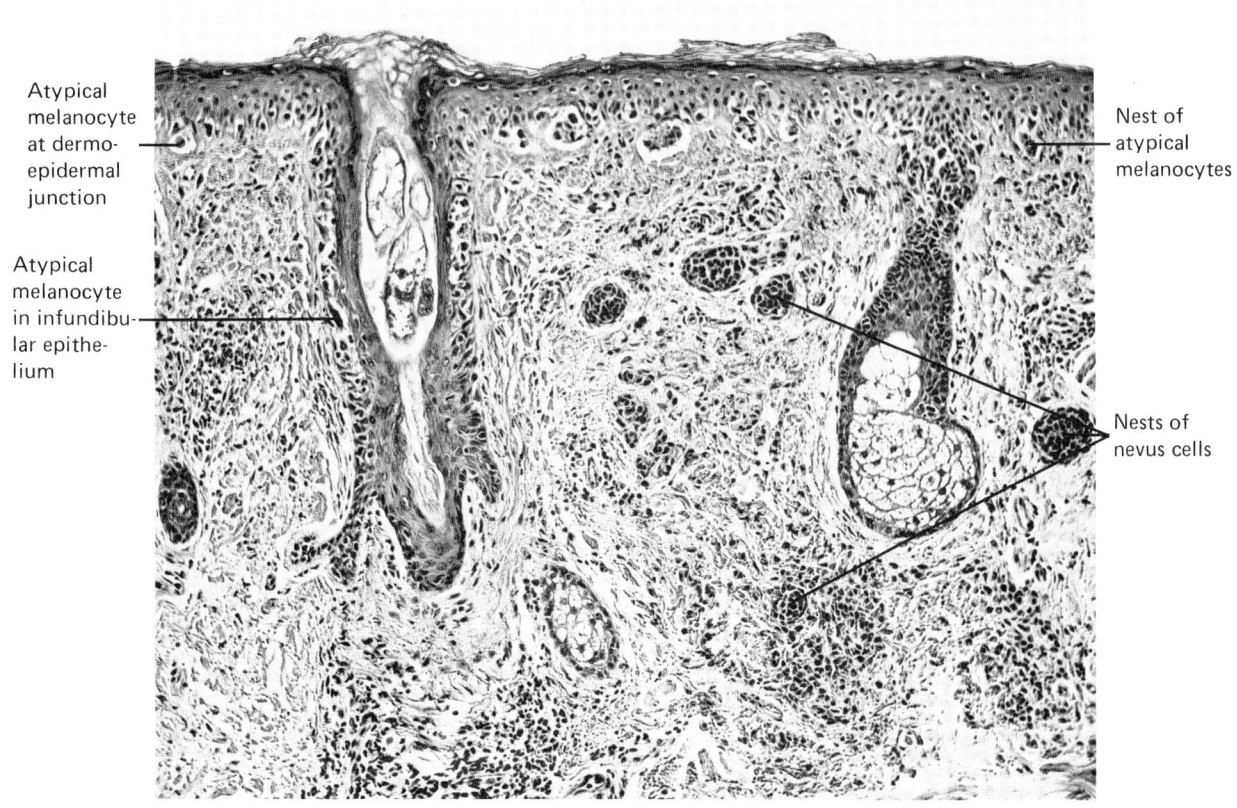

FIGURE 106B. **Lentigo maligna in association with an intradermal melanocytic nevus.** *In this higher-power view of Fig. 106A, the atypical melanocytes can be seen to have extended down the epithelium of follicular infundibula, as well as across the epidermis. Some nests of nevocytes are found episodically in lentigo maligna and lentigo maligna melanoma, but much less often than in superficial spreading malignant melanoma. (Reduced from ×155)*

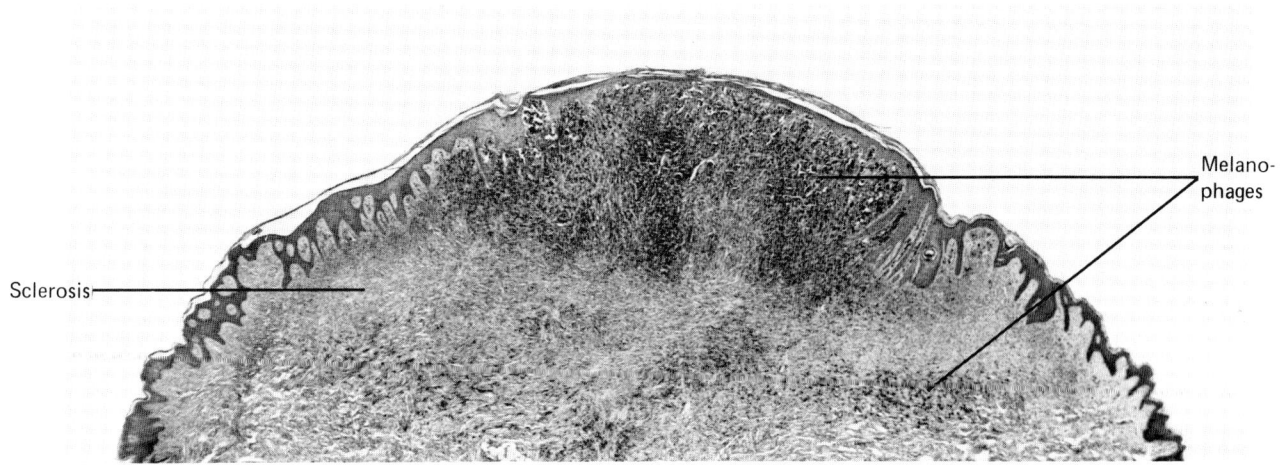

FIGURE 107A. ***Desmoplastic malignant melanoma masquerading as a blue nevus.*** *Among the many variants of blue nevi is the spindle-sclerotic type, which must be differentiated from some desmoplastic malignant melanomas, such as the one pictured here. All of the heavily pigmented cells seen in this view with scanning magnification are melanophages. Atypical melanocytes are present at the dermoepidermal junction and throughout the dermis where they have elicited a fibrotic (desmoplastic) response. (Reduced from ×21)*

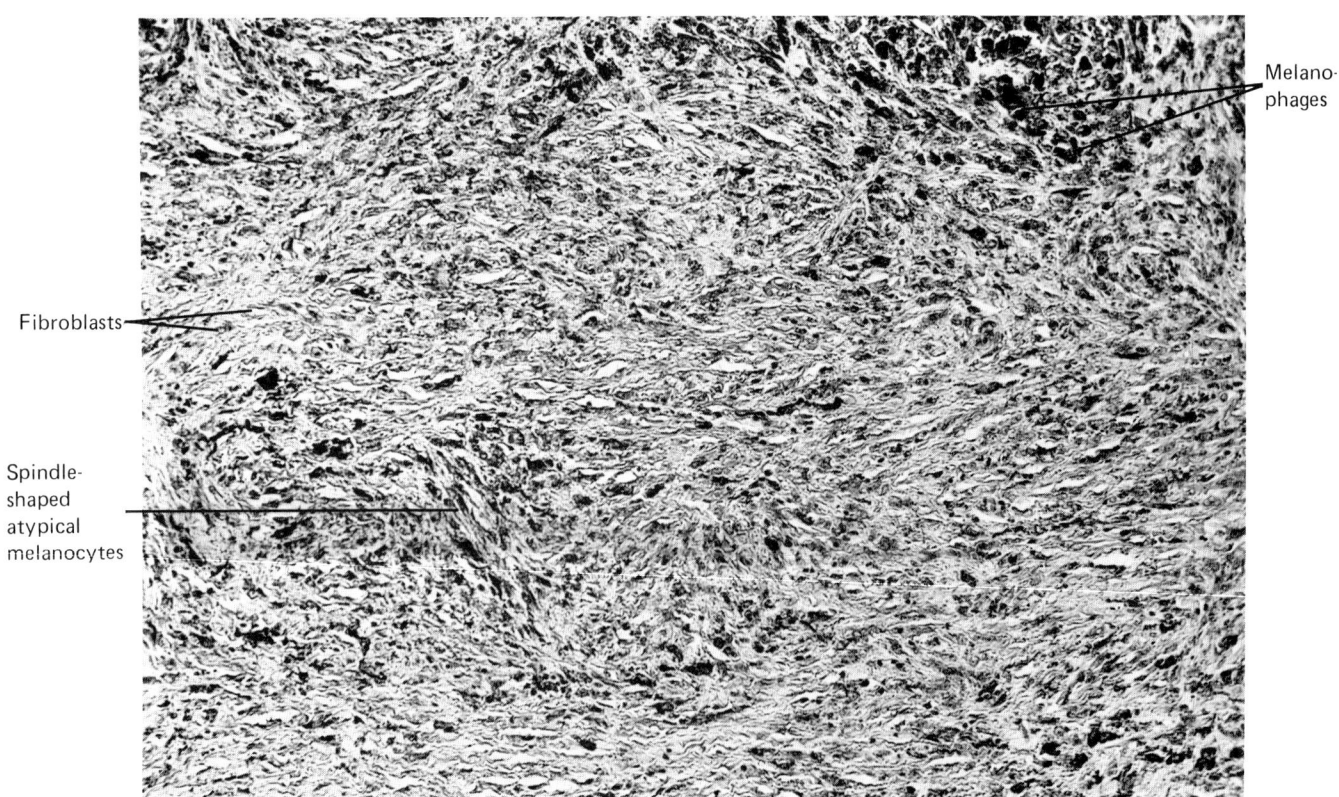

FIGURE 107B. ***Desmoplastic malignant melanoma masquerading as a blue nevus.*** *This higher magnification of a field within Fig. 107A shows a dense infiltrate of melanophages (melanosis), atypical spindle-shaped melanocytes (malignant melanoma), and thin spindle-shaped fibroblasts (desmoplasia). (Reduced from ×173)*

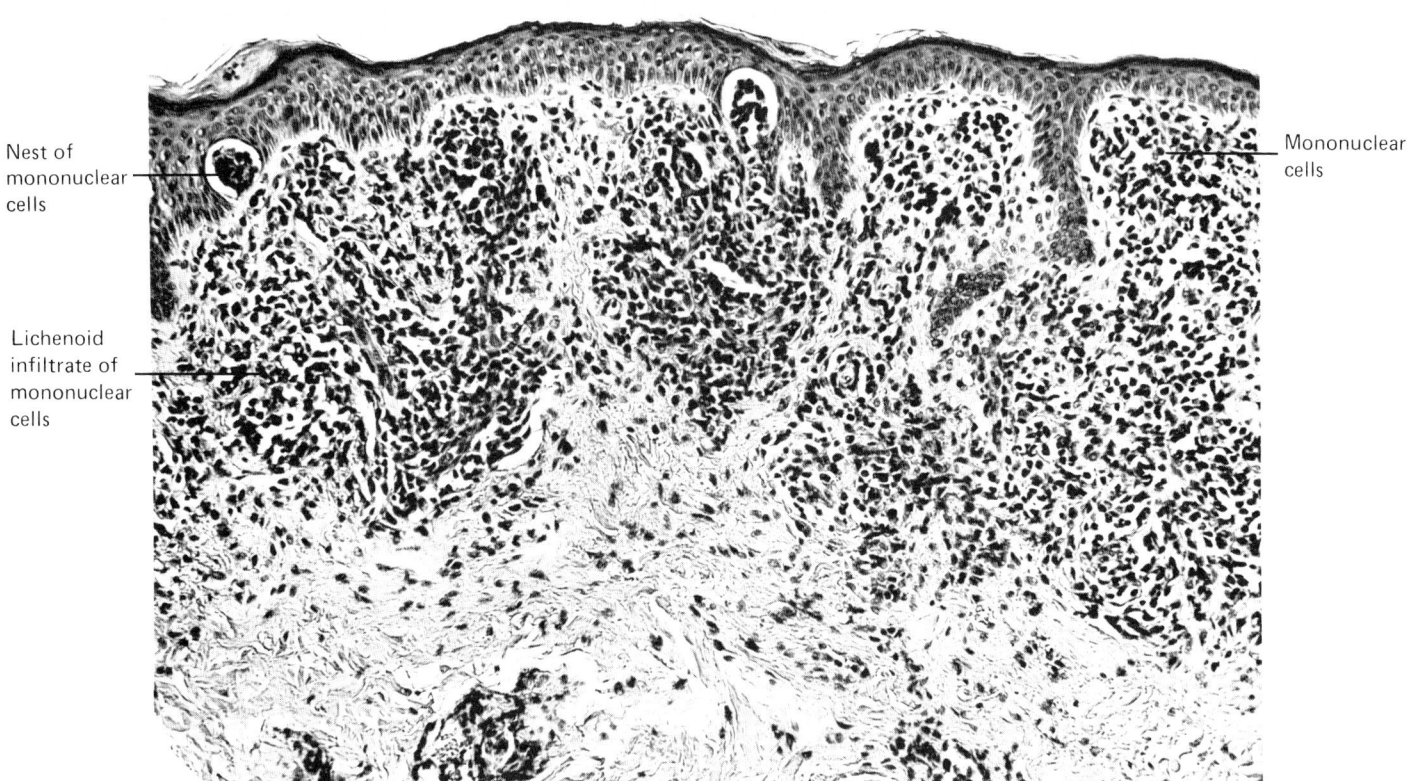

FIGURE 108. **Mycosis fungoides.** *At first glance, the nests of atypical cells at the dermoepidermal junction and in the dermis could be confused with atypical melanocytes of malignant melanoma. In fact, this is the plaque stage of mycosis fungoides and the infiltrate within the dermis and the epidermis consists mostly of atypical T lymphocytes. When nests of these cells form in the epidermis, they are often referred to as Pautrier's microabscesses, a misnomer. (Reduced from ×180)*

"Atypical melanocytic hyperplasia" is a wholly descriptive, rather than definitive, diagnosis that, like "active junctional nevus," evades acknowledging that one simply does not know for sure whether the melanocytic lesion is benign or potentially malignant. Some pathologists use the phrase as a euphemism for malignant melanoma *in situ* (level I). "Atypical melanocytic hyperplasia" can apply equally to the intraepidermal changes of a recurrent melanocytic nevus following partial surgical removal, a junction type of nevus of large spindle and/or epithelioid cells, and to a malignant melanoma *in situ*, just as atypical keratinocytic hyperplasia may describe a hyperplastic solar keratosis as well as the changes in the epidermis associated with granular-cell tumors, some infections by deep fungi and atypical mycobacteria, and halogenodermas. Therefore, if the descriptive diagnosis of "atypical melanocytic hyperplasia" is made, it should be followed in every instance by an explanatory note in which the pathologist conveys that the lesion is probably benign or potentially malignant, or that he simply does not know for sure.

What has been written about junctional activity and atypical melanocytic hyperplasia, applies equally to the euphemism "borderline" malignant melanoma, a term used by some authors for melanocytic lesions that cannot be diagnosed by them as a melanocytic nevus or a malignant melanoma. To us, "borderline" implies that the lesion lies somewhere in between a melanocytic nevus and a malignant melanoma rather than being one or the other, as it actually is. For that reason we advocate acknowledging uncertainty directly, without diagnoses such as "borderline melanoma," "minimal deviation melanoma," and "melanocytic dysplasia."

In our experience of studying malignant melanomas by step sections through the entire specimen, we find remnants of nevus cells within the dermis in about 50% of lesions of superficial spreading malignant melanoma. The higher

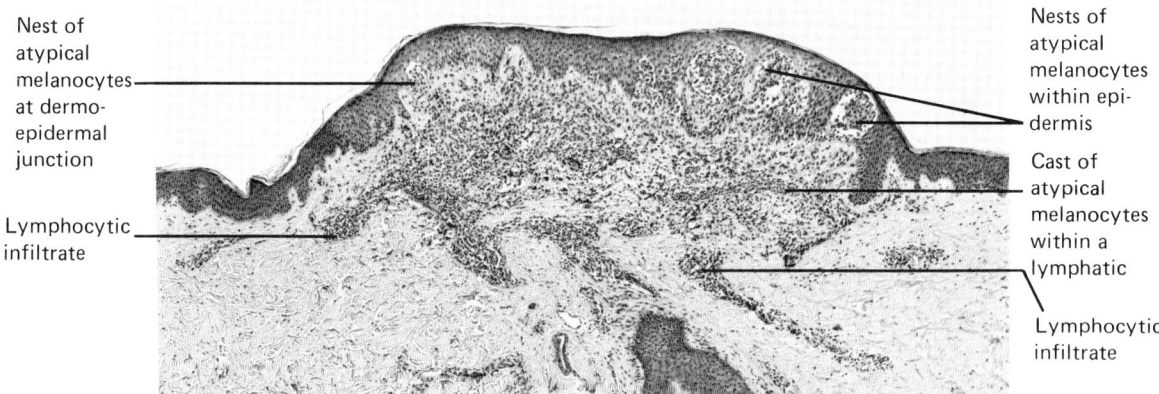

FIGURE 109A. *Epidermotropically metastatic malignant melanoma.* This small dome-shaped papule consists of large nests of atypical melanocytes within the epidermis and nests of atypical melanocytes within the thickened papillary dermis. Note the dense predominantly lymphohistiocytic infiltrate around the vessels of the superficial plexus and the absence of atypical melanocytes within the epidermis to the sides of the nodule. (Reduced from ×53)

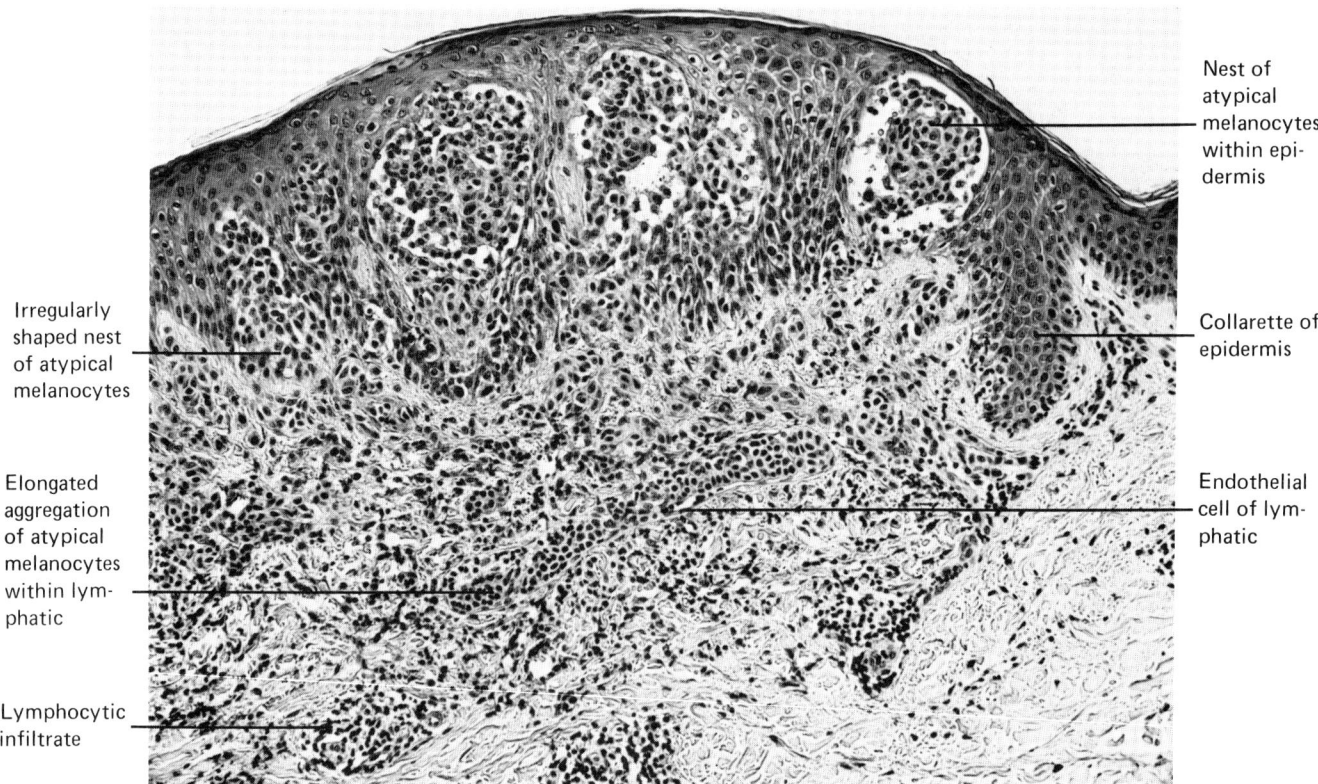

FIGURE 109B. *Epidermotropically metastatic malignant melanoma.* This higher magnification of Fig. 109A again shows the atypical melanocytes within the epidermis and the papillary dermis such as in a superficial spreading malignant melanoma. However, at an angle in the papillary dermis is an endothelial-lined vessel filled with atypical melanocytes, unequivocal evidence of metastatic malignant melanoma. That this is malignant melanoma metastatic to the skin rather than malignant melanoma primary in skin that secondarily involved cutaneous vessels may also be inferred from the small size of the lesion, its superficiality, and the failure of the atypical melanocytes to extend laterally much beyond the bounds of the bulk of the intraepidermal component of the neoplasm. (Reduced from ×164)

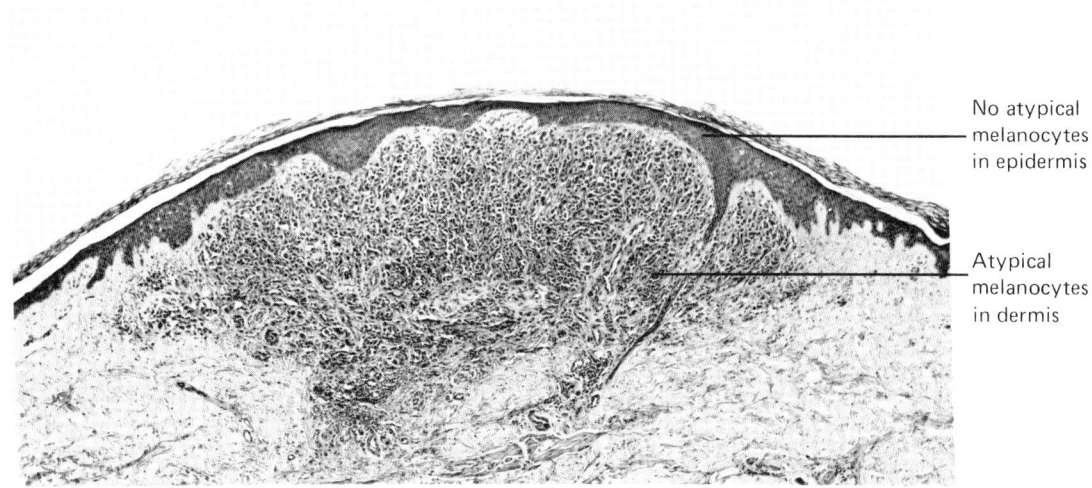

FIGURE 110A. **Malignant melanoma metastatic to the dermis.** *Unlike primary cutaneous malignant melanoma in which atypical melanocytes are found within the epidermis, a metastasis to skin of a malignant melanoma tends to involve the dermis, as pictured here, and/or the subcutaneous fat and to spare the epidermis. Note that the atypical melanocytes are not always evident within vascular channels, may have little or no melanin with their cytoplasms, and may be arranged in small well-circumscribed aggregates. (Reduced from ×50)*

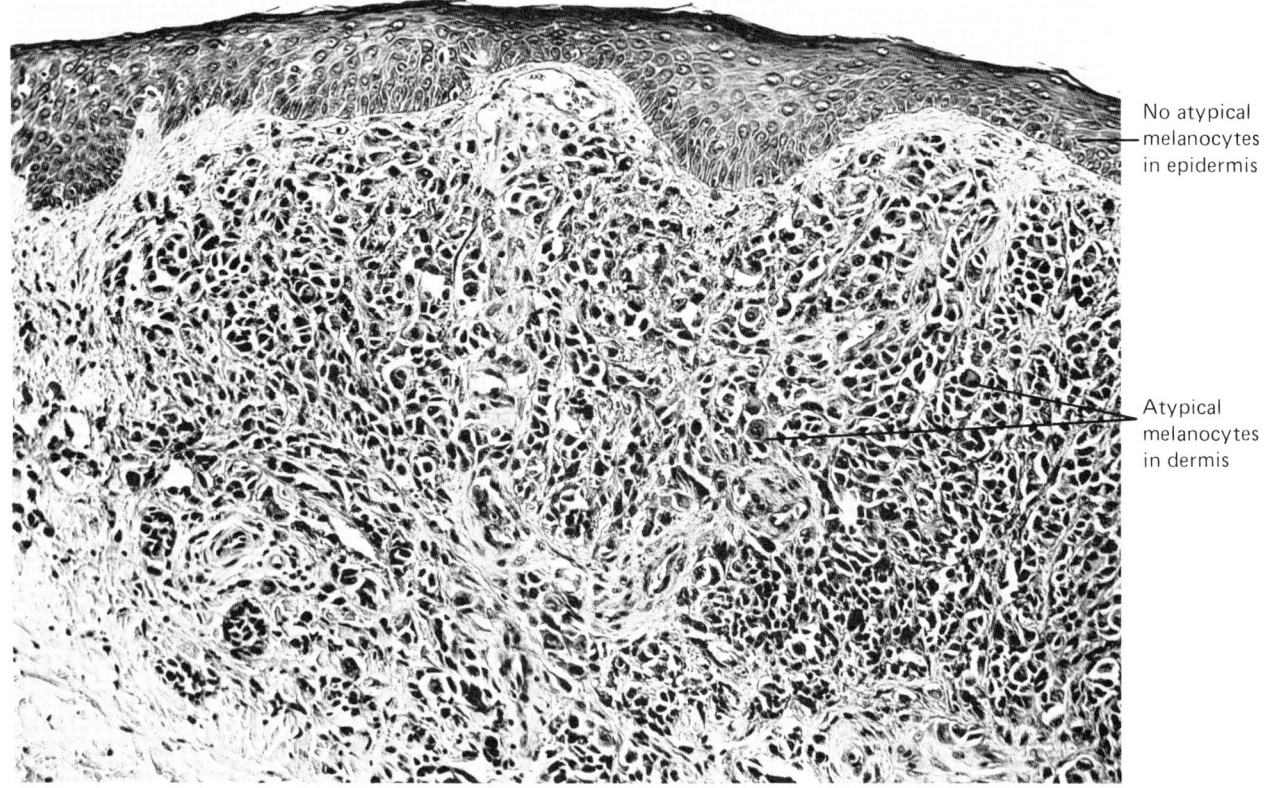

FIGURE 110B. **Malignant melanoma metastatic to the dermis.** *Atypical melanocytes are seen to fill the upper portion of the dermis in this higher magnification of Fig. 110A. The epidermis is devoid of atypical melanocytes in most instances of malignant melanoma that is metastatic in the skin. (Reduced from ×185)*

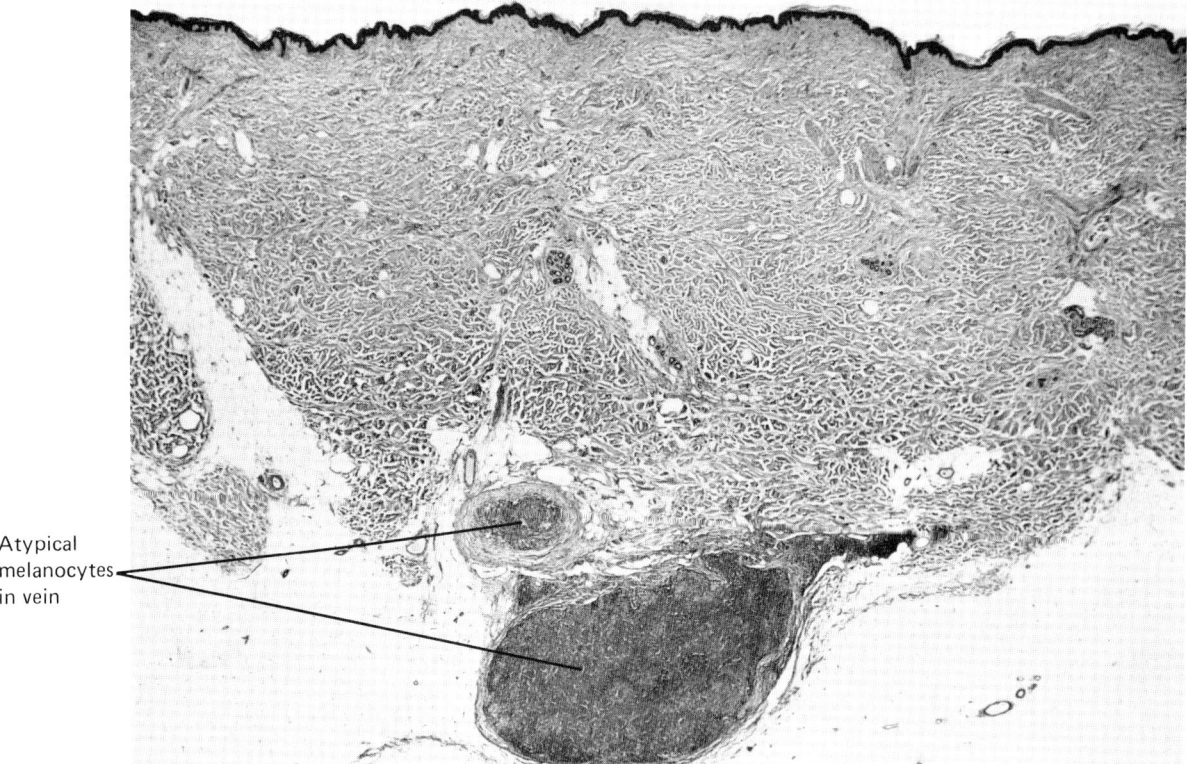

FIGURE 111A. **Metastatic malignant melanoma within a large vein in the subcutis.** *The lumina of the segments of this large vessel are filled with atypical melanocytes from a primary cutaneous malignant melanoma that has metastasized to the skin. In some instances such as this, the metastases of malignant melanoma may be confined wholly to the subcutaneous fat. In other instances, metastases may go to the subcutis and the dermis, sometimes to the dermis alone, and, rarely to the dermis and the epidermis (epidermotropically metastatic malignant melanoma). (Reduced from ×17)*

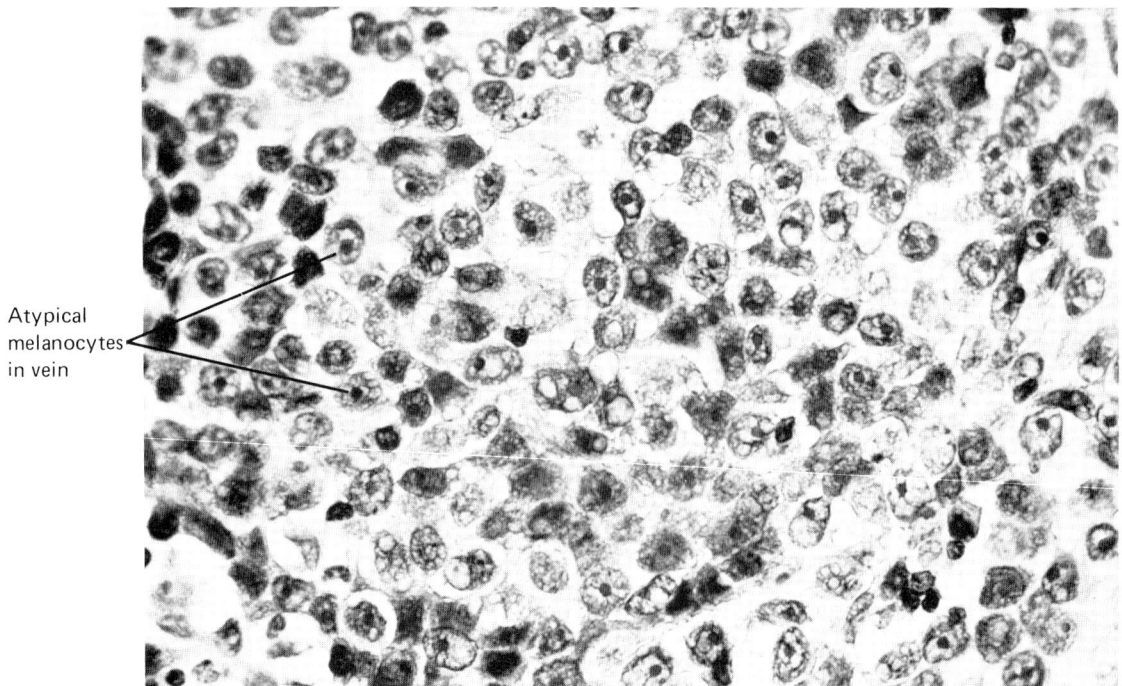

FIGURE 111B. **Metastatic malignant melanoma within a large vein in the subcutis.** *This higher magnification of Fig. 111A shows atypical melanocytes with prominent nucleoli within the lumen of the vein. Note the uniformity of the nuclei in this metastatic malignant melanoma, in contrast to the pleomorphism in primary lesions. (Reduced from ×666)*

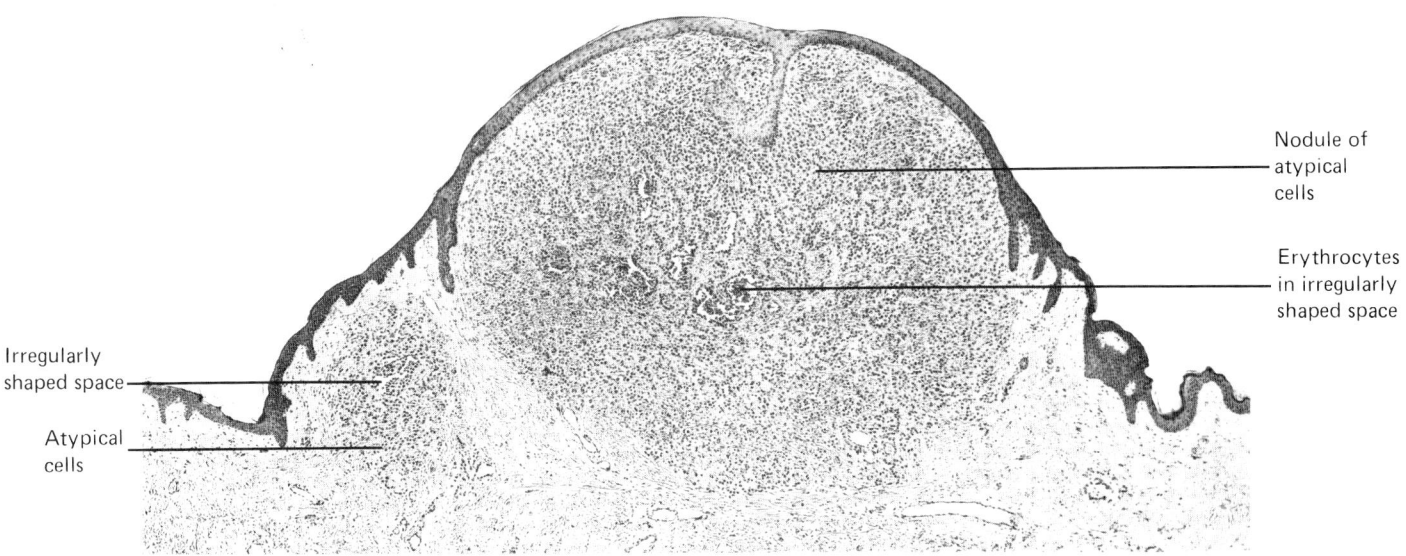

FIGURE 112A. **Metastatic malignant melanoma simulating angiosarcoma.** *The two nodules of atypical cells pictured have irregularly shaped spaces within them that resemble bizarre lumena of blood vessels. In fact, the spaces are curious clefting artifacts within nodules of metastatic malignant melanoma. (Reduced from ×45)*

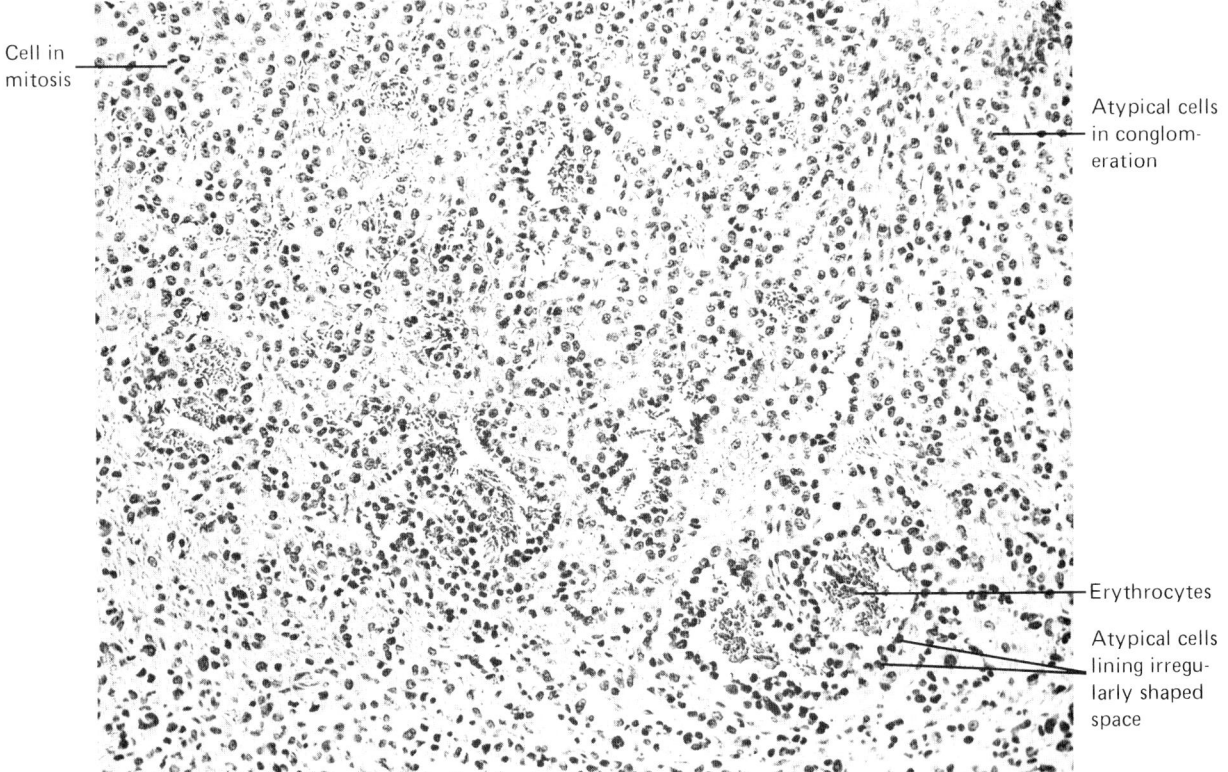

FIGURE 112B. **Metastatic malignant melanoma simulating angiosarcoma.** *In this higher-power magnification of Fig. 112A, the spaces containing erythrocytes can be seen to be lined by atypical cuboidal cells like those in the rest of the small nodule. This patient had many nodules of metastatic malignant melanoma and no clinical evidence whatever of angiosarcoma. (Reduced from ×164)*

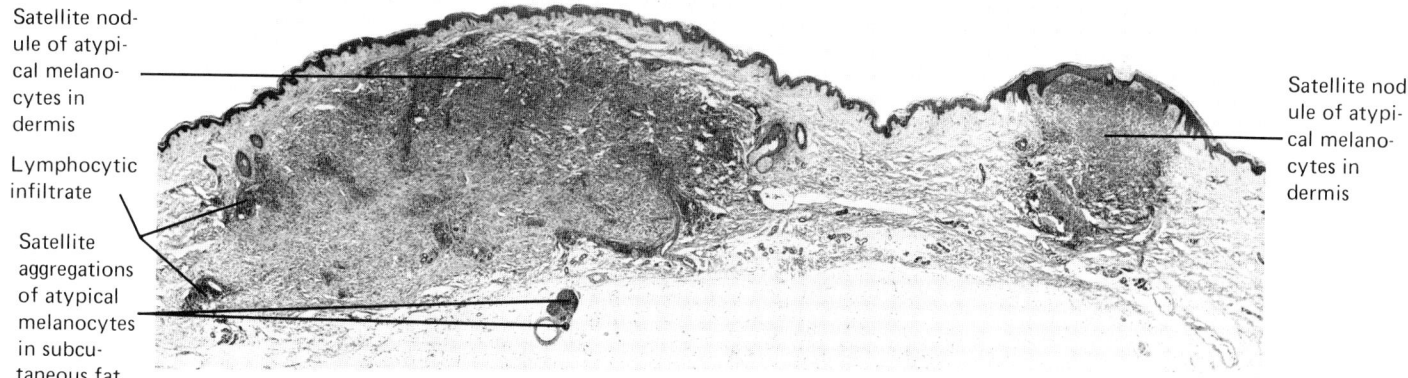

FIGURE 113A. **Satellite (locally metastatic) nodules of malignant melanoma in the dermis and the subcutis.** *Two large foci of metastatic malignant melanoma to the skin may be seen within the dermis, and smaller aggregates are present around the large vessel in the subcutaneous fat. (Reduced from ×13)*

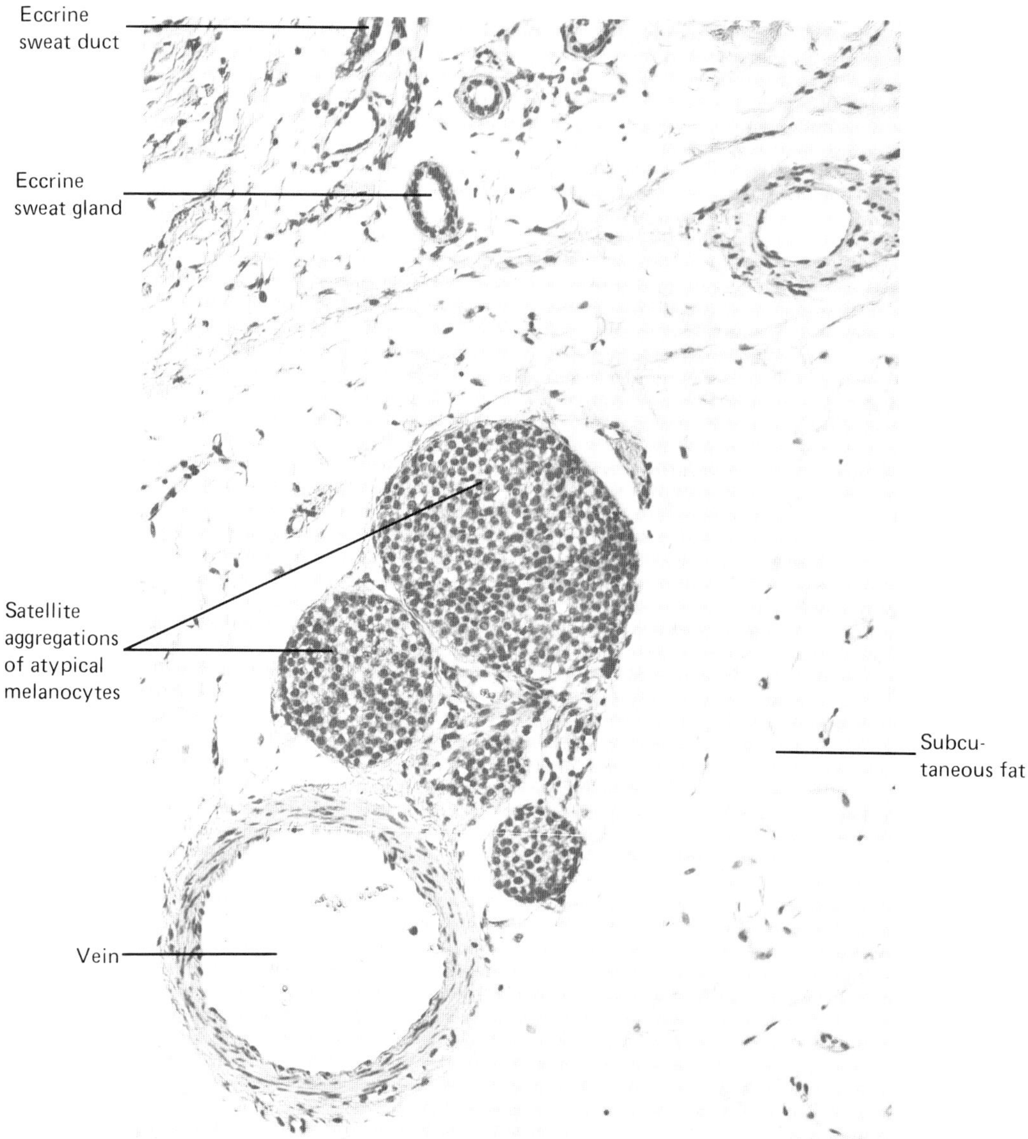

FIGURE 113B. **Satellite nodules of malignant melanoma in the subcutis.** *This higher magnification of Fig. 113A shows endothelial-lined spaces filled completely by atypical melanocytes.* Malignant melanoma metastasizes by both blood and lymph vessels. *(Reduced from ×173)*

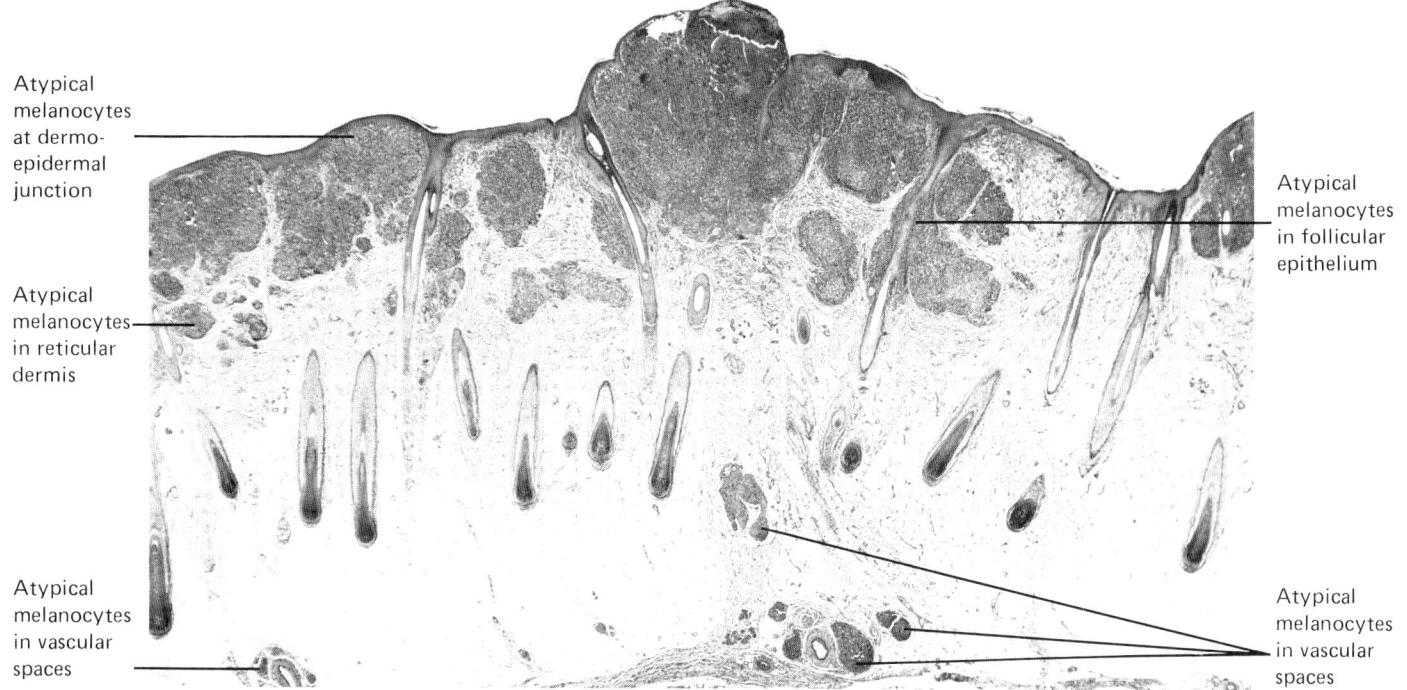

FIGURE 114A. **Malignant melanoma with in-transit metastases.** *This is a primary malignant melanoma because there are many atypical melanocytes at the dermoepidermal junction and within epidermis of this very large lesion. Note the irregularly shaped aggregates of atypical melanocytes within the subcutaneous fat. They are situated within blood vessels there, evidence of metastatic spread. (Reduced from ×14)*

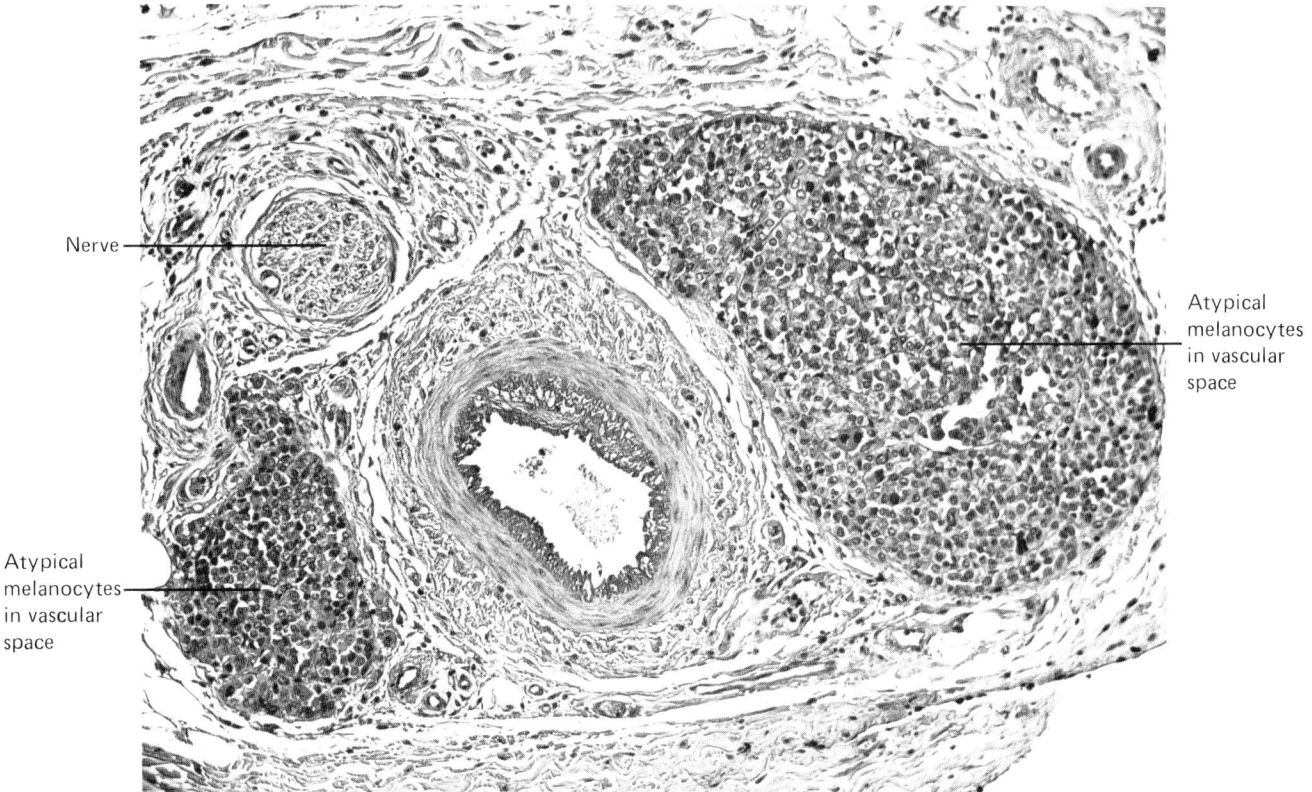

FIGURE 114B. **Malignant melanoma with in-transit metastases.** *Higher magnification of Fig. 114A showing complete occlusion of blood vessels in the subcutis by atypical melanocytes. (Reduced from ×164)*

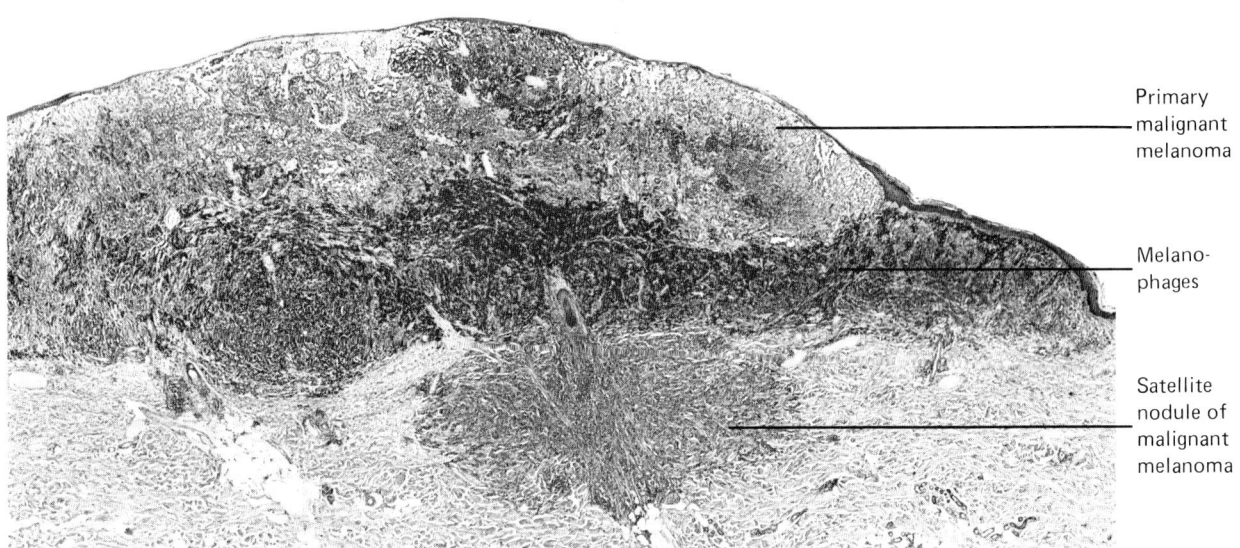

FIGURE 115A. **Satellitosis beneath a primary cutaneous malignant melanoma.** *There are three tiers of distinct histologic features within this lesion, namely, a superficial spreading malignant melanoma, a zone of melanophages, and a nodule that represents a local metastasis of the primary malignant melanoma. That the nodule is truly metastatic can be inferred from the starburst arrangement of the atypical melanocytes, i.e., the cells are interposed between collagen bundles in cords and strands. (Reduced from ×17)*

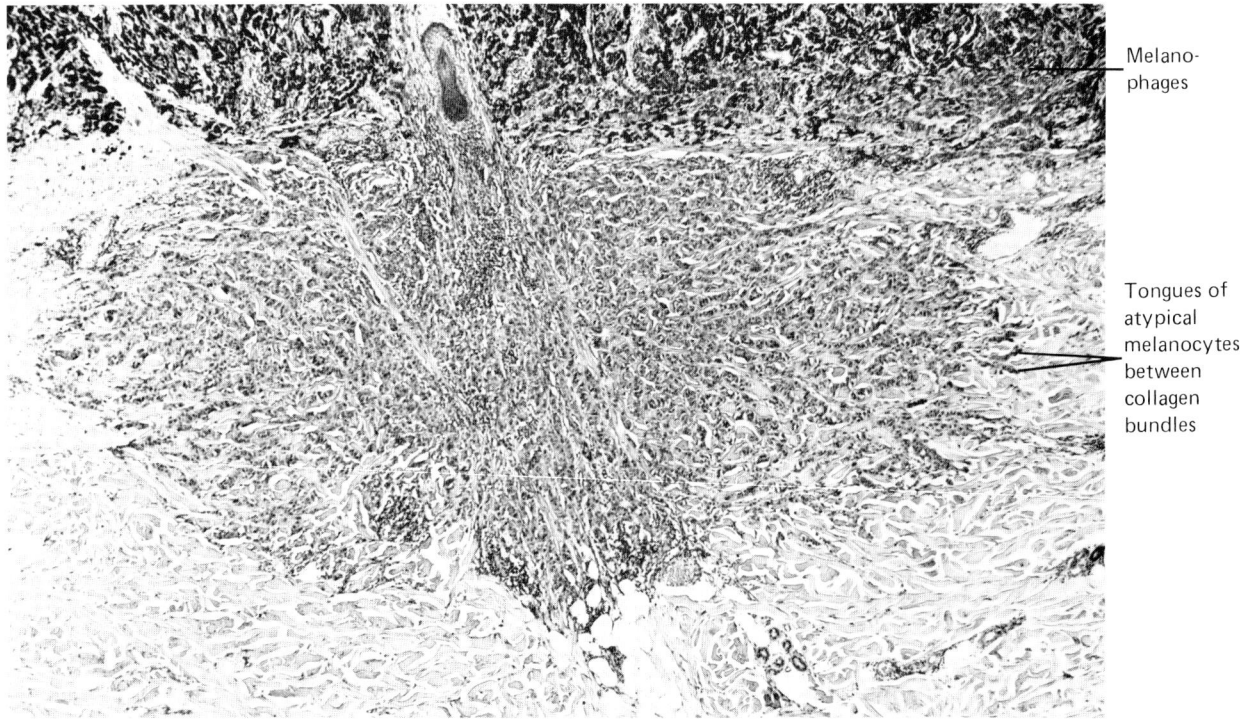

FIGURE 115B. **Satellitosis beneath a primary cutaneous malignant melanoma.** *The "starburst" appearance characteristic of metastatic neoplasms in the skin is well seen in this higher-power view of the malignant melanoma pictured in Fig. 115A. (Reduced from ×47)*

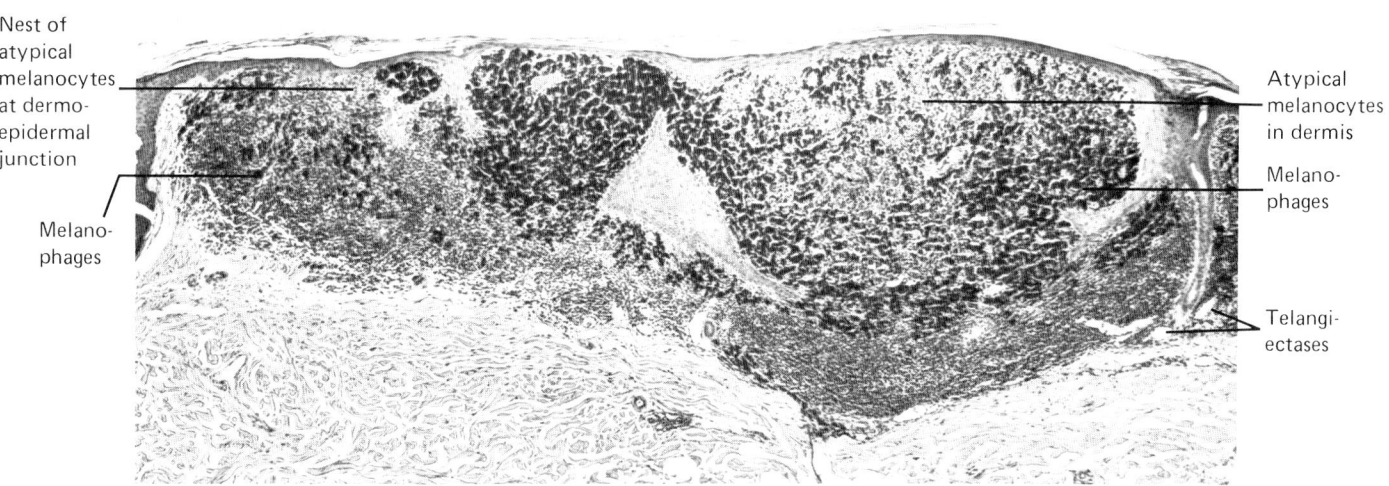

FIGURE 116A. ***Malignant melanoma, superficial spreading type, with extensive melanosis.*** *Most of the pigmented cells pictured in this photomicrograph are melanophages rather than atypical melanocytes. The diagnosis of malignant melanoma is made on the basis of changes within the epidermis and the dermis, namely, atypical melanocytes there. The presence of melanophages per se is not helpful in differentiating benign from malignant melanocytic lesions. Numerous melanophages may be present in benign melanocytic processes, such as blue nevi and some forms of Spitz's nevus, as well as in malignant melanomas. (Reduced from ×55)*

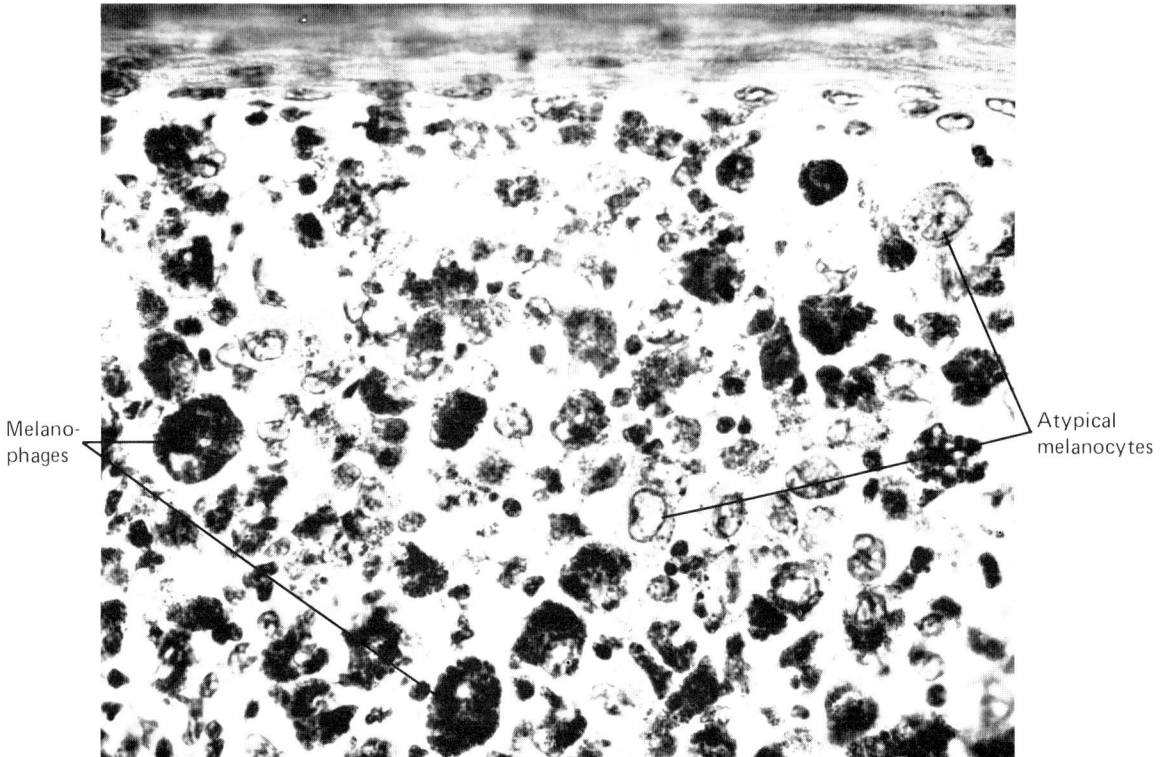

FIGURE 116B. ***Malignant melanoma, superficial spreading type, with extensive melanosis.*** *Higher magnification of Fig. 116A shows atypical melanocytes that are relatively unpigmented as well as heavily pigmented macrophages. If nuclear detail cannot be discerned in heavily pigmented lesions such as this, the specimen should be bleached with potassium permanganate. Then more accurate cytologic judgments can be made about melanocytes and macrophages. (Reduced from ×655)*

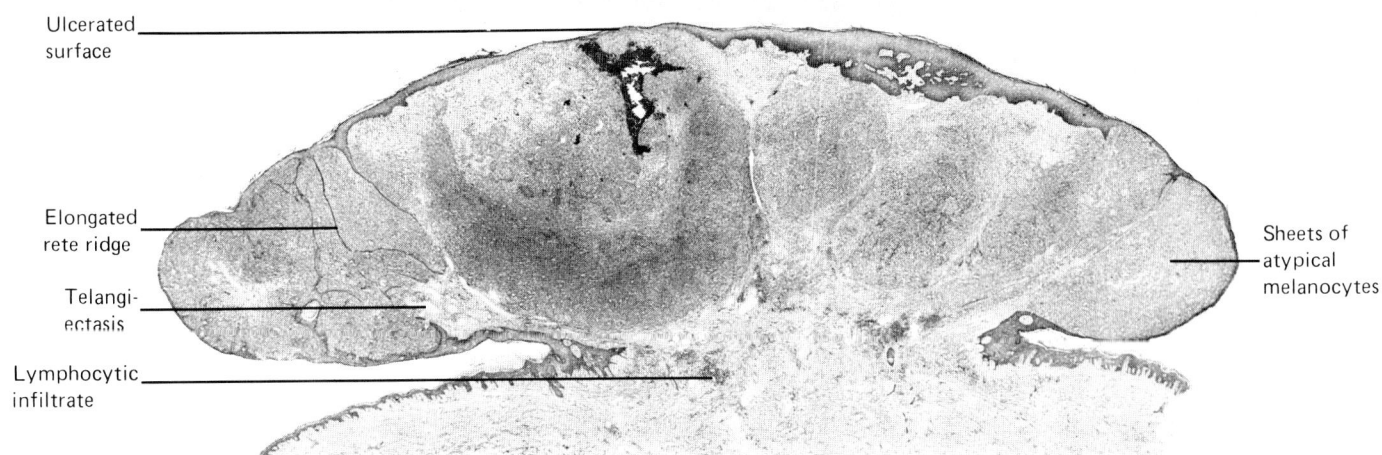

FIGURE 117A. **Sessile malignant melanoma.** *All the atypical melanocytes within the specimen in this exophytic variant of malignant melanoma are situated above the skin surface. Such a lesion offers problems for assigning a level according to the criteria of Clark because the melanocytes are wholly above the normal papillary dermis (above level II) and yet a neoplasm such as this one carries a grave prognosis. (Reduced from ×9.5)*

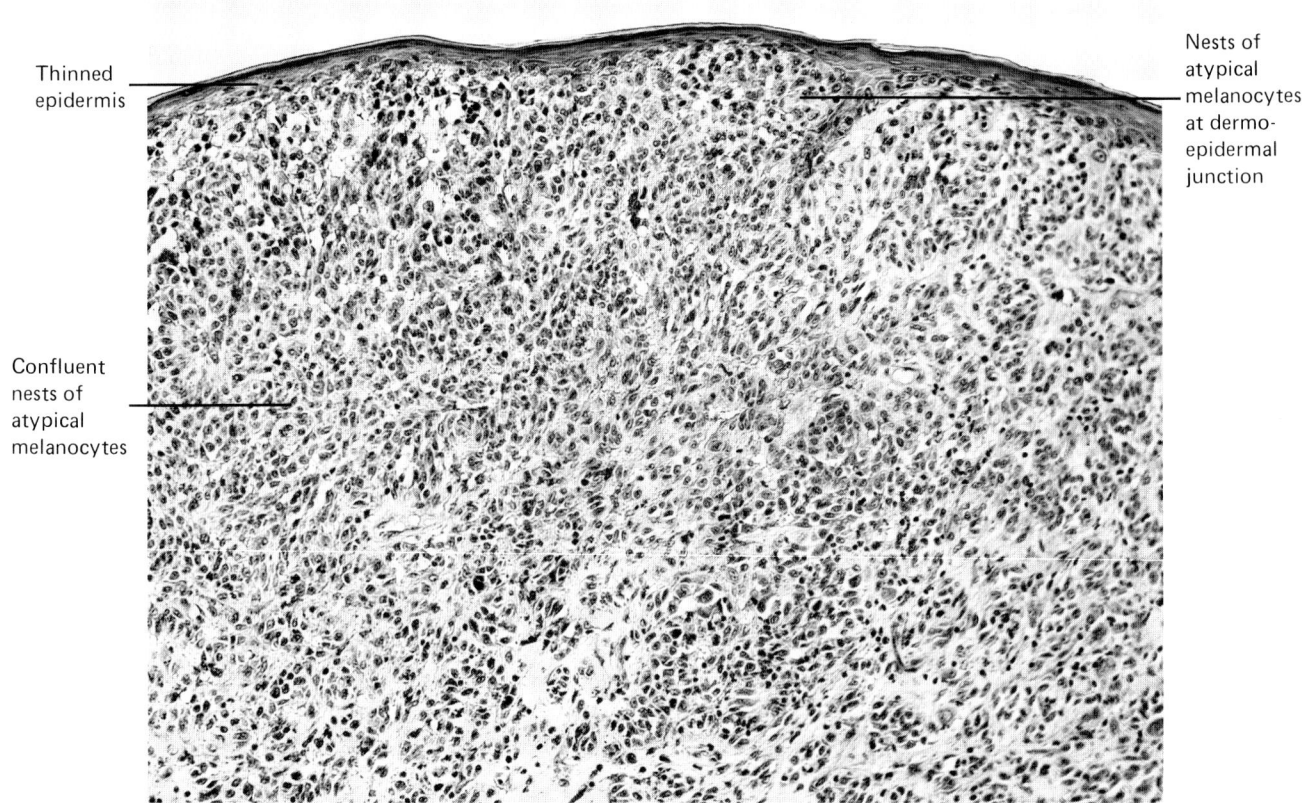

FIGURE 117B. **Sessile malignant melanoma.** *Higher-power view of Fig. 117A showing atypical melanocytes at the dermoepidermal interface and in nests and sheets throughout the dermis. (Reduced from ×164)*

incidence of our series than that of others may be the result of our practice of cutting numerous sections through specimens or because many of the malignant melanomas we see are early ones that have not yet obliterated preexisting nevi. What is the meaning of this association and why is there so rarely a junction nevus conjoined with a malignant melanoma in our material, which now consists of thousands of cases of malignant melanomas? There must be something special about the melanocytes in the epidermis overlying an intradermal nevus, something different from the melanocytes in normal skin. How else can one explain the fact that so many malignant melanomas, especially of the superficial spreading type, arise within the epidermis above the geographic boundaries of intradermal nevi? Perhaps these melanocytes possess particular inherent biologic urges or perhaps messages are transmitted to them by the subjacent nevus cells. In any case, the uniqueness of this population of melanocytes within the epidermis above an intradermal nevus must be recognized. Connective tissue altered by sunlight (solar elastosis), radiotherapy, vaccinations, and genetics (e.g., xeroderma pigmentosum) also may induce melanocytes within the epidermis to transform into malignant melanoma.

As a corollary to these observations about the relationship of atypical melanocytes within the epidermis to nevus cells, it should be mentioned once again that the evolution of malignant melanoma begins with proliferation of individual melanocytes situated in the basal layer of the epidermis or at the dermoepidermal junction. Malignant melanomas do not arise from nests of melanocytes that comprise a junction nevus. In our view, the cells in the nests of junction nevi do not convert into malignant melanomas, any more than the sebaceous glands in a nevus sebaceus of Jadassohn become basal-cell carcinomas. Malignant melanomas germinate in the soil of some intradermal nevi, just as basal-cell carcinomas develop in the terrain of some lesions of nevus sebaceus.

Unusual appearing melanocytic nevi, often large junction or compound types, do occur from time to time in women during pregnancy, in patients who have a concurrent malignant melanoma elsewhere in the skin, and in individuals with family histories of malignant melanomas. These unusual melanocytic nevi must be differentiated histologically from authentic malignant melanomas that may also develop during pregnancy, in more than one cutaneous location in the same patient at the same time, or in persons whose blood relatives have had malignant melanomas. The unusual melanocytic nevi and superficial spreading malignant melanomas share features in common, namely, both may be broad, contain nests of melanocytes within the epidermis that vary in size and shape and that tend to confluence, involve hair follicles and eccrine ducts, and show alterations of the papillary dermis, such as thickening by coarse or lamellar collagen and by an inflammatory-cell infiltrate. The epidermis of these unusual melanocytic nevi is often hyperplastic, but the nuclei of the melanocytes are not significantly atypical and their cytoplasms are not pagetoid, i.e., are not abundant, pale staining, and replete with "dusty" melanin. Whether such lesions are actually wholly benign melanocytic nevi, precursors of malignant melanomas, or even evolving malignant melanomas is still to be learned (Fig. 121). In any event, if doubt about the diagnosis exists, the dubious lesion should be completely excised.

How can one explain the remarkable variations in the appearances of cells of malignant melanomas—small, cuboidal (epithelioid), pagetoid, balloon, spindle-shaped, mucin-containing, and dendritic? And how is it that, as a rule, the intraepidermal melanocytes in lentigo maligna melanoma are spindle-shaped, in superficial spreading melanoma pagetoid, in nodular melanoma cuboidal, and in acral lentiginous melanoma dendritic? The answers to these questions are not really known, but perhaps are related to subtle cytologic differences in the normal melanocytes in different regions of the normal skin. For example, the ratio of keratinocytes to melanocytes on the skin of the face is relatively low; the melanocytes are crowded together there and are somewhat spindle-shaped, like those in lentigo maligna melanoma which occurs mostly on the face. Melanocytes on the palms and soles tend to be dendritic, like those in acral lentiginous melanoma. In addition, the cytologic appearance and biologic behavior of the keratinocytes have a telling effect on their neighboring melanocytes. Thus, sunburn, which causes keratinocytes to divide more rapidly, will inevitably affect the melanocytes not only directly, but also indirectly by the affects upon them of sun-damaged keratinocytes. Sunlight, which has a profound effect on the epidermis and papillary dermis, especially of the face, has practically no impact on the skin of the palms and soles. Therefore, the role of sunlight upon the structure of melanocytes, directly and indirectly by alterations in keratinocytes and in the connective tissue of the papillary dermis, may be a factor in the different appearances of melanocytes in malignant melanomas on different body sites.

For decades, surgeons have justified the use of wide (5 cm of normal skin around the circumference of a malignant melanoma) and deep (to and often including the fascia) excisions as necessary for the possible cure of malignant melanomas. To do less than a "wide and deep" procedure,

The Histology of Cutaneous Malignant Melanoma

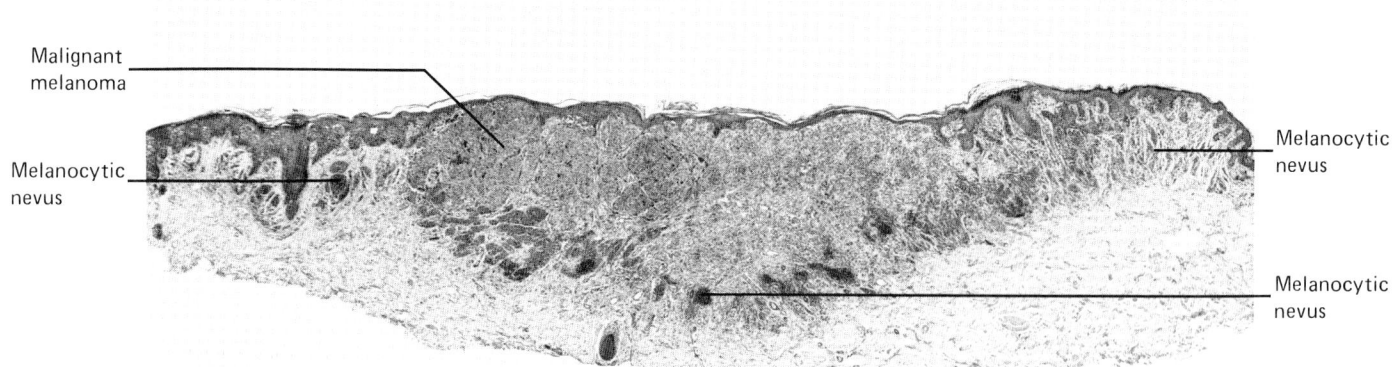

FIGURE 118A. **Malignant melanoma, superficial spreading type, in which there is an intermingling of atypical melanocytes and cells of a melanocytic nevus.** Under scanning power, as in this photomicrograph, it is often easier to differentiate the melanocytes of a malignant melanoma from those of a melanocytic nevus than it is with high power. The paler cells that tend to confluence in the center of the specimen are atypical melanocytes of a malignant melanoma, whereas the darker-staining cells in discrete nests at the periphery are those of a benign melanocytic nevus. (Reduced from ×22)

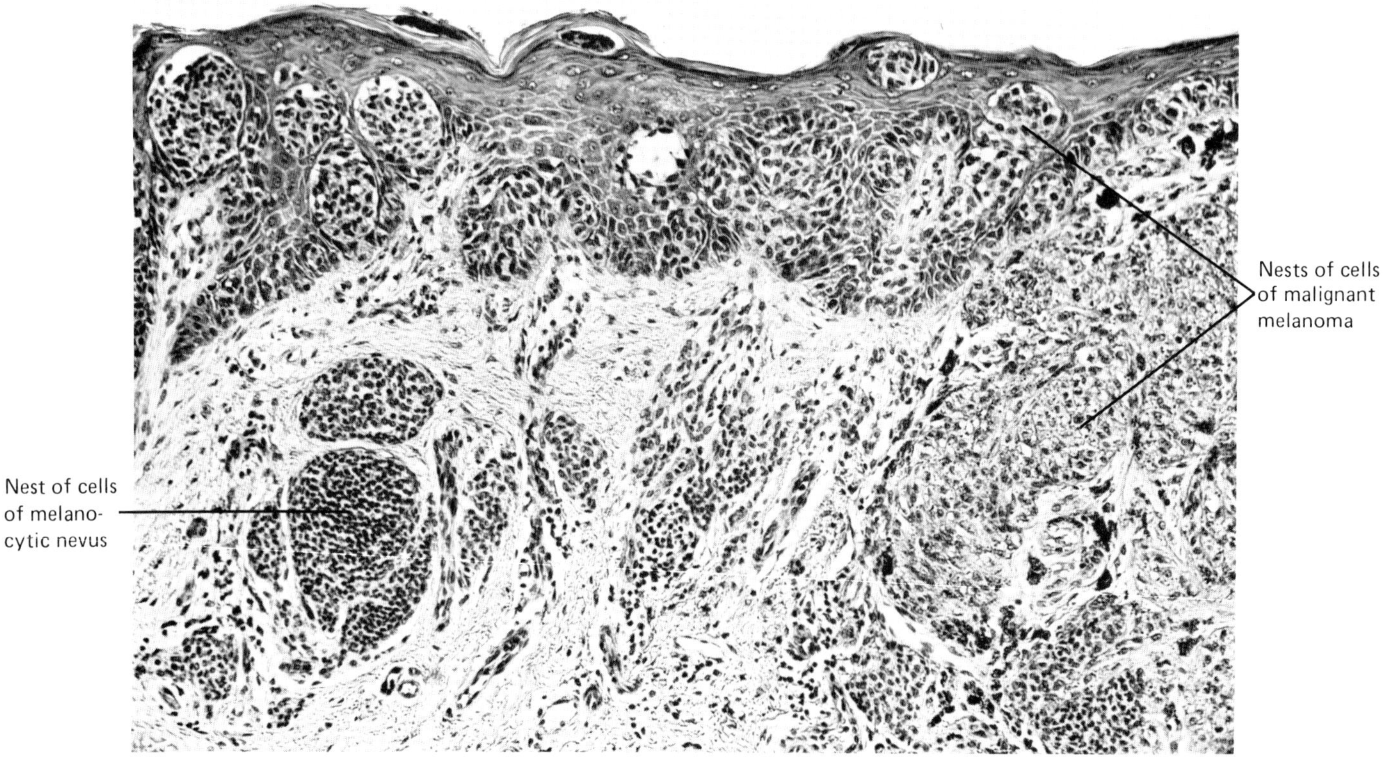

FIGURE 118B. **Malignant melanoma, superficial spreading type, in which there is an intermingling of atypical melanocytes and cells of a melanocytic nevus.** Higher magnification of Fig. 118A shows atypical melanocytes of a malignant melanoma in the epidermis and in the dermis on the right of this photomicrograph and nests of cells of a melanocytic nevus in the dermis on the left. (Reduced from ×180)

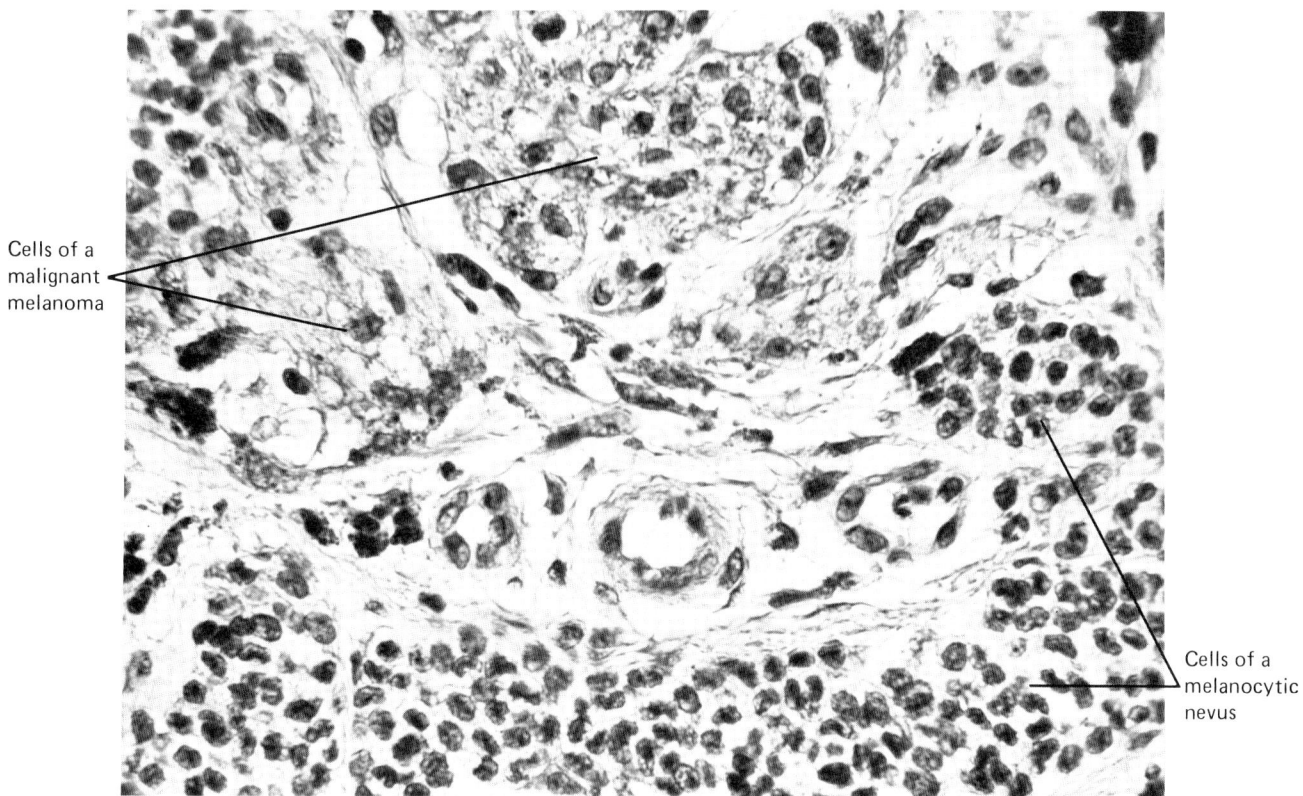

FIGURE 118C. **Malignant melanoma, superficial spreading type, in which there is an intermingling of atypical melanocytes and cells of a melanocytic nevus.** *In the upper left portion of this still higher magnification of Fig. 118B are atypical melanocytes and to the right and in the lower half are cells of a melanocytic nevus. Sometimes it is difficult to differentiate finely between the two cell types, which complicates accurate measurement of the thickness of a malignant melanoma with an ocular micrometer. (Reduced from ×700)*

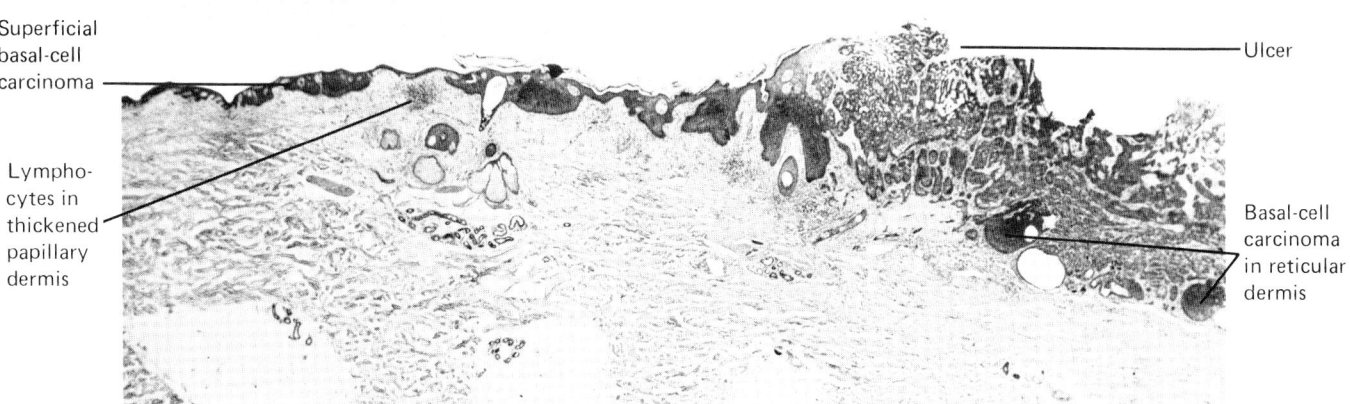

FIGURE 119. **Basal-cell carcinoma, superficial type.** *This photomicrograph illustrates the analogy between basal-cell carcinoma of the superficial type and malignant melanoma of the superficial spreading type. On the left-hand portion of this photomicrograph the superficial basal-cell carcinoma is comparable to a malignant melanoma in situ, whereas on the right, the ulcerated-nodular basal-cell carcinoma is comparable to a nodule of malignant melanoma. The principles that pertain to these basal-cell carcinomas and to malignant melanomas apply equally to the relationship between solar keratoses and squamous-cell carcinomas. (Reduced from ×18)*

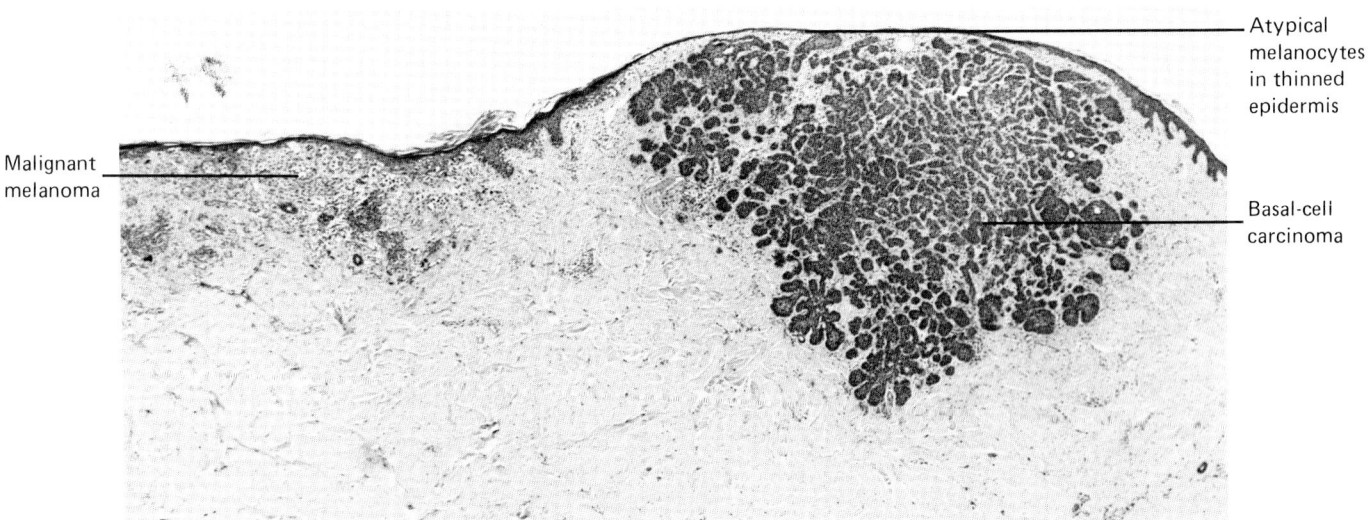

FIGURE 120A. **Malignant melanoma contiguous with basal-cell carcinoma (collision lesion).** *On the left-hand portion of this photomicrograph there is a superficial spreading malignant melanoma. On the right there is a typical basal-cell carcinoma. (Reduced from ×30)*

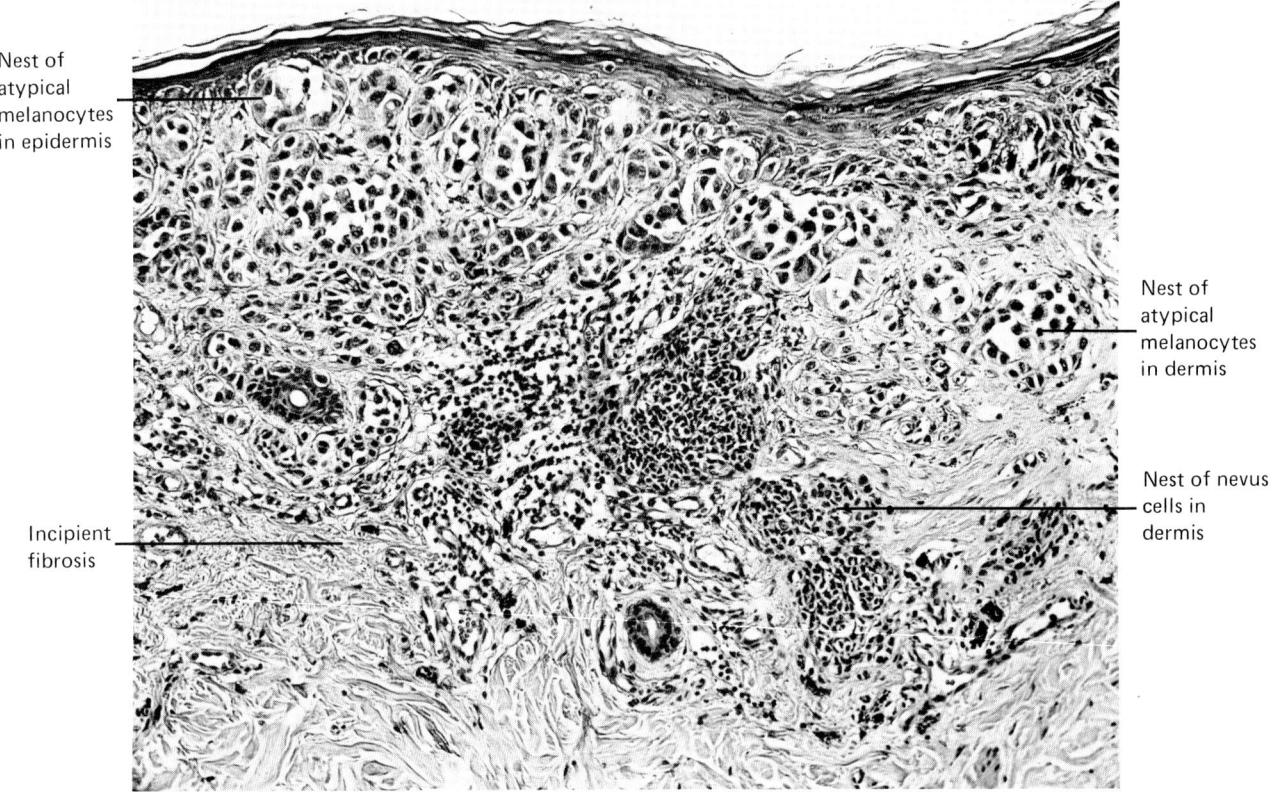

FIGURE 120B. **Malignant melanoma contiguous with basal-cell carcinoma (collision lesion).** *This higher-power view of a portion of Fig. 120A shows pagetoid melanocytes, singly and in nests, within the epidermis and within the papillary dermis where there is a dense lymphohistiocytic infiltrate. Note the different cytologic features in the malignant melanoma and the subjacent intradermal melanocytic nevus. (Reduced from ×164)*

according to many surgeons, risks the possibility of local recurrence at the scar from primary closure or at the margin of the skin graft. The logic for doing wide and deep excisions of malignant melanomas when anatomically feasible is said to be the attempt to catch in transit and satellite metastases before more widespread dissemination has taken place. The fact that some narrowly excised malignant melanomas have recurred in surgical scars or at the margins of skin grafts does not necessarily prove that the method of spread was by metastases within the skin. It could be that not all of the atypical melanocytes that extended horizontally within the epidermis had been completely removed. These biologically malignant melanocytes often extend many rete ridges beyond what is appreciated clinically as pigmentation. Therefore, it is incumbent upon the surgeon to carry his excision beyond the zone of detectable pigmentation of a malignant melanoma and for the pathologist to review the sections with particular attention to the presence of increased number of melanocytes (not all of them necessarily atypical) in the zone of what was clinically normal skin in order to ensure complete removal of the neoplastic cells.

So far as the depth of the surgical excision is concerned, surely some of the subcutaneous fat should be taken, but to include the fascia or even tissue near it for a thin malignant melanoma (one that measures less than 0.76 mm and possibly up to 1.5 mm in thickness) seems excessive. In any event, careful studies should be undertaken jointly by surgeons and pathologists to clarify these issues of breadth and depth of excisions of malignant melanomas.

Some groups interested in malignant melanoma have recommended that all congenital nevi, irrespective of size, be excised early in life in order to prevent possible supervention of malignant melanoma within them. We are not impressed by the evidence of others or by our own experience that there is a significant incidence of malignant melanoma developing in small congenital nevi (less than about 5 cm in diameter). Furthermore, it our impression that malignant melanomas that do arise in congenital melanocytic nevi do so first within the epidermis, just as do all other malignant melanomas that are primary in the skin. Many malignant melanomas that are said to begin within the population of nevus cells in the dermis or the subcutaneous fat, are actually pigmented malignant schwannomas and others may in reality be satellite metastases, rather than primary malignant melanomas. In hairy congenital nevi, both small and large, it would perhaps be preferable to shave the hairs periodically and to study the lesions for clinical signs of evolving malignant melanomas rather than attempt to remove all congenital nevi. Suspicious pigmentary changes within a congenital nevus should certainly be biopsied.

We cannot write about malignant blue nevus because we have so little personal experience with it. Such lesions must be exceedingly rare. A pathologist who entertains a diagnosis of malignant blue nevus should also consider that the lesion may be a metastatic malignant melanoma, a nodular melanoma in which no atypical melanocytes can be discerned within the epidermis, or a desmoplastic malignant melanoma. Search for indubitable evidence of a typical blue nevus in the very same lesion should be undertaken before a diagnosis of malignant blue nevus is rendered with finality.

Lastly, there is the enigmatic presence of focal acantholytic dyskeratosis (Fig. 122) and/or epidermolytic hyperkeratosis within the epidermis to the sides of malignant melanomas in about 5% of step-sectioned superficial spreading melanomas. These distinctive histologic features that reflect alterations in epidermal metabolism are usually confined to only one or two rete ridges. Perhaps when associated with malignant melanoma, they represent a response to some diffusable soluble product elaborated by the atypical melanocytes.

XII. LABORATORY PROCEDURES RELEVANT TO MALIGNANT MELANOMA

A. Biopsy

A crucial consideration in the attempt at definitive diagnosis of malignant melanoma and accurate measurement of thickness or level of invasion is an adequate biopsy specimen for histopathologic examination. Although there is no certain evidence that incisional or punch biopsy of a malignant melanoma has a detrimental effect on the future biological behavior of a malignant melanoma or on the survival rate of patients (Jones et al., 1968; Epstein et al., 1969; Knutson et al., 1971), it is preferable that biopsy be excision *in toto* when possible on all lesions suspected of being malignant melanoma. Occasionally, the lesion may be too large or situated anatomically in such a way that total excision is impractical or impossible. Then, an attempt should be made to take a thoroughly adequate specimen for histologic examination. We cannot emphasize too strongly that for diagnostic and prognostic purposes shave biopsies are often unsatisfactory for lesions suspected of being malignant melanoma (Fig. 123). Should there be involvement of the deeper part of the dermis, the pathologist may not be able to make the correct diagnosis and cannot measure the entire thickness of the lesion (Fig. 124). As a consequence, the clinician will be deprived of precise guidelines for best management of the patient. In our experience, misinterpretations of melanocytic lesions have, in almost every in-

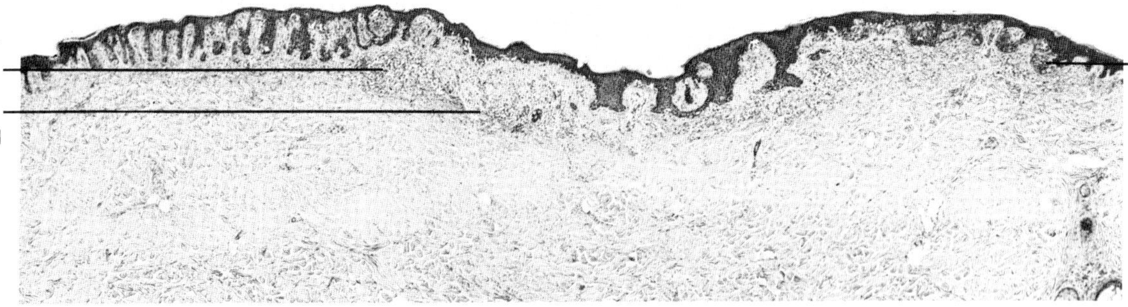

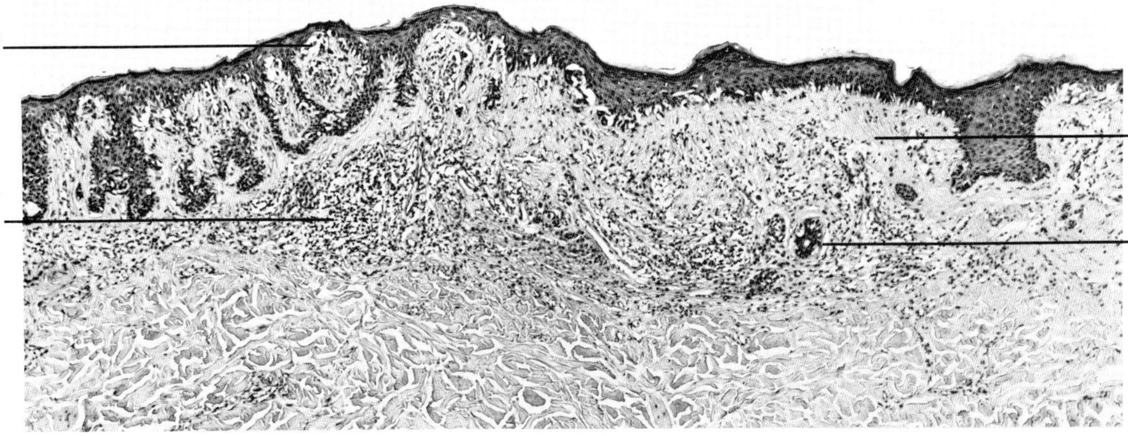

FIGURE 121A & B. **Unusual proliferation of melanocytes, in situ.** *The early histologic changes of malignant melanoma are often very subtle and may be mistaken for a junction nevus. Clues to the more likely potentially malignant nature of this lesion are its breadth, the variation in size and shape of the nests of melanocytes and their tendency to confluence, the extension of the melanocytes into epithelium of adnexal structures, and the papillary dermis, which is thickened by coarse laminated collagen and an inflammatory-cell infiltrate. This patient, it happens, previously had an indubitable malignant melanoma. Lesions with similar proliferations of melanocytes may occur in persons with family histories of malignant melanoma. (Reduced from ×65)*

FIGURE 121D. **Unusual proliferation of melanocytes, in situ.** *This large, peculiarly shaped aggregate of melanocytes surrounds an eccrine sweat duct. The crucial question about the melanocytic process pictured in Figs. 121A to 121D is whether it is simply an unusual melanocytic nevus of the junction type or a true malignant melanoma in situ. It is in instances such as this that an absolute judgment cannot always be made with utter confidence and the better part of wisdom is to advise conservative, but complete, excision. (Reduced from ×400)* See bottom figure face page.

stance, occurred in specimens that were removed by shave excisions. The shave procedure deprives the pathologist of the lateral and deep margins of the pigmented lesion where the crucial histologic features for the differentiation of a melanocytic nevus from a malignant melanoma are found (Fig. 125). We suggest that when feasible the biopsies of suspected malignant melanomas be fusiform with an approximately 3 to 5 mm margin around the lesion and deep enough to include some of the subcutaneous tissue (Fig. 81).

B. Sectioning and Processing of a Specimen Suspected of Being Malignant Melanoma

A biopsy specimen suspected of being a malignant melanoma should be placed into a solution of 10% neutral

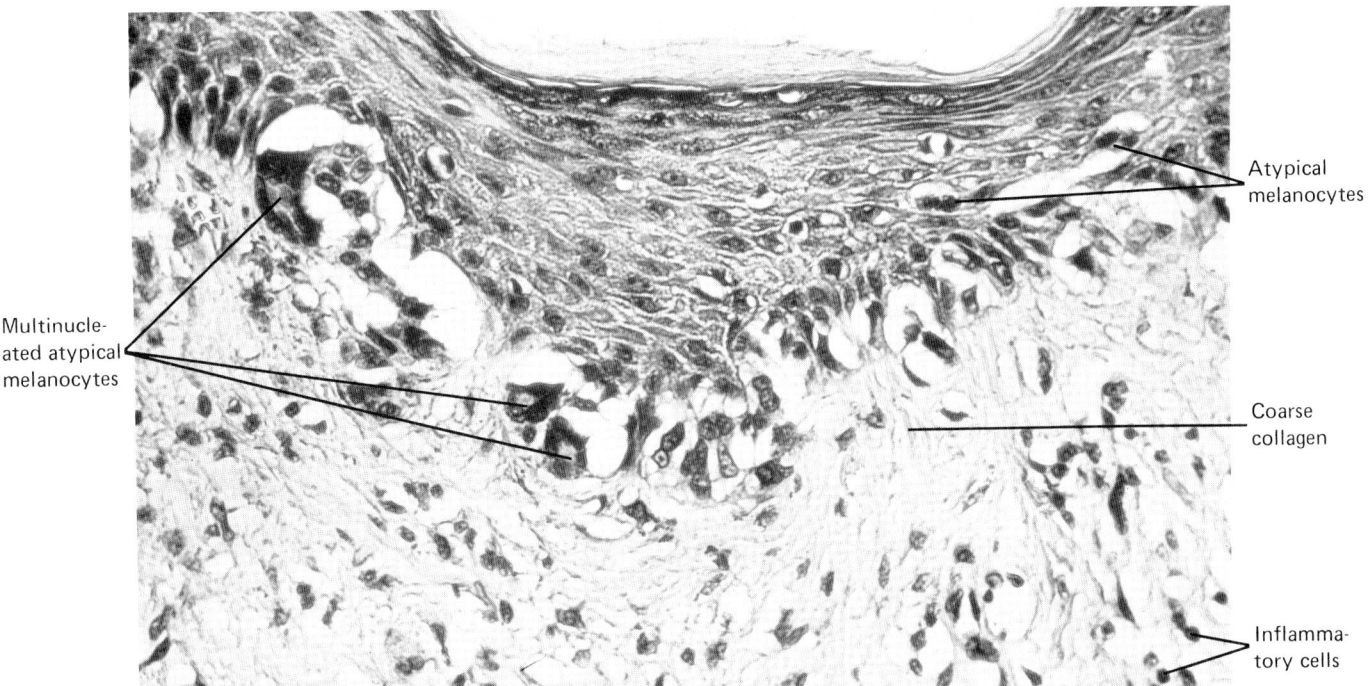

FIGURE 121C. *Unusual proliferation of melanocytes*, **in situ**. *Not only is there hyperplasia of melanocytes at the dermoepidermal junction, singly and in nests, but there are some melanocytes in the mid-spinous zone. Other melanocytes are multincleated. Note also the marked alteration of the collagen in the thickened papillary dermis. (Reduced from ×443)*

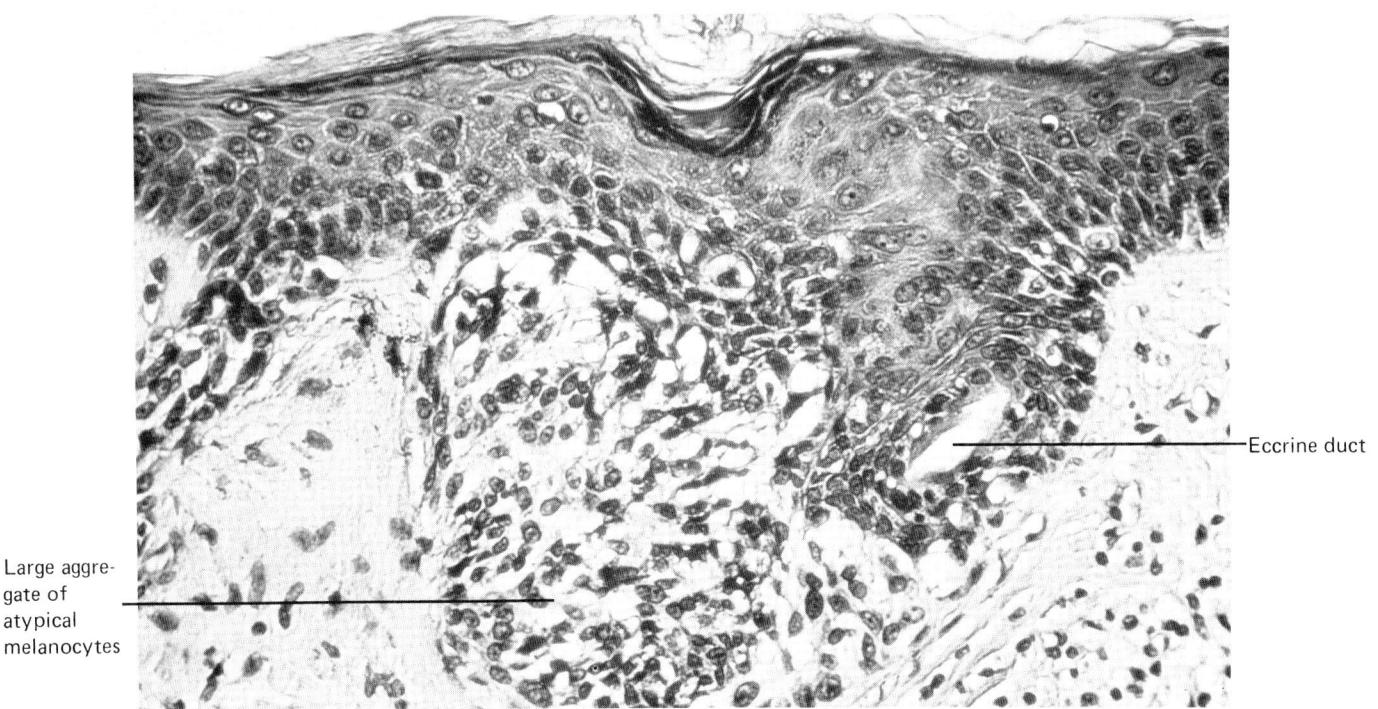

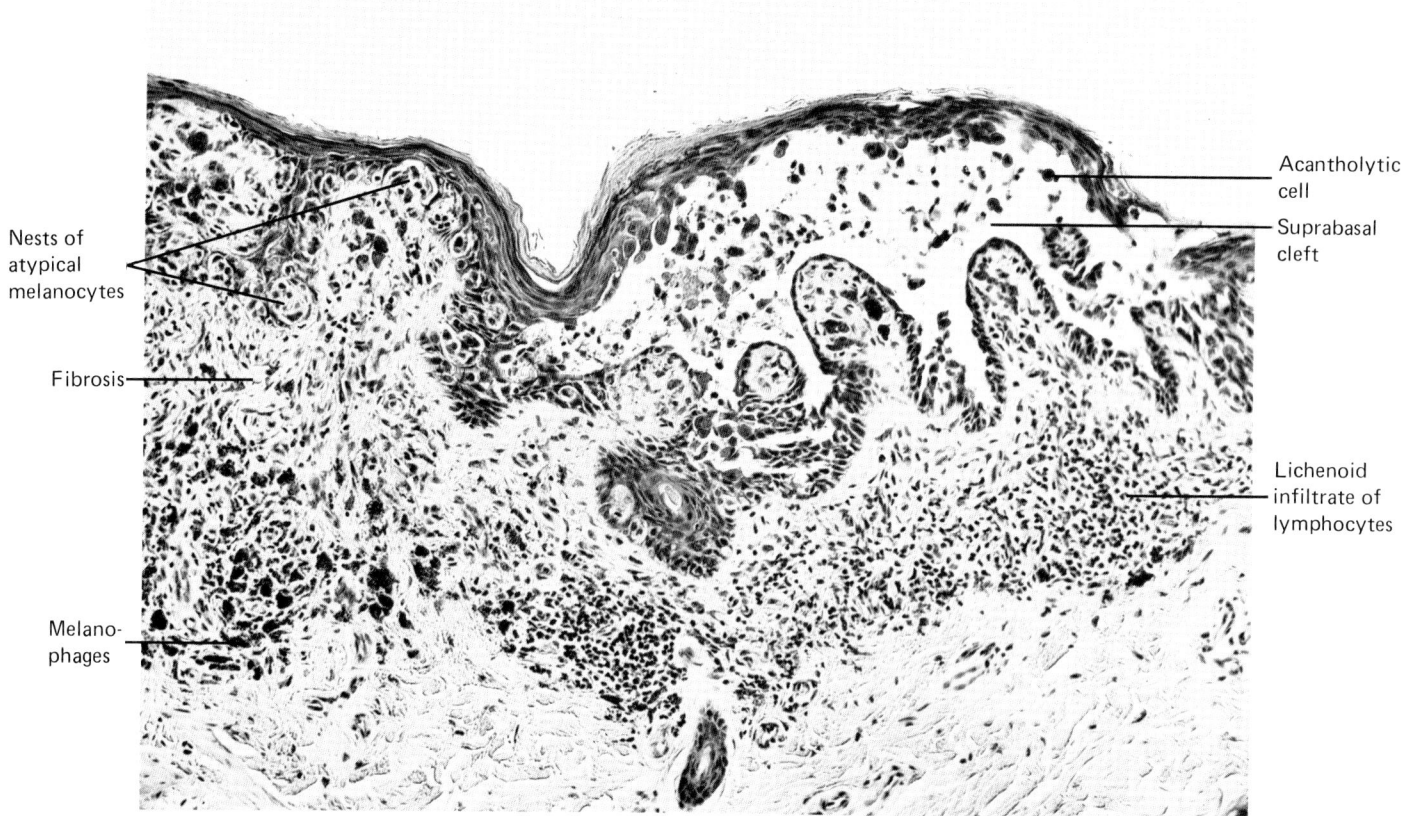

FIGURE 122. **Focal acantholytic dyskeratosis in association with malignant melanoma.** *On the left-hand portion of this photomicrograph there is a superficial spreading malignant melanoma, and on the right there is focal acantholytic dyskeratosis, namely, suprabasal clefts above which there are acantholytic and dyskeratotic cells. This histologic finding is not uncommonly associated with superficial spreading malignant melanoma. Focal acantholytic dyskeratosis is also seen in a variety of other diseases such as keratosis follicularis (Darier's disease) and transient acantholytic dermatosis (Grover's disease). (Reduced from ×173)*

buffered formalin (or, if electron microscopy is also contemplated, in modified Milonig's fixative, which is also effective for sections visualized by conventional microscopy). If the specimen is large, it should be placed in a container whose volume of fixative is at least 20 times that of the biopsy specimen in order to assure adequate fixation. When the laboratory receives the specimen, the tissue should be grossed in such a way that cross sections are taken at approximately 3 mm intervals at right angles to the long axis of the specimen as shown in Fig. 126. Each piece of cross-sectioned tissue should then be labeled and put into a different cassette for processing. In specimens not suspected clinically of being malignant melanoma, both halves of the bisected tissue should be processed for eventual histologic examination (Fig. 127). In almost every instance, a precise diagnosis can be made on sections stained by hematoxylin and eosin. Sometimes in heavily pigmented lesions it may be necessary to bleach the specimen with potassium permanganate in order to better study nuclear detail. In neoplasms suspected of being amelanotic malignant melanoma, the Fontana-Masson stain may be helpful in revealing melanin within the neoplastic cells. Electron microscopy may also be useful in these cases by revealing melanosomes within the cytoplasms of atypical cells. Special stains, such as the reticulin, are said (McGovern, 1975) to be helpful in differentiating malignant melanomas from unusual melanocytic nevi, but we have come to a contrary conclusion about their value.

C. ROLE OF FROZEN SECTIONS

Little and Davis (1974) reviewed the experience at Princess Alexandra Hospital in Brisbane, Australia re-

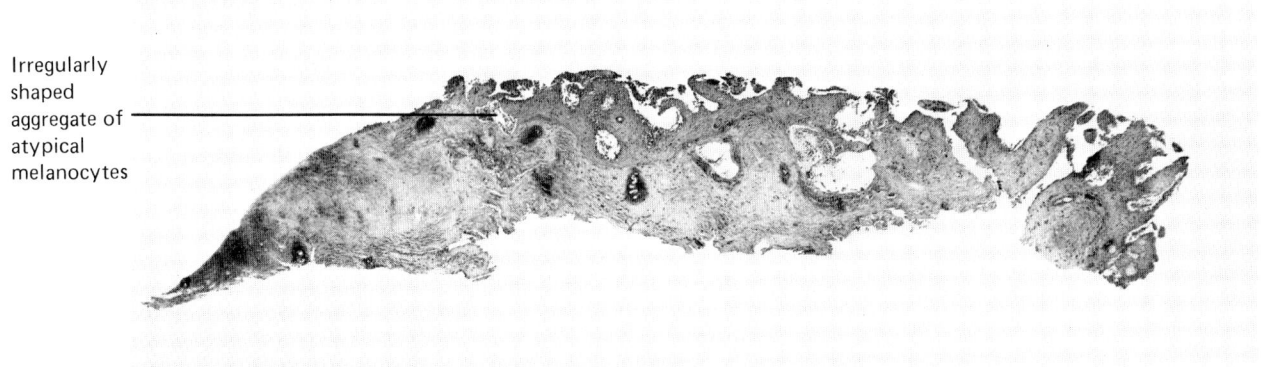

FIGURE 123A. ***Specimen of malignant melanoma removed by shave excision.*** *This thin specimen from a hand consists wholly of epidermis within which there are diffusely scattered atypical melanocytes, diagnostic of malignant melanoma in situ. The depth to which atypical melanocytes extend cannot be determined in a specimen such as this one that was taken by merely shaving the lesion (Reduced from ×18)*

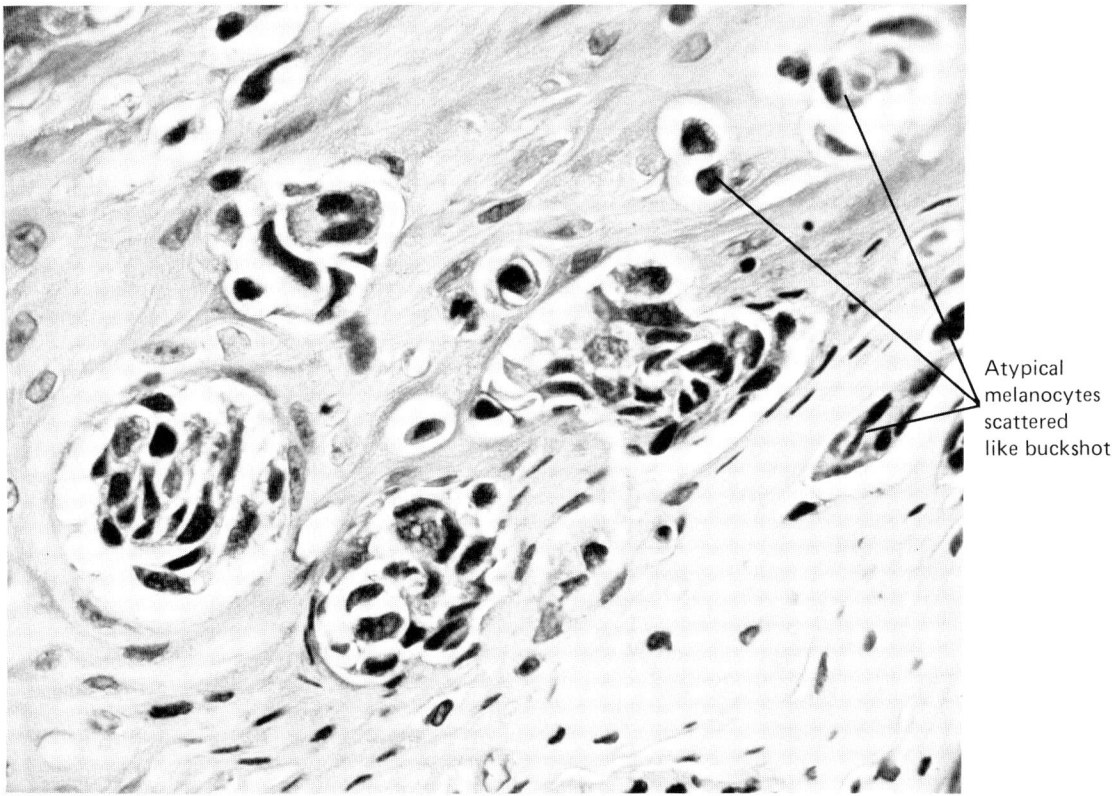

FIGURE 123B. ***Specimen of malignant melanoma removed by shave excision.*** *Higher magnification of Fig. 123A shows "buckshot" scatter of atypical melanoyctes throughout the cornified layer of this malignant melanoma. (Reduced from ×660)*

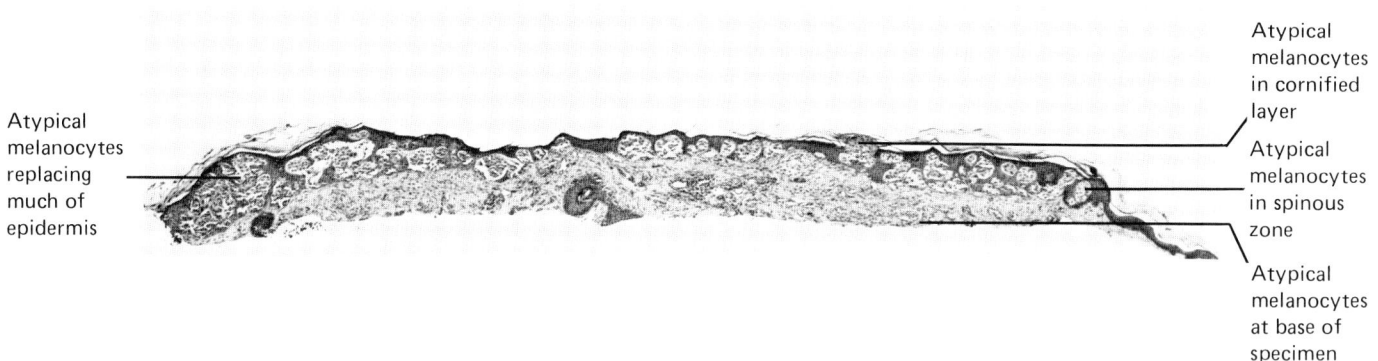

FIGURE 124A. **Shave excision biopsy of a malignant melanoma, superficial spreading type.** *With scanning magnification, it can be seen that this specimen was removed by shave excision and that the atypical melanocytes extend to at least one lateral margin and to the deep margin. (Reduced from ×32)*

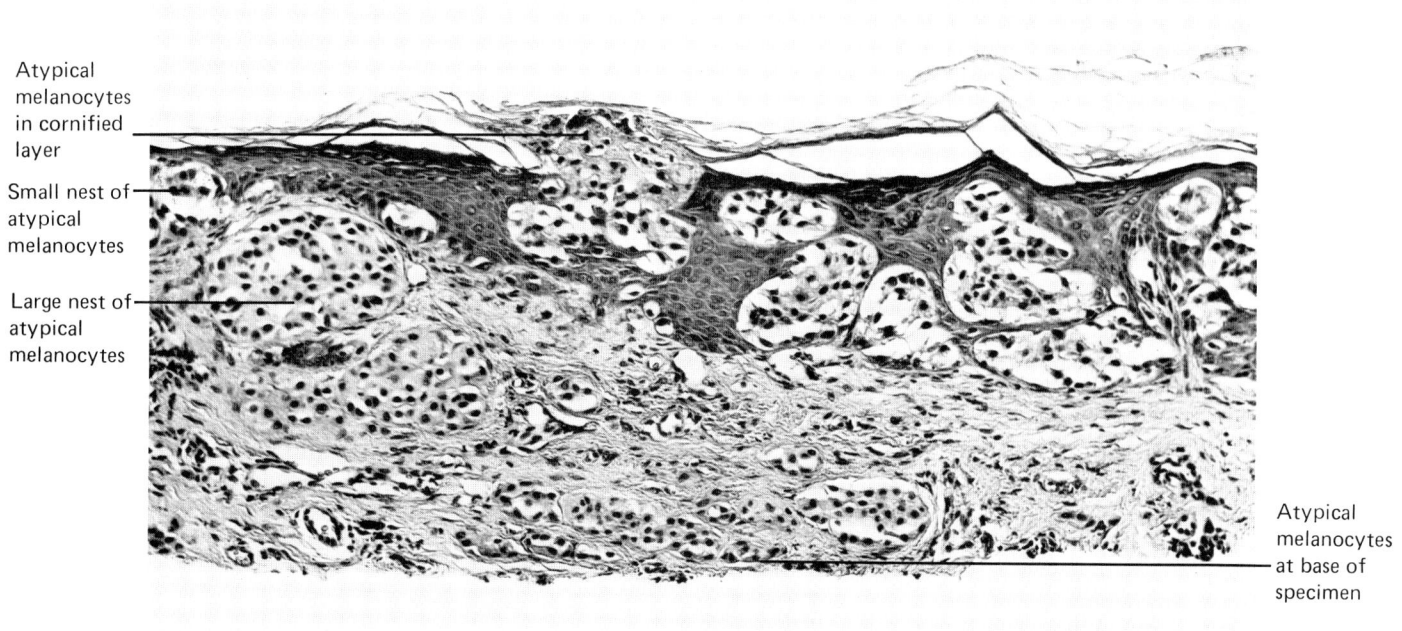

FIGURE 124B. **Shave biopsy specimen of a malignant melanoma, superficial spreading type.** *In this higher magnification of Fig. 124A, pagetoid melanocytes are present at all levels of the epidermis including the cornified layer and throughout the papillary dermis to the base of the specimen. This is surely a malignant melanoma of the superficial spreading type, but no judgment can be made about the exact depth of extension (thickness) and therefore the clinician (and patient) cannot be well advised about prognosis or subsequent therapy. (Reduced from ×175)*

garding the use of frozen sections in the diagnosis of 329 pigmented skin lesions suspected of being malignant melanomas. There were errors in four neoplasms (1.2%) as a result of differences in interpretation of the frozen sections and paraffin sections. In each instance, the error was a false diagnosis of malignancy. Two of the patients had unnecessary surgery as a consequence of the misdiagnosis of malignant melanoma by frozen sections. Little and Davis nevertheless concluded that diagnosis of malignant melanoma by frozen section in experienced hands is reliable and is of value to the surgeon. Hirst and his associates (1972) at the Mayo Clinic reported that 18 out of 215 cases (8.3%)

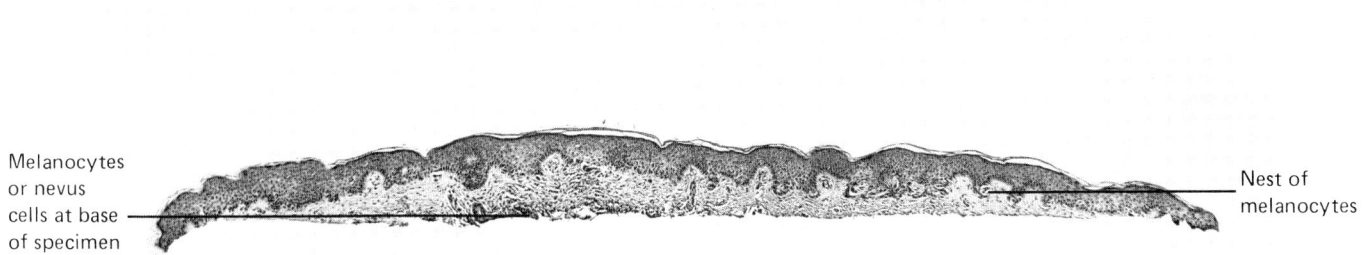

FIGURE 125A. ***Shave excision biopsy of a melanocytic lesion.*** *With scanning magnification one can see that this melanocytic process involves the epidermis and the papillary dermis and extends to all margins. (Reduced from ×50)*

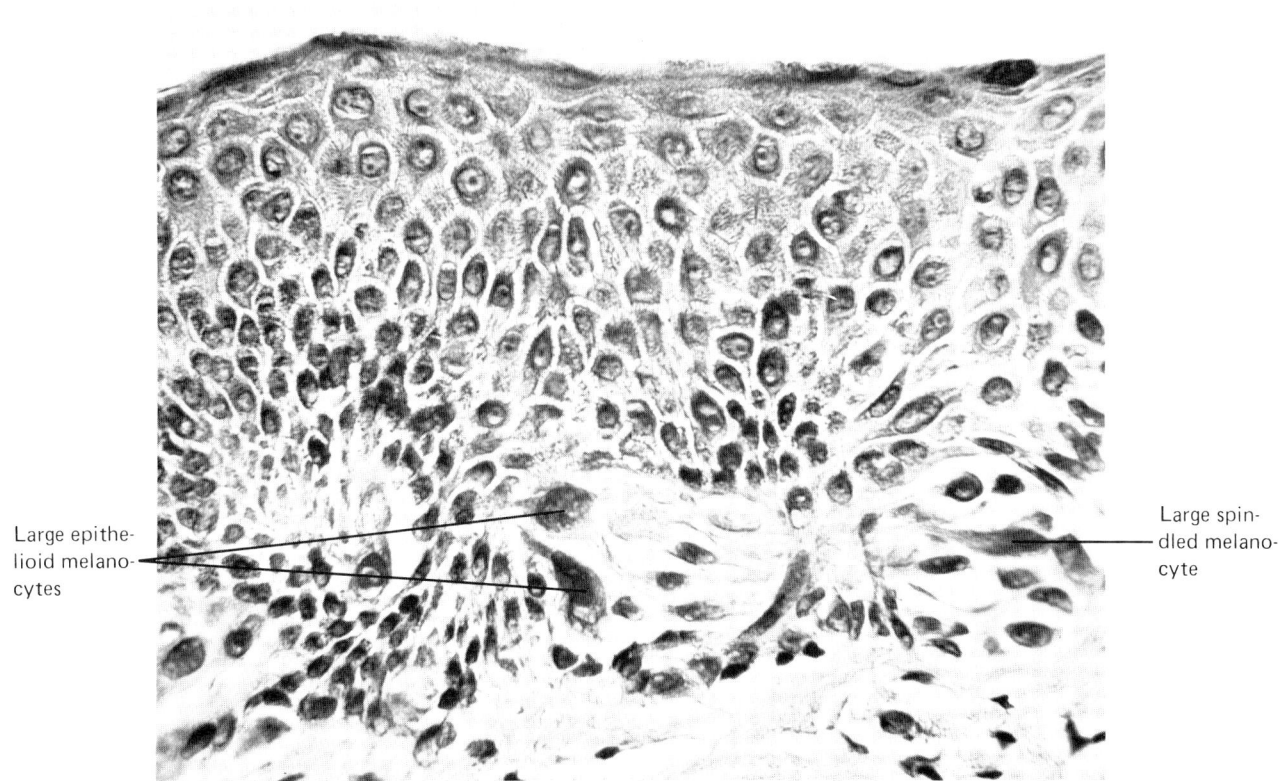

FIGURE 125B. ***Shave excision biopsy of a melanocytic lesion.*** *This higher magnification of Fig. 125A shows nests of melanocytes at the dermoepidermal junction that are both spindled and epithelioid and have large nuclei. The most likely diagnosis in this specimen is the nevus of large spindle and/or epithelioid cells. However, because this shaved specimen is inadequate, the clinician should be advised that the entire lesion must be completely excised. It is important to strongly urge clinicians to completely excise pigmented lesions rather than to partially excise them by shave procedure. (Reduced from ×655)*

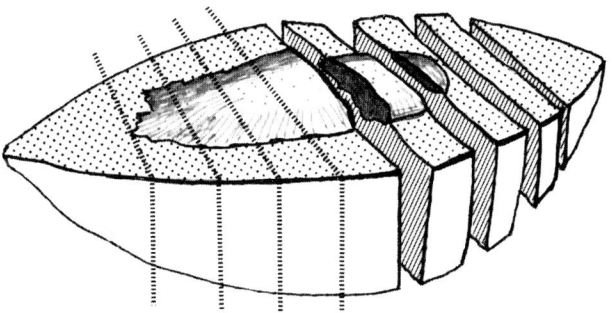

FIGURE 126. ***Proper sectioning of a lesion suspected of being malignant melanoma.*** *Many sections cut at about 3 mm intervals at right angles to the long axis should be taken through all specimens suspected of being a malignant melanoma. Only by this technique can the pathologist be certain of the actual thickness of the neoplasm and can other valuable information, such as the presence of a preexisting melanocytic nevus, be obtained.*

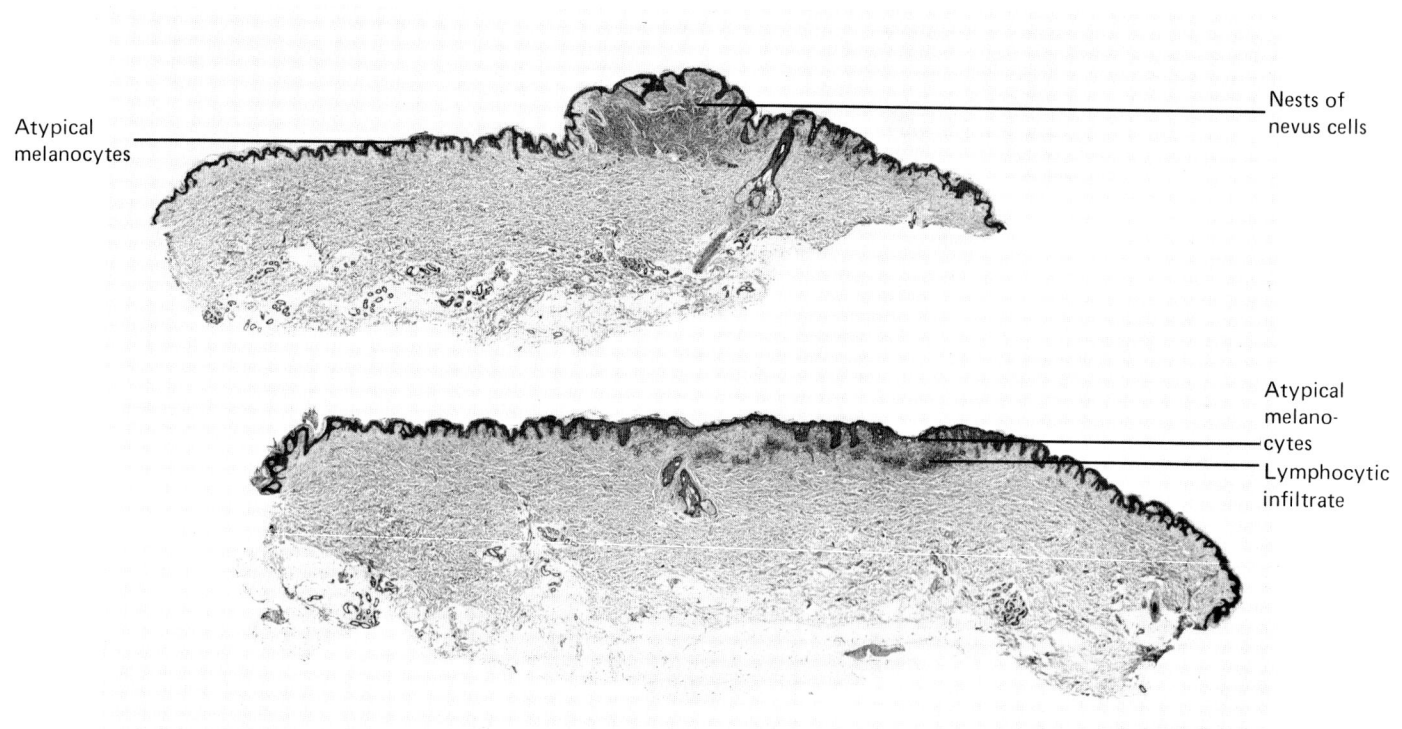

FIGURE 127A. ***Malignant melanoma, superficial spreading type, in association with an intradermal melanocytic nevus.*** *If only the upper portion of this bisected specimen had been submitted for histologic examination, the lesion could easily have been misinterpreted as a simple intradermal melanocytic nevus. (Reduced from ×11)*

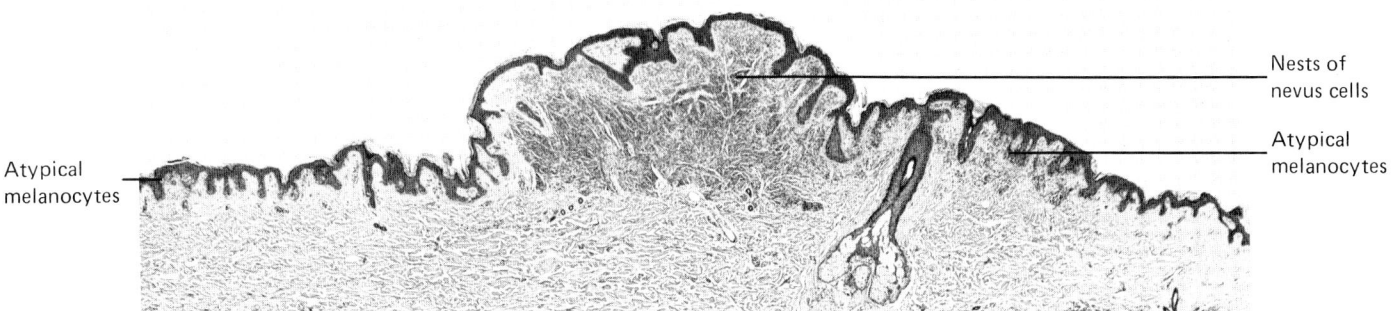

FIGURE 127B. *Malignant melanoma, superficial spreading type, in association with an intradermal melanocytic nevus.* This higher-power view of the upper portion of the bisected specimen pictured in Fig. 127A shows horizontal extension of atypical melanocytes within the epidermis to the side of the melanocytic nevus, an evidence of superficial spreading malignant melanoma in situ. *(Reduced from ×23)*

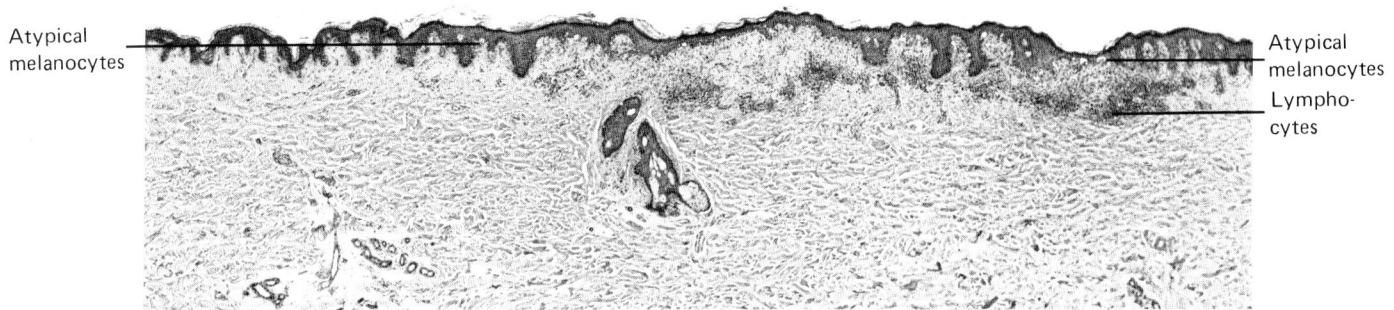

FIGURE 127C. *Malignant melanoma, superficial spreading type, in association with an intradermal melanocytic nevus.* This higher magnification of the lower portion of the bisected specimen pictured in Fig. 127A shows diagnostic features of superficial spreading malignant melanoma in situ, *namely,* an increased number of atypical melanocytes singly and in irregularly shaped and sized nests at all levels of the epidermis of this broad lesion. *(Reduced from ×23)*

of malignant melanoma were misdiagnosed as a result of frozen sections alone. Others have also told of misdiagnosis of pigmented nevi as malignant melanomas owing to faulty interpretation of frozen sections resulting in unnecessarily wide excisions and lymph node resections (Hirst et al., 1969). We do not advocate frozen section examinations of lesions suspected of being malignant melanoma. When melanin is present in large amounts, nuclear detail is often obscured even under optimal circumstances, let alone in frozen sections. Furthermore, mitoses in malignant melanoma, in contrast to other forms of malignancy, are very difficult to identify in frozen sections (Pack, 1962; Hirst et al., 1972).

In sum, erroneous diagnoses may be made on examination of pigmented lesions processed by the frozen section method. Such errors could be avoided by waiting but a few hours for the study of permanent sections.

D. Reporting a Malignant Melanoma Histopathologically

In our pathology report the clinician receives the following information:

1. Diagnosis: malignant melanoma.
2. The histologic type of malignant melanoma: lentigo maligna, acral lentiginous, superficial spreading, nodular, or unclassified.
3. The measurement of the thickness of the neoplasm and the level of invasion.
4. Presence or absence of a preexisting melanocytic nevus.
5. Additional histopathologic information which might have some prognostic or therapeutic significance for the patient, e.g., the presence of
   a. ulceration,

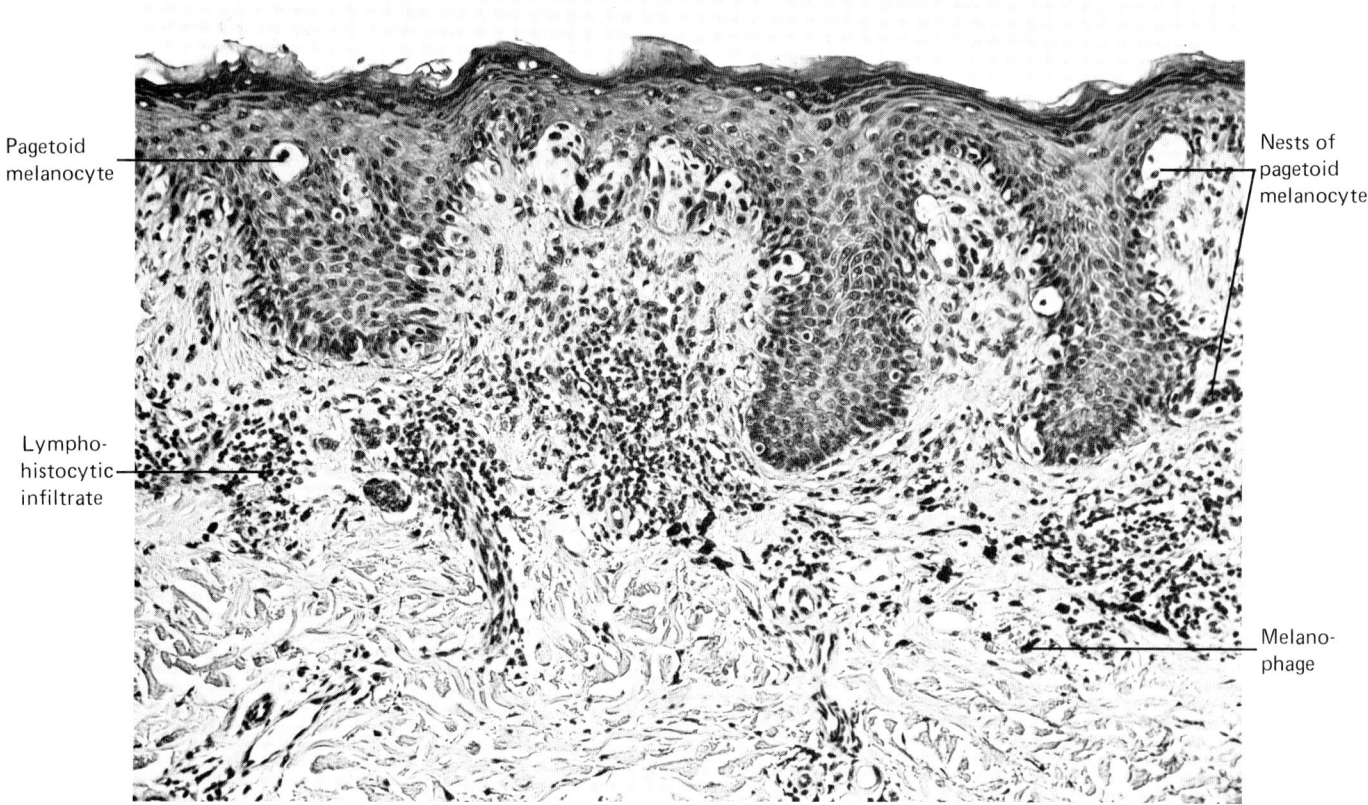

FIGURE 127D. *Malignant melanoma, superficial spreading type, in association with an intradermal melanocytic nevus. Still higher-power view of Fig. 127C to illustrate the atypical pagetoid melanocytes within the epidermis. These are early histologic changes of superficial spreading malignant melanoma. (Reduced from ×179)*

    b. nodularity or pedunculation,
    c. invasion of blood vessels or lymphatics,
    d. mitotic figures and number per high-power field,
    e. more than one type of neoplastic melanocyte,
    f. inflammatory-cell infiltrate and its density,
    g. neoplastic cells at the margins of the specimen.

We also telephone the clinician as soon as the diagnosis of malignant melanoma has been made in order to facilitate prompt management of the patient.

In difficult cases, for instance, in a malignant melanoma which simulates a Spitz's nevus or vice versa, the report always includes the reasons the decision for benignity or malignancy was reached.

Occasionally, a melanocytic lesion will be beyond one's ability to recognize it with certainty as being benign or malignant. In such cases, it is advisable to seek the opinion of one or more respected colleagues knowledgeable about the vagaries of melanocytic neoplasms. Their opinions should be forwarded to the patient's physician.

ACKNOWLEDGMENTS

Photomicrography was by William Atkinson and illustrations were by Howard B. Goldstein, M.D.

REFERENCES

Ackerman, L. V. Malignant melanoma of the skin: Clinical and Pathologic analysis of 75 cases. Am. J. Clin. Pathol. 18:602–624, 1948.

Allen, A. C. Survey of pathologic studies of cutaneous disease during World War II. Arch. Dermat. Syph. 57:19–56, 1948.

Allen, A. C., and Spitz, S. Malignant melanoma. A clinicopathological analysis of the criteria for diagnosis and prognosis. Cancer 6:1–45, 1953.

Anderson, W. A. D., and Scotti, T. M. Synopsis of Pathology, 9th ed. St. Louis, C. V. Mosby Co., 1976. Chap. 24, p. 1019.

Arao, T., Kuwahara, H., and Inone, S. Clinico-pathological and electronmicroscopical studies on melanotic freckle Hutchinson and malignant melanoma arising from the melanotic freckle. Jpn. J. Dermatol., Series B., 81:444-453, 1971.

Arrington, J. H., III, Reed, R. J., Ichinose, H., and Krementz, E. T. Plantar lentiginous melanoma: A distinctive variant of human cutaneous malignant melanoma. Am. J. Surg. Path. 1:131-143, 1977.

Balch, C. M., Murad, T., Soong, A., Griffin, A. L., Halpern, N., and Maddox, W. A. A multifactorial analysis of melanoma: I. Prognostic histopathologic features comparing Clark's and Breslow's staging methods, In press.

Becker, S. W. Cutaneous melanoma. Arch. Dermat. Syph. 21:818-840, 1930.

Becker, S. W. Critical evaluation of the so-called junction nevus. J. Invest. Dermat. 22:217-223, 1954.

Bodenham, D. C. A study of 650 observed malignant melanomas in the South-West region. Ann. R. Coll. Surg. Engl. 43:218, 1968.

Bodenham, D. C. Malignant melanoma. Proc. R. Soc. Med. 62:1090-1092, 1969.

Booher, R. J., and Pack, G. T. Malignant melanoma of the feet and hands. Surg. 42:1084-1121, 1957.

Breslow, A. Thickness, cross-sectional areas and depth of invasion in the prognosis of cutaneous melanoma. Ann. Surg. 172:902-908, 1970.

Breslow, A. Tumor thickness, level of invasion and node dissection in stage I cutaneous melanoma. Ann. Surg. 182:572-575, 1975.

Breslow, A., Cascinelli, V., van der Esch, E. P., and Marabito, A. Stage I melanoma of the limbs: assessment of prognosis by levels of invasion and maximum thickness. In press.

Breslow, A., and Macht, S. D. Optimal size of resection margin for thin cutaneous melanoma. Surg. Gynecol. Obstet. 145:691-692, 1977.

Breslow, A., and Macht, S. D. Evaluation of prognosis in stage I cutaneous melanoma. Plas. Reconstr. Surg. 61:342-346, 1978.

Callen, J. P., Chanda, J. J., and Stowiski, M. A. Malignant melanoma. Arch. Dermatol. 114:369-370, 1978.

Caro, M. R. Diagnostic pitfalls in dermal pathology. Arch. Derm. 67:18-29, 1953.

Carswell, R. Pathological Anatomy, Part 9, "Melanoma." Longman, London, 1838.

Clark, W. H. Jr. A classification of malignant melanoma in man correlated with histogenesis and biologic behavior. In Advances in Biology of Skin, Montagna, W. and Hu, F., eds. New York, Pergamon Press, 1966, pp. 621-647.

Clark, W. H., Jr., Ainsworth, A. M., Bernardino, E. A., Yang, C. H., Mihm, M. C., Jr., and Reed, R. J. The developmental biology of primary human malignant melanomas. Semin. Oncol. 2:83-103, 1975.

Clark, W. H., Jr., From, L., Bernardino, E. H., and Mihm, M. C. The histogenesis and biologic behavior of primary human malignant melanomas of the skin. Cancer Res. 29:705-727, 1969.

Clark, W. H., Jr., Reimer, R. R., Greene, M., Ainsworth, A. M., and Mastrangelo, M. F. Origin of familial malignant melanomas from heritable melanocytic lesions: The B-K mole syndrome. Arch. Dermatol. 1978 (in press.)

Cochrane, A. J. Histology and prognosis in malignant melanoma. J. Path. 97:459, 1969.

Conley, J., Lattes, R., and Orr, W. Desmoplastic malignant melanoma (a rare variant of spindle cell melanoma). Cancer 28:914-93, 1971.

Corsi, H. Three cases of melanose circonscrite precancereuse. Proc. Roy. Soc. Med. 32:261-263, 1938-1939.

Costello, M. J., Fisher, S. B., and DeFeo, C. P. Melanotic freckle: Lentigo maligna. A. M. A. Arch. Derm. 80:753, 1959.

Couperus, M., and Rucker, R. C. Histopathologic diagnosis of malignant melanoma. Arch. Dermat. 70:199-216, 1954.

Das Gupta, T., and Brasfield, R. Subungual melanoma: 25-year review of cases. Ann. Surg. 161:545-552, 1965.

Davis, J., Pack, G. T., and Higgins, G. K. Melanotic freckle of Hutchinson. Am. J. Surg. 113:457-463, 1967.

Davis, N. C., McLeod, G. R., Beardmore, G. L., Little, J. H., Quinn, R. L., and Holt, J. Primary cutaneous melanoma: a report from the Queensland melanoma project. CA 26:80-107, 1976.

Deckner, K. Zur Klinik der Melanome. Beitr. Z. Klin. Chir. 154:159-166, 1931.

Dubreuilh, M. W.: Lentigo malin des vieillards. Société de Dermatologie, 4 août, 1894.

Dubreuilh, M. W. De la mélanose circonscrite précancéreuse. Ann. Dermat. Syph. 3:129, 205, 1912.

Duhring, L. A. A Practical Treatise on Diseases of the Skin. Philadelphia, J. B. Lippincott Co., 1882, pp. 559-560.

Eiselt, T. Ueber pigment Krebs. Viertegjahrsch. f. d. praktische Heilkunde 70:87, 197, 1861; 76:26, 1862.

Epstein, E., Bragg, K., and Linden, G. Biopsy and prognosis of malignant melanoma. J.A.M.A. 208:1369-1371, 1969.

Fitzpatrick, P. J., Brown, T. C., and Reid, J. Malignant melanoma of the head and neck: A clinicopathological study. Can. J. Surg. 15:90-101, 1972.

Franklin, J. D., Reynolds, V. H., and Page, D. L.: Cutaneous melanoma: a twenty-year retrospective study with clinico-pathologic correlation. Plas. Reconstr. Surg. 56:227-285, 1975.

Frolow, G. R., Englewood, N. J., Shaprio, L., and Brownstein, M. H. Desmoplastic malignant melanoma. Arch. Derm. 111:753-754, 1975.

Gibson, S. H., Montgomery, H., Woolner, L. B., and Brunsting, L. A. Melanotic whitlow (subungual melanoma). J. Invest. Dermat. 29: 119-129, 1957.

Gordon, D., and Silverstone, H. Worldwide epidemiology of premalignant and malignant cutaneous lesions. In Cancer of the Skin, Andrade, R. et al., eds. Philadelphia, Saunders, 1976, p. 423.

Graham, W. P. Sunungual melanoma. Pennsylvania Med. 76:56, 1973.

Gromet, M. A., Sagebiel, R. W., and Epstein, W. L. The regressing thin malignant melanoma: A distinctive lesion with metastatic potential. Cancer 42:2282-2292, 1978.

Gumport, S. L., and Harris, M. H. Melanoma of the skin, in Cancer of the Skin, Andrade, R., et al., eds. Philadelphia, Saunders, 1976, pp. 950-971.

Hansen, M., and McCarten, A. B. Tumor thickness and lymphocytic infiltration in malignant melanoma of the head and neck. Am. J. Surg. 128:557-561, 1974.

Hazen, H. H. Malignant moles. South. M. J. 13:345, 1920.

Helwig, E. B. Malignant melanoma of the skin of man. Natl. Cancer Inst., Monograph 10, 287:95, 1963.

Helwig, E. B. In Neoplasms of the Skin and Malignant Melanoma, Chicago, Year Book Medical Publishers, Inc., 1975.

Hermanek, P., Hornstein, O. P., Tonak, J., and Weidner, F. Malignant melanoma: Depth of invasion and histologic typing. Beitr. Pathol., 157:269-282, 1976.

Hertzler, A. E. Melanoblastoma of the nail-bed (melanotic whitlow). Arch. Dermat. Syph. 6:701-708, 1922.

Hirst, E., Cains, G. D., Bale, P. M., Palmer, A. A., and Hambly, C. K. Diagnosis by frozen section examination, II: Results in skin lesions. Aust. N.Z. J. Surg. 38:216-220, 1969.

Hirst, E., McCarthy, S. W., and Bale, P. M. Frozen section diagnosis of cutaneous malignancy. In Melanoma and Skin Cancer (Proceedings of the International Cancer Conference, Sydney, 1972). McCarthy, W. H., ed. Sydney, V.C.N. Blight, 1972, pp. 185-192.

Hutchinson, J. Melanosis often not black: melanotic whitlow. Br. Med. J. 1:491, 1886.

Hutchinson, J. On cancer. Arch. Surg. 4:61-65, 1892.

Hutchinson, J. On tissue dotage. Arch. Surg. (London) 3:315-322, 1892.

Hutchinson, J. Lentigo-melanosis. A further report. Arch. Surg. (London) 5:253-256, 1894.

Hutchinson, J.: President's address at the Third International Congress of Dermatology. Arch. Surg. (London) 7:297-317, 1896.

Huvos, A. G., Mike, V., Donnellan, M. J., Seemayer, T., and Strong, W. E. Prognostic factors in cutaneous melanoma of the head and neck. Am. J. Pathol. 71:33-48, 1973.

Huvos, A. G., Shah, J. P., and Goldsmith, H. S. A clinicopathologic study of amelantic melanoma. Surg. Gynecol. Obstet. 135:917-920, 1972.

Huvos, A. G., Shah, J. P., and Mike V. Prognostic factors in cutaneous malignant melanoma. Hum. Pathol. 5:347-357, 1974.

Hyde, J. N., and Montgomery, F. H. A Practical Treatise on Diseases of the Skin. Philadelphia and New York, Lea Brothers & Co., 1901, pp. 693-694, 711-712.

Jackson, G. T. The Ready Reference Handbook of Diseases of the Skin. New York and Philadelphia, Lea Brothers & Co., 1899, p. 487.

Jackson, R. Myths of cutaneous malignant melanoma. Laval. Med. 42: 921-925, 1971.

Jackson, R., Williamson, G. S., and Beattie, W. G.: Lentigo maligna and malignant melanoma. Can. Med. Assoc. J. 95:846-851, 1966.

Jones, W. M., Jones Williams, W., Roberts, M. M., and Davies, K. Malignant melanoma of the skin: Prognostic value of clinical features and the role of treatment in 111 cases. Br. J. Cancer 22:437-451, 1968.

Jones Williams, W., Davies, K., Jones, W. M., and Roberts, M. M. Malignant melanoma of the skin: Prognostic value of histology in 89 cases. Br. J. Cancer 22:452-460, 1968.

Kaposi, M.: Pathologie und Therapie der Hautkrankheiten. Wein und Leipzig, Urban & Schwarzenberg, 1887, p. 881.

Klauder, J. V. and Beerman, H.: Melanotic freckle (Hutchinson) Mélanose circonscrite précancéreuse (Dubreuilh). A. M. A. Arch. Derm. 71:2-10, 1955.

Knutson, C. O., Hori, J. M., and Spratt, J. S., Jr. Melanoma. Curr. Probl. Surg. December 1971, pp. 1-55.

Konrad, K., and Wolff, K. Pathogenesis of diffuse melanosis secondary to malignant melanoma. Br. J. Derm. 91:635-655, 1974.

Kopf, A. W., Bart, R. S., and Rodriguez-Sains, R. Malignant melanoma: A review. J. Dermat. Surg. Oncol. 3:41-125, 1977.

Kornberg, R., and Ackerman, A. B. Pseudomelanoma: Recurrent melanocytic nevus following partial surgical removal. Arch. Dermatol. 111:1588-1590, 1975.

Kornberg, R., Harris, M., and Ackerman, A. B. Epidermotropically metastatic malignant melanoma. Arch. Dermatol. 114:67-69, 1978.

Kumer, L., and Lang, F. J.: Die bösartigen Geschwulst der Haut. In Artz, L., and Zieler, K., eds. Die Haut- und Geschlechtskrankheiten, Vol. 2. Berlin, Urban & Schwarzenberg, 1935.

Labrecque, P. G., Hu, C. H., and Winkelmann, R. K. On the nature of desmoplastic melanoma. Cancer 38:1205-1213, 1976.

Lane, N., Lattes, R., and Malm, J. Clinicopathological correlations in a series of 117 malignant melanomas of the skin of adults. Cancer 11: 1025-1043, 1958.

Leppard, B., Sanderson, K. V., and Behan, F. Subungual malignant melanoma: Difficulty in diagnosis. Br. Med. J. 1:310-312, 1974.

Lever, W. F. Histopathology of the Skin. Philadelphia, J. B. Lippincott Co., 1949, pp. 398-404.

Lever, W. F.: Pigmented nevi and malignant melanoma. In Histopathology of the Skin. 2d ed. Philadelphia, J. B. Lippincott Co., 1954, Chap. 25, p. 458.

Lever, W. F. Histopathology of the Skin, 3d ed. Philadelphia, J. B. Lippincott Co., 1961, pp. 582-589.

Lever, W. F. Histopathology of the Skin, 4th ed. Philadelphia, J. B. Lippincott Co., 1967, pp. 715-724.

Lever, W. F. Histopathology of the Skin, 5th ed. Philadelphia, J. B. Lippincott Co., 1975, pp. 664-677.

Lewis, M. G. Malignant melanoma in Uganda. Br. J. Cancer 21:483-495, 1967.

Lewis, M. G., and Kiryabwire, J. W. M. Aspects of behavior and natural history of malignant melanoma in Uganda. Cancer 21:876-887, 1968.

Little, J. H. Histology and prognosis in cutaneous malignant melanoma. In McCarthy, W. H., ed. Melanoma and Skin Cancer, Proceedings of the International Cancer Conference, Sydney, 1972. Sydney, V. C. N. Blight, 1972, pp. 107-120.

Little, J. H., and Davis, N. C.: Frozen section diagnosis of suspected malignant melanoma of the skin. Cancer 34:1163-1172, 1974.

Lund, R., and Ihned, M. Malignant melanoma, clinical and pathologic analysis of 93 cases—Is prophylactic lymph node dissection indicated? Surgery 38:652, 1955.

Lupulescu, A., Pinkus, H., Birmingham, D. J., et al. Lentigo maligna of the fingertip. Arch. Derm. 107:717, 1973.

Mackie, R. M., Carfrae, D. C., and Cochran, A. J. Assessment of prognosis in patients with malignant melanoma. Lancet 2:455-456, 1972.

MacLeod, J. M. H. and Muende, I.: Practical Handbook of the Pathology of the Skin: An Introduction to the Histology, Pathology, Bacteriology, and Mycology of the Skin with Special Reference to Technique, 2nd ed. Hagerstown, Maryland, Paul B. Hoeber, 1940, p. 321.

Masson, P. My conception of cellular nevi. Cancer 4:9-38, 1951.

McCarthy, L. Histopathology of Skin Diseases. St. Louis, C. V. Mosby Co., 1931, pp. 408-418.

McGovern, V. J., Caldwell, R. A., Duncan, C. A., et al. Moles and malignant melanoma: terminology and classification. Med. J. Aust. 1: 123-125, 1967.

McGovern, V. J. Malignant Melanoma, Clinical and Histologic Diagnosis, New York, John Wiley and Sons, 1976.

McGovern, V. J. The classification of melanoma and its relationship with prognosis. Pathology 2:85-98, 1970.

McGovern, V. J., Mihm, M. C., Jr., Bailly, C., et al.: The classification of malignant melanoma and its histologic reporting. Cancer 32: 1446-1457, 1973.

McLeod, G. R., Beardmore, G. L., Little, J. H., Quinn, R. L., and Davis, N. C. Results of treatment of 361 patients with malignant melanoma in Queensland. Med. J. Aust. 1:1211-1216, 1971.

Mehnert, J. H., and Heard, J. L. Staging of malignant melanoma by depth of invasion. Am. J. Surg. 110:168-176, 1965.

Miescher, G. Die Entstehung der bosartigen Melanome der Haut. Virchows Arch. 264:86, 1927.

Miescher, G. Präceröses Vorstadium des Melanoms, präcanceröse Melanose. In Jadassohn, J., ed. Handbuch der Haut und Geschlechtskrankheiten, Vol. 12, Pt. 3, Berlin, Springer-Verlag, 1933, p. 1085.

Miescher, G., Haberlin, L., and Guggenheim, L. Über fleckförmige Alterspigmenterungen: Ihre Beziehungen zur melanotischen Präcancerose und zur senilen Warze. Arch. Dermat. Syph. 174:105-125, 1936.

Mihm, M. C. Melanoma cure possible if detected in its intraepidermal proliferative phase. Dermat. News 10(8):8, 1977.

Mihm, M. C., Clark, W. H., Jr., and Reed, R. J. The clinical diagnosis of malignant melanoma. Semin. Oncol. 2:105–118, 1975.

Mihm, M. C., Jr., and Fitzpatrick, T. B. Early detection of malignant melanoma. Cancer 37:597–603, 1976.

Mihm, M. D., Jr., Fitzpatrick, T. B., Lane Brown, M. M., et al. Early detection of primary cutaneous malignant melanoma: A color atlas. N. Engl. Med. J. 289:989–996, 1973.

Milne, J. A. An Introduction to the Diagnostic Histopathology of the Skin. Baltimore, The Williams and Wilkins Co., 1972, pp. 291–316.

Mishima, Y. Melanosis circumscripta precancerose (Dubreuilh). A non-nevoid premelanoma distinct from junction nevus. J. Invest. Dermat. 34:361–375, 1960.

Niven, J., and Lubin, J. Pedunculated malignant melanoma. Arch. Dermatol. 111:755–756, 1975.

Ollstein, R. N., Kaplan, H. S., and Crikelair, G. F. Is there a malignant freckle? Cancer 19:767–775, 1966.

Ormsby, O. S., and Montgomery, H. Diseases of the Skin, 8th ed. Philadelphia, Lea and Febiger, 1954, pp. 864–898.

Pack, G. T. Functions and dysfunctions of the surgical pathologist. Surgery 52:752–755, 1962.

Pack, G. T., Gerber, D. M., and Scharnagel, I. M. End results in the treatment of malignant melanoma: A Report of 1,190 cases. Ann. Surg. 136:905:911, 1952.

Pack, G. T., and Oropeza, R. Subungual melanoma. Surg. Gynecol. Obstet. 124:571–582, 1967.

Pemberton, O. Observations on the History, Pathology and Treatment of Cancerous Disease, Part I, Melanosis. London, J. Churchill, 1858.

Peterson, N. C., Bodenham, D. C., and Lloyd, O. C. Malignant melanomas of the skin. Br. J. Plast. Surg. 15:45–94, 1962.

Pinkus, H., and Mehregan, A. H. A Guide to Dermatohistopathology. New York, Appleton-Century-Crofts, Meredity Corp., 1969, pp. 362–366.

Price, N. M., Rywlin, A. M., and Ackerman, A. B. Histologic criteria for the diagnosis of superficial spreading malignant melanoma: Formulated on the basis of proven metastatic lesions. Cancer 38:2434–2441, 1976.

Reed, R. J. Acral lentiginous melanoma. In New Concepts in Surgical Pathology of the Skin. Wiley, New York, 1976, pp. 89–90.

Reimer, R. R., Clark, W. H., Jr., Greene, M. H., Ainsworth, A. M., and Fraumeni, J. F. Precursor lesions in familial melanoma: A new genetic preneoplastic syndrome. J.A.M.A. 239:744–746, 1978.

Sachs, W., MacKee, G. M., Schwartz, O. D., and Pierson, H. S. Junction nevus-nevocarcinoma (the so-called melanoma group). J.A.M.A. 135:216–218, 1947.

Schmoeckel, C., and Braun-Falco, O. The prognostic index in malignant melanoma, Arch. Dermatol. 114:871–873, 1978.

Shoemaker, J. V. A Practical Treatise on Diseases of the Skin. F. A. Davis Co., Philadelphia, 1909, pp. 766–767.

Silberberg, I., Kopf, A. W., and Gumport, S. L. Diffuse melanosis in malignant melanoma, Arch. Derm. 97:671–677, 1968.

Sinha, B. K., and Buntine, D. W. Prognosis of cutaneous malignant melanoma: a clinicopathological study. Can. J. Surg. 17:328–334, 1974.

Solly, E. Melanotic carcinoma and melanomata of doubtful character. Trans. Pathol. Soc. Lond. 41:315–319, 1890.

Stout, A. P. Relationship of malignant melanoma (nevocarcinoma) to extramammary Paget's disease. Am. J. Cancer 33:196–204, 1938.

Suffin, S. C., Waisman, J., and Clark, W. H., Jr. Congruence of diagnosis of malignant melanoma. Lab. Invest. 32:436, 1975.

Sulzberger, M. B., Kopf, A. W., and Witten, V. H. Pigmented nevi, benign juvenile melanoma and circumscribed precancerous melanosis. Postgrad. Med. 26:617–631, 1959.

Sutton, R. L. Diseases of the Skin. St. Louis, C. V. Mosby Co., 1928, pp. 828–832.

Trapl, J., Palecek, L., Ebel, J., and Kucara, M. Origin and development of skin melanoblastoma on the basis of 300 cases. Acta Derm. Venereol. 44:377–380, 1964.

Trapl, J., Palecek, L., Ebel, J., and Kucera, M. Tentative new classification of melanoma of the skin. Acta. Derm. Venereol. (Stockholm) 46: 443–446, 1966.

Unna, P. G. The Histopathology of the Disease of the Skin. New York, MacMillan and Co., 1896, pp. 745–755.

Urteaga, B., and Pack, G. T. On the antiquity of melanoma. Cancer 19: 607–619, 1966.

Veronesi, U., Cascinelli, N., and Preda, F. Prognosis of malignant melanoma according to regional metastases. Am. J. Roentgenol. Radium Ther. Nucl. Med. 111:301–309, 1971.

Virchow, R. Die pathologischen pigmente. Arch. Pathol. Anat. Physiol. Virchows 1:379–404, 1847.

Voglino, A. La melanosi de Dubreuilh. Osservazioni su due casi a localizzazione rara. Chronica Dermatol. 2:728–730, 1971.

Wanebo, H. J., Fortner, J. G., Woodruff, J., Maclean, B., and Binkowski, E. Selection of the optimum surgical treatment of stage I melanoma by depth of microinvasion: use of the combined microstage technique (Clark-Breslow). Ann. Surg. 182:302–315, 1975.

Wanebo, H. J., Woodruff, J., and Fortner, J. G. Malignant melanoma of the extremities: a clinicopathologic study using levels of invasion (microstage). Cancer 35:666–676, 1975.

Wayte, D. M., and Helwig, E. B. Melanotic freckle of Hutchinson. Cancer 21:892–911, 1968.

Webster, J. P., Stevenson, T. W., and Stout, A. P. The surgical treatment of malignant melanomas of the skin. Surg. Clin. N. Am. 24:319, 1944.

Chapter 5

Familial Malignant Melanoma

We have recently reviewed the subject of familial malignant melanoma (Kopf et al., 1976) and much of what follows has been abstracted from that paper (also see Fig. 128).

The mode of inheritance of the predisposition to human malignant melanoma has been studied by a number of investigators. In a recent review of the literature, Anderson (1971) found 74 pedigrees of familial malignant melanoma. In comparing this group with non-familial malignant melanomas, he reported that there is a tendency in the familial variety for the tumors: (1) to begin earlier in life, (2) to have a higher frequency of multiple primary lesions, and (3) to have a higher survival rate compared to non-familial melanomas. The genetic aspects are complex and probably involve several autosomal loci. Anderson suggests there may be a cytoplasmic component transmitted through affected or carrier females.

Sutherland et al. (1975) identified 18 families in Louisiana that had more than one patient with melanoma in an estimated patient population of 1050 patients with malignant melanomas. They report that the initial data suggest that an autosomal dominant gene with incomplete penetrance could account for the patterns.

Wallace et al. (1973) reported 42 pedigrees of familial malignant melanoma in Queensland, Australia, and concluded that familial melanoma shows many features found in polygeneic inheritance, the result of added contributions of a number of alleles at separate loci. They also noted that the inheritance pattern could not be classified as dominant, recessive or sex-linked. Such patients had no greater sun exposure than did controls. Familial melanomas tended to spare the face and were randomly distributed elsewhere, whereas non-familial cases clustered on the face, back, shoulder and legs. Familial malignant melanomas were not the result of larger families. In their series, families with familial malignant melanomas had a higher incidence of cancers of all types and of multiple primary malignant melanomas. In an earlier study, Wallace et al. (1971) evaluated genetic factors in malignant melanoma in Queensland, Australia. These authors concluded that heredity accounts for about one-tenth of the causative factors resulting in the development of malignant melanomas in Queensland (Davis, 1976).

Mukherji et al. (1973) studied HL-A phenotypes in malignant melanoma. All of their 33 patients with malignant melanomas failed to reveal the HL-A5 locus whereas 9 of 62 normals and 5 of 25 patients with cancers other than malignant melanomas were positive for the HL-A5 locus. Since the parents of one patient had an HL-A5 locus, acquired deletion or genetic crossing over was suggested. Singal et al. (1974) could not confirm these findings. Thus, data did not show any significant difference in HL-A antigen frequency in melanoma patients as compared to normal controls. Tarpley et al. (1975) reported evaluation of HL-A8 histocompatibility antigen in patients with malignant melanoma. Both Chen (1973) and Berger et al. (1973) have shown chromosomal abnormalities in patients with malignant melanomas. Certain minor blood group determinants have been shown to have a higher incidence in malignant melanoma (Jorgensen and Lal, 1972).

Schultheis et al. (1975) found no significant difference in Gm allotypes between sera from melanoma patients and normal controls.

Reimer et al. (1978) have recently described distinctive melanocytic nevi in families who show clustering of malignant melanomas. Clinically the syndrome consists of numerous nevocytic nevi scattered principally on the trunk and limbs. The moles show marked variability in size, color, and outline. Histologically, the nevi have atypical mela-

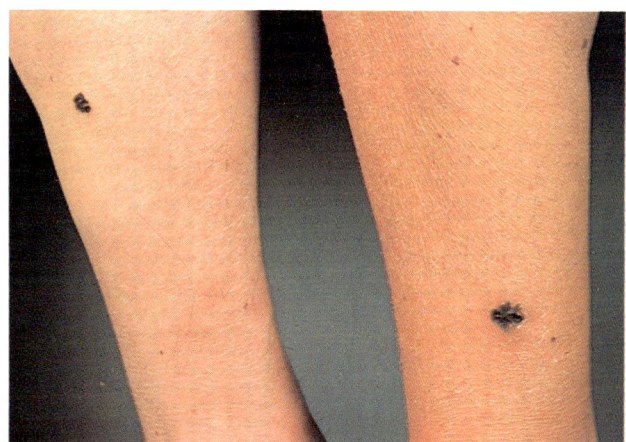

FIGURE 128A. **Familial malignant melanoma.** *Legs of two sisters, shown side-by-side.*

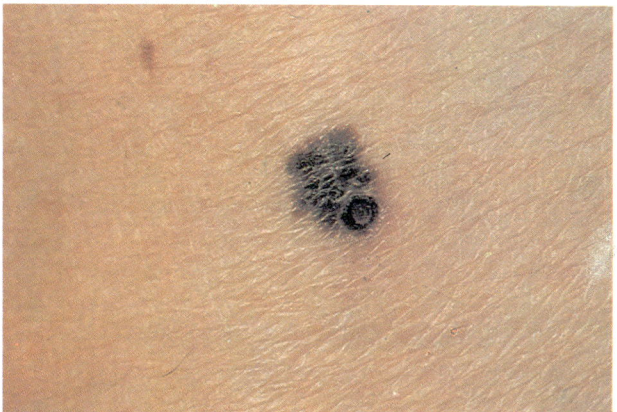

FIGURE 128B. *Close-up view of superficial spreading melanoma of one sister.*

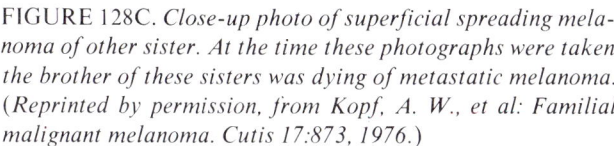

FIGURE 128C. *Close-up photo of superficial spreading melanoma of other sister. At the time these photographs were taken the brother of these sisters was dying of metastatic melanoma. (Reprinted by permission, from Kopf, A. W., et al: Familial malignant melanoma. Cutis 17:873, 1976.)*

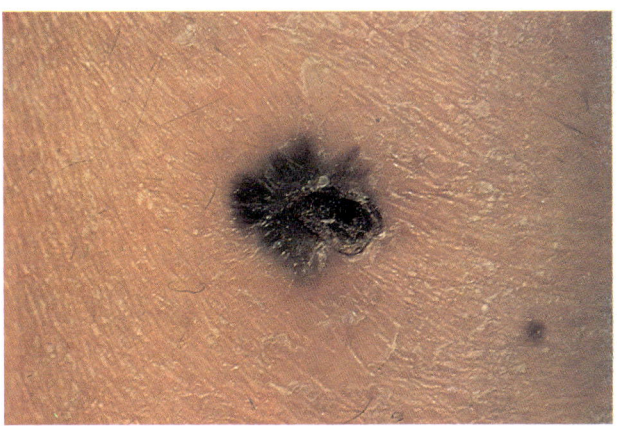

nocytic hyperplasia, delicate dermal fibroplasia, lymphocytic infiltration, and neovascular formation. In the seven melanoma-prone families, these distinctive clinical and histologic lesions occurred in 18 of 20 patients who developed melanomas and in 24 of 43 first-degree relatives. Identification of these "mole syndrome" lesions led to the diagnosis of six early melanomas in these families. It appears to be an autosomal dominant trait and is a marker for the identification of individuals at high risk to develop melanomas. Clark (personal communication, 1978) has also referred to this condition as the "B-K mole syndrome."

Animal models of genetically determined malignant melanoma have been studied. In the classical work of Gordon (1953) hybrids of platyfish and swordtails developed malignant melanomas whereas pure strains of either fish did not. Knutson et al. (1971) report a heard of miniature swine at the University of Missouri in which 21% developed melanocytic lesions, and 11% malignant melanomas. It is also well known that melanomas occured in certain genetic strains of grey horses (Hadwen, 1931). Moreover, the strains of pigs and horses that do develop malignant melanomas often develop widespread loss of pigment of their skins and hair implying a relationship between malignant melanocytic tumors and vitiligo, a phenomenon also seen in man.

Several mechanisms other than direct genetic effects have been postulated to explain familial melanomas. First, there are certain phenotypic features which predispose to malignant melanoma (Gellin et al., 1969) and these factors are known to be familial traits. Thus, there is a statistically significant propensity for patients with malignant melanoma to have light complexions, light eyes (blue, grey or green), and light hair (blond or red) when compared to patients in a control group. Pack (1962) observed that only 11% of the American white population is red-haired, sandy complexioned and freckled but 80% of patients with melanoma in his series had these features.

A second possible explanation that has been suggested

to explain familial malignant melanomas is that environmental factors could be responsible. Such factors are becoming more prominent in our understanding of the pathogenesis of these tumors. A considerable amount of data has been accumulated (Lee et al., 1970, 1971; Magnus, 1973; Movshovitz et al., 1973) to indicate that a high degree of sun exposure plays a distinct role in the development in certain types of malignant melanoma (see chapter on Sunlight and Melanoma). Thus, certain families may be more exposed and/or more susceptible to the carcinogenic effects of solar radiation than others. This could trigger neoplastic changes in susceptible melanocytes. Afflicted members of families who have xeroderma pigmentosum are susceptible to malignant melanomas and other cancers of the skin when such individuals are exposed to sunlight.

A third possible cause of malignant melanoma which might be considered in the familial form of this disease is the recent evidence that viruses may cause malignant melanoma in man (Birkmayer et al., 1972; Balda and Birkmayer, 1973; Balda et al., 1973; Birkmayer et al., 1974; Balda et al., 1975). An infectious cause for malignant melanoma in man is supported by the work of Spitler (1975) who found that both related and non-related individuals living with patients who develop melanoma have a higher prevalence of anti-melanoma cell-mediated immunologic responses than do members of the general population. The interesting reports of malignant melanomas occurring in a husband and wife and among stepbrothers add further evidence for the possibility of an infectious cause for these malignancies (Bauman, 1971; Mintzis et al., 1978; Robertson, 1971; Robinson, 1972; Smart, 1975).

Obviously, much more information is required in order to determine the importance, if any, of these explanations for the familial clustering of malignant melanomas. Of practical importance is the fact that some families who have more than one person afflicted with malignant melanoma may be prone to develop cancers of other organs (especially breast, gastrointestinal tract, lung and the reticuloendothelial system) (Lynch et al., 1975).

REFERENCES

Anderson, D. E. Clinical characteristics of the genetic variety of cutaneous melanoma in man. Cancer 21:721–725, 1971.

Balda, B.-R., and Birkmayer, G. D. Further evidence of viral etiology of human melanoma. Naturwissenschaften, 60:304–1973.

Balda, B.-R., Birkmayer, G. D., and Braun-Falco, O. Particle associated RNA-directed DNA polymerase and 70S RNA in the hamster melanoma A Mel 3. Arch. Dermatol. Forsch. 248:229–236, 1973.

Balda, B.-R., Hehlmann, K., Cho, J.-R., and Spiegelman, S. Oncornavirus-like particles in human skin cancers. Proc. Nat. Acad. Sci. 72: 3697–3700, 1975.

Bauman, L. Melanoma in relatives. J.A.M.A. 218:1300–1301, 1971.

Berg, O., and Gordon, M. Relationship of atypical pigment cell growth to gonadal development in hybrid fishes. In: Gordon, M. ed. Pigment Cell Growth, New York, Academic Press, 1953, pp. 43–72.

Berger, R., and LaCour, J. Estrude chromatosomique de melanomes malins. Biomedicine [Express] 19:22–27, 1973.

Birkmayer, G. D., Balda, B.-R., and Miller, F. Oncorna-viral information in human melanoma. Europ. J. Cancer 10:419–424, 1974.

Birkmayer, G. D., Balda, B.-R., Miller, F., and Braun-Falco, O. Virus-like particles in metastases of human malignant melanoma. Naturwissenshaften, 59:369–370, 1972.

Chen, T. R., and Shaw, M. W. Stable chromosome changes in a human malignant melanoma. Cancer Res. 33:2042–2047, 1973.

Davis, N. C. Cutaneous melanoma: the Queensland experience. Curr. Probl. Surg. 13:1–63, 1976.

Gellin, G. A., Kopf, A. W., and Garfinkel, L. Malignant melanoma—a controlled study of possibly associated factors. Arch. Dermatol. 99: 43–48, 1969.

Hadwen, S. The melanomata of grey and white horses. Can. Med. Assoc. J. 25:519–530, 1931.

Jörgensen, G., and Lal, V. B. Serogenetic investigations on malignant melanomas with reference to the incidence of ABO system, Rh system, Gm, Inv, Hp and Gc systems. Humangenetik 15:227–231, 1972.

Kakati, S., Song, S. Y., and Sandberg, A. A. Chromosomes and causation of human cancer. XXII. Karyotypic changes in malignant melanoma. Cancer 40:1173–1181, 1977.

Knutson, C. O., Hori, J. M., and Spratt, J. S. Melanoma. Curr. Probl. Surg. Dec.:1–55, 1971.

Kopf, A. W., Mintzis, M., Grier, W. R. N., Silvers, D. N., and Bart, R. S. Familial malignant melanoma. Cutis 17:873–876, 1976.

Lamm, L. U., Kissmeyer-Nielsen, F., Kjerbye, K. E. et al. HL-A and ABO antigens and malignant melanoma. Cancer 33:1458–1461, 1974.

Lee, J. A. H., and Merrill, J. N. Sunlight and the etiology of malignant melanoma: a synthesis. Med. J. Aust. 2:846–851, 1970.

Lee, J. A. H., and Yongchaiyudha, S. Incidence of and mortality from malignant melanoma by anatomical site. J. Natl. Cancer Inst. 47: 253–263, 1971.

Lynch, H. T., Frichot, B. C., Lynch, P., Lynch, J., and Guirgis, H. A. Family studies of malignant melanoma and associated cancer. Surg. Gynecol. Obstet. 141:517–522, 1975.

Magnus, K. Incidence of malignant melanoma of the skin in Norway, 1955–1970. Cancer 32:1275–1286, 1973.

Mintzis, M. J., Berger, A. P., Greenwald, E., Greenwald, E., and Golomb, F. Malignant melanoma in spouses. Cancer 42: 804–807, 1978.

Movshovitz, M., and Modan, B. Role of sun exposure in the etiology of malignant melanoma: epidemiologic inference. J. Natl. Cancer Inst. 51:777–779, 1973.

Mukherji, B., Nathanson, L., and Clark, D. A. Studies of humoral and cell-mediated immunity in human melanoma. Yale J. Biol. Med. 46: 681–692, 1973.

Pack, G. T. The pigmented mole and the malignant melanoma. CA 12: 11–26, 1962.

Parsons, P. G., Klucis, E., Goss, P. D., Pope, J. H., Little, J. H., and Davis, N. C. Oncornavirus-like particles in malignant melanoma and control biopsies. Int. J. Cancer 18:757–763, 1976.

Reimer, R. R., Clark, W. H., Greene, M. H., Ainsworth, A. M., and Fraumeni, J. F. Precursor lesions in familial melanoma: A new genetic preoplastic syndrome. J.A.M.A. 239:744–746, 1978.

Robertson, M. G. Malignant melanoma in husband and wife. J.A.M.A. 217:1553, 1971.

Robinson, M. J. Familial melanomas. J.A.M.A. 220:277, 1972.

Schultheis, W., Peter, H. H., and Deicher, H. Gm(1) and Gm(2) immunoglobulin allotypes in patients with malignant melanoma. Humangenetik 28:177–181, 1975.

Siciliano, M. J., and Perlmutter, A. Maternal effect on development of melanoma in hybrid fish of the Genus *Xiphophorous*. J. Natl. Cancer Inst. 49:415–421, 1972.

Singal, D. P., Bent, P. B., McCulloch, P. B., Blajchman, M. A., and MacLaren, R. G. C. HL-A antigens in malignant melanoma. Transplantation 18:186, 1974.

Smart, C. R., and Carle, B. N. Malignant melanoma in husband and wife. J.A.M.A. 232:705–706, 1975.

Spitler, L. Personal communication, February, 1975.

Sutherland, E. M., Klopfer, H. W., Mausell, P. W. A., and Krementz, E. T. Familial melanoma. In: Proceedings of the IX International Pigment Cell Conference, Houston, 1975, p. 60.

Tarpley, J. L., Chretien, P. B., Rogentine, N., Twomey, P. L., and Dellon, A. L. Histocompatibility antigens and solid malignant neoplasms. Arch. Surg. 110:269–271, 1975.

Wallace, D. C., Exton, L. A., and McLeon, G. R. C. Genetic factor in malignant melanoma. Cancer 27:1262–1266, 1971.

Wallace, D. C., Beardmore, G. L., and Exton, L. A. Familial malignant melanoma. Ann. Surg. 177:15–20, 1973.

Chapter 6

Malignant Melanomas in Children

Prepuberal malignant melanomas are very uncommon. When they occur they may arise de novo, result from transplacental metastases, or originate in giant nevocytic nevi. Recent evidence indicates that the prognosis of definite pre-puberal malignant melanomas (i.e., those which have metastasized) is as poor, if not worse, than melanomas of adults. Great confusion exists in the older literature because benign juvenile melanomas were included in the general category of "malignant melanoma" of children (for discussion, see Kopf and Andrade, 1966). Thus, the reader should be aware that some optimistic statements made in the past about the prognosis of prepuberal melanomas must be discounted in the light of newer knowledge.

A recent report concerning prepuberal metastatic malignant melanoma by Trozak et al. (1975) is an excellent review of this subject. These authors discuss only those cases which have reached Stage II (regional metastases) and Stage III (distant mestastases). They suggest the following classification for prepuberal metastatic malignant melanomas:

Type I: Congenital transplacentally acquired malignant melanoma.
Type II: Metastatic malignant melanoma with onset before puberty.
Type III: Metastatic malignant melanoma with onset before puberty in a nevus pigmentosus giganticus (giant congenital nevocytic nevus).

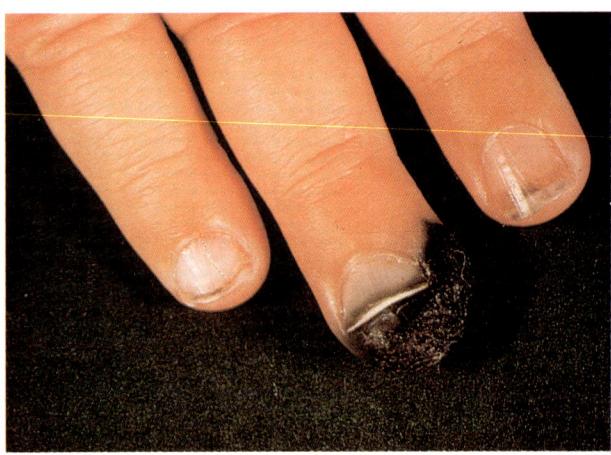

FIGURE 129. **Primary malignant melanoma of fingertip in an 11-month-old infant boy.** *The lesion had been present since birth and thus represents an exceedingly rare variety of congenital malignant melanoma that was not transferred placentally since, in this instance, the mother had no evidence of melanoma. The malignancy metastasized to the axillary lymph nodes in this infant. Treatment consisted of amputation of the finger and a radical axillary lymph node dissection. No further metastases occurred. This case was reported by Lyall (1967). Reprinted by permission from J.A.M.A. 201:1153, 1976. Copyright 1967, American Medical Association.*

TABLE 8.

Five-Year Survival of Metastatic Malignant Melanoma in Prepuberal Patients*

Type†	Number of patients	Alive after five years	Five-year survival (%)
I (Transplacental)	3	0	0
II	35	12	34
III (In Giant Nevus)	20	0	0
All types	58	12	21

* After Trozak et al. (1975).
† See text for explanation of types.

Table 8 summarizes their findings. From this review of the literature, it becomes apparent that Type I and Type III lesions have been inevitably fatal. The survival for the entire group is 20.7%, which is comparable to, or somewhat lower than, the survival for metastatic malignant melanomas in postpuberal individuals. This conclusion was previously arrived at by Skov-Jensen et al. (1966) who calculated from a review of the literature that the three-year survival rate in children is similar to a five-year survival rate in adults in comparable stages of the disease.

Regarding Type I lesions, Stevenson et al. (1971) reported that malignant melanoma is the most common malignancy to metastasize to the placenta. In their review of the literature there were 18 cases of metastases to the placenta from all kinds of cancer. Of these, seven were placental metastases from malignant melanomas. There were two cases of transplacental metastases of maternal cancers to the fetus, both malignant melanomas.

A very rare case of congenital primary malignant melanoma, not transplacentally acquired, was published from our institution by Lyall (1967) (Fig. 129). (See section on Congenital Nevocytic Nevi and Malignant Melanomas.)

REFERENCES

Kopf, A. W., and Andrade, R. Benign juvenile melanoma. In: Year Book of Dermatology, Chicago, Year Book Medical Publishers, pp. 7–52, 1966.

Lyall, D. Malignant melanoma in infancy. J.A.M.A. 202:1153, 1967.

Skov-Jensen, T., Hastrup, J., and Lambrethsen, E. Malignant melanoma in children. Cancer 19:620–626, 1966.

Stevenson, H. E., Terry, C. W., Lukens, J. N., Shively, J. A., Busby, W. E., Stoeckle, H. E., and Esterly, N. A. Immunologic factors in human melanoma "metastatic" to products of gestation (with exchange transfusion of infant to mother). Surgery 69:515–522, 1971.

Trozak, D. J., Rowland, W. D., and Hu, F. Metastatic malignant melanoma in prepubertal children: Pediatr. Clinician 55:191–204, 1975.

Chapter 7

Congenital Nevocytic Nevi and Malignant Melanomas

A congenital nevocytic (melanocytic) nevus may be both a cosmetic problem and a medical problem. The seriousness of the cosmetic problem increases with the size of the nevus and its location. As a medical problem the risk of malignant melanoma developing in a congenital nevus may be roughly proportional to its size.

Pigmented nevi are unusual at birth; they were found in about 2.5% of newborn babies by Pack (1960). Congenital pigmented nevi have a tendency to be larger than those acquired later in life (Mark et al., 1973), some being large enough to be considered "giant." If one accepts 30 as the average number of pigmented nevi per young adult (Nicholls, 1973), then for every 1,000 nevi in young adults there is only one congenital nevus, an incidence of about 0.1%. The prevalence of truly giant congenital pigmented nevi is, of course, much smaller.

Walton et al. (1975) examined 1,058 newborn infants and found that 41 (3.9%) had discernible pigmented lesions. On biopsy of 34 of the 41 lesions, 11 proved to be nevocytic nevi, representing 1% of the infants. Only 2 of the 11 had histologic features of giant nevocytic nevi and only 5 of the 11 biopsy proved nevocytic nevi were 1.5 cm or greater in diameter (i.e., 0.5% of the newborns in this series). We calculated, based on these figures, that the 3,000,000 babies born each year in the United States would therefore have 15,000 nevocytic nevi 1.5 cm or larger.

Even the smaller congenital nevocytic nevi tend to be larger than acquired nevi, that is, they are often more than 1.5 cm in greatest diameter (Mark et al., 1973). Furthermore, they differ histologically from the more common acquired variety. In their more superficial parts, congenital nevocytic nevi show features similar to those of acquired compound or intradermal nevi. However, they may have deep involvement which is absent from the usual acquired nevus (Mark et al., 1973). Characteristically, there are spindle or fusiform cells that extend to or into the subcutaneous tissue and also surround the adnexa, vessels and nerves. Thus, the congenital nevus may have elements that are like those of junctional nevocytic nevi, blue nevi, and neurofibromas. Melanophages may also be present. The features of benign juvenile melanoma are sometimes found and, most importantly, malignant melanoma may be found in congenital nevi.

When a large congenital nevus involves the head and neck, there may be an associated meningeal melanocytosis (Touraine), sometimes complicated by hydrocephalus and/or malignant melanoma (Kaplan et al., 1975).

The incidence of malignant melanoma developing in small congenital nevi is unknown. However, Kaplan (1974) suggests that all congenital nevi, regardless of size, "be viewed with suspicion," and some observers have suggested that the frequency of malignant melanoma developing in small congenital nevi warrants the routine excision of all congenital nevi. No convincing data, however, is presented to support the idea. In our extensive experience, we can recall only a few instances in which malignant melanomas were known to have arisen in smaller congenital nevocytic nevi (Fig. 130).

The reported incidence of malignant melanomas developing in so-called giant congenital pigmented (giant hairy, garment, bathing trunks) nevi varies. In some series it is as high as 42% (Bergfeld and Helwig, 1972) but the average is probably closer to 15% (Kaplan, 1974). There are two obvious problems when one considers the reported rates of melanomas developing in giant congenital pigmented nevi. First, there is no uniformly accepted definition of a giant nevus. Greely et al. (1965) suggest that a lesion greater than 144 sq. inches (900 sq. cm) or smaller (if it involves the major portion of an anatomic area) be termed giant. Second, there is probably a bias toward reporting nevi associated with malignant melanomas, since undoubtably many large congenital nevi would never be brought to the attention of the medical profession unless some untoward event occurred. The role of giant congenital pigmented nevi in the genesis of malignant melanomas is emphasized by the fact that malignant melanomas are rare before puberty and yet almost 40% of the malignant melanomas seen in children occur in "large congenital nevi" (Fish et al., 1966).

Pers (1963) collected 110 cases of giant pigmented nevocytic nevi. Of the 80 adult patients who responded to a questionnaire, 43 (54%) stated they had psychological "depression" and/or persistent desire for treatment. Furthermore, this group would want their children treated should they be born with similar giant nevi. The author suggests treatment for large congenital nevocytic nevi when they are obviously visible, verrucous, and, in women, hairy. Only total excision and plastic surgical repair provided satisfactory results and operation in childhood was advocated.

Orkin et al. (1974) report on three patients who presented cerebriform intradermal nevi of the scalp appearing as cutis verticis gyrata. After a review of the literature, they concluded that "the most urgent reason for surgical intervention is the potential for malignant melanoma, which has occurred in two of 50 patients (4%).

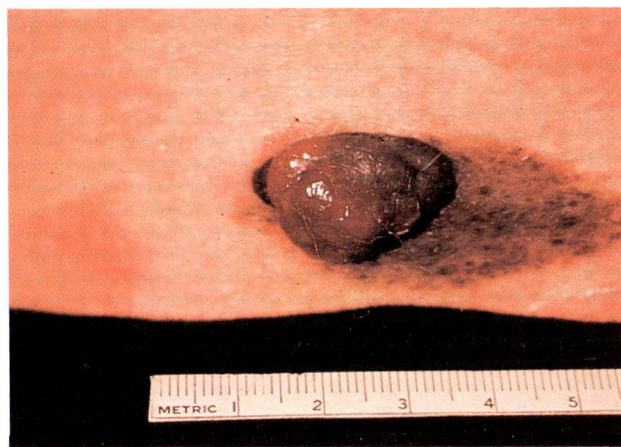

FIGURE 130. *Malignant melanoma arising in a small, congenital nevocytic nevus.* In our experience this is a rare occurrence.

MANAGEMENT OF CONGENITAL NEVOCYTIC NEVI: AN APPROACH

How does a physician decide on a course of action when confronted with a patient bearing a congenital nevocytic nevus? If the lesion is small and can be excised with an acceptable cosmetic result (especially if the cosmetic appearance after surgery can be anticipated to be superior to that of the nevus), it is easy to recommend surgical excision.

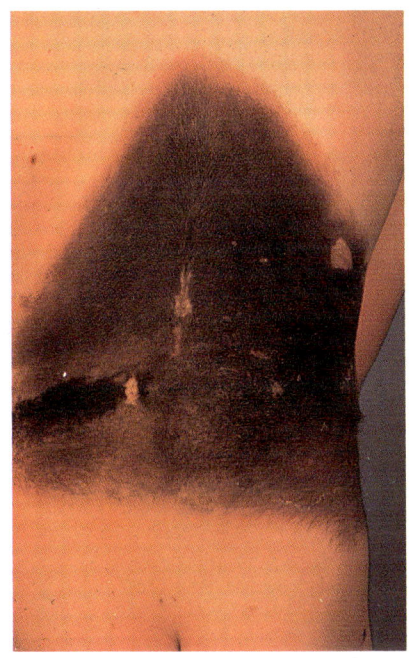

FIGURE 131A. *Giant congenital nevocytic nevus.* Nevus prior to excision.

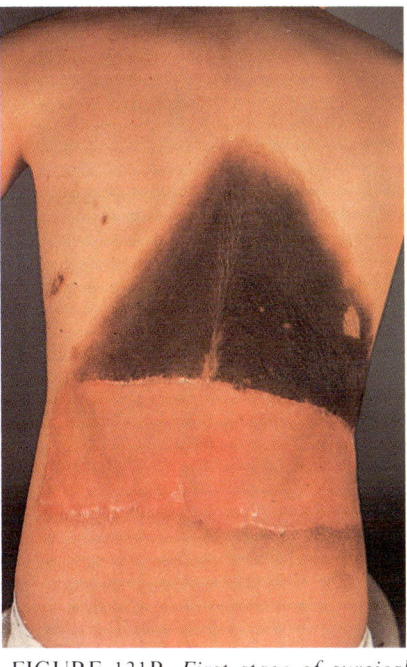

FIGURE 131B. *First stage of surgical removal of the lesion seen in (A).*

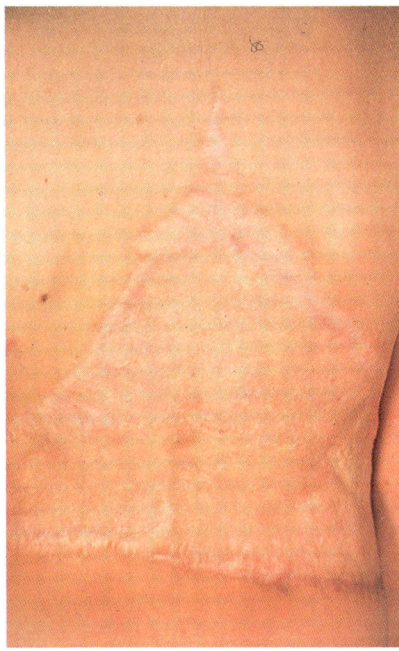

FIGURE 131C. *Appearance after total surgical excision of the lesion.*

If the surgery necessary to remove such a lesion is difficult, or if the cosmetic appearance after surgery can be anticipated to be significantly inferior to that of the nevus, the choice is much more difficult. Were it substantiated that there is a significant incidence of malignant melanoma developing in a small lesion, the judgment for removal would be easier. But, we are unaware of cogent data substantiating that small congenital nevi have a significant risk of giving rise to malignant melanomas.

As a matter of fact, if, as we calculated, there are 18,000 newborns in the United States each year who have congenital nevocytic nevi 1.5 cm or larger, it is probable that the risk of melanoma developing in such lesions is small, since it is unusual to see malignant melanomas arise in such lesions clinically.

There is little doubt, however, that if truly giant congenital nevi such as bathing trunks or garment types were completely excised during childhood the incidence of malignant melanoma in such patients would decrease from its figure of approximately 15% of reported cases. Since more than half the malignant melanomas reported occurred during the first decade of life, the earlier the excision, the better. Unfortunately, such removals usually require multiple surgical procedures over months and years, are expensive, and are emotionally and physically taxing for parents and children alike. Furthermore, it is sometimes technically impossible to excise nevi of garment size. The potential donor sites of the split-thickness skin grafts that could be used to cover the excised areas are frequently studded with the numerous pigmented nevi characteristically associated with large congenital nevi; or feasible donor sites may be too small. More coverage can be obtained by using mesh-grafts, but this further reduces the possibility of a good cosmetic result.

Thus, when one considers both the cosmetic and the medical problems, it would seem that the greatest good can be done for the greatest number of patients by removing those cosmetically disfiguring small nevi that may be eradicated by non-mutilating surgical procedures and by removing as much as possible of giant nevi without undue mutilation. Such decisions should usually be made in consultation with a plastic surgeon. At times, truly gratifying results may be achieved even for large nevi (Fig. 131). Kaplan (1974) has suggested that biopsies may be of predictive value in deciding areas with the highest risk for developing malignant melanoma, since, in his experience, superficial intradermal nevi do not seem to have malignant potential in contrast to junctional nevi, deep-dermal (neural) nevi and cellular blue nevi.

In summary, insufficient data are currently available to establish the prevalence of giant nevocytic nevi and to determine the risk of such lesions giving rise to malignant melanomas. However, the reports of some investigators indicate that the risk may be around 15% which, of course, far exceeds the risk of developing malignant melanoma in a lifetime for persons in the general population.

REFERENCES

Bergfeld, W., and Helwig, W. B. Exhibit at Academy of Dermatology, Miami Beach, December, 1972.

Dellon, A. L., Edelson, R. L., and Chretien, P. B. Defining the malignant potential of the giant pigmented nevus. Plastic Reconstr. Surg. 57: 611–618, 1976.

Demian, S. D. E., Donnelly, W. H., Frias, J. L., and Monif, G. R. G. Placental lesions in congenital giant pigmented nevi. Am. J. Clin. Path. 61:438–442, 1974.

Fish, J., Smith, E. B., and Canby, J. P. Malignant melanoma in childhood. Surgery 59:309–315, 1966.

Greeley, P. W., Middleton, A. G., and Curtin, J. W. Incidence of malignancy in giant pigmented nevi. Plast. Reconstr. Surg. 36:26–37, 1965.

Kaplan, A. M., Itabashi, H., Hanelin, L. G., and Lu, A. T. Neurocutaneous melanosis with malignant leptomeningeal melanoma. Arch. Neurol. 32:669–671, 1975.

Kaplan, E. N. The risk of malignancy in large congenital nevi. Plast. Reconstr. Surg. 53:421–428, 1974.

Lamas, E., Lobato, R. D., Sotelo, T., Ricoy, J. R., and Castro, S. Neurocutaneous melanosis. Report of a case and review of the literature. Acta Neurochirugica 36:93–105, 1977.

Lanier, V. C., Pickrell, K. L., and Georgiade, N. G. Congenital giant nevi: Clinical and pathological considerations. Plast. Reconstr. Surg. 58: 48–54, 1976.

Mark, G. J., Mihm, M. C., Liteplo, M. G., Reed, R. J. and Clark, W. H. Congenital melanocytic nevi of the small and garment type: clinical, histologic and ultrastructural studies. Hum. Pathol. 4:395–418, 1973.

Nicholls, E. M. Development and elimination of pigmented moles and the anatomical distribution of primary malignant melanoma. Cancer 32: 191–195, 1973.

Orkin, M., Frichot, B. C., and Zelickson, A. S. Cerebriform intradermal nevus. Arch. Derm. 110:575–582, 1974.

Pack, G. T., and Davis, J. The pigmented mole. Post-Grad. Med. 27: 370–382, 1960.

Pers, M. Nevus pigmentosa giganticus. Indications for removal. Ugeskr. Laeger 125:613–619, 1963.

Reed, W. B., Becker, S. W., Sr., Becker, S. W., Jr., and Nickel, W. R. Giant pigmented nevi, melanoma, and leptomeningeal melanocytosis. Arch. Dermatol. 91:100–119, 1965.

Walton, R. G., Jacobs, A. H., and Cox, A. J. Pigmented lesions in newborn infants. Brit. J. Derm. 95:389–396, 1976.

Chapter 8

Multiple Primary Malignant Melanomas

Multiple primary malignant melanomas are not rare. In non-familial cases of melanoma reported occurrences range between 1 and 4%. Out of 1,250 patients with malignant melanoma reviewed by Booher (1969), 16 had multiple primaries, an incidence of 1.28%. Beardmore and Davis (1975) report that 57 of 1,444 patients with primary cutaneous malignant melanoma developed more than one primary lesion, an incidence of 3.95%.

Cascinelli et al. (1975) report that 20 (3.8%) of their series of 521 patients with malignant melanomas had multiple primary lesions. They attribute their high rate to the policy in their institution of removing all apparently benign pigmented lesions presenting with any change and the removal of any pigmented lesions regarded as cutaneous metastases. Bellet et al. (1977) also found the prevalence (3.4%) of additional primary melanomas to be significantly greater than the expected number calculated on the basis of patient years at risk.

Within the general population of the United States, the annual incidence of primary melanoma is 4.2 per 100,000 (.0042%). It can be seen, then, that a patient with a malignant melanoma has a much higher risk of developing another primary malignant melanoma than has an individual in the general population of developing a primary malignant melanoma.

Multiple primary melanomas occur in 19% of patients with a familial history of malignant melanoma as compared to 1–4% in non-familial cases (Luce et al., 1973). Wallace et al. (1973) also found an increased occurrence of multiple primary malignant lesions in patients with a familial history of malignant melanomas. Furthermore, Reimer et al. (1978) reported multiple primary malignant melanomas in the "mole syndrome."

A distinction has to be made between multiple primary cutaneous malignant melanomas and multiple cutaneous metastases. Histologically, one finds junctional activity in the overlying epithelium in primary malignant melanoma but usually not in metastatic melanoma (Allen and Spitz, 1953). Rarely, however, metastases to the skin may be at the dermal-epidermal junction and may even invade the epidermis and thus appear as though they were primary lesions (see Chapter 4).

The number of primary lesions found in patients with multiple melanomas is usually less than five. Kahn and Donaldson (1970) describe a 34-year-old white man who developed more than 100 widely separated pigmented lesions of his skin within a three-year period. Of these, 48 were excised and all were found to be primary malignant melanomas. It was also found that the addition of the patient's serum to his tissue-cultured malignant melanoma cells caused more rapid growth and reduced contact inhibition of the cells. Thus, the authors postulated the presence of an "activating-factor" or the lack of an "inhibitory-factor" in the patient's serum. Several other investigators have considered the possibility of some intrinsic factor stimulating the growth of cells of preexisting nevi. Both Allen and Spitz (1953) and Pack (1959) observed that patients with proved cutaneous malignant melanomas are likely to show histologic evidence of "active" junctional change in coexisting nevi. Greenhalgh et al. (1971) postulate that the host may possess some intrinsic factor(s), possibly familial, which favor the formation of multiple nevi and of malignant melanoma.

A 27-year-old woman seen at the N.Y.U. Medical Center had three primary cutaneous melanomas removed within an 11-year-period. She had 61 other pigmented lesions excised, all of which turned out to be junctional or compound nevi. It was of particular interest that most of these nevi had moderate lymphocytic infiltrates beneath them but no clear-cut evidence of malignant melanoma.

Patients with malignant melanoma are not only more likely to develop other primary malignant melanomas than individuals in the general population but may also have a greater tendency to develop other cancers (Fletcher, 1973). For other reports of malignancies of multiple organs, including malignant melanomas, readers are referred to Gunz and Angus (1965), Moertel (1966), Berg (1967), and Fraser et al. (1971).

The pathogenesis of multiple primary malignant melanomas is unknown. Theories such as induction by sunlight, genetic susceptibility and viral cause all have some observations to support them.

Skibba et al. (1972) report a patient who developed multiple primary malignant melanomas following levodopa administration for Parkinson's disease. There are other reports of a possible relationship between levodopa and malignant melanoma (Robinson et al., 1973; Lieberman and Shupack, 1974).

SUMMARY

Patients with malignant melanoma are at a higher risk of developing other primary malignant melanomas than persons in the general population of developing a single malignant melanoma. This is especially so for patients with a familial history of melanoma. There is some evidence that patients who have melanomas have a more than average chance of developing other types of cancers as well. Clark et al. (1975) suggest that when a patient develops malignant melanoma during the first three decades of life or when the patient had multiple primary malignant melanomas, the clinician should be suspicious of the possibility of hereditary malignant melanoma and the blood relatives of the patient, as well as the patient himself, should be followed closely.

REFERENCES

Allen, A. C., and Spitz, S. Malignant melanoma: a clinicopathological analysis of the criteria for diagnosis and prognosis. Cancer 6:1–45, 1953.

Beardmore, G. L., and Davis, N. C. Multiple primary cutaneous melanomas. Arch. Dermatol. 111:603–609, 1975.

Bellet, R. E., Vaisman, I., Mastrangelo, M. J., and Lustbader, E. Multiple primary malignancies in patients with cutaneous melanoma. Cancer 40:1974–1981, 1977.

Berg, J. W. The incidence of multiple primary cancers. Development of further cancers in patients with lymphomas, leukemias and myeloma. J. Natl. Cancer Inst. 38:741–752, 1967.

Booher, R. J. Recognition and treatment of melanoma. Surg. Clin. North Am. 49:389–405, 1969.

Cascinelli, N., Fontana, V., Cataldo, I., and Balzarini, G. P. Multiple primary melanoma. Tumori 61:481–486, 1975.

Clark, W. H., Jr., Ainsworth, A. M., Bernardino, E. A., Yang, C. H., Mihm, M. C., Jr., and Reed, R. J. The developmental biology of primary human malignant melanomas. Semin. Oncol. 2:83–103, 1975.

Clinicopathologic conference: multiple malignancies: chronic lymphocytic leukemia, malignant melanoma, multiple myeloma, and acute myelomonocytic leukemia. Am. J. Med. 58:408–416, 1975.

Fraser, D. G., Bull, J. G., and Dunphy, J. E. Malignant melanoma and coexisting malignant neoplasms. Am. J. Surg. 122:169–174, 1971.

Fletcher, W. S. In: Riley, V. ed., "Pigment Cell: Mechanisms in Pigmentation," Vol. 1, Basel, S. Karger, 1973, pp. 255–260.

Greenhalgh, R. M., Talbot, I. C., and Calnan, J. S. Multiple malignant melanoma. Report of a patient with four primary malignant cutaneous melanomas. Br. J. Plast. Surg. 24:301–306, 1971.

Gunz, F. W., and Angus, H. B. Leukemia and cancer in the same patient. Cancer 18:145–152, 1965.

Kahn, L. B., and Donaldson, R. C. Multiple primary melanoma. Case report and study of tumor growth in vitro. Cancer 25:1162–1169, 1970.

Korsch, A., Gartmann, H., and Steigleder, G. K. Primar multiple maligne Melanome mit ungewohnlich langem Verlauf. Z. Hautkr, 51:949–956, 1976.

Lieberman, A. N., and Shupack, J. L. Levodopa and melanoma. Neurology 24:340–343, 1974.

Luce, J. K., McBride, C. M., and Frei, E. Melanoma. In: Holland, J. F. and Frei, E., eds. Cancer Medicine, Philadelphia, Lea & Febiger, 1973, pp. 1823–1843.

Moertel, C. G. Multiple Primary Malignant Neoplasms: Their Incidence and Significance. Recent Results in Cancer Research. (7), New York, Springer, 1966.

Pack, G. T. End results in the treatment of malignant melanoma: a later report. Surgery 46:447–460, 1959.

Reimer, R. R., Clark, W. H., Green, M. H., Ainsworth, A. M., and Fraumeni, J. F. Precursor lesions in familial melanoma: A new genetic preneoplastic syndrome. J.A.M.A. 239:744–746, 1978.

Robinson, E., Wajsbort, J., and Hirshowitz, B. Levodopa and malignant melanoma. Arch. Pathol. 95:213, 1973.

Robinson, E., Wajsbort, J., and Hirshowitz, B. Levodopa and malignant melanoma. Arch. Pathol. 95:213, 1973.

Skibba, J. L., Pinckley, J., Gilbert, E. F., and Johnson, R. O. Multiple primary melanoma following administration of levodopa. Arch. Pathol. 93:556–561, 1972.

Wallace, D. C., Beardmore, G. L., and Exton, L. A. Familial malignant melanoma. Ann. Surg. 177:15–20, 1973.

Chapter 9

Subungual Malignant Melanoma

Subungual malignant melanoma was first clearly described as "melanotic whitlow" by Sir Jonathan Hutchinson in 1886. The name was inspired by its resemblance, excepting pigmentation, to ordinary infections of whitlow.

In order that readers may appreciate the rarity of subungual malignancies in general, we reviewed 5,727 lesions suspect of malignancy seen in the Oncology Section of the Skin and Cancer Unit. There were only eight subungual malignant lesions, four on fingers and four on toes. Of these eight lesions, only one was a malignant melanoma.

One of the largest series of subungual melanomas published is that of Pack and Oropeza (1967) and it serves as the source of much of the information in this chapter. These authors described 72 patients with histologically proved melanotic whitlows. These 72 lesions represented 2.6% of 2,824 malignant melanomas treated by the Pack Medical Group up to 1967.

About half of all subungual malignant melanomas occur under fingernails and half occur under toenails. By far the most common locations are the nails of thumbs and great toes.

The majority of patients who develop subungual malignant melanomas are in the fifth, sixth and seventh decades of life with a mean age of about 55 years. The incidence in men and women is almost equal.

Although malignant melanomas occur much less commonly in American Negroes than in Caucasians, when they do occur in Negroes the subungual position is relatively frequent. Compared to the 2 to 3% in Caucasians, approximately 15 to 20% of malignant melanomas that occur in Negroes appear in subungual locations.

Most subungual malignant melanomas produce little discomfort. The patient often seeks consultation because of the appearance of the lesion. Usually no history of a preceding pigmented lesion is given by the patient. Frequently the lesion comes to the patient's attention because of trauma to the affected digit. Symptoms and signs then are of pain, discomfort, deformity of the nail, ulceration, swelling, and bleeding from the nail bed and surrounding tissues.

The diagnosis of subungual malignant melanoma is often delayed because of procrastination by the patient or because of a mistaken diagnosis by the physician. For example, Gibson et al. (1975) report that two-thirds of their cases had some form of minor surgical procedure performed before the true diagnosis was suspected. In only one-half of their cases was the correct diagnosis made within two years after onset of symptoms. At least one-third of the cases had detectable metastases by the time the diagnosis was made. Others have also pointed out the many errors which occur in the clinical diagnosis of malignant melanomas under nails (Leppard et al., 1974; Pack and Oropeza, 1967).

Subungual melanomas often begin as brown to black discolorations in the nail bed that frequently become bands or streaks of pigmentation. Thickening, splitting, distortion, or complete destruction of the nail plate may occur (Fig. 132). The nail bed and surrounding tissue may also show variable degrees of hyperpigmentation, inflammation, pain, discomfort, and purulent discharge. An almost pathognomonic sign described by Hutchinson (1886) is macular, mottled, tan to brown to black discoloration of the tissue around the affected site (Fig. 133). The primary lesion of subungual malignant melanoma is a great imitator of benign conditions such as bacterial and fungal infections, hematomas, and vascular tumors.

Approximately one-fifth of subungual malignant melanomas are amelanotic. Thus, that most important clinical feature, hyperpigmentation, is lacking in a significant percentage of these malignant melanomas.

We have encountered several patients who have had

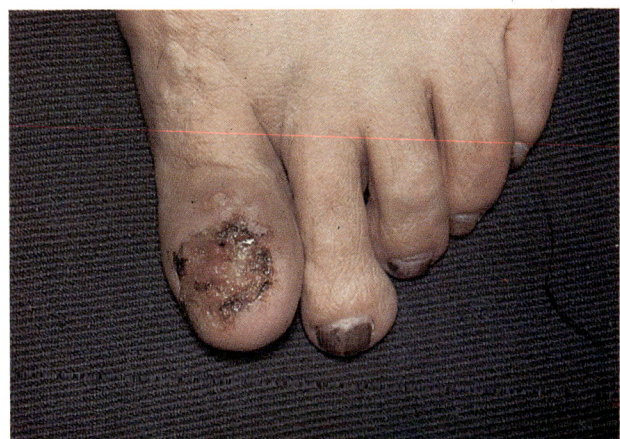

FIGURE 132. **Subungual malignant melanoma.** *This advanced lesion has caused complete destruction of the nail plate. The discoloration of the neighboring nail plates was caused by potassium permanganate soaks used by the patient for the treatment of a presumed bacterial or fungal paronychia, and is not related to the malignancy.*

macular pigmented lesions of the digits that were at first read histologically as benign. Some such biopsies were read as "benign melanocytic hyperplasia," others as "atypical melanocytic hyperplasia" and still others as "lentigo maligna-like" lesions (also see Lupulescu et al., 1973). Recently a concept of "acral-lentiginous melanomas" has been published by Clark et al. (1975) and by Reed (1976). Included in this group are subungual malignant melanomas.

They are characterized by a radial-growth phase which simulates but is differentiable from lentigo maligna. Abnormal (large and spindled) melanocytes are situated in the nail bed. Pagetoid cells are not prominent. When the vertical-growth phase ensues, such lesions act biologically like superficial spreading malignant melanomas (Fig. 134).

DIFFERENTIAL DIAGNOSIS

No neoplasm of the skin can mimic more conditions than can subungual melanomas. A partial list includes: nevocytic nevus, keratoacanthoma, Bowen's disease, squamous-cell carcinoma, hematoma, glomus tumor, granuloma pyogenicum (telangiectaticum), foreign body granuloma, Kaposi's sarcoma, subungual exostosis, epidermoid inclusions (Lewin, 1967), onychia and paronychia secondary to microbial infections, ingrowing nails, onychodystrophies, and pigmentation secondary to adrenalectomy for Cushing's disease (Bondy and Harwich, 1969). It is important to stress that melanotic bands in subungual position that are not malignant melanoma are not unusual in blacks and Orientals (Higashi, 1968; Leyden et al., 1972.) but are very uncommon in whites (Allyn et al., 1963).

TREATMENT

While it is preferable to do a conservative biopsy in toto in order to obtain a specimen for histologic examination for most malignant melanomas, this is usually not feasible for

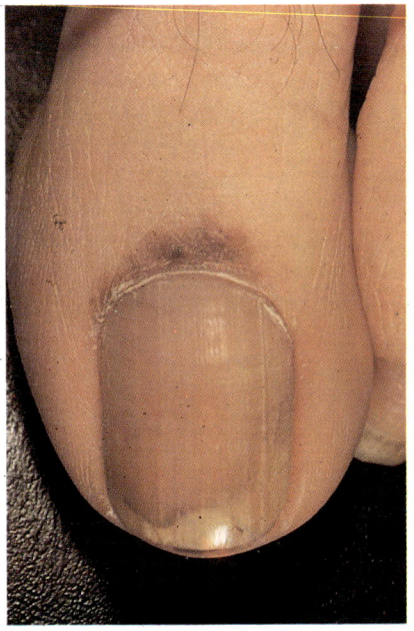

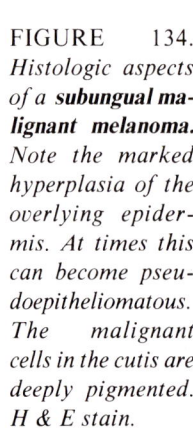

FIGURE 133. **Hutchinson's sign of subungual malignant melanoma.** *Acquired periungual melanotic pigmentation in a Caucasian is suggestive of subungual malignant melanoma.*

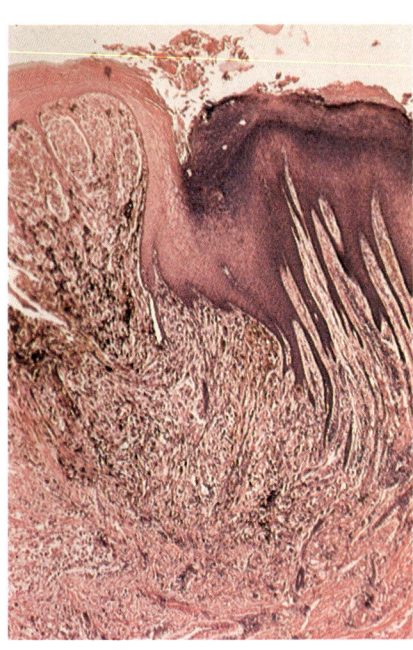

FIGURE 134. *Histologic aspects of a* **subungual malignant melanoma.** *Note the marked hyperplasia of the overlying epidermis. At times this can become pseudoepitheliomatous. The malignant cells in the cutis are deeply pigmented. H & E stain.*

subungual lesions. Accordingly, in this anatomical site, biopsy of a portion of the lesion is usually practised. Once the diagnosis has been histologically established, the recommended form of treatment is amputation of the digit and all, or the distal portion of, the corresponding metacarpal or metatarsal bone. However, disarticulation at the metacarpal-phalangeal joint may be preferred if reconstruction of a thumb is planned.

There is considerable controversy concerning treatment of the local lymph nodes in patients who have subungual malignant melanomas. Those who advocate elective removal do so on the basis of observations that microscopic foci of tumor are found in approximately one-fourth of those dissections in patients whose nodes are clinically negative. According to Das Gupta and McNeer (1964) regional metastases occurred in half their cases of subungual malignant melanomas under finger and toenails in nearly equal proportion.

Some surgeons advocate clinical observation of the lymph nodes with removal only if they become clinically involved. If there is clinical involvement of lymph nodes and if there are no contraindications such as distant metastases, the consensus is that these nodes should be removed by radical lymphadenectomy. Most surgeons do not do elective epitrochlear or popliteal lymph node dissections because of the rarity of involvement of these nodes.

Satellitosis can be managed by excision and graft, amputation of the extremity, isolation perfusion with hyperthermic chemotherapeutic agents (Stehlin et al., 1975), and/or intralymphatic injections of radioactive isotopes such as Yttrium^{90} in the form of microspheres (Ariel et al., 1964). Today it is generally recognized that heroic surgical procedures such as hemipelvectomy are rarely life-saving but are occasionally indicated for extreme pain, massive hemorrhage or other complications.

PROGNOSIS

Since malignant melanomas of subungual areas are relatively rare tumors, the statistics on survival are not conclusive. In five-year survival rates, Booher and Pack (1957) reported 21% in 29 subungual malignant melanomas of the hands and feet seen in an 18-year span (1917-1935); Pack and Oropeza (1967) reported 35% (Stage I, II and III lesions); Das Gupta and Brasfield (1965) reported 38% (Stage I and II lesions); and Graham (1973) reported 50%.

SUMMARY

In Caucasians it is probable that an acquired subungual melanotic lesion is more likely to be a malignant melanoma than a benign nevocytic nevus. All such lesions should be considered malignant melanomas until proved otherwise by histologic examination of biopsy material. If one biopsy is inconclusive, more should be done. Recently, the concept of acral-lentiginous melanomas has been described, but no analyses of "level" and "thickness" have yet been published to guide the physician in the more sophisticated management of these lesions.

Treatment of the primary lesion of subungual malignant melanoma is amputation of the digit and at least part of its associated metacarpal or metatarsal bone. Some exceptions exist (e.g., metacarpal-phalangeal joint disarticulation for melanomas on the thumb if plastic reconstruction is being considered).

The value of elective lymphadenectomy, isolation perfusion and other procedures are not yet firmly established.

REFERENCES

Allyn B., Kopf, A. W., Kahn, M., and Witten, V. H. Incidence of pigmented nevi. J.A.M.A. 186:890-893, 1963.

Ariel, I. M., Resnick, M. I., and Galey, D. The intralymphatic administration of radioactive isotopes and cancer chemotherapeutic drugs. Surgery 55:355-363, 1964.

Bondy, P. K., and Harwick, H. J. Longitudinal banded pigmentation of nails following adrenalectomy for Cushing's syndrome. N. Engl. J. Med. 281:1056-1057, 1969.

Booher, R. J., and Pack, G. T. Malignant melanoma of the feet and hands. Surgery 42:1084-1121, 1957.

Clark, W. H. Jr., Ainsworth, A. M., Bernardino, E. A., Yang, C. H., Mihm, M. C., and Reed, R. J. The developmental biology of primary human malignant melanomas. Semin. Oncol. 2:83-103, 1975.

Das Gupta, T., and Brasfield, R. Subungual melanoma: 25-year review of cases. Ann. Surg. 161:545-552, 1965.

Gibson, S. H., Montgomery, H., Woolner, L. B., and Brunsting, L. A. Melanotic whitlow (subungual melanoma). J. Invest. Dermatol. 29: 119-129, 1957.

Graham, W. P. Subungual melanoma. Pennsylvania Med. 76:56, 1973.

Higashi, N. Melanocytes of nail matrix and nail pigmentation. Arch. Dermatol. 97:570-574, 1968.

Hutchinson, J. Melanosis often not black: melanotic whitlow. Br. Med. J. 1:491, 1886.

Leppard, B., Sanderson, K. V., and Behan, F. Subungual malignant melanoma: difficulty in diagnosis. Br. Med. J. 1:310-312, 1974.

Lewin, K. Subungual epidermoid inclusions. Br. J. Dermatol. 81:671-675, 1969.

Leyden, J. J., Spott, D. A., and Goldschmidt, H. Diffuse and banded melanin pigmentation in nails. Arch. Dermatol. 105:548-550, 1972.

Lupulescu, A., Pinkus, H., Birmingham, D. J., Usndek, H. E., and Posch, J. L. Lentigo maligna of the fingertip. Arch. Dermatol. 107:717-722, 1973.

Pack, G. T., and Oropeza, R. Subungual melanoma. Surg. Gynecol. Obstet. 124:571-582, 1967.

Stehlin, J. S., Giovanella, B. C., Ipolyi, P. D., Muenz, L. R., and Anderson, R. F. Results of hyperthermic perfusion for melanoma of the extremities. Surg. Gynecol. Obstet. 140:339-348, 1975.

Chapter 10

Leukoderma and Malignant Melanomas

One of the most fascinating clinical phenomena in oncology is the development of leukoderma around cutaneous tumors. In 1965, Kopf et al. reported on neuroectodermally derived tumors associated with circumferential leukoderma, namely, nevocytic nevus, neuroid nevus, blue nevus, benign juvenile melanoma, and malignant melanoma (Fig. 135). Recently, Ridley (1975) reported a giant nevocytic nevus that developed a halo of depigmentation and then underwent spontaneous involution. The mechanism of the usual "halo nevus" phenomenon, in which melanocytic cells are destroyed, is unknown, but presumably the dense inflammatory reaction occurring around them is somehow involved. Shapiro and Kopf (1965) published a report of a nine-year-old girl who developed a depigmented halo around a pigmented tumor of her shoulder. Subsequently she developed widespread metastases and died of her disease. Histologically, the primary tumor, as well as the metastases, was malignant melanoma. Review of the literature at that time indicated that there were about a dozen reports of association of leukoderma and malignant melanoma.

Since our summary in 1965, other reports appeared relating malignant melanomas with depigmentary processes of the skin. Of particular interest are (1) leukoderma around benign nevocytic nevi in patients with malignant melanoma, (2) "halo melanoma" in which the leukoderma encircles the cutaneous tumor, and (3) widespread vitiligo and/or leukoderma distant from cutaneous tumors bearing leukodermic halos.

One of the most provocative reports is that by Copeman et al. (1973) in which the authors indicate that patients who have halo nevi have circulating antimelanoma antibodies which react with the cytoplasm of homologous cells of malignant melanoma. They found such antibodies in 15 patients with actively resolving halo nevi. Once resolution of the nevus was complete, or after the tumor has been completely excised, the antibodies disappeared. Such anti-melanoma antibodies were not demonstrable in patients who had ordinary nevocytic nevi, vitiligo or benign juvenile melanoma. The authors speculated that the leukodermic phenomenon in a halo nevus represents rejection of nevus cells that are undergoing malignant change. In a more recent report Copeman and Elliott (1976) tested 800 sera taken from patients with various pigmented lesions. One-third of the sera of patients with early cutaneous malignant melanomas and all halo nevi in process of resolution had significant titers of anti-melanoma antibody. In contrast sera from patients with various other pigmented benign skin lesions were negative. These authors suggest the possibility of using the anti-melanoma antibody test (1) to diagnose pigmented lesions, (2) to prognosticate and continuously monitor the course of malignant melanomas, and (3) to alert the physician to the development of malignant melanomas in high risk patients such as those who have giant nevocytic nevi or a familial history of malignant melanoma.

Epstein et al. (1973) reported five patients who, following removal of their primary malignant melanomas, developed multiple halo nevi. Immunologically these patients reacted with cell-mediated anti-melanoma immune responses as determined by lymphocyte stimulation and migration-inhibitory factor (MIF) responses against melanoma "antigens." They concluded that the development of halo nevi in association with malignant melanoma is likely to represent an immunologic reaction in which the patient reacts to antigens in the cells of melanomas and related antigens in nevus cells and in melanocytes.

Not only is leukoderma associated with human malignant melanomas but leukoderma and leukotrichia have been

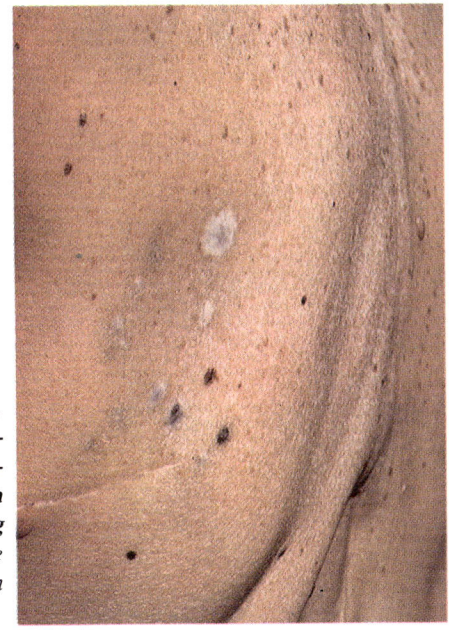

FIGURE 135A. *Cutaneous metastases of malignant melanoma with surrounding leukoderma. The primary site in the lumbar area.*

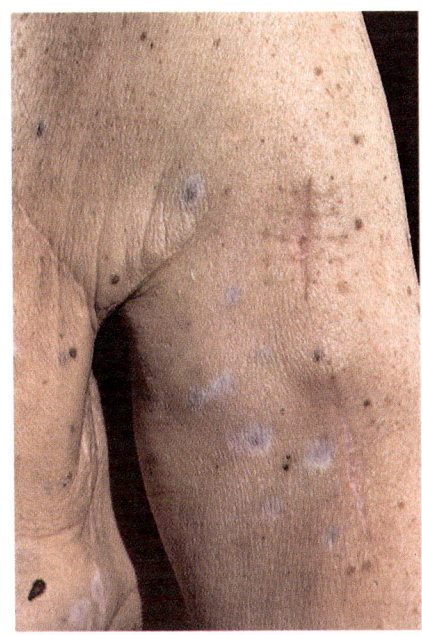

FIGURE 135B. **Metastatic lesions on the arm and chest of the same patient.** *It should be noted that the leukodermatous areas are in relation to metastatic lesions only.*

reported in animals bearing melanomas. Examples are genetic strains of horses (Hadwen, 1931) and pigs (Millikan et al., 1973) that spontaneously develop malignant melanomas and "vitiligo." Chimpanzees immunized against human melanoma have also developed "vitiligo" (Hornung and Krementz, 1974).

Leukoderma within malignant melanomas occurs frequently. Colors seen in many melanomas include "red, *white* and blue." The histologic correlate of this clinical whiteness (leukoderma) is a relative lack of epidermal melanin associated with a dermal lymphohistiocytic infiltrate and melanophages. Such regressive phenomena are seen often both clinically and histopathologically. If totally successful, the outcome of this host-tumor interaction is the complete disappearance of the lesion (see Chapter 11 on "Occult Primary and Spontaneous Regression of Malignant Melanomas"). In examining patients who had had spontaneous involution of primary and/or secondary malignant melanomas it is not unusual to observe clinical hypo- or depigmentation at the site (e.g., Maurer et al., 1974).

Roenigk et al. (1974) report "inflammatory vitiligo" occurring after treatment of malignant melanoma with vaccinia; Herrman et al. (1970) reported a patient who developed leukoderma following immunotherapy with smallpox vaccine and Freund's adjuvant; McPeak (1971) described depigmented areas at sites of cutaneous metastases after immunotherapy with intralymphatic administration of immune lymphocytes; Donaldson et al. (1974) reported two patients who developed uveitis and vitiligo after treatment of malignant melanomas with BCG.

Sumner (1953) and later Sumner and Foraker (1960) reported a woman who had a "mole" on her ankle that became "infected and dropped off," leaving an area of depigmentation three years prior to the development of disseminated melanoma. Some of these metastases disappeared spontaneously leaving zones of leukoderma similar to that at the presumed primary site of what is thought to have been the primary malignant melanoma on her ankle. Remarkably, transfusion of whole blood from this patient into a man with metastatic malignant melanoma was followed by disappearance of all of his lesions. Following regression, hair over a site on the scalp where a tumor nodule had been present became depigmented, whereas the rest of the hair remained black. Everson (1964) reported a similar case of a man who experienced spontaneous involution of multiple cutaneous and pulmonary metastases and in whom the cutaneous sites of previous malignant melanomas were described as "bone-white depigmented" scars.

It has been demonstrated that amelanotic malignant melanomas have a prognosis worse than melanotic malignant melanomas (Huvos et al., 1972). Nonetheless, it appears that the peritumoral leukodermatous changes associated with any particular stage of malignant melanoma generally foretell a better prognosis even if the tumor becomes depigmented in the process. Thus, it may be that amelanotic melanomas without peritumoral leukoderma develop by a different mechanism, perhaps by emergence of clones of highly malignant cells which do not produce pigment. (For further discussion see Chapter 4.)

Other observations concerning the association of leukoderma and malignant melanoma include:

—Maurer et al. (1974) presented photographic documentation of depigmentation surrounding a regressing metastatic cutaneous lesion. The metastatic nodule was 3 cm in diameter at the start of observation and eventually resolved completely. The patient lived eight years with other persistent metastatic malignant melanoma lesions.

—Berger and Voorhees (1971) described a patient who had multiple congenital giant nevocytic nevi, all with leukodermic halos. The nevi did not regress.

—Krebs et al. (1976) studied lymphocytes from 11 patients with halo nevi (leukoderma acquisitum centrifugum) for lymphocyte cytoxicity against allogeneic melanoma cells. The six patients who had actively regressing nevi had significant cytotoxicity whereas the four patients with "unchanged" central nevi had evidence of a serum "blocking factor" and low cytotoxicity. The remaining patient had low cytotoxicity, no blocking, and clinical nonregression of the central nevus.

—Roth (1968) reported vitiligo following x-ray therapy of multiple metastases from a malignant melanoma. He suggests that this result may have been caused by massive disturbance of the malignant cells resulting in the development of anti-melanin antibodies.

—Little (1972) found a 13% prevalence of partial regression of primary cutaneous malignant melanomas and McGovern (1975) reported that histologic signs of regression occurred in 12% of primary cutaneous melanomas. They found that among the various ways that regressive phenomena can manifest themselves clinically is leukoderma.

—A dramatic case of multiple primary malignant melanomas with leukodermatous halos was reported by Messeritsch (1972).

—Smith and Stehlin (1965) reviewed their experience with spontaneous regression of melanomas which included several associated with leukodermas.

—Frenk (1969) reported a patient with extensive vitiligo associated with a fatal malignant melanoma. In a review of the literature up to the time of his writing, he found only eight other cases of vitiliginous depigmentation during the evolution of malignant melanoma and he questioned if this could be coincidental.

—Milton et al. (1967) reported on light and electron microscopic studies of leukoderma in a patient with an occult primary malignant melanoma.

—Gerner and Moore (1976) reported that generalized depigmentation occurred in three patients inoculated with microbial antigens plus melanoma cells in an experimental immunotherapy protocol. In two patients destruction of malignant cells occurred.

—Hertz et al. (1977) describe antibodies to melanin-producing cells in patients with autoimmune vitiligo. These IgG antibodies bind *in vitro* specifically to human melanocytes, nevus cells, and melanoma cells. Among the many potential uses for such specific antibodies would be a radioactively tagged probe to ferret out distant metastases; an immunochemotherapeutic agent, in which a melanoma-cidal chemotherapeutic agent could be coupled with the specific anti-pigment-cell antibodies; and a diagnostic tool for differentiating melanoma from other histologically similar tumors.

SUMMARY AND COMMENT

The observation of the association of leukoderma and vitiligo with malignant melanomas has now been made repeatedly. These hypo- and depigmentary phenomena are due to impairment or destruction of melanocytes at the dermal-epidermal interface. The not infrequent association of leukodermas with partial or complete regression of malignant melanomas suggests a common mechanism. However, further study is needed in order to elucidate the precise mechanisms responsible for this dramatic association.

REFERENCES

Berger, R. S., and Voorhees, J. J. Multiple congenital giant nevocellular nevi with halos. Arch. Dermatol. 104:515–521, 1971.

Copeman, P. W. M., and Elliott, P. G. Melanoma cytoplasmic humoral antibody test. Br. J. Dermatol. 94:565–568, 1976.

Copeman, P. W. M., Lewis, M. G., Phillips, T. M., and Elliott, P. G. Immunological associations of the halo naevus with cutaneous malignant melanoma. Br. J. Dermatol. 88:127–137, 1973.

Donaldson, R. C., Cannan, S. A., McLean, R. B., and Ackerman, L. V. Uveitis and vitiligo associated with BCG treatment for malignant melanoma. Surgery 76:771–778, 1974.

Editorial: the halo naevus and malignant melanoma. Lancet 1:982, 1973.

Epstein, W. L., Sagebeil, R., Spitler, L., Wybran, J., Reed, W. B., and Blois, M. S. Halo nevi and melanoma. J.A.M.A. 225:373–377, 1973.

Everson, T. C. Spontaneous regression of cancer. Ann. N.Y. Acad. Sci. 114:721–735, 1964.

Fishman, H. C. Malignant melanoma arising with two halo nevi. Arch. Derm. 112:407–408, 1976.

Fodor, J., and Bodrogi, I. Vitiligo and malignant melanoma. Neoplasma 22:445–446, 1975.

Frenk, E. Dépigmentations vitiligineuses chez des patients atteints de mélanomes malins. Dermatologica 139:84–91, 1969.

Gerner, R. E., and Moore, G. E. Feasibility study of active immunotherapy in patients with solid tumors. Cancer 38:131-143, 1976.

Hadwen, S. The melanomata of grey and white horses. Can. Med. Assoc. J. 25:519-530, 1931.

Happle, R., Schotola, I., and Macher, E. Spontanregression and Leukoderm bein malignen Melanom. Der. Hautarzt 26:120-123, 1975.

Hermann, W. P., Tritsch, H., and Gartmann, H. Rückbildung von Melanom-Metastasen nach Injektion von Freundschem Adjuvans. Hautarzt 21:181-183, 1970.

Hertz, K. C., Gazze, L. A., Kirkpatrick, C. H., and Katz, S. I. Autoimmune vitiligo. New Engl. J. Med. 297:634-637, 1977.

Hornung, M. O., and Krementz, E. T. Specific tissue and tumor responses of chimpanzees following immunization against human melanoma. Surgery 75:477-486, 1974.

Huvos, A. G., Shah, J. P., and Goldsmith, H. S. A clinicopathologic study of amelanotic melanoma. Surg. Gynecol. Obstet. 135:917-920, 1972.

Kopf, A. W., Morrill, S. D., and Silberberg, I. Broad spectrum of leukoderma acquisitum centrifugum. Arch. Dermatol. 92:14-35, 1965.

Krebs, J. A., Roenigk, H. H., Deodhar, S. D., and Barna, B. Halo nevus: Competent surveillance of potential melanoma. Cleveland Clinic Quart. 43:11-15, 1976.

Lerner, A. B., and Nordlund, J. J. Should vitiligo be induced in patients after resection of primary melanoma? Arch Derm 113:421, 1977.

Lewis, M. G., and Copeman, P. W. M. Halo naevus—a frustrated malignant melanoma? Br. Med. J. 2:47-48, 1972.

Little, J. H. Histology and prognosis in cutaneous malignant melanoma. In: McCarthy, W. H., ed. Melanoma and Skin Cancer, Proceedings International Cancer Conference, Sydney, 1972. V.C.N., Blight, Government Printer, pp. 107-120.

Maurer, L. H., McIntyre, O. R., and Rueckert, F. Spontaneous regression of malignant melanoma: pathologic and immunologic study in a ten year survivor. Am. J. Surg. 127:397-403, 1974.

McGovern, V. J. Melanoma-growth patterns, multiplicity and regression. In: McCarthy, W. H., ed. Melanoma and Skin Cancer. Proceedings International Cancer Conference, Sydney, 1972. V. C. N. Blight, Government Printer, pp. 95-106.

McGovern, V. J. Spontaneous regression of melanoma. Pathology 7:91-99, 1975.

McPeak, C. J. Intralymphatic therapy with immune lymphocytes. Cancer 28:1126-1128, 1971.

Messeritsch, H. Multiple Primäre Melanome. Hautarzt 23:289, 1972.

Millikan, L. E., Hook, R. R., and Manning, P. J. Gross and ultrastructural studies in a new melanoma model: the Sinclair swine. Yale J. Biol. Med. 46:631-645, 1973.

Millikan, L. E., Boylon, J. L., Hook, R. R., and Manning, P. J. Melanoma in Sinclair swine: a new animal model. J. Invest. Dermatol. 62:20-30, 1974.

Milton, G. W., Lane Brown, M. M., and Gilder, M. Malignant melanoma with an occult primary lesion. Br. J. Surg. 54:651-658, 1967.

Perrot, H., Ortonne, J. P., and Schmitt, D.: Vitiliginous achromia with malignant melanoma. Arch. Dermatol. Res. 257:247-253, 1977.

Ridley, C. M. Giant halo naevus with spontaneous resolution. Trans. St. Johns Hosp. Dermatol. Soc. 60:54-58, 1974.

Roenigk, H. H., Deodhar, S., St. Jacques, R., and Burdick, K. Immunotherapy of malignant melanoma with vaccinia virus. Arch. Dermatol. 109:668-673, 1974.

Roth, W. G. Vitiligo nach Röntgenbestrahlung Multipler Melanommetastasen. Hautarzt 19:178-180, 1968.

Shapiro, L., and Kopf, A. W. Leukoderma acquisitum centrifugum. Arch. Dermatol. 92:64-68, 1965.

Smith, J. L., and Stehlin, J. S. Spontaneous regression of primary malignant melanomas with regional metastases. Cancer 18:1399-1415, 1965.

Sumner, W. C. Spontaneous regression of melanoma. Cancer 6:1040-1043, 1953.

Sumner, W. C., and Foraker, A. G. Spontaneous regression of human melanoma. Cancer 13:79-81, 1960.

Chapter 11

Occult Primary Malignant Melanomas and Spontaneous Regression of Malignant Melanomas

Everson and Cole (1966) define spontaneous regression of a malignant neoplasm as partial or complete disappearance in the absence of any or indubitably inadequate therapy. Cases of either partial and complete spontaneous regression of malignant melanomas have been reported. Failure to find a primary malignant melanoma in a patient with metastatic disease has many possible explanations, one of which may be spontaneous regression of the primary tumor. Spontaneous regression of metastatic visceral melanomas has rarely been reported (Milton et al., 1967).

OCCULT PRIMARY MALIGNANT MELANOMA

The occurrence of occult primary melanomas reported by different observers varies from 1 to 15% of patients included in their series. Brownstein and Helwig (1972) reported from the Armed Forces Institute of Pathology that a review of their files of more than 1000 patients with metastatic malignant melanoma revealed that 15% had undeterminable primary sites. A rate of 15% was also reported by Einhorn et al. (1974). Most of their 426 patients had subcutaneous or nodal metastases. Das Gupta et al. (1963) reviewed 992 cases of malignant melanoma and found that 37 had metastatic lesions from unknown primary sites, an incidence of about 3.7%. These authors thought that in some cases the cutaneous sites where primary malignant melanomas had once been were then hypopigmented areas. Histologic examination of such leukodermatous areas revealed melanophages and mild chronic inflammatory infiltrates, but no malignant cells. They found that the prognosis for patients in whom a primary lesion is undeterminable is the same as that for patients with known primary lesions in the same stage of disease.

Baab and McBride (1975) reported that 4% of 2,446 patients with malignant melanoma they reviewed did not have a known primary site. The 5- and 10-year survivals for those patients with occult primary melanomas were higher than for similar patients with known primary lesions. They speculated that if a primary lesion spontaneously regresses, the immunity, of which that regression is an expression, might be the reason for unexpectedly longer survival. In contrast, Milton et al. (1977) report that their patients with occult primary melanomas had a poor outlook.

Other explanations for occult primary malignant melanomas are: (1) they were destroyed by trauma, (2) they actually exist in the skin but are indistinguishable from other pigmented lesions, (3) they are too small and/or deeply placed in the skin to be recognized, (4) their origin is not in the skin but in an internal organ (e.g., gastrointestinal tract, adrenal gland, meninges) (Milton et al., 1967), or, (5) they arose de novo within lymph nodes (Das Gupta et al., 1963). Concerning the last, McCarthy et al. (1974) reported that in non-melanoma bearing subjects 6.2% of specimens from axillary nodes and 4% of inguinal nodes contained nevus cells. In a somewhat different study Ridolfi et al. (1977) found aggregates of nevus cells in 0.33% of axillary lymph node specimens removed from patients with mammary carcinomas, and in 3% of lymph node specimens removed from patients who underwent radical lymph-node dissections for malignant melanomas. Thus, there is the remote possibility that melanomas may arise from nevus cells within the nodes themselves.

The sex ratio, age distribution, family history and survival rates of patients with unknown primary malignant melanomas are similar to those of patients with obvious malignant melanomas in the skin. (Baab and McBride, 1975).

SPONTANEOUS REGRESSION OF MALIGNANT MELANOMAS

The occurrence of spontaneous regression of melanomas in different reports varies from 0.08% to about 13%. Most spontaneous regressions in malignant melanoma are of cutaneous or lymphatic tumors. The first histologically proved case of spontaneous regression in a case of visceral metastatic disease was reported by Bulkley et al. (1975). The presence and subsequent absence of visceral metastases were substantiated by open liver biopsies. Histologic examination of metastatic hepatic lesions revealed extensive necrosis of the tumor and infiltration of the tumor by lymphocytes and plasma cells. Retrospective evaluation of the patient's immune status after regression of the melanoma showed a strongly positive delayed hypersensitivity response to dinitrochlorobenzene, to bacterial and fungal antigens, and to two of four potassium-chloride solubilized extracts of allogeneic human melanoma cells. The patient's leukocytes exhibited a slightly increased level of migration inhibition when reacted with one of these melanoma extracts. Eleven years following remission, the patient's lymphocyte response to stimulation by phytohemagglutinin did not exceed the normal range. Cell- and serum-mediated cytotoxicity against tissue-cultured allogeneic melanoma cells slightly exceeded the normal range.

Maurer et al. (1974) reported on pathologic and immunologic studies on a patient who had survived eight years with metastatic malignant melanoma. During this time repeated tests showed a gradual decrease in the stimulation of cultured lymphocytes by malignant cells obtained from several metastatic nodules and the eventual emergence of a cell line from a metastasis in the intestine that did not cause lymphocyte stimulation. The authors speculated that the visceral metastases were derived from a new cell line less antigenic then the original subcutaneous metastatic tumors. As further evidence they found that metastases to the stomach showed substantially less round-cell infiltrate than in the subcutaneous nodules, and they observed disappearance of a serum factor which augmented lymphocytotoxicity once the visceral metastases occurred.

Doyle et al. (1973) reported a patient whose remission was not traceable to immunological, hormonal or other mechanisms.

McGovern (1975) claims that cutaneous malignant melanomas have a tendency to disappear spontaneously. He found that of 437 primary cutaneous malignant melanomas, 54 (12.3%) showed histological features of partial regression. These features were characterized by a dense lymphocytic infiltrate similar to that found around nevi that disappear spontaneously. He concluded that the process may cease after partial regression or may continue until the tumor has been completely destroyed. Once the regression process stops, the lymphocytes disappear, leaving scar tissue with a variable number of melanophages and increased vasculature. He stated that all tumors exhibiting the regression phenomenon were malignant melanomas of the superficial-spreading type. Certain clinical patterns of this process can be recognized, namely, (1) an inflammatory nodule with or without pigmentation, (2) scarring in the tumor, (3) several foci of malignancy simulating multicentricity, (4) a pigmented lesion with a depigmented halo, (5) a pigmented scar with surviving malignant cells, (6) a pigmented scar without surviving tumor cells, (7) metastatic melanoma with no demonstrable cutaneous primary lesion.

Bodurtha et al. (1976) reported a case of metastatic malignant melanoma that underwent spontaneous regression. Using a microcytotoxicity assay in which melanoma target cells were used, the authors demonstrated a significant increase in lymphocyte cytotoxicity during the clinical course of regression. The clinical and histologic features were also consistent with an immunologic explanation for the spontaneous remission of the metastases.

Nathanson (1976) reviewed the pertinent literature and reported on the incidence, clinical features, and possible mechanisms of spontaneous regression of melanomas. He concluded that there were 33 patients who had total regression of their primary melanomas and 40 patients (13 of whom were somewhat doubtful) with regression of melanoma metastases. Cutaneous lesions were the most common metastases to regress, followed by lymphatic, pulmonary, and hepatic metastases. About 40% of patients with spontaneous regression had "spontaneous cure," i.e., no relapse of melanoma during a long period of follow-up or until death from other causes. Based on this literature the average incidence of partial regression of primary melanoma was 14.9%, of unknown (cryptic) primary melanomas 5.4%, and of spontaneous regression of metastatic melanoma 0.22%.

REFERENCES

Baab, G. H., and McBride, C. M. Malignant melanoma. The patient with an unknown site of primary origin. Arch. Surg. 110:896–900, 1975.

Bodenham, D. C. A study of 650 observed malignant melanomas in the south-west region. Ann. R. Coll. Surg. Engl. 43:218–239, 1968.

Bodurtha, A. J., Berkelhammer, J., Kim, Y. H., Laucius, J. F., and Mastrangelo, M. J. A clinical, histologic, and immunologic study of a case of metastatic malignant melanoma undergoing spontaneous remission. Cancer 37:735–742, 1976.

Booher, R. J. Recognition and treatment of melanoma. Surg. Clin. North. Am. 49:389-405, 1969.

Boyd, W. The Spontaneous Regression of Cancer. Springfield, Charles C. Thomas, 1966.

Brownstein, M. H., and Helwig, E. B. Patterns of cutaneous metastasis. Arch. Dermatol. 105:862-868, 1972.

Bulkley, G. B., Cohen, M. H., Banks, P. M., Char, D. H., and Ketcham, A. S. Long-term spontaneous regression of malignant melanoma with visceral metastases. Report of a case with immunologic profile. Cancer 36:485-494, 1975.

Das Gupta, T., Bowden, L., and Berg, J. W. Malignant melanoma of unknown primary origin. Surg. Gynecol. Obstet. 117:341-345, 1963.

Doyle, J. C., Bennett, R. C., and Newing, R. K. Spontaneous regression of malignant melanoma. Med. J. Aust. 2:551-552, 1973.

Einhorn, L. H., Burgess, M. A., Vallejos, C., et al. Prognostic correlations and response to treatment in advanced metastic malignant melanoma. Cancer Res. 34:1995-2004, 1974.

Everson, P. C., and Cole, W. H. Spontaneous Regression of Cancer. Philadelphia, W.B. Saunders, 1966.

Maurer, H., McIntyre, O. R., and Rueckert, F. Spontaneous regression of malignant melanoma. Pathologic and immunologic study in a ten year survivor. Am. J. Surg. 127:397-403, 1974.

McCarthy, S. W., Palmer, A. A., Bale, P. M., and Hirst, E. Naevus cells in lymph nodes. Pathology 6:351-358, 1974.

McGovern, V. J. Spontaneous regression of melanoma. Pathology 7:91-99, 1975.

Milton, G. W., Lane Brown, M. D., and Gildes, M. Malignant melanoma with an occult primary lesion. Br. J. Surg. 54:651-658, 1967.

Milton, G. W., McGovern, V. J., and Lewis, M. G. Malignant Melanoma of the Skin and Mucous Membrane. Edinburgh London, and New York, Churchill Livingston, 1977.

Nathanson, L.: Spontaneous regression of malignant melanoma: A review of the literature on incidence, clinical features, and possible mechanisms. Natl. Cancer Inst. Monogr. 44:67-76, 1976.

Ridolfi, R. L., Rosen, P. P., and Thaler, H. Nevus cell aggregates associated with lymph nodes: Estimated frequency and clinical significance. Cancer 39:164-171, 1977.

Chapter 12

Extra-regional Metastases from Malignant Melanomas

No malignancy metastasizes more widely than malignant melanoma, which is known to be able to involve every organ of the human body. If one excludes regional metastases (i.e., satellitosis, in-transit metastases and metastases to regional lymph-nodes), it is impossible to predict to what organ metastases will go, since extra-regional metastases are usually via the hematogenous route. Das Gupta and Brasfield (1964) concluded that multiple cutaneous and/or subcutaneous metastases limited to a single area, which are usually lymphatic in origin, are characterized by longer patient survival than those of hematogenous dispersion. They assume that bilateral cutaneous and/or subcutaneous nodules, either diffuse or solitary, are usually the result of hematogenous spread; such spread, when diffuse, is often associated with metastatic disease of the heart. Einhorn and co-workers (1974) analyzed the areas of metastatic spread from melanomas arising in different anatomical sites. The only primary site that had a consistent anatomical pattern was in the eyes wherefrom hepatic metastases frequently were detected as the initiation of metastatic disease. They also found that levels of lactic dehydrogenase (LDH) were elevated in almost every case of metastatic melanoma in the liver, that usually the elevation was greater than twice the range of normal, and that if the levels of LDH were normal the likelihood of hepatic metastases was remote.

According to Einhorn et al. (1974) patients with disseminated metastatic melanoma limited to the skin and subcutaneous tissues when treated by chemotherapy had an average survival of 11 months. Although the average survival for patients with visceral involvement was but 4.7 months, patients whose only detectable visceral involvement was pulmonary had a median survival of ten months. Women with disseminated melanoma lived somewhat longer than men with disseminated melanoma.

Das Gupta and Brasfield (1964) and Einhorn and his co-workers (1974) reported on the incidence of metastases to various organs in two large series of autopsies, 125 patients and 96 patients respectively. Many of these data are summarized in Table 9. The lungs, skin and subcutaneous tissue, and the liver are among the commonest extra-regional sites of metastatic involvement found at autopsies.

TABLE 9
Extra-Regional Metastases Found at Autopsy

Site*	Percentage in 125 autopsies[†]	Percentage in 96 autopsies[‡]
Skin and subcutis	75	54
Brain	39[§]	54[¶]
Thyroid	39	21
Lungs	70	87
Pleura	24	15
Heart	49	55
Liver	68	76
Pancreas	53	38
Spleen	36	43
Lymph nodes	65	74
Bone	42	23
Adrenals	50	54
Kidneys	45	58
Stomach	26	7
Small bowel	58	26
Large bowel	22	14
Peritoneum	13	27
Urinary bladder	18	14

* Other sites showed rates of metastases varying from 0 to 20% in the two reports.[1,2]
[†] Das Gupta and Brasfield, 1964.   [‡] Einhorn et al., 1974.
[§] Studied in 105 cases.   [¶] Studied in 85 cases.

REFERENCES

Das Gupta T., and Brasfield, R. Metastatic melanoma: a clinicopathological study. Cancer 17:1323–1339, 1964.

Einhorn, L. H., Burgess, M. A., Vallejos, C. et al. Prognostic correlations and response to treatment in advanced metastatic malignant melanoma. Cancer Res. 34:1955–2004, 1974.

Chapter 13

Staging of Malignant Melanoma

There are several staging classifications in use for malignant melanoma. Thus, the practitioner must know the classification used by the authors of articles he reads and by oncologists to whom he refers his patients (Figs. 136 and 137).

Table 10 is the staging system currently used by the NYU Melanoma Cooperative Group. Even this classification will probably undergo revision as the factors which significantly influence outcome are identified.

There is no accepted Tumor-Node-Metastases (TNM) classification for malignant melanoma at this time. One has been proposed (Veronesi et al., 1971), but is not yet agreed upon.

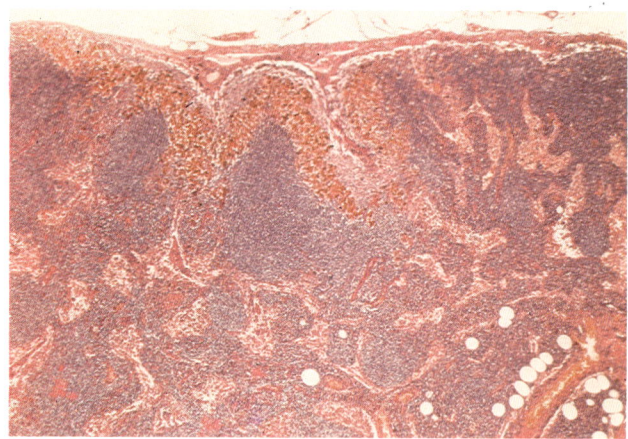

FIGURE 137A. *Histology of malignant melanoma metastatic to lymph node.* The pigmented malignant cells are primarily on the peripheral area of the node. H & E stain.

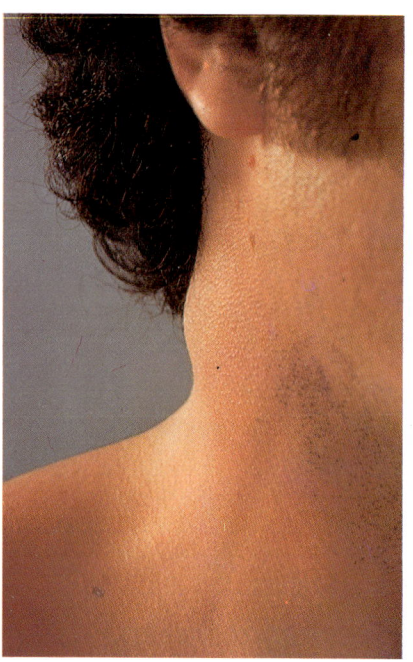

FIGURE 136. *Metastatic malignant melanoma to a lymph node.* If, in addition to the primary tumor, this were the only other finding on clinical examination, the patient would be classified as Stage IIA malignant melanoma by the staging criteria used by the NYU Melanoma Cooperative Group.

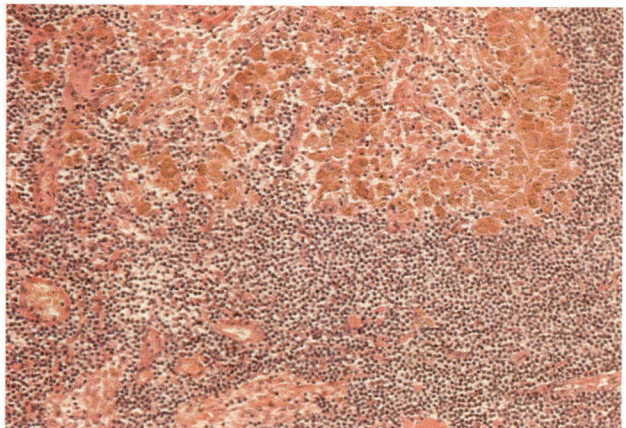

FIGURE 137B. *Higher magnification of same node showing deeply pigmented metastatic cells destroying the normal architecture of the node. H & E stain.*

TABLE 10
NYU Melanoma Cooperative Group Staging System

Stage I—Local disease
   IA Primary lesion alone
   IB Primary and satellites within 5 cm
   IC Local recurrence within 5 cm of primary site
   ID Spread more than 5 cm from primary site but within primary lymphatic drainage area
Stage II—Nodal disease (regional draining nodes)
   IIA Regional lymph nodes; clinically positive, histology not done
   IIB Regional lymph nodes; clinically negative, histology positive
   IIC Regional lymph nodes; clinically positive, histology positive
Stage III—Disseminated disease
   IIIA Remote cutaneous/subcutaneous melanoma
   IIIB Remote nodal involvement only
   IIIC *Both* of above
   IIID Visceral spread

REFERENCES

Goldsmith, H. S., Shah, J. P., and Kim, D. H. Prognostic significance of lymph node dissection in the treatment of malignant melanoma. Cancer 26:606–609, 1970.

Luce, J. K., McBride, C. M., and Frei, E. Melanoma. In: Holland, J. F., and Frei, E., eds., Cancer Medicine. Philadelphia, Lea & Febiger, 1973, p. 1834.

McNeer, G., and Das Gupta, T. Prognosis in malignant melanoma. Surgery 56:512–518, 1964.

Veronesi, U., Cascinelli, N., and Preda, F. Prognosis of malignant melanoma according to regional metastases. Am. J. Roentgenol. Radium Ther. Nucl. Med. 111:301–309, 1971.

Chapter 14

Prognostication of Behavior of Malignant Melanoma

The age and sex of the patient, the anatomic site of the neoplasm, the type, level of invasion, thickness and surface area of the lesion, the presence or absence of metastases to the regional lymph nodes or beyond, and the presence or absence of pigment in the tumor are some of the factors that not only directly affect the prognosis but which also must be taken into account when deciding on the type and extent of treatment. Although we often think in terms of 5-year "cure" rates, it is important to realize that about 13 to 20% of patients destined to have recurrent melanomas do so after the fifth year from the time of diagnosis (Mundth et al., 1965; Luce et al., 1973).

Clark and co-workers (1969) and McGovern (1970) reported that survival rates in patients with malignant melanoma are inversely related to the level of cutaneous invasion of the malignant cells. This relationship has been confirmed by other investigators. In the study of Clark et al. (1969) each lesion was classified according to its depth of invasion in the skin as follows: level I—is entirely intraepidermal; level II—reaches into the papillary dermis; level III—fills the papillary dermis and abuts on the junction of the papillary and reticular dermis; level IV—reaches into the reticular dermis; level V—invades into the subcutaneous tissue. The Clark group found that level II melanomas were attended by an 8.3% mortality; level III, 35.2%; level IV, 46.1%; and level V, 52%. Lentigo maligna melanoma was the type found to have the best survival rate, 89.7%, followed by superficial spreading melanoma which had a rate of 68.5%. Nodular melanoma showed the worst survival rate, 43.9%.

A link between prognosis and thickness of the neoplasm measured histologically with an ocular micrometer was reported by Breslow (1970). In the 98 patients studied, no recurrences or metastases were found if the thickness was less than 0.76 mm. Patients with lesions 0.76 to 1.5 mm thick sometimes developed metastases; this range of thickness was judged prognostically to be a "gray area."

When lesions were thicker than 1.5 mm, metastases were found to be frequent. Clark's levels and Breslow's thicknesses are more or less dependent criteria, but the determination of thicknesses may identify those level II and III lesions which have relatively good or poor prognoses (e.g., less or more than 0.76 mm thick).

Bodenham (1968, 1969) found the following factors prognostically ominous: rapid growth rate, marked elevation, ulceration or bleeding, little pigment, satellitosis, and location on the trunk. Histologically, Bodenham found three types of malignant cells. Lesions on males more often had a spindle cell-type, and females a round cell-type. A mixed cell-type was also found in both sexes, and this type was attended by the best prognosis whereas the worst prognosis was associated with the round cell-type. If the malignancy was not surrounded by lymphocytes, if it invaded deeply into the dermis, or if the lymphatics were involved, the prognosis was the poorer. Fitzpatrick et al. (1972) and Hansen and McCarten (1974) also reported that malignant melanomas with a lymphocytic infiltrate at the base of the tumor had a more favorable prognosis than lesions without this feature.

Jones Williams et al. (1968) reveiwing the five-year survival rate of 89 patients with malignant melanoma found that depth of involvement and the number of mitoses (if greater than one per five high-power fields) were the only features that were of prognostic value. McGovern (1972) also found an inverse relationship between survival and the prevalence of mitoses among the melanoma cells. Furthermore, he states that tumors of similar degrees of mitotic activity have similar survival rates whatever their histogenetic mode of development, and concludes that pathologists should grade melanomas according to mitotic activity in their reports. He concludes that mitotic activity and depth of invasion are the two most important histologic parameters in determining the prognosis of melanomas.

Jones et al. (1968) stated that malignant melanomas on

the trunk are commonest in men, those on the lower limbs commonest in women and those on the head and neck commonest in aged women. These authors found that prognosis is best when malignancies are situated on the lower limbs, worst when on the trunk, and intermediate when on the head and neck. If the primary lesion was greater than 3 cm in diameter there was a 9% five-year survival rate while if the lesion was less than 3 cm in diameter the five-year survival rate was 49%. The clinical state of the disease was also found to be valuable in prognostication: Stage I patients had a 41% five-year survival rate as compared to an 18% rate for Stage II patients.

Veronesi et al. (1971) found that prognosis was favorable in lentigo maligna melanomas, slow-growing malignant melanomas situated on the lower limbs of women, and "ring" melanomas (malignant melanomas with very slow growth that expanded centrifugally and simultaneously regressed in the center). A bad prognosis was associated with amelanotic melanomas, ulcerating neoplasms, satellitosis, and marked elevation on the skin. The authors found the highest survival rate was for malignant melanomas on the head and neck.

Sinha and Buntine (1974), in a retrospective study of 112 patients with malignant melanoma, found that neoplasms in women, in young patients, and those tumors situated on upper extremities had relatively good prognoses (provided the melanomas had not spread beyond the primary site). The authors stated, however, that the clinical stage and depth of invasion of the tumor appeared to be the most valuable indicators of prognosis. A retrospective study by Franklin et al. (1975) on 296 patients with malignant melanoma also indicated that women had better prognoses than men. These authors found that the level of dermal invasion of the lesion correlated with metastases to regional nodes, and with prognosis. Of patients with level II lesions, 7.4% developed positive nodes; with level III, 42%; with level IV, 52.7%; and with level V, 93.5%.

Cady (1975) found a reciprocal relationship between level and 6-year disease-free survival: namely, level II, 86%; level III, 67%; level IV, 67%; and level V, 11%. Also the larger the diameter, the poorer the 6-year disease-free survival: namely, 0 to 0.49 cm diameter, 83%; 0.5 to 0.99 cm, 37%; 1.0 to 1.99 cm, 37%; 2.0 or more cm, 18%.

Huvos et al. (1973) studied 119 patients with malignant melanomas of the head and neck and found significant correlation between the depth of invasion and the type. Nodular melanomas were the most deeply penetrating (and had the worst prognosis) whereas melanomas arising in Hutchinson's melanotic freckles were the most superficial (and had the best prognosis). Sober et al. (1974) found that for patients with lentigo maligna melanoma, the death rate at five years was 15%. For superficial spreading melanoma the death rate at five years was 35% and for nodular melanoma, 60%.

Huvos et al. (1974) seeking prognostic signs compared 100 patients with malignant melanomas who died within five years after diagnosis with 100 patients who were free of disease for 10 years or longer. They found the prognosis to be poorer if the lesion were in a male; if the size were more than 1 cm in diameter; if ulceration, deep dermal penetration, blood vessel invasion, lack of lymphocytic response around the primary tumor were present; if the duration were longer than six months; if there were lack of pigmentation; and finally if there were giant cells. Factors that did not make a statistically significant difference in prognosis were origin in a preexisting mole, elevation, satellitosis, epidermal hyperplasia, cell morphology, high mitotic rate, or junctional activity. That amelanotic malignant melanoma behaves in a biologically more aggressive manner and has a worse prognosis than its melanotic counterpart was previously reported by Huvos et al. (1972). These authors further found a striking preponderance of amelanotic melanomas in women.

Wanebo et al. (1975) confirmed others' findings that the histologic type of the melanoma is an important measure of survival and that nodular melanoma carries the worst prognosis. They stated, however, that microstaging by depth of invasion and Clark's levels showed better prognostic correlation than the histologic type of melanoma. The authors found a positive correlation between Clark's levels and the incidence of metastases to nodes. In their data, level II lesions had a 5% rate of metastases to nodes and level V lesions, a 75% rate. High risk lesions, according to these investigators, were Clark's levels III to V, lesions 0.9 mm or greater in thickness, and all nodular melanomas. Das Gupta (1977) compared level with prognosis in 150 melanoma patients followed 5 years or more. No evidence of disease at 5 years was noted, as follows: level II, 100%; level III, 95%; level IV, 50%; level V, 37%; all levels, 76%.

Davis et al. (1976) found lesions situated on the limbs to carry the best prognosis; those on the head and neck next best; and those on the trunk worst. Other factors indicating a favorable prognosis were found to be size less than 2 cm in diameter, flatness (as opposed to pedunculated or polypoid), absence of ulceration, and age of women (better if premenopausal). The depth of invasion was found to be one of the most important factors in prognosis.

Mackie et al. (1972) report on a Prognostic Score Sheet (Table 10A) devised by Cochran in which various features are given a weighted score. Those features are sex of the

TABLE 10A
Prognostic Score-Sheet*

Clinical features		Pathological features	
Feature	Score	Feature	Score
Sex:		*Relation to epidermal*	
Female	1	*appendages:*	
Male	6	Above	1
Site:		Below	4
Head and neck	1	*Mitotic rate:*	
Lower limb	3	Less than 1 per high	
Trunk	6	power field	1
Upper limb	2	1 per high power field	
Anogenital	6	or more	3
Occult	8	*Ulceration:*	
Subungual	4	No	1
Mucosal	8	Yes	4
Size:		*Invasion of lymphatics or*	
Less than 2 cm diameter	1	*vessels:*	
2 cm or larger diameter	4	No	1
Duration of symptoms:		Yes	4
Less than 2 yr	1		
2 yr or more	2		
Exposed site	1		
Non-exposed site	5		
Nodal involvement:			
No	1		
Yes	10		
Disseminated disease	15		

* Mackie et al. (1972).

patient, anatomic site of the lesion, and whether exposed or unexposed, duration of symptoms, absence or presence of positive nodes, dissemination, depth of invasion, mitotic rate, ulceration, and invasion of lymph or blood vessels. A low-risk patient would be one with a total prognostic score less than 20, and a high-risk patient one whose score was greater than 25. In their review of 85 patients the authors noted that of those whose total prognostic score was less than 20, 6% died of melanoma, for scores between 20 and 25, 37% of these patients succumbed to their disease; and for those patients with scores greater than 25, the death rate was 78%. Barclay et al. (1977), using the prognostic index of Cochran observed almost identical results.

Claudy et al. (1975) found the active E-rosette count drops significantly below 15% among patients whose tumors grow rapidly.

For predicting the behavior of malignant melanomas Cohen et al. (1977) place emphasis on the number of histologically positive nodes found in the surgical specimens. These authors report a 5-year postoperative survival rate of 73% if lymph nodes were histologically negative, 55% if one to three nodes were involved, and 26% if four or more nodes had tumor. However, the 10-year survival in patients with one to three histologically positive nodes *or no positive nodes* was 50–55% compared to an 8-year survival of 25% in patients with four or more histologically positive nodes. Utilizing multivariate analyses they found the most important prognostic factors in decreasing order of importance to be: (1) the number of lymph nodes involved histologically, (2) node palpability (poorer prognosis if nodes clinically involved), and (3) site—both upper and lower extremity melanomas had better survival than axial (trunk or head and neck) melanomas. They found that level and thickness (divided into <1.50 mm and >1.50 mm) had some prognostic significance at 5 years but less pronounced differences at 10 years following node dissection.

Balch et al. (1978) conducted a multifactorial analysis of features that might influence the outcome of malignant melanomas. Of the 13 factors they simultaneously compared, only five independently influenced survival, namely:

pathological stage, thickness, ulceration, surgical treatment, and anatomical location.

Schmoeckel and Braun-Falco (1978) developed a Prognostic Index based on the product of the tumor thickness (in millimeters) and the number of mitoses per square millimeter. For Indices greater than 12, a very high risk of metastases (91%) was observed.

THE INFLUENCE OF PREGNANCY ON THE PROGNOSIS OF MELANOMA

Shiu and his co-workers (1976) attempted to resolve some of the conflicting evidence concerning the effect of pregnancy on malignant melanomas. They studied patients who had been treated between 1950 and 1969 at Memorial Sloan-Kettering Cancer Center. Only women for whom there was accurately recorded data concerning pregnancy and whose melanomas were other than "in-situ" or "superficial" were included. There were 165 patients with primary melanoma (Stage I) and 86 patients with histologically proved metastases confined to the regional lymph nodes (Stage II). The patients were divided into four groups: nulliparous women; parous women with no activation of the lesion during previous pregnancies; parous women with definite activation of the lesion during previous pregnancies; and women with malignant melanomas admitted and treated during pregnancy. The five-year survival rate for Stage I was 84%, with little difference among the various groups. For Stage II cases the overall survival rate was 42%. It was better for nulliparous patients (55%) and for parous women (57%) who had not had activation of their lesions in previous pregnancies. In contrast, only 22% of those who had activation in a previous pregnancy survived five years, and of those who were admitted and treated during pregnancy, the survival rate was 29%. If one combines the data, 28 of 54 patients (52%) in the first two groups were alive after five years, whereas only 8 of 32 patients (25%) in the last two groups were alive after five years. It was found that in the Stage II patients, 33% of the lesions were on the trunk in the first two groups and 44% in the second two groups. It is generally accepted that lesions on the trunk have a prognosis worse than that of lesions on the extremities.

Shiu and his associates concluded "There is no evidence to indicate that termination of pregnancy, oophorectomy, adrenalectomy, or hypophysectomy can offer any benefit to the pregnant woman with a malignant melanoma. Advice to patients regarding the risk of pregnancy after treatment of melanoma has always been difficult, owing to the lack of sufficient clinical data substantiating the mere suspicion that pregnancy might be deleterious. Observations made in the present study now permit some guidelines to be offered. For Stage II melanoma, because of the great disparity in survival rates noted, it can be concluded that pregnancy after treatment would be hazardous. For Stage I disease, however, no such disparity was found so that categorically denying all these patients the opportunity of pregnancy and childbirth would not be justified. Still, for patients who have experienced activation of the lesion in a previous gestation, it would seem wise to refrain from having another pregnancy." The authors suggested that, although there was insufficient information to support the contention that oral contraceptive agents are harmful to patients with nevi or melanomas, alternative methods of contraception be used, particularly for patients who have been treated for Stage II disease.

Hersey et al. (1977) concluded that women with pregnancies before the development of melanoma have a better survival rate from this cancer than do women without previous pregnancies. They speculate that the reason for this is that melanoma cells are known to express fetal antigens. Exposure to fetal antigens during pregnancy may thus protect against metastases of melanoma cells bearing similar fetal antigens, leading to the increase in survival.

SUMMARY AND COMMENTS

Of the many factors that seem to influence the prognosis of patients with melanomas, the ones that seem to carry the most weight are the depth of invasion and thickness of the malignancy in the skin, the type of malignant melanoma, the sex of the patient, the location of the melanoma, involvement of regional nodes, and dissemination beyond the regional lymph nodes.

The physician and the patient may be able to improve the prognosis and overall survival by suspecting and establishing the diagnosis of melanoma at an early phase. As pointed out by Clark et al. (1975), the three types of melanoma have different patterns of growth and clinical behavior. The radial-growth phase of superficial spreading melanoma (associated with metastatic disease in less than 5% of patients) probably lasts from five to ten years before the vertical growth phase appears (associated with metastases in 35% to 75% of cases). Thus, one may have between five and ten years to recognize and treat superficial spreading melanoma during a phase when most cases of the malignancy are curable.

REFERENCES

Balch, C. M., Murad, T. M., Soong, S.-J., Griffin, A. L., Halpern, N. B., and Maddox, W. A. A multifactorial analysis of melanoma: I. Prognostic histopathological features comparing Clark's and Breslow's staging methods. Ann. Surg., in press.

Barclay, T. L., Crockett, D. J., Eastwood, D. S., Eastwood, J., and Giles, G. R. Assessment or prognosis in cutaneous malignant melanoma. Brit. J. Surg. 64:54–58, 1977.

Bodenham, D. C. Malignant melanoma. Proc. R. Soc. Med. 62:1090–1092, 1969.

Bodenham, D. C. A study of 650 observed malignant melanomas in the south-west region. Ann. R. Coll. Surg. Engl. 43:218–239, 1968.

Breslow, A. Thickness, cross-sectional areas and depth of invasion in the prognosis of cutaneous melanoma. Ann. Surg. 172:902–908, 1970.

Breslow, A. Tumor thickness, level of invasion and node dissection in stage I cutaneous melanoma. Ann. Surg. 182:572–575, 1975.

Cady, B. Changing concepts in malignant melanoma. Med. Clinics North Am. 59:301–308, 1975.

Clark, W. H., Jr., From, L., Bernardino, E. A., and Mihm, M. C. The histogenesis and biologic behavior of primary human malignant melanomas of the skin. Cancer Res. 29:705–727, 1969.

Clark, W. H. Jr., Ainsworth, A. M., Bernardino, E. A., Yang, C. H., Mihm, M. C., Jr., and Reed, R. J. The developmental biology of primary human malignant melanomas. Semin. Oncol. 2:83–103, 1975.

Claudy, A. L., Viac, J., Pelletier, N., Fouad-Wassef, N., Alario, A., and Thiovolet, J. Prognostic correlations in malignant melanoma. Europ. J. Cancer 2:821–827, 1975.

Cohen, M. H., Ketchem, A. S., Felix, E. L., Li, S-H., Tomaszewski, M-M., Costa, J., Rabson, A. S., Simon, R. M., and Rosenberg, S. A. Prognostic factors in patients undergoing lymphadenectomy for malignant melanoma. Ann. Surg. 186:635–642, 1977.

Das Gupta, T. K. Results of treatment of 269 patients with primary cutaneous melanoma. Ann. Surg. 186:201–209, 1977.

Elias, E. G., Didolkar, M. S., Goel, I. P., Formeister, J. F., Valenzuela, L. A., Pickren, J. L., and Moore, R. H. A clinicopathologic study of prognostic factors in cutaneous malignant melanoma. Surg. Gynecol. Obstet. 144:327–334, 1977.

Davis, N. C., McLeod, G. R., Beardmore, G. L., Little, J. H., Quinn, R. L., and Holt, J. Primary cutaneous melanoma: a report from the Queensland melanoma project. CA 26:80–107, 1976.

Fitzpatrick, P. J., Brown, T. C., and Reid, J. Malignant melanoma of the head and neck: a clinicopathological study. Can. J. Surg. 15:90–101, 1972.

Franklin, J. D., Reynolds, V. H., and Page, D. L. Cutaneous melanoma: a twenty-year retrospective study with clinicopathologic correlation. Plast. Reconstr. Surg. 56:277–285, 1975.

Hansen, M. G., and McCarten, A. B. Tumor thickness and lymphocytic infiltration in malignant melanoma of the head and neck. Am. J. Surg. 128:557–561, 1974.

Hersey, P., Morgan, G., Stone, D. E., McCarthy, W. H., and Milton, G. W. Previous pregnancy as a protective factor against death from melanoma. Lancet 1:451–452, 1977.

Huvos, A. G., Shah, J. P., and Goldsmith, H. S. A clinicopathologic study of amelanotic melanoma. Surg. Gynecol. Obstet. 135:917–920, 1972.

Huvos, A. G. Miké, V., Donnellan, M. J., Seemayer, T., and Strong, E. W. Prognostic factors in cutaneous melanoma of the head and neck. Am. J. Pathol. 71:33–48, 1973.

Huvos, A. G., Shah, J. P., and Miké, V. Prognostic factors in cutaneous malignant melanoma. Hum. Pathol. 5:347–357, 1974.

Ironside, P., Pitt, T. T. E., and Rank, B. K. Malignant melanoma: Some aspects of pathology and prognosis. Aust. N. Z. J. Surg. 47:70–75, 1977.

Jones, W. M., Jones Williams, W., Roberts, M. M., and Davies, K. Malignant melanoma of the skin: prognostic value of clinical features and the role of treatment in 111 cases. Br. J. Cancer 22:437–451, 1968.

Jones Williams, W., Davies, K., Jones, W. M., and Roberts, M. M. Malignant melanoma of the skin: prognostic value of histology in 89 cases. Br. J. Cancer 22:452–460, 1968.

Luce, J. K., McBride, C. M., and Frei, E. Melanoma. In: Holland, J. F., and Frei, E. eds. Cancer Medicine. Philadelphia, Lea & Febiger, 1973, pp. 1823–1843.

Mackie, R. M., Carfrae, D. C., and Cochran, A. J. Assessment of prognosis in patients with malignant melanoma. Lancet 2:455–456, 1972.

McGovern, V. J. The classification of melanoma and its relationship with prognosis. Pathology 2:85–98, 1970.

McGovern, V. J.: Melanoma-growing patterns, multiplicity and regression. In: McCarthy, W. H., ed. Melanoma and Skin Cancer. Proceedings International Cancer Conference, Sydney, 1972, V.C.N. Blight, Government Printer, pp. 95–106.

McGovern, V. J., Mihm, M. C., Jr., Bailly, C., Booth, J. C., Clark, W. H., Jr., Cochran, A. J., Hardy, E. G., Hicks, J. D., Levene, A., Lewis, M. G., Little, J. H., and Milton, G. W. The classification of malignant melanoma and its histologic reporting. Cancer 32:1446–1457, 1973.

Milton, G. W., McGovern, V. J., and Lewis, M. G. Malignant Melanoma of the Skin and Mucous Membrane. Edinburgh, London, and New York, Churchill Livingston, 1977.

Mundth, E. D., Guralnick, E. A., and Raker, J. W.: Malignant melanoma: A clinical study of 427 cases. Ann. Surg. 162:15–28, 1965.

Schmoeckel, C., and Braun-Falco, O. Prognostic index in malignant melanoma. Arch. Dermatol. 114:871–873, 1978.

Shiu, M. H., Schottenfeld, D., Maclean, B., and Fortner, J. G. Adverse effect of pregnancy on melanoma: a reappraisal. Cancer 37:181–187, 1976.

Sinha, B. K., and Buntine, D. W. Prognosis of cutaneous malignant melanoma: a clinicopathological study. Can. J. Surg. 17:328–334, 1974.

Veronesi, U., Cascinelli, N., and Preda, F. Prognosis of malignant melanoma according to regional metastases. Am. J. Roentgenol. Radium Ther. Nucl. Med. 111:301–309, 1971.

Wanebo, H. J., Fortner, J. G., Woodruff, J., MacLean, B., and Binkowski, E. Selection of the optimum surgical treatment of stage I melanoma by depth of microinvasion: use of the combined microstage technique (Clark-Breslow). Ann. Surg. 182:302–315, 1975.

Chapter 15

Biopsy of Malignant Melanoma

Accurate histologic diagnosis of the type, level and thickness of a malignant melanoma is essential for prognosis and for determination of the extent of necessary surgery.

The clinical diagnosis of a malignant melanoma is based on the appearance of the lesion and on the history of a change in size, color, elevation, surface characteristics, surroundings, consistency, and symptoms. The importance of having histologic verification prior to attempt at definitive radical surgery for malignant melanoma was emphasized in a study of Kopf and co-workers (1975), in which the accuracy of the physicians in the Oncology Section of the Skin and Cancer Unit (N.Y.U.) in diagnosing malignant melanomas was found to be only 64%. Thus, in about one of every three histologically proved malignant melanomas, an error in clinical diagnosis was made.

The concern expressed by some that an incisional biopsy (i.e., partial removal) of a melanoma might disseminate the tumor and worsen the patient's prognosis has not been borne out. Epstein et al. (1969) reported that there was no evidence to indicate that incomplete removal of malignant melanomas, when followed by adequate surgery, decreases the rate of survival. In a review of 111 cases of malignant melanoma, Jones et al. (1968) found no decrease in the five-year survival rate of those patients who had had incisional biopsies of their lesions. Using actuarial life-table analyses, Knutson et al. (1971) compared patients with malignant melanomas who had had excisional and incisional biopsies. They, too, found no evidence that incisional biopsies of malignant melanomas before definitive treatment have a detrimental influence on the patients' survival.

The diagnosis of malignant melanoma is best confirmed by means of an excisional biopsy unless the lesion is so large or is so situated anatomically that biopsy in toto would be impractical, in which case an incisional biopsy is appropriate. A total biopsy is usually fusiform in shape with a 3-to-10 mm border around the lesion. It should be deep enough to include some subcutaneous fat but should not reach the underlying fascia. In most sites the biopsy scar should be positioned so that it points toward the regional lymph nodes. If only a portion of the lesion is removed for the biopsy specimen, it should be taken through what is judged to be the deepest portion of the lesion (Harris and Gumport; 1973; 1975). Total excision better enables the pathologist, by means of step sections, to define the type, level and deepest thickness of the melanoma. These are important factors that influence the extent of surgery for the primary lesion and help to determine whether or not a regional lymph node dissection is warranted.

A somewhat different concept is expressed by Cady (1975) who advocates dermal punch biopsies of lesions suspected of being malignant melanomas. Since the procedure is simple, safe, and reliable, many more physicians are apt to use it, resulting in a higher yield of early melanomas. If the widespread use of punch biopsies is to be advocated, it is important to stress that the thickest portion of the tumor should be selected since levels are so important in deciding definitive therapy. It will frequently be necessary to do a conservative excision biopsy of a punch-biopsy-proved melanoma in order to level it accurately prior to definitive surgery.

SUMMARY

All lesions suspected of being malignant melanomas should be biopsied. Histologic examination is essential for a definitive diagnosis and to determine the type, level and thickness of a malignant melanoma. Definitive radical surgery should not be undertaken prior to obtaining a histologic diagnosis since the clinical diagnostic accuracy, even of very experienced physicians, is surprisingly low and errors cannot be avoided. A properly performed conservative excisional or incisional biopsy will obviate unnecessary radical surgery should the lesion prove to be not malignant or if malignant of a type not requiring a radical approach.

REFERENCES

Cady, B. Changing concepts in malignant melanoma. Med. Clin. North Am. 59:301–308, 1975.

Epstein, E., Bragg, K., and Linden, G. Biopsy and prognosis of malignant melanoma. J.A.M.A. 208:1369–1371, 1969.

Harris, M. N., and Gumport, S. L. Total excisional biopsy for primary malignant melanoma. J.A.M.A. 226:354–355, 1973.

Harris, M. N., and Gumport, S. L. Biopsy technique for malignant melanoma. J. Dermatol. Surg. 1:24–27, 1975.

Jones, N. M., Jones, Williams, W., Roberts, M. M., and Davies, K. Malignant melanoma of the skin: prognostic value of clinical features and the role of treatment in 111 cases. Br. J. Cancer 22:437–451, 1968.

Knutson, C. O., Hori, J. M., and Spratt, J. S. Melanoma. Curr. Probl. Surg. December, 1971, pp. 1–55.

Kopf, A. W., Mintzis, M., and Bart, R. S. Diagnostic accuracy in malignant melanoma. Arch. Dermatol. 111:1291–1292, 1975.

Lee, Y. T. N. Malignant melanoma: to biopsy or not to biopsy. CA 24:104–105, 1974.

Chapter 16

Surgical Management of Malignant Melanomas

The treatment of malignant melanomas is primarily surgical. Decisions concerning the type and extent of surgery depend, among other factors, on the type, level and thickness of the primary tumor and the stage of disease. The current surgical approaches for malignant melanomas used by the Melanoma Cooperative Group at New York University Medical Center are described below.

Prior to the Clark classification of primary malignant melanomas into the three major types (lentigo maligna, superficial spreading, and nodular) and their microstaging (determination of level of invasion and thickness), most malignant melanomas were considered to be of utmost seriousness, bearing grave prognoses. Therefore, the surgical approaches were generally radical for practically all lesions. We now know that certain malignant melanomas have excellent prognoses and therefore require less radical surgery. Specifically, elective lymph node dissections are no longer performed by our group for level I or level II lesions and for melanomas less than 0.76 mm thick. This spares approximately 25% of patients who have superficial spreading melanomas (the most common variety of malignant melanoma) from elective lymph node dissection. This decision has been based on the fact that the five-year survival rate for patients with levels I and II superficial spreading melanomas is over 95%.

The present status of surgical management of malignant melanoma was recently reviewed by Harris and Gumport (1976) in the *Journal of Dermatologic Surgery*. We here borrow extensively from that paper.

WORK-UP PRIOR TO DEFINITIVE SURGERY

Whenever possible total excision biopsy of a lesion suspected of being a malignant melanoma is recommended. If the lesion is situated in anatomical areas where total removal would be disfiguring or would make primary closure impossible, incisional biopsy is recommended. The specimen should be submitted to a histopathologist well versed in the modern classification of malignant melanomas, including determinations of types, levels, and thicknesses. The specimen should be processed with "step" sections throughout. This is very important since only by examining the entire lesion can one confidently identify that portion which penetrates deepest into the underlying tissues or is the thickness area.

The patient should undergo a complete work-up for metastatic malignant melanoma which includes a thorough physical examination, x-ray examination of the chest, complete blood count, and an SMA-12. Liver-spleen scans are not done routinely at our medical center.

DEFINITIVE SURGICAL TREATMENT OF STAGE I MALIGNANT MELANOMAS

The following, largely abstracted from the previously cited article by Harris and Gumport, outlines the current principles for surgical management of malignant melanomas as performed at New York University Medical Center. These principles were originally outlined in the "N.Y.U. Melanoma Newsletter" and they represent the consensus of the surgeons who deal with these types of malignancies at our medical center.

LENTIGO MALIGNA MELANOMA

Level I or II lesions are excised with a 1 cm or greater margin beyond the clinically visible perimeter of the lesion or scar from the original biopsy, provided that such excision does not result in sacrifice of a major structure such as an eye. Level III, IV or V lesions are excised more radically with margins up to 5 cm, when technically feasible. When present, the underlying fascia is included in the surgical specimen. Grafts, as needed, are placed following excision. Lymph node dissections are usually not done unless the nodes are clinically involved or the clinical and histologic features of the tumor indicate a poor prognosis.

SUPERFICIAL SPREADING MELANOMA

Level I lesions ("atypical melanocytic hyperplasia") are treated by conservative excision, with primary closure when feasible. The lesion should be step-sectioned throughout by the pathologist to insure that no dermal invasion has occurred. Level I lesions, once removed, are considered biologically benign in terms of metastases.

Level II lesions are excised with a 3- to 5-cm margin from the perimeter of the lesion or from the biopsy scar. The width of the margin often depends on the anatomical site. The underlying fascia is included if present. Skin grafts are applied as needed. Elective lymph node dissections are not done for level II lesions less than 0.76 mm thick.

Level III, IV and V superficial spreading melanomas are treated aggressively with a 5-cm margin taken from the edge of the lesion or from the biopsy scar, if anatomically feasible. Underlying fascia, where present, is included in the surgical specimen. A graft is almost always required. For lesions 1.5 mm or thicker elective lymph node dissections are performed if the lymphatic drainage from the lesion is to a single major node group and, rarely, if two predictable major node groups drain the site. If possible, an "incontinuity" operation is performed in which the primary site, intervening lymphatics and regional lymph nodes are removed en bloc. If this is not feasible, a discontinuous lymph node dissection is done at the time of the definitive local operation or is deferred for several weeks. Recently, much consideration has been given to the thickness of the lesion in determining whether or not elective lymph node dissections are to be done. According to Breslow (1970, 1975), Wanebo et al. (1975) and Hansen and McCarten (1974), lesions 0.75 mm and less in thickness have an excellent prognosis. Since some level III malignant melanomas (so-called "thin" level III's) fall within this group, there is much discussion and controversy concerning whether excision of such level III lesions should or should not be combined with elective lymph node dissections. Breslow (1975) believes tumor thickness should be used to select patients for elective node dissections; patients with lesions less than 0.76 mm should not be subjected to elective lymphadenectomy, whereas those with lesions greater than 1.50 mm should. Indications for elective node dissections for lesion thicknesses between 0.76 and 1.50 mm depend on the largely subjective judgment of the surgeon; there is not enough data for more objective decision at this time. It seems likely that in the future much more emphasis will be given to the thickness of a malignant melanoma than to its level.

In operable cases, clinically positive lymph nodes are managed by dissection.

NODULAR MELANOMA

Such lesions almost invariably invade to levels III, IV and V. Whenever feasible, a 5-cm margin beyond the perimeter of the lesion or the biopsy scar is excised. The underlying fascia is included in the surgical specimen. An elective lymph node dissection is performed if the lesion drains to one major lymph node basin or sometimes if two predictable lymph node groups drain the site. If the lymph nodes are clinically involved radical lymphadenectomy is done.

OTHER SURGICAL CONSIDERATIONS

The publication of Breslow and Macht (1977) should be of great interest to those who treat cutaneous melanomas. These authors studied a series of 62 patients who had melanomas of the skin measuring less than 0.76 mm in thickness. Such lesions were excised with margins (on the *in vitro* specimens) of as little as 1 mm up to 3 cm or more. All survived over 5 years disease free and none had local recurrences or metastases. The authors concluded that melanomas less than 0.76 mm thick can be treated by conservative excision with primary closure. In most instances, they suggest, skin grafting should not be necessary.

Until recently a "radical groin dissection" included both superficial and deep inguinal nodes. Since involvement of deep lymph nodes almost invariably means incurable disease, McCarthy et al. (1974) have challenged the concept of removing such nodes especially because the more radical procedure fails significantly to increase cure rates. The concept is that if such nodes are not involved the operation is unnecessary; if they are involved, the operation does not favorably affect chances for cure. Based on these and other considerations, most of the surgeons at New York University Medical Center no longer routinely do deep (iliac-obturator) lymph node dissections in the inguinal area; they do superficial dissections only. Holmes et al. (1977) recommend frozen section studies of any suspicious nodes in the surgical specimens obtained from elective superficial inguinal node dissections and, if any node is found to be positive, to proceed with an iliac-obturator node dissection.

Digital malignant melanomas are usually treated by "ray amputation" which includes the entire digit plus the distal portion of the corresponding metatarsal or metacarpal bone. For lesions of the thumb, an amputation through the metacarpal-phalangeal joint allows for the possibility of reconstruction later.

Despite the frequency of malignant melanomas of the trunk, these tumors rarely occur on the breast. Perhaps the reason for this is that in women this is an anatomical site not often exposed to sun. Jochimsen et al. (1977) recommend total mastectomy with or without lymphadenectomy for such lesions. At NYU the surgeons treat most melanomas of the breast by the same surgical procedures used in other sites and do not routinely perform radical mastectomies (Roses et al., 1977).

Mucosal malignant melanomas have very poor prognoses. Therefore, removal, even though radically performed, usually is followed by recurrence, metastases and death. Consultation with surgeons in other specialites (otorhinolaryngologic, oral, ophthalmic, gynecologic, proctologic, etc.) is important to plan surgical procedures in muscosal areas. Cryosurgery has been used with some success for treating mucosal melanomas of the head and neck (Barton, 1975).

The surgical management of metastatic malignant melanomas is beyond the scope of this chapter, except to note that localized metastatic lesions may be surgically excised, although such procedures rarely cure. They are performed mainly for palliation.

The recent report of Veronesi et al. (1977) concludes that elective lymph node dissections for malignant melanomas of the extremities do not improve prognosis (see Chapter 17—Elective Lymph Node Dissections for Malignant Melanoma). This report, particularly if the conclusions hold up after further follow-up of patients by the WHO Melanoma Group and if they are confirmed by others, could significantly influence the surgical approach in many institutions, including our own.

OTHER SELECTED REFERENCES

The literature on the surgical management of malignant melanoma is voluminous. Some surgical approaches in other institutions are at variance with those used at our medical center. However, space does not permit enumeration of many controversial issues. References for additional reading are included in the bibliography.

Other surgical aspects such as elective lymphadenectomy and isolation-perfusion techniques utilizing chemotherapy will be reviewed in other chapters.

REFERENCES

Barton, R. T. Muscosal melanomas of the head and neck. Larynogoscope 85:93–99, 1975.

Booher, R. J. Recognition and treatment of melanoma. Surg. Clin. North Am. 49:389–405, 1969.

Breslow, A. Thickness, cross-sectional area and depth of invasion in the prognosis of cutaneous melanoma. Ann. Surg. 172:902–908, 1970.

Breslow, A. Tumor thickness, level of invasion and the node dissection on stage I cutaneous melanoma. Ann. Surg. 182:572–575, 1975.

Breslow, A., and Macht, S. D. Optimal size of resection margin for thin cutaneous melanoma. Surg. Gynec. Obstet. 145:691–692, 1977.

Clark, W. H., Jr., Lynn, F., Bernardino, E. A., and Mihm, M. C., Jr. The histogenesis and biologic behavior of primary human malignant melanomas of the skin. Cancer Res. 29:705–715, 1969.

Das Gupta, T. K., Bowden, L., and Berg, J. W. Malignant melanoma of unknown primary origin. Surg. Gynecol. Obstet. 117:341–345, 1963.

Das Gupta, T. K., and McNeer, G. P. The incidence of metastasis to accessible lymph nodes from melanoma of the trunk and extremities—its therapeutic significance. Cancer 17:897–911, 1964.

Davis, N. C. Cutaneous melanoma: the Queensland experience. Curr. Probl. Surg. 13:1–63, 1976.

Davis, N. C., and McLeod, G. R. The surgery of primary melanoma problems and practice. Med. J. Aust. 2:778–782, 1972.

Everall, J. D., and Dowd, P. M. Diagnosis, prognosis, and treatment of melanoma. Lancet 2:286–289, 1977.

Fortner, J. G., Booher, R. J., and Pack, G. T. Results of groin dissection for malignant melanoma in 220 patients. Surgery 55:485–494, 1964.

Goldsmith, H. S., Shah, J. P., and Kim, D. H. Prognostic significance of lymph node dissection in the treatment of malignant melanoma. Cancer 26:606–609, 1970.

Graham, G. F., and Stewart, R. Cryosurgery for unusual cutaneous neoplasms. J. Derm. Surg. Oncol. 3:437–444, 1977.

Gumport, S. L., and Harris, M. N. Results of regional node dissection for melanoma. Ann. Surg. 179:105–108, 1974.

Gumport, S. L., Lyall, D., and Zimany, A. A radical axillary lymph node dissection for malignancy. Arch. Surg. 83:227–230, 1961.

Gumport, S. L., and Meyer, H. W. An improved technique for an adequate radical groin dissection for malignancy. Surgery 38:660–666, 1955.

Gumport, S. L., and Meyer, H. W.: Treatment of 126 cases of malignant melanoma. Ann. Surg. 150:989–992, 1959.

Hansen, M. G., and McCarten, A. B. Tumor thickness and lymphocytic infiltration in malignant melanoma of the head and neck. Am. J. Surg. 128:557–561, 1974.

Harris, M. N., and Gumport, S. L. Biopsy technique for malignant melanoma. J. Dermatol. Surg. 1:24–27, 1975.

Harris, M. N., and Gumport, S. L. Present status of surgical management of malignant melanoma. J. Dermatol. Surg. 2:129–133, 1976.

Harris, M. N., Gumport, S. L., Berman, I. R., and Bernard, R. W. Ilioinguinal lymph node dissection for melanoma. Surg. Gynecol. Obstet. 136:33–39, 1973.

Harris, M. N., Roses, D. F., Culliford, A. T., and Gumport, S. L. Melanoma of the head and neck. Ann. Surg. 182:86–91, 1975.

Holmes, E. C., Clark, W., Morton, D. L., Eilber, F. R., and Bochow, A J. Regional lymph node metastases and the level of invasion of primary melanoma. Cancer 37:199–201, 1976.

Holmes, E. C., Moseley, H. S., Morton, D. L., Clark, W., Robinson, D., and Urist, M. M. A rational approach to the surgical management of melanoma. Ann. Surg. 186:481–490, 1977.

Jochimsen, P. R., Pearlman, N. W., Lawton, R. L., and Platz, C. E. Melanoma of the skin of the breast: Therapeutic considerations based on six cases. Surgery 81:583–587, 1977.

Lane, N., Lattes, R., and Malm, J. Clinicopathological correlations in a series of 117 malignant melanomas of the skin of adults. Cancer 11:1025–1043, 1958.

Lee, Y. N., Sparks, F. C., and Morton, D. L. Primary melanoma of the breast region. Ann. Surg. 185:17–22, 1977.

Lerman, R. I., Murray, D., O'Hara, J. M., Booher, R. J., and Foote, F. W. Jr. Malignant melanoma of childhood. A clinicopathologic study and a report of 12 cases. Cancer 25:436–449, 1970.

Lorenc, E., Wooldridge, W. E., and Huewe, D. A. The melanotic freckle of Hutchinson: Preliminary report. Cutis 16:485–486, 1975.

McCarthy, J. G., Haagensen, C. D., and Herter, F. P. The role of groin dissection in the management of melanoma of the lower extremity. Ann. Surg. 179:156–159, 1974.

Meyer, H. W., and Gumport, S. L. Malignant melanoma: Appraisal of the disease and analysis of 105 cases. Surgery 138:643–660, 1953.

Pack, G. T., Gerber, D. M., and Scharnagel, I. M. End results of the treatment of malignant melanoma: a report of 1190 cases. Ann. Surg. 136:905–911, 1952.

Reed, R. J. New Concepts in Surgical Pathology of the Skin. New York, John Wiley, 1976, p. 89–90.

Roses, D. F., Harris, M. N., Stern, J. S., and Gumport, S. L. Cutaneous melanoma of the breast. Unpublished.

Seigler, H. F., and Fetter, B. F. Current management of melanoma. Ann. Surg. 186:1–12, 1977.

Shah, J. P., and Goldsmith, H. S. Incontinuity versus discontinuous lymph node dissection for malignant melanoma. Cancer 26:610–614, 1970.

Shingleton, W. W. Perfusion chemotherapy for recurrent melanoma of extremity: a progress report. Ann. Surg. 169:969–973, 1969.

Shingleton, W. W., Seigler, H. F., Stocks, L. H., and Downs, R. W. Management of recurrent melanoma of the extremity. Cancer 35:574–579, 1975.

Stehlin, J. S., Jr. Malignant melanoma: an appraisal. Surgery 64:1149–1157, 1968.

Stehlin, J. S., Smith, J. L., Jing, B. S., and Sherrin, D. Melanomas of the extremities complicated by in-transit metastases. Surg. Gynecol. Obstet. 122:3–14, 1966.

Sugarbaker, E. V., and McBride, C. M. Melanoma of the trunk: the results of surgical excision and anatomic guidelines for predicting nodal metastasis. Surgery 80:22–30, 1976.

Veronesi, V., et al. Inefficacy of immediate node dissection in Stage I melanoma of the limbs. New Engl. J. Med. 297:627–630, 1977.

Wanebo, H. J., Woodruff, J. and Fortner, J. G. Malignant melanoma of the extremities; a clinicopathologic study using levels of invasion (microstage). Cancer 35:666–676, 1975.

# Chapter 17

Elective Lymph Node Dissection in the Management of Malignant Melanoma

Whether or not elective (prophylactic) lymph node dissections should be done for patients with malignant melanoma who do not have clinically involved regional nodes remains one of the most controversial issues about the treatment of this malignancy. There are those who favor the frequent use of the procedure and those who consider the procedure rarely justified (Sinha and Buntine, 1974; McCarthy et al., 1974; Lane et al., 1958; Jones et al., 1968; Goldsmith et al., 1970; McLeod et al., 1966; Wilkinson and Paletta, 1969; Gumport and Harris, 1974; Stehlin, 1968; Davis, 1972; Polk and Linn, 1971; Davis and McLeod, 1972; Bodenham, 1968, 1969). Those who favor dissections of clinically uninvolved nodes cite as evidence for their practice the fact that a high percentage (e.g., 30%, Gumport and Harris, 1974) of clinically uninvolved nodes are found to be microscopically involved with malignant melanoma.

Some information is accumulating which may be helpful in deciding whether or not to do an elective lymph node dissection for a particular malignant melanoma. For example, Gumport and Harris (1974), who believe strongly in the benefits of elective regional lymph node dissections, nevertheless list six circumstances in which the procedure need not be done, namely, (1) the malignancy is entirely superficial (i.e., level I or II and/or thickness less than 0.76 mm); (2) it arose in a melanotic freckle of Hutchinson; (3) the primary site is so situated that the lymphatic drainage is to several different groups of regional lymph nodes; (4) the presence of serious concurrent disease; (5) the patient is very old (70 years of age or older) and debilitated; (6) there already are distant metastases. The first three circumstances given are similar to those put forth by Davis (1972).

In recent years, many investigators have clarified the situation in which malignant melanomas are sufficiently superficial to make elective regional lymph node dissections seem unnecessary. Thus, Holmes and co-workers (1976) and Wanebo et al. (1975) advocate abandoning the practice for level I and level II malignant melanomas, and Breslow (1970; 1975) considers the procedure unnecessary for lesions less than 0.76 mm in thickness, since lymph node metastases are unusual from these lesions. Breslow (1970, 1975) found that all patients with lesions less than 0.76 mm in thickness were free of disease five or more years after treatment whether or not elective lymph node dissections had been done. Hansen and McCarten (1974) found that elective node dissection seemed to improve survival for lesions 1.5 mm or greater. Breslow (1975) and Geehoed et al. (1977) concluded that patients with melanomas less than 0.76 mm thick should not be subjected to node dissections; patients with melanomas more than 1.5 mm thick in their series appeared to benefit by elective node dissections; and their patients with melanomas 0.76 to 1.50 mm thick had no proven benefit from node dissection. However, possible bias in patient selection was subsequently reported by Breslow (1978) which may negate the seeming advantage of elective lymph node dissection for lesions more than 1.5 mm thick. Wanebo and co-workers (1975) reported increased survival rates for patients with level III lesions of the extremities when elective lymph node dissections were done. Holmes et al. (1977), using a combination of the Clark (level) and Breslow (thickness) methods of categorizing malignant melanomas, recommend regional lymphadenectomies for lesions that are Clark level III (if greater than 0.76 mm thick), IV, and V, and for any lesion greater than 1.5 mm thick.

In Breslow's study (1975) tumor thickness seemed a more reliable index of prognosis than tumor level. For example, 25% of level III lesions in this series of patients were less than 0.76 mm thick. Lesions less than this thickness rarely metastasized. Accepting Breslow's data, one might conclude that if one were to do lymph node dissections on all patients who have level III lesions (in which the distribution of thicknesses were as he found them), then 25% of such patients would have unnecessary surgery.

Among surgeons who consider that elective lymph node dissections should be employed for all malignant melanomas of sufficient depth or thickness, there is still disagreement as to what should be done in the case of a malignant melanoma that is situated so that it could drain to two or more groups of regional lymph nodes. Some advise that no lymph node dissection be done and that the patient be followed very carefully in order that immediate dissection be done at the first sign of clinical involvement of a particular group of nodes. Others advise elective lymph node dissections of that group of nodes most likely to become involved, and if they prove to be positive, they advise further dissection of other groups that could be involved. Still others advocate doing multiple elective lymph node dissections at once in the situation where more than one lymph node group may become involved (Das Gupta and McNeer, 1964). Southwick (1976) concludes from reviewing his cases that elective discontinuous node dissections are not indicated in the primary treatment of malignant melanomas, whereas in-continuity excision of the primary site, intervening lymphatics, and the lymph nodes achieved a significant increase in 5-year disease-free rate.

The report of Das Gupta and McNeer (1964) describes the locations of lymph node metastases from various anatomic sites on the trunk and extremities in patients who were still alive with malignant melanoma and also in patients who had died from metastatic malignant melanoma. In general, metastases to lymph nodes tend to be widespread in patients who die from metastatic malignant melanoma, and therefore the findings from autopsies are not very helpful to the surgeon facing the clinical situation in which the possibility of drainage is to more than one group of nodes. However, the sites of metastases found clinically, and at operation in patients not yet riddled with metastases are of help to those faced with making a decision as to which lymph nodes may be involved for a particular malignant melanoma of the trunk or an extremity.

The report of Sugarbaker and McBride (1976) is helpful for prediction of which lymph node groups may become involved with metastases originating from primary malignant melanomas on the trunk. Since the vast majority of the patients in this study were treated with local excision alone (without elective lymph node dissections), the artifact of lymphatic blockage resulting in aberrant metastases secondary to lymph node dissections (a possible influence in the study of Das Gupta and McNeer, 1964) was not present.

Fortner and colleagues (1977) compared the 10-year cure rates of 259 Stage I patients treated by wide excision of the primary plus elective lymph node dissection with 145 Stage I patients treated by wide excision alone. In the elective-node-dissection group 15% were found to have microscopically positive nodes. The 10-year cure rate of this group was found to be profoundly affected by the extent of node involvement: 67% survived if only a microscopic focus of involvement was found; 50% survived if one node was involved by melanoma larger than a microscopic focus; and 15% survived if more than one node was involved. In contrast, in the group treated initially by wide excision alone without elective node dissection 18% subsequently required *therapeutic* lymphadenectomies with a 10-year cure rate of 6%. The authors conclude that these data support the concept of doing elective lymph node dissections, since the earlier one removes regional node metastases the better is the 10-year survival: 67% if one microscopic focus; 50% if one node larger than a microscopic focus; 15% if multiple nodes; 6% if lymphadenectomy is postponed until the nodes become clinically positive.

Those who are opposed to elective lymph node dissections argue that the appropriate study for proving the worth of such dissections has not been done and that the benefit from such dissections is likely to be small; they cite possible complications of elective lymph node dissections, both operative and postoperative as negating possible benefit. Such complications include operative or anesthetic deaths, paralyses (as in cases of facial nerve injury during parotid dissections), and postoperative edema with the added risk of chronic or recurrent bacterial cellulitis. Polk (1971), on the basis of certain mathematical calculations of the probability of complications concluded that more harm than good is done by elective lymph node dissections. Gumport and Harris (1974) strongly disagree. Their argument seems to be that in the absence of evidence to the contrary, one must assume that patients are benefitted by the removal of microscopically involved regional lymph nodes. They have had no operative deaths and morbidity from operations has been acceptable. On the other hand, Papachristou and Fortner (1977) report that approximately two-thirds of their patients developed lymphedema and two-fifths had wound complications following inguinal lymphadenectomies. They were unable to demonstrate any significant differences in complications in the group treated with discontinuous as compared to in-continuity groin dissections, but noted a lower local recurrence rate of melanoma with the in-continuity surgical approach.

In our recent publication (Kopf, Bart and Rodriguez-Sains, 1977) upon which this book is largely based, we concluded this section with the comment, "What is obviously needed is a proper, prospective, randomized study . . . ." Since our comment, a report has recently appeared in the *New England Journal of Medicine* (Veronesi et al., 1977) by the World Health Organization Melanoma Group. Treatment was prospectively randomized in 553 patients who had Stage I malignant melanomas of the upper or lower limbs. Of the total, 267 patients had excision of their primary melanomas and immediate elective regional lymph node dissections, and 286 had excisions of their primary melanomas and regional lymph node dissections only if nodal metastases subsequently appeared clinically. Patients were followed at monthly intervals. Statistical analyses revealed no significant differences in survival rates between the two groups whether the data were analyzed by sex, site of origin, maximum diameter of the tumors, Clark's levels, or Breslow's thickness. These authors conclude that elective lymph node dissection for melanoma of the limbs does not improve prognosis and is therefore not recommended for patients who can be closely followed. A report on such a study has been long awaited but many questions have been raised concerning this report (Krementz, 1977; Dubin and Pasternack, 1978; Frazier, 1978; Roses et al., 1978; Wanebo, 1978). After carefully reviewing the publication of Veronesi et al., we believe much more data from their study are needed before we can accept their conclusion that elective lymph node dissections for malignant melanoma of the extremities should be abandoned (Kopf et al., 1978).

Sim et al. (1978) also conducted a prospective randomized study of the efficacy of routine elective lymphadenectomy for malignant melanomas. The 173 patients were divided into three groups: no lymphadenectomy, delayed (2 to 4 months after primary excised) lymphadenectomy, and immediate lymphadenectomy. None of these regimens differed significantly from the others in terms of survival or interval to metastases. Their preliminary conclusion is that elective lymph node dissection is not beneficial in the treatment of melanoma. However, the fact that 103 of 110 patients who underwent elective lymphadenectomy did not have evidence of lymph node involvement microscopically indicates they were dealing with a group of patients with relatively good prognosis to begin with. In our experience, about 30% of patients selected for elective node dissections have microscopic evidence of nodal metastases.

Only with further data and analysis will this very important debate be brought to an end. In the meanwhile each surgeon must decide in his own mind the appropriateness of elective lymphadenectomy for his patient.

REFERENCES

Bodenham, D. C. A study of 650 observed malignant melanomas in the south-west region. Ann. R. Coll. Surg. 43:218–239, 1968.

Bodenham, D. C. Malignant melanoma: the problem of lymph-node metastases. Proc. R. Soc. Med. 62:1090–1092, 1969.

Breslow, A. Thickness, cross-sectional areas and depth of invasion in the prognosis of cutaneous melanoma. Ann. Surg. 172:902–908, 1970.

Breslow, A. Tumor thickness, level of invasion and node dissection in stage I cutaneous melanoma. Ann. Sur. 182:572–575, 1975.

Breslow, A. Melanoma thickness and elective node dissection. Arch. Dermatol. 114: 1399, 1978.

Cady, B., Legg, M. A., and Redfern, A. B. Contemporary treatment of malignant melanoma. Am. J. Surg. 129:472–482, 1975.

Das Gupta, T. and McNeer, G. The incidence of metastases to accessible lymph nodes from melanoma of the trunk and extremities: its therapeutic significance. Cancer 17:897–911, 1964.

Davis, N. C. Elective lymph node dissection—yes or no? In: McCarthy, W. H., ed., Melanoma and Skin Cancer. Sydney, V. C. N. Blight, 1972, pp. 407–416.

Davis, N. C., and McLeod, G. R. The surgery of primary melanoma: problems and practice. Med. J. Aust. 2:778–782, 1972.

Dubin, N., and Pasternack, B. S. Letter to the Editor. New Engl. J. Med. 298:223–224, 1978.

Fortner, J. G., Woodruff, J., Shottenfeld, D., and Maclean, B. Biostatistical basis of elective node dissection for malignant melanoma. Ann Surg. 186:101–103, 1977.

Frazier, T.-G. Letter to the Editor. New. Eng. J. Med. 298:223, 1978.

Geehoed, G. W., Breslow, A., and McCune, W. S. Malignant melanoma: Correlation of long-term follow-up with clinical staging, level of invasion and thickness of the primary tumor. Am. Surgeon 43: 77–85, 1977.

Goldman, L. I., Clark, W. H., Bernardino, E. A., and Ainsworth, A. M. The accuracy of predicting lymph node metastases in malignant melanoma by clinical examination and microstaging. Ann. Surg. 184: 537–540, 1976.

Goldsmith, H. S., Shah, J. P., and Kim, D.-H. Prognostic significance of lymph node dissection in the treatment of malignant melanoma. Cancer 26:606–609, 1970.

Gumport, S. L., and Harris, M. N. Results of regional lymph node dissection for melanoma. Ann. Surg. 179:105–108, 1974.

Hansen, M. G., and McCarten, A. B. Tumor thickness and lymphocytic infiltration in malignant melanoma of the head and neck. Am. J. Surg. 128:557–561, 1974.

Holmes, E. C., Clark, W., Morton, D. L., Eilber, F. R., and Bochow, A. J. Regional lymph node metastases and the level of invasion of primary melanoma. Cancer 37:199–201, 1976.

Holmes, E. C., Moseley, H. S., Morton, D. L., Clark, W., Robinson, D., and Urist, M. M. A rational approach to the surgical management of melanoma. Ann. Surg. 186:481–490, 1977.

Jones, W. M., Jones Williams, W., Roberts, M. M., and Davies, K. Malignant melanoma of the skin: prognostic value of clinical features and the role of treatment in 111 cases. Br. J. Cancer 22:437–450, 1968.

Kopf, A. W., Bart, R. S., and Rodriguez-Sains, R. S. Malignant melanoma: A review. J. Derm. Surg. Oncol. 3:41–125, 1977.

Kopf, A. W., et al., To do or not to do elective lymph-node dissections for certain malignant melanomas. J. Derm. Surg. Oncol. 4: 493 and 497–498, 1978.

Krementz, E. T.; Node dissection for extremely melanoma? New Eng. J. Med. 297:627–730, 1977.

Lane, N., Lattes, R., and Malm, J. Clinicopathological correlations in a series of 117 malignant melanomas of the skin of adults. Cancer 11: 1025–1043, 1958.

McCarthy, J. G., Haagensen, C. D., and Herter, F. P. The role of groin dissection in the management of melanoma of the lower extremity. Ann. Surg. 179:156–159, 1974.

McLeod, R., Davis, N. C., Herron, J. et al. A retrospective surgery of 498 patients with malignant melanoma. Surg. Gynecol. Obstet. 12:99–108, 1968.

Milton, G. W., McGovern, V. J., and Lewis, M. G. Malignant Melanoma of the Skin and Muscous Membrane. Churchill Livingston, Edinburgh London and New York, 1977.

Mohs, F. E. Chemosurgery for melanoma. Arch. Derm. 113:285–291, 1977.

Norvell, S. T., McCleave, J. J., Bodurtha, A. J., and Irwin, A. C. Prophylactic node dissection for malignant melanoma. Canad. J. Surg. 20: 429–435, 1977.

Papachristov, D., and Furtner, J. G. Comparison of lymphedema following incontinuity and discontinuity groin dissection. Ann. Surg. 185:13–16, 1977.

Polk, H. C., Jr., and Linn, B. S. Selective regional lymphadenectomy for melanoma: a mathematical aid to clinical judgment. Ann. Surg. 174: 402–413, 1971.

Roses, D. F., Harris, M. N., and Gumport, S. L. Letter to the Editor, New Eng. J. Med. 298:223, 1978.

Sim, F. H., Taylor, W. F., Ivins, J. C., Pritchard, D. J., and Soule, E. H. A prospective randomized study of the efficacy of routine prophylactic lymphadenectomy in management of malignant melanoma: Preliminary results. Cancer 41: 948–956, 1978.

Sinha, B. K., and Buntine, D. W. Prognosis of cutaneous malignant melanoma: a clinicopathological study. Can. J. Surg. 17:328–334, 1974.

Southwick, H. W. Malignant melanoma. Role of node dissection reappraisal. Cancer 37:202–205, 1976.

Stehlin, J. S., Jr. Malignant melanoma: an appraisal. Surgery 64: 1149–1157, 1968.

Sugarbarker, E. V., and McBride, C. M. Melanoma of the trunk: the results of surgical excision and anatomic guidelines for predicting nodal metastasis. Surgery 80:22–30, 1976.

Veronesi, V., et al. Inefficacy of immediate node dissection in Stage I melanoma of the limbs. New Engl. J. Med. 297:627–630, 1977.

Wanebo, H. J. Letter to the Editor. New Eng. J. Med. 298:222, 1978.

Wanebo, H. J., Woodruff, J., and Fortner, J. G. Malignant melanoma of the extremities: a clinicopathologic study using levels of invasion (microstage). Cancer 35:666–676, 1975.

Wilkinson, T. S., and Paletta, F. X. Malignant melanoma: current concepts. Am. Surg. 35:301–309, 1969.

Chapter 18

CHEMOTHERAPY

PART ONE
Systemic Chemotherapy of Malignant Melanomas

Systemic chemotherapy of malignant melanoma is at present used in hope of palliation; it is not yet curative. Thus, chemotherapeutic agents are used mostly in patients who develop dissemination of the malignant melanomas.

In general, chemotherapeutic agents are more effective against small tumor burdens and against dividing cells than against resting cells. Good vascular supply and consequently better delivery of drugs to cells is more likely with small tumor deposits. One purpose of surgery, then, is to reduce the tumor volume allowing for more effective action of the chemotherapeutic agents. It is hoped that following surgery and chemotherapy the patient's immunologic defense mechanisms will be successful in destroying the remaining tumor. But, many chemotherapeutic agents are also potentially immunosuppressive and may actually impair host defenses.

Other side effects of these agents have also to be considered. The range of toxicity of systemic chemotherapy is wide. Among the many potential adverse effects are nausea, vomiting, diarrhea, alopecia, rashes, bone marrow suppression, fever, hepatotoxicity, and cystitis. Chemotherapy may result in prolongation of life, but the quality of that life, while on chemotherapy, may be disagreeable.

Patients can be benefited most by chemotherapy if the natural history of the disease, tumor-cell kinetics, pharmacology of the drugs and response rates are known and applied so that optimal benefit with the least toxicity is obtained.

Upon reviewing the literature on the chemotherapy of melanoma one is struck by the fact that numerous investigators have conducted many trials of different chemotherapeutic agents, both singly and in combination, yet one finds little consistency in dosages, scheduling of drug administration, populations of patients studied, and statistical treatment of data. Consequently there are differences in interpretation of data and arguable conclusions. Another uncertainty occurs when results in animal models are extrapolated to human disease. For example, many drugs tested cause greater inhibition of B16 murine melanoma than of human malignant melanoma. This may stem from biological differences between the tumors or the hosts, from different routes of administration and schedules of drugs used, or from relative differences in tumor size (Luce, 1975).

With present knowledge of the human melanoma cell cycle, it should be possible to improve effectiveness of chemotherapy by scheduling according to the kinetics of cell division. As described by Luce (1975) such scheduling arrests the melanoma cells at some stage of the cycle, releases them more or less simultaneously (synchronization), and then delivers the chemotherapeutic agent at a time when the synchronized cells are sensitive to a likely effective drug. Both the antimetabolites and the vinca alkaloids, because of their phase-specific effects, will probably be more widely used in future clinical trials in schedules conforming to cell kinetics.

DRUGS

As used throughout this Chapter, an objective response is defined as a reduction of between 50 and 100% of all discernible tumors for at least one month.

Cell-cycle times of human malignant melanomas (see Fig. 138) have been worked out by various investigators. Shirakawa et al. (1970) found a cell-cycle time of 72 hours with G-2 phase of 5.3 hours and synthesis phase of 21 hours. Subsequently Hagemann and Schiffer (1971) found the cell-cycle time to be 36 hours with G-1 phase of 16.3 hours

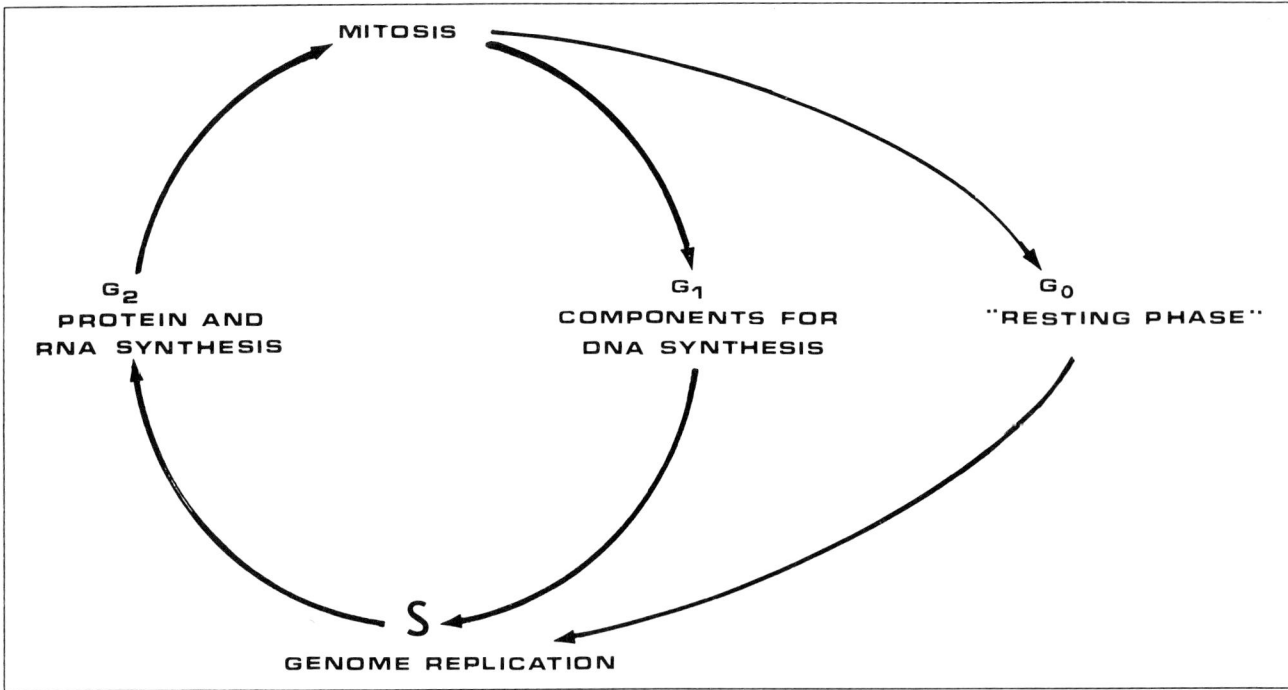

FIGURE 138. *The cell cycle.* "S" indicates DNA synthesis.

and synthesis phase of 14.5 hours. Marked variability in doubling times (*in vitro*) for tissue cultured human melanoma cells ranged from 34 to 106 hours in a report by Giovanella et al. (1976). Similarly, in a study of the doubling times of metastatic pulmonary lesions, a range of from 4 to 295 days was found (average doubling time 43 days) (Spratt, 1976). These variations may be explained, at least in part, by a newly presented concept in tumor cell proliferation, which postulates that cycling cells can arrest in three points in the cell cycle: in early G_1, in late G_1, and in late G_2 (Gelfant, 1977).

Modern chemotherapeutic drugs may be classified as follows:

1. *Alkylating agents:* These generally act at any phase of the cell cycle. They have greatest toxicity for rapidly multiplying cells. They cause cross-linking and abnormal base-pairing in DNA. In this group are mechlorethamine, cyclophosphamide, phenylalanine mustard, chlorambucil, and busulfan.

These drugs generally are not satisfactorily effective against malignant melanoma. Objective response rates are less than 10%. Except for phenylalanine mustard (Melphalan), which is used for perfusion of extremities, this class of agents has been surpassed by newer and more effective drugs, and they are currently not used often to treat melanomas.

2. *Antimetabolites:* These agents act during the S phase (DNA synthesis) of the mitotic cycle. They are subdivided into:

(a) *Folate antagonists:* methotrexate.
(b) *Pyrimidine analogs:* 5-fluorouracil, cytosine arabinoside.
(c) *Purine analogs:* 6-mercaptopurine.

These agents have not been widely used and are not very effective against malignant melanoma. Objective response rates have been less than 10%.

3. *Vinca Alkaloids:* These act on phase G2 (protein and RNA synthesis) and M (mitosis) of the cell cycle. Vinblastine and vincristine, the two agents in this group, have shown fair activity against melanoma and are generally used in combination with other agents.

4. *Antibiotics:* (actinomycin-D, bleomycin, adriamycin) Bleomycin has not shown anti-tumor activity against malignant melanoma (Blum et al., 1973). This and other antibiotics have also been tried in combination with other agents, but again without much success.

5. *Enzymes:* substances as L-aspariginase have not been widely used against malignant melanoma.

6. *Hormones:* various reports in the literature indicate that malignant melanoma may be hormone-dependent, but objective response rates with hormones have not been encouraging.

TABLE 12
Summary Table of Objective Response Rates for Various Clinical Trials Using DTIC

Dosage	No. responding/ No. evaluable	Response rate (%)	Reference
3.5 or 5.5 mg/kg/day × 10 q 3 wks.	3/15	20	Gerner and Moore, 1973
150 mg/m^2/day × 5	9/51	18	Constanza et al., 1972
2.0 mg/kg/day × 10 various courses	19/57	33	Nathanson et al., 1971
4.5 mg/kg/day × 10 various courses	13/58	22	Nathanson et al., 1971
300 mg/m^2/day × 6	6/25	24	Moon et al., 1975
100 mg/m^2/8 hr × 18 q 30 days	6/21	29	Moon et al., 1975
4.5 mg/kg/day × 10 q 6-8 wks.	18/62	29	Hill et al., 1974
250 mg/m^2/day × 5 q 21 days	19/113	17	Einhorn et al., 1974

7. *Other:*

(a) DTIC (dimethyl-triazeno-imidazole-carboxamide). This is probably an alkylating agent and is currently the most extensively used chemotherapeutic agent against malignant melanoma and the one with the most encouraging results. The objective response rates for this drug have ranged from 17% to 33% with an average of about 25%. It is paradoxical that in trials comparing 2.0 mg/kg/day with 4.5 mg/kg/day for ten days, higher objective response rates and longer responses were obtained with the smaller dosages (Nathansen et al., 1971). Moon et al. (1975) found a better response rate to three doses daily than to a single dose daily with the same total amount (300 mg/day for six days). Einhorn and co-workers (1974) reported that patients with non-visceral disease respond much better to DTIC than do patients with visceral (lung, liver, brain) metastases. The studies of Johnson and Jacobs (1971) and Nathanson et al. (1971) have shown that DTIC has a greater effect in females than in males. On the negative side, Hill et al. (1974) studied 107 patients after surgery for malignant melanoma by random assignment to receive or not to receive DTIC. No significant difference was found in the average survival times between the treated and the untreated groups.

Table 12 is a summary of various clinical trials with DTIC. It shows not only varying response rates reported by different investigators but also the diversity in dosage schedules typical of the way most drugs are being tested.

(b) *Nitrosoureas* (BCNU, CCNU, MeCCNU): These are alkylating agents and also inhibit DNA synthesis. They have been extensively used singly and in combination with other drugs against malignant melanoma. Ahman et al. (1974) found the highest response rate (26%) for MeCCNU. The results of trials with single nitrosoureas against malignant melanoma are summarized in Table 13. Various investigators have observed a better response rate in patients with melanoma metastases to the central nervous system treated with BCNU (singly or in combination) than in those treated without BCNU (Constanza et al., 1972; Einhorn et al., 1974).

(c) *Hydroxyurea* inhibits DNA synthesis. Results with this agent used by itself have been discouraging. In a small series of patients, Larson and Hill (1971) found a response rate of 14%, which is one of the best obtained by this agent. It is now used mainly in combination with other drugs.

(d) *TIC mustard* has not been found to be very effective against malignant melanoma. Response rates have been much poorer than for DTIC, the parent compound.

(e) Some investigational drugs which have been shown to have inhibitory effects against malignant melanoma in experimental animals may give us clues to newer agents that may be effective against malignant melanoma in man. Lippman et al. (1975) report good results with macromomycin B against B16 mouse melanoma. Pyran co-polymer has also been found to be very effective against this malignancy (Morahan et al., 1974). Bart et al. (1975) reported that polyinosinic-polycytidylic acid (PIC) inhibits the growth of B16 mouse melanoma but that the mechanism of this inhibition remains obscure, perhaps involving induced interferon.

TABLE 13*
Objective Response Rates of Melanoma Using Various Nitrosoureas

Drugs	No. responding/ No. evaluation	Response rate (%)
BCNU	22/123	18
CCNU	17/136	13
MeCCNU	15/124	12

* Adapted from Wasserman et al. (1975).

TABLE 14
Objective Response Rates of Melanomas Treated With Drug Combinations

Drugs	No. responding/ No. evaluable	Response rate (%)	Reference
BCNU/Vincristine	8/51	16.0	Moon et al., 1975
DTIC/Vincristine	4/19	21.0	Ahman et al., 1972, 1974
DTIC/BCNU	12/61	19.5	Constanza et al., 1972
DTIC/Procarbazine	10/62	16.0	Einhorn et al., 1974
DTIC/Dactinomycin	14/69	20.0	Gerner et al., 1973
BCNU/Vincristine/DTIC	21/106	19.0	Einhorn et al., 1974
BCNU/Vincristine/DTIC	10/16	62.5	Cohen et al., 1972
BCNU/Hydroxyurea/DTIC	24/89	27.0	Constanzi et al., 1975
BCNU/Hydroxyurea/DTIC/Vincristine	27/89	30.0	Constanzi et a., 1975

COMBINATION DRUG THERAPY

With the knowledge that chemotherapeutic combinations have been used with considerable success in the treatment of leukemia and lymphomas, many investigators have tried combining two or more drugs against melanoma. Table 14 is a summary of some of the drug combinations tried. As previously mentioned, these trials unfortunately suffer from diversity of dosage schedules, lack of randomization, and problems with statistical interpretation.

DTIC has been combined with many other agents; some such combinations produced greater toxicity. For example, both Gerner et al. (1973) and Gams and Carpenter (1974) report on the possibility of serious complications in the central nervous system (seizures, hemorrhage) following treatment with the combination of DTIC and dactinomycin.

BCNU has also been used extensively in combination with DTIC and other agents. The triple combination of BCNU, vincristine and DTIC has generally produced response rates of less than 20%. Cohen et al. (1972), however, report a response rate of 62.5% in a series of 16 patients. They attribute this unusually high rate to the fact that drug doses used by them, especially with respect to BCNU, were much higher than dosages used by other investigators.

Response rates equal or superior to those obtained with DTIC alone have been reported with the combinations of BCNU, hydroxyurea and DTIC and BCNU, hydroxyurea, DTIC and vincristine (Constanzi et al., 1975). The authors cited note that if cases of early deaths (within 28 days of drug treatment) are removed from their study the overall response rate for the drug combinations becomes 38%, a result superior to that obtained with DTIC alone.

An increase in remission rates, prolongation of remission and prolonged survival have been observed in patients treated with DTIC and BCG as compared to DTIC alone (Gutterman et al., 1974). Wood et al. (1978) also report a reduced number of early recurrences of malignant melanomas using chemoimmunotherapy (combined DTIC and BCG) in patients predicted to have high risk for recurrences.

SUMMARY AND COMMENTS

An overview of the present practice of chemotherapy against malignant melanoma reveals that currently DTIC is the one agent most used. The nitrosoureas when combined with DTIC and other agents show more promising objective response rates than does DTIC alone. The phase-specific vinca alkaloids and antimetabolites may have a greater role in the future as cytokinetic principles are further applied in chemotherapy.

Chemotherapeutic agents have also been used for malignant melanoma by local perfusion so that a limited tumor burden becomes maximally exposed to the drug. This topic is covered in Part Two, Regional Chemotherapy.

BCG used in combination with DTIC has been reported to raise the efficacy of DTIC (Gutterman et al., 1974, Wood et al., 1978).

It is expected that kinetic scheduling and synchronization of chemotherapeutic combinations along with additional animal and clinical trials will produce chemotherapeutic and chemoimmunotherapeutic regimens that are more useful against malignant melanomas in man.

REFERENCES

Ahmann, D. L., Hahn, R. G., and Bisel, H. F. A comparative study of 1-(2-chloroethyl)-3-cyclohexyl-1-nitrosourea (NSC 79037) and imidazole carboxamide (NSC 45388) with viscristine (NSC 67574) in the palliation of disseminated malignant melanoma. Cancer Res. 32: 2432-2434, 1972.

Ahmann, D. L., Hahn, R. G., and Bisel, H. F. Evaluation of 1-(2-chloroethyl-3,4-methylcyclohexyl)-1-nitrosourea (methyl-CCNU, NSC 95441) versus combined imidazole carboxamide (NSC 45388) and vincristine (NSC 67574) in palliation of disseminated malignant melanoma. Cancer 33:615-618, 1974.

Ahmann, D. L., Hahn, R. G., Bisel, H. F., Eagan, R. T., and Edmonson, J. H. Comparative study of methyl-CCNU (NSC-95441) with cyclophosphamide (NSC-2671) and 5-(3,3-dimethyl-1-triazeno) imidazole-4-carboxamide (NSC-45388) with vincristine (NSC-67574) in patients with disseminated malignant melanoma. Cancer Chemother. Rep. 59:451-453, 1975.

Balda, B.-R., and Birkmayer, G. D. Drug effects in melanoma: Tumor-specific interactions of proflavine and ethidiumbromide. Yale J. Biol. Med. 46:464-470, 1973.

Bart, R. S., Lam, S., Cooper, J. S., and Kopf, A. W. Retention of antimelanoma effect of polyinosinic-polycytidylic acid in neonatally thymectomized, irradiated, leukopenic mice. J. Invest. Dermatol. 65: 285-289, 1975.

Birkmayer, G. D., Balda, B. R., and Miller, F. The inhibitory effect of proflavine and ethidiumbromide on the cell-free transmission and the growth of the hamster melanoma A Mel 3. Eur. J. Cancer 9:859-864, 1973.

Blum, R. H., Carter, S. K., and Agre, K. A clinical review of bleomycin—a new antineoplastic agent. Cancer 31:903-914, 1973.

Cohen, S. M., Greenspan, E. M., Weiner, M. J., and Kabakow, B. Triple combination chemotherapy of disseminated melanoma. Cancer 29: 1489-1495, 1972.

Constanza, M. E., Nathanson, L., Lenhard, R., Wolter, J., Colsky, J., Oberfield, R. A., and Schilling, A. Therapy of malignant melanoma with an imidazole carboxamide and bis-chloroethyl nitrosourea. Cancer 30:1457-1461, 1972.

Constanzi, J. J., Vaitkevicius, V. K., Quagliana, J. M., Hoogstraten, B., Coltman, C. A., Jr., and Delaney, F. C. Combination chemotherapy for disseminated malignant melanoma. Cancer 35:342-346, 1975.

Dowell, K. E., Armstrong, D. M., Aust, J. B., and Cruz, A. B. Jr., Systemic chemotherapy of advanced head and neck malignancies. Cancer 35: 1116-1120, 1975.

Einhorn, L. H., Burgess, M. A., Vallejos, C., Bodey, G. P., Sr., Gutterman, J., Mavligit, G., Hersh, E. M., Luce, J. K., Frei, E., III, Freireich, E. J., and Gottlieb, J. A. Prognostic correlations and response to treatment in advanced metastatic malignant melanoma. Cancer Res. 34:1995-2004, 1974.

Falkson, G., van der Merwe, A. M., and Falkson, H. C. Clinical experience with 5-[3,3-bis(2-chloroethyl)-1-triazeno)] imidazole-4-carboxamide (NSC-82196) in the treatment of metastatic malignant melanoma. Cancer Chemother. Rep. 56:671-677, 1972.

Gams, R. A., and Carpenter, J. T. Central nervous system complications after combination treatment with adriamycin (NSC-123127) and 5-(3,3-dimethyl-1-triazeno) imidazole-4-carboxamide (NSC-45388). Cancer Chemother. Rep. 58:753-754, 1974.

Gelfant, S. A new concept of tissue and tumor cell proliferation. Cancer Res. 37:3845-3862, 1977.

Gerner, R. E., and Moore, G. E. Study of 5-(3,3-dimethyl-1-triazeno) imidazole-4-carboxamide (NSC 45388) in patients with disseminated melanoma. Cancer Chemother. Rep. 57:83-84, 1973.

Gerner, R. E., Moore, G. E., and Didolkhar, M. S. Chemotherapy of disseminated malignant melanoma with dimethyl triazeno imidazole carboxamide and Dactinomycin. Cancer 32:756-760, 1973.

Gerner, R. E., Moore, G. E., and Dickey, C. Combination chemotherapy in disseminated melanoma and other solid tumors in adults. Oncology 31:22-30, 1975.

Giovanella, G., et al. Human neoplastic and normal cells in tissue culture. I. Cell lines derived from malignant melanoma and normal melanocytes. J. Natl. Cancer Inst. 56:1131-1142, 1976.

Gottlieb, J. A., Frei, E., III, and Luce, J. K. Dose-schedule studies with hydroxyurea (NSC-32065) in malignant melanoma. Cancer Chemother. Rep. 55:277-280, 1971.

Gutterman, J. U., Mavligit, G., Gottlieb, J. A., Burgess, M. A., McBride, C. E., Einhorn, L., Freireich, E. J., and Hersh, E. M. Chemoimmunotherapy of disseminated malignant melanoma with dimethyl trizeno imidazole carboxamide and Bacillus Calmette-Guérin. N. Engl. J. Med. 291:592-597, 1974.

Hagemann, R. E., and Schiffer, L. M. Cell kinetic analysis of a human melanoma *in vitro* and *in vivo-vitro*. J. Natl. Cancer Inst. 47:519-526, 1971.

Hill, G. J., II, Ruess, R., Berris, R., Philpott, G. W., and Parkin, P. Chemotherapy of malignant melanoma with dimethyl triazeno imidazole carboxamide (DTIC) and nitrosourea derivatives (BCNU, CCNU). Ann. Surg. 180:167-174, 1974.

Johnson, F. D., and Jacobs, E. M. Chemotherapy of metastatic malignant melanoma. Experience with 73 patients. Cancer 27:1306-1312, 1971.

Larsen, R. R., and Hill, G. J., II. Improved systemic chemotherapy for malignant malanoma. Am. J. Surg. 122:36-41, 1971.

Lippman, M. M., Laster, W. R., Abbott, B. J., Venditti, J., and Baratta, M. Antitumor activity of macromomycin B (NSC 17015) against murine leukemias, melanoma, and lung carcinoma. Cancer Res. 35: 939-945, 1975.

Livingston, R. B., Einhorn, L. H., Bodey, G. P., Burgess, M. A., Freireich, E. J., and Gottlieb, J. A. COMB (cyclophosphamide, oncovin, methyl-CCNU, and bleomycin): a four-drug combination in solid tumors. Cancer 36:327-332, 1975.

Luce, J. K. Chemotherapy of malignant melanoma. Cancer 30:1604-1615, 1972.

Luce, J. K. Chemotherapy of melanoma. Semin. Oncol. 2:179-186, 1975.

McKelvey, E. M., Luce, J. K., Talley, R. W., Hersh, E. M., Hewlett, J. S., and Moon, T. E. Combination chemotherapy with bischloroethyl nitrosurca (BCNU), vincristine and dimethyl triazeno imidazole carboxamide (DTIC) in disseminated malignant melanoma. Cancer 39: 1-4, 1977.

Mitchell, M. S., Mokyr, M. B., and Davis, J. M. Effect of chemotherapy and immunotherapy on tumor-specific immunity in melanoma. J. Clin. Invest. 59:1017-1026, 1977.

Moon, J. H., Gailani, S., Cooper, M. R., Hayes, D. M., Rege, V. E., Blom, J., Falkson, G., Maurice, P., Brunner, K., Glidewell, O., and Holland, J. F. Comparison of the combination of 1,3-bis(2-chloroethyl)-1-nitrosourea (BCNU) and vincristine with two dose schedules of 5-(3,3-dimethyl-1-triazeno) imidazole 4-carboxamide (DTIC) in the treatment of disseminated malignant melanoma. Cancer 35:368-371, 1975.

Morahan, P. S., Munson, J. A., Baird, L. G., Kaplan, A. M., and Regelson, W. Antitumor action of pyran copolymer and tilorone against Lewis lung carcinoma and B-16 melanoma. Cancer Res. 34:506-511, 1974.

Nathanson, L., Wolter, J., Horton, J., Colsky, J., Schnider, B. I., and Schilling, A. Characteristics of prognosis and response to an imidazole carboxamide in malignant melanoma. Clin. Pharmacol. Ther. 12: 955–962, 1971.

Perlin, E., Engeler, J., Reid, J. W., Lokey, J. L., and Kostinas, J. Treatment of malignant melanoma with vinblastine (NSC-49842), procarbazine (NSC-77213), and actinomycin D (NSC-3053). Cancer Chemother. Rep. 59:767–768, 1975.

Shirakawa, S., Luce, J. K., Tannock, I., and Frei, E., III. Cell proliferation in human melanoma. J. Clin. Invest. 49:1188–1199, 1970.

Stolinsky, D. C., Jacobs, E. M., Braunwald, J., and Bateman, J. R. Further study of trimethylcolchicinic acid, methyl ether, d-tartrate (TMCA: NSC-36354) in patients with malignant melanoma. Cancer Chemother. Rep. 56:263–265, 1972.

Spratt, J. S. Symposium on melanoma. Contemporary Surg. 9:45–72, 1976.

Vogel, C. L., Comis, R., Ziegler, J. L., and Kiryabwire, J. W. M. Clinical trials of 5-(3,3-dimethyl-1-triazeno) imidazole-4-carboxamide (NSC-45388) given intravenously in the treatment of malignant melanoma in Uganda. Cancer Chemother. Rep. 55:143–149, 1971.

Wasserman, T. H., Slavik, M., and Carter, S. K. Clinical comparison of the nitrosoureas. Cancer 36:1258–1268, 1975.

Wood, W. C., Cosimi, A. B., Carey, R. W., and Kaufman, S. D. Randomized trial of adjuvant therapy for "high risk" primary malignant melanoma. Surgery 83:677–681, 1978.

Young, R. C., Cavellos, G. P., Chabner, B. A., Schein, P. S., Brereton, H. D., and DeVita, V. T. Treatment of malignant melanoma with methyl CCNU. Clin. Pharmacol. Ther. 15:617–622, 1974.

Part Two
Regional Chemotherapy of Malignant Melanomas

Regional chemotherapy by isolation perfusion, or by infusion, maximally exposes a limited tumor-cell burden to cytotoxic drugs and minimizes systemic toxicity. Its place in the treatment of melanoma is as an adjuvant to surgery and its main use is in those patients with lesions confined to the extremities.

The indications for regional chemotherapy vary but the modality is thought useful for patients with high-risk limb lesions ("thick" level III, level IV, and level V), for patients exhibiting local metastatic disease (in-transit metastases, satellitosis, clinically involved nodes); and as a last recourse for patients in whom repeated surgery, radiation, and other means have not been successful in eradicating the malignancy.

Unfortunately, evaluation of the results of perfusion by various techniques and various drugs compared with other means of treatment is difficult because of a lack of suitable controls in most studies (Luce, 1972). As is true for systemic chemotherapy, trials of regional chemotherapy also suffer from diversity in dosage schedules, lack of randomization, and little consistency in statistical manipulation of the data obtained, which makes, at times, for differences in interpretation of results.

Golomb (1975) defines regional perfusion as a technique designed to isolate a limited area by mechanically controlling its arterial inflow and venous outflow (via an extracorporeal circuit) and thus allowing for a high concentration of cytotoxic drugs to be delivered to cancer-bearing sites. The duration of the perfusion is generally less than two hours. Infusion is the technique of administering drugs into the arterial supply of an area without cutting off its blood supply from the general circulation. A high drug concentration can be delivered to the area of malignancy with this method. The infusion is continued for several days to several weeks in order to expose each tumor cell to the chemotherapeutic agent as it enters its vulnerable stage in the mitotic cycle.

For perfusions, phenylalanine mustard and other short-acting alkylating agents are most commonly used. For infusions, methotrexate in high doses is commonly used, sometimes with citrovorum factor (Leukovorin) as an antidote against systemic effects.

Local complications of regional chemotherapy include tissue necrosis, thrombophlebitis, wound infection and dehiscence, edema, and arterial and venous thrombosis. Systemically, leukopenia, alopecia and pulmonary emboli are possible side effects depending on the drugs used.

(a) *Infusion.* Oberfield (1975) reported that arterial infusion for regionally confined malignant melanomas and for localized lesions limited to the extremities has given favorable results. He also noted that infusion chemotherapy (via catheterization of the common carotid artery mainly) has resulted in enhanced antitumor responses and prolongation of survival in locally recurrent advanced cancers of the head and neck.

A group of 169 patients with head and neck cancers (nine of them with malignant melanoma) who received regional intra-arterial infusion chemotherapy was reported by Freckman (1972). Six of the nine patients with malignant melanomas responded to infusion chemotherapy, and the combination of 5-fluorouracil (5-FU), cyclophosphamide and vinblastine was the most effective form of chemotherapy in such patients. Table 15, adapted from Freckman's article, shows the doses of chemotherapeutic agents used. Fluorouracil and methotrexate are anti-metabolites and kill cells during the S phase (DNA synthesis) of the mitotic cycle, while vinblastine acts on the G2 and M (mitosis) phases of the cell cycle and commonly causes metaphase

TABLE 15

Regional Infusion: Dosage of Chemotherapeutic Agents per Course

Drug	Dose (mg/24 hr)	Duration (days)
5-Fluorouracil	250–500	10–14
Cyclophosphamide	100–200	5–10
Vinblastine	1–2	5–10

* From Freckman (1972). Three or more courses were given at monthly intervals.

arrest. Cyclophosphamide, an alkylating agent, acts on all phases of the cell cycle.

Intra-arterial infusions of DTIC were used by Savlov et al. (1971) to treat six patients who had recurrent melanomas localized to body areas served by a major artery. Good results were obtained in two of the six patients. The authors point out two distinct advantages of infusion chemotherapy, namely, (1) higher drug concentrations are delivered to the tumor-bearing areas, and (2) less systemic toxicity.

DTIC intra-arterial infusions were also used by Einhorn et al. (1973) to treat 17 patients with advanced regional malignant melanoma. The response rate, i.e., greater than 50% reduction in observable tumor, was found to be 41%. There was a greater response rate in women than in men (54%:17%). Similarly, the studies of Johnson and Jacobs (1971) and Nathanson et al. (1971) have shown that systemic administration of DTIC also has a better effect in women than in men. These investigators found that the toxicity of DTIC by infusion was less than by systemic administration. They concluded that intra-arterial therapy is preferable to systemic therapy for isolated, inoperable lesions of malignant melanoma.

Ariel (1974) and Edwards (1974) reported on treatment of patients with malignant melanoma by a combination of surgery and infusions of endolymphatic radioactive isotopes. Both authors report five-year survival rates of about 80% for Stage I patients and 28.5% and 21.4%, respectively, for Stage II (positive regional nodes) patients.

(b) *Perfusion.* Isolation-perfusion chemotherapy for cancer was first reported by Creech et al. (1958). Krementz and Ryan (1972) reported that chemotherapy by perfusion as an adjuvant to conventional surgical therapy for Stage I disease adds approximately 15% to the five-year survival rate for invasive malignant melanoma, reduces the incidence of regional recurrences, and eliminates the need for major amputations. In Stage II disease the survival rates are doubled in most categories, according to these authors.

They consider chemotherapy by perfusion the therapy of choice for satellitosis.

Shingleton (1969) reported encouraging results with Melphalan perfusion for recurrent malignant melanoma of the limbs. Control of malignancies for two years or longer was achieved in 40% of his patients. Golomb (1972) reported a five-year survival rate of 72% for patients with primary malignant melanoma treated by perfusion as an adjunct to surgical excision. For patients with recurrent malignant melanoma of the extremities who were perfused the five-year survival rate was 35%. This is comparable or better than the five-year survival rates for the same class of patients who undergo amputations. Golomb (1975) reported that of 35 patients treated with surgery and perfusion for Stage I malignant melanoma of the extremities, 23 or 66% survived more than five years, and the five-year survival rate for patients with Stage II disease (lymph node metastases) was 42%.

McBride and Clark (1971) treated 240 patients with malignant melanoma by isolation perfusion with phenylalanine mustard. They found that compared to previous patients treated by conventional surgery, the five-year survival rate was increased (62% versus 51%), that the necessity for skin grafts or amputations was reduced, and that in-transit metastases were reduced.

McBride et al. (1975) reported on 202 patients with malignant melanoma who had Stage I disease and at least level III lesions and who underwent isolation perfusion with phenylalanine mustard. The 10-year survival rate for this group of patients was found to be 83%. For 71 historical controls treated only by wide and deep excision (with and without lymphadenectomy) the 10-year survival rate was but 57%. Eighteen percent of the perfused patients developed clinical disease in the regional lymph nodes after isolation perfusion compared to 38% of patients treated by surgery alone. Forty-three percent of these with metastases to lymph nodes after perfusion were salvaged by a second perfusion, which indicated in the authors' opinion, that regional lymph-node dissections are unnecessary in patients undergoing isolation-perfusion.

Fontaine and Jamieson (1974) reported a series of 56 patients with malignant melanomas of limbs treated by surgery and perfusion with phenylalanine mustard in which the five-year survival rate was 67%. Wagner (1976) reported on a series of 245 patients with malignant melanoma treated by regional perfusion with phenylalanine mustard in whom regional perfusion improved cure rates of conventional surgery by at least 10–15%. In another series, excision of the primary lesion and isolation-perfusion with phenylalanine mustard was the treatment in 199 patients with invasive Stage I malignant melanoma of the extremities. Survival rates were 88% at five years and 84% at 10 years. For patients treated by wide excision alone the five-year survival rate was 68%. A decrease in the rate of regional lymph-node metastases was also found in the excision-perfusion group as compared to the non-perfused groups (Sugarbaker and McBride, 1976).

Stehlin et al. (1975) reported on a seven-year experience with 185 hyperthermic perfusions (temperature of 43.3°C) for malignant melanomas of the extremities. For 70 patients with Stage I disease, the projected five-year survival rate was 83.5%. For 30 patients with in-transit metastases, the projected five-year survival was 71.8%. This compares to a 22.2% five-year survival for a group of 27 patients with in-transit metastases who did not receive hyperthermic perfusion. These authors claim that survival rates for the heated perfusion groups are 300% better than for non-heated perfusions. They point out that the activity of the plasma and lymphocytes of patients against autologous cells of malignant melanoma increases after hyperthermic perfusion. Of interest, however, is the report of Harris (1976) that showed that cytolytic activity of T-lymphocytes against allogeneic cells of mastocytoma was greatly reduced when the lymphocytes were exposed to heat. He found that 45 minutes at 43°C decreased lymphocytic activity by 99%.

Hersh et al. (1973) found that for patients with malignant melanoma of the extremities treated by perfusion with phenylalanine mustard, actinomycin-D or nitrogen mustard, there was an irreversible inhibitory effect on the lymphocytes circulating within the perfusion circuit (i.e., the lymphocyte blastogenic responses became impaired). No systemic immunologic effects of the perfusion therapy were found.

From our institution Golomb (1977) concludes that isolated perfusion is established as an effective modality for the treatment of recurrent melanoma, particularly of the limbs. He performed 105 perfusions in 92 patients. Of 44 treated for recurrent melanoma 10 (22%) were free of disease 7 to 124 months after perfusion, with a 5-year survival of 35%. Of 39 patients perfused as an adjunct to surgical excision 27 (69%) are free of disease with a 73% 5-year survival.

SUMMARY AND DISCUSSION

Regional chemotherapy seems to have a useful role in the treatment of some localized malignant melanomas.

A cause of failure of surgical treatment for melanomas of the extremities is local or regional recurrence, presumably secondary to occult microscopic metastases at the time of surgery. By instilling a high concentration of cytotoxic drug in a local area, regional chemotherapy may destroy these microscopic metastases and improve the chances of prolongation of life of these patients. The minimization of systemic toxicity, the avoidance of amputations, as well as improved survival are other positive aspects of regional chemotherapy. The procedure must be carried out, however, with meticulous attention to details and by persons who are experienced in its use and have knowledge of its potentially serious complications.

Perhaps with the application of cytokinetic principles, better drugs, hyperthermia, and more sophisticated methods, regional chemotherapy may become even more useful.

For details as to techniques of isolation perfusion and infusion, readers are referred to Krementz and Ryan (1972), Golomb (1975, 1977), and Oberfield (1975).

REFERENCES

Ariel, I. M. Results of treating malignant melanoma intralymphatically with radioactive isotopes. Surg. Gynecol. Obstet. 139:726–730, 1974.

Brown, A. S., Wallack, M. K., Horstmann, J. T., Hamilton, R. W., Johnson, J. L., and Rosato, F. E. Perfusion therapy for extremity melanoma. Arch. Surg. 111:961–963, 1976.

Creech, O., Jr., Krementz, E. T., Ryan, R. F., and Winblad. J. N. Chemotherapy of cancer: regional perfusion utilizing an extracorporeal circuit. Ann. Surg. 148:616–632, 1958.

Cox, K. R. Survival after regional perfusion for limb melanoma. Aust. N. Z. J. Surg. 45:32–36, 1975.

Edwards, J. M. Treatment of melanoma by endolymphatic therapy. Proc. R. Soc. Med. 67:97–99, 1974.

Einhorn, L. H., McBride, C. M., Luce, J. K., Caoili, E., and Gottlieb, J. A. Intra-arterial infusion therapy with 5-(3,3-dimethyl-1-triazeno) imidazole-4-carboxamide (NSC 45388) for malignant melanoma. Cancer 32:749–755, 1973.

Fontaine, C. J., and Jamieson, C. W. Perfusion in limb melanoma: indications and results. Proc. R. Soc. Med. 67:99–100, 1974.

Freckman, H. A. Results in 169 patients with cancer of the head and neck treated by intra-arterial infusion therapy. Am. J. Surg. 124:501–509, 1972.

Golomb, F. Perfusion of melanoma; 105 isolated perfusions in 92 patients. Oncology 26:197–205, 1972.

Golomb, F. M. Perfusion therapy for skin cancer. J. Dermatol. Surg. 1(4):39–48, 1975.

Golomb, F. M., Solowey, A. C., Postel, A., Gumport, S. L., and Wright, J. C. Induced remission of malignant melanoma with Actinomycin D. Cancer 20:656–662, 1967.

Goss, P., and Parsons, P. G. The effect of hyperthermia and melphalan on survival of human fibroblast strains and melanoma cell lines. Cancer Res. 37:152–156, 1977.

Hansson, J. A., Simert, G., and Vang, J. The effect of regional perfusion treatment on recurrent melanoma of the extremities. Acta. Chir. Scand. 143:33–39, 1977.

Harris, J. W. Effects of tumor-like assay conditions, ionizing radiation, and hyperthermia on immune lysis of tumor cells by cytotoxic T-lymphocytes. Cancer Res. 36:2733–2739, 1976.

Hersh, E. M., McBride, C. M., and Gschwind, C. Local and systemic immunologic effects of perfusion therapy for malignant melanoma. Surg. Gynecol. Obstet. 137:461–464, 1973.

Hill, G. J., II, Johnson, R. O., Metter, G., Wilson, W. L., Davis, H. L., Grage, T., Fletcher, W. S., Golomb, F. M., and Cruz, A. B. Multimodal surgical adjuvant therapy for a broad spectrum of tumors in humans. Surg. Gynecol. Obstet. 142:882–892, 1976.

Johnson, F. D., and Jacobs, E. M. Chemotherapy of metastatic malignant melanoma: experience with 73 patients. Cancer 27:1306–1312, 1971.

Koops, H. S., et al. Regional perfusion for recurrent malignant melanoma of the extremities. Am. J. Surg. 133:221–224, 1977.

Krementz, E. T., and Ryan, R. F. Chemotherapy of melanoma of the extremities by perfusion: fourteen years clinical experience. Ann. Surg. 175:900–917, 1972.

Luce, J. K. Chemotherapy of malignant melanoma. Cancer 30:1604–1615, 1972.

McBride, C. M., and Clark, R. L. Experience with 1-phenylalanine mustard dihydrochloride in isolation-perfusion of extremities for malignant melanoma. Cancer 28:1293–1296, 1971.

McBride, C. M., Sugarbaker, E. V., and Hickey, R. C. Prophylactic isolation-perfusion as the primary therapy for invasive malignant melanoma of the limbs. Ann. Surg. 182:316–324, 1975.

Nathanson, L., Wolter, J., Horton, J., Colsky, J., Schneider, B. I., and Schilling, A. Characteristics of prognosis and response to an imidazole carboxamide in malignant melanoma. Clin. Pharmacol. Ther. 12:955–962, 1971.

Oberfield, R. A. Current status of regional arterial infusion chemotherapy. Med. Clin. North Am. 59:411–424, 1975.

Savlov, E. D., Hall, T. C., and Oberfield, R. A. Intra-arterial therapy of melanoma with dimethyl triazeno imidazole carboxamide (NSC-45388). Cancer 28:1161–1164, 1971.

SchraffordtKoops, H., Oldhoff, J., van der Ploeg, E., Vermey, A., Eibergen, R., and Beekhuis, H. Some aspects of the treatment of primary malignant melanoma of the extremities by isolated regional perfusion. Cancer 39:27–33, 1977.

Shingleton, W. W. Perfusion chemotherapy for recurrent melanoma of extremity: a progress report. Ann. Surg. 169:969–973, 1969.

Stehlin, J. S., Giovanella, B. C., de Ipolyi, P. D., Muenz, L. R., and Anderson, R. F. Results of hyperthermic perfusion for melanoma of the extremities. Surg. Gynecol. Obstet. 140:339–348, 1975.

Sugarbaker, E. V. and McBride, C. M. Survival and regional disease control after isolation-perfusion for invasive stage I melanoma of the extremities. Cancer 37:188–198, 1976.

Wagner, D. E. A retrospective study of regional perfusion for melanoma. Arch. Surg. 111:410–413, 1976.

Chapter 19

Radiotherapy of Malignant Melanoma

It is generally held that malignant melanoma is relatively radioresistant and not curable with x-ray therapy. The consensus is that treatment for the primary tumor is surgical. However, in those instances where surgery cannot be used, radiation may be helpful (Pearson, 1974).

In reviewing the recent literature on the radiotherapy of malignant melanoma it becomes clear that many of the reports lack sufficient information and proper controls. First, many patients received radiotherapy for "malignant melanomas" without confirmation by biopsy. Since an error in clinical diagnosis is made in about one of every three melanomas (Kopf et al., 1975), it is likely that some of the lesions irradiated were not malignant melanomas and therefore the cure rates do not accurately reflect those for malignant melanomas. Second, the techniques and dosage schedules used for treating malignant melanoma vary widely from report to report. Third, long term follow-ups are often not found in such reports. Fourth, most reports do not include analyses of the types, levels, and thicknesses of the "malignant melanomas" treated. Last, no randomized studies have been done to prove the value of radiation therapy compared to surgery. Nonetheless, as previously indicated, if surgery cannot be used for treatment of a primary or metastatic malignant melanoma serious consideration may be given to radiotherapy.

SELECTED REPORTS

Lissner and Von Lieven (1974) in a review of the literature compared results from among surgery, radiotherapy, and combinations of both in terms of five-year, symptom-free, follow-ups for Stage I malignant melanomas. Results for surgery alone were 50%; radiotherapy alone, 67%; radiotherapy followed by surgery, 69%; and surgery followed by radiotherapy, 48%.

Sharmer (1976) in his review of radiotherapy of malignant melanoma concluded that the malignancy is relatively radioresistant, but that treatment of malignant malanoma by radiotherapy is not useless.

Hellriegel (1963) reported on 259 malignant melanomas treated with radiation and followed for five years or longer. Only 68% of the cases were histologically proved. The overall five-year survival rate for Stage I primary melanoma treated with radiation was 62%. Those treated by radiation alone had a 68% survival rate; those treated by local excision followed by radiation had a 54% survival rate; and those treated with radiation followed by local excision had an 82% survival rate. This encouraged the authors to advise preoperative radiation therapy followed by local excision. The technique recommended was radiation delivered to the primary tumor, to the surrounding skin, and to the regional lymph nodes. Late radiation sequelae were observed in a significant proportion of patients. He concluded that malignant melanoma can be successfully treated with radiotherapy, but that very high dosages are required.

Dewey (1971) studying the biology of cultured cells of malignant melanoma irradiated with a single dose of x-rays concluded that there is no evidence of any intrinsic cellular resistance to x-rays. He conjectured that difficulties in curing malignant melanomas probably result from factors other than radio-resistance of the cells themselves. However, Hornsey (1972) interpreted Dewey's data differently and concluded that excessively high doses of radiation would be required to treat malignant melanomas. Others, have used specialized techniques such as (1) "split course" radiotherapy in which three courses are given with a two-week interval between the first and second courses and a three-week interval between the second and third courses (Konecny and Krenarova, 1969); (2) the additional use of hyperbaric oxygen (Sealey et al., 1974) on the theory that rapidly growing malignancies contain within them areas of poor vasculization and thereby relatively radioresistant hypoxic cells may be oxygenated by exposure of patients to hyperbaric oxygen; (3) the use of fast neutrons (Catterall, 1974) whose cancericidal effect is independent of the degree of oxygenization of malignant cells (Castro et al., 1973); and (4) intralymphatic injection of radioactive colloids (Edwards, 1969).

Apparently one important reason for failure in the radiotherapy of malignant melanomas is the amount of x-rays given per dose, according to Habermalz and Fischer (1976). In reviewing their records they concluded that high doses per fraction (≥ 600 rads) are required to destroy metastatic melanomas. Individual doses of 200 to 500 rads failed to cause involution of such lesions, even though in some cases the total doses were greater than 5000 rads. On the other hand, treating brain metastases with large doses per fraction commonly leads to severe late effects (Withers and Harter, 1976).

For metastases of malignant melanomas to the brain, Withers and Harter (1976) report increased survivals by giving radiation treatments twice per day five days per week for two weeks rather than once daily. This schedule permitted increase of the total tumor dose to as much as 4800 rads.

Treatment by radiotherapy has been reported to be especially useful for lentigo maligna and conjunctival melanoma and for palliation. Melanomas arising in the oral cavity, nasal cavity, and larynx may also be radiosensitive according to Levene (1972). Although our original report (Petratos et al., 1972) generally supported the use of the Meischer technique that employs soft x-rays for the treatment for lentigo maligna, we subsequently abandoned the method at the Skin and Cancer Unit of the New York University Medical Center because further experience showed an unacceptable recurrence rate and an inability to control metastases (Kopf et al., 1976).

Precancerous melanosis of the conjunctiva and cancerous melanosis of the conjunctiva are reported to be curable by radiotherapy (Lederman, 1961). Such conditions on the palpebral conjunctiva are less radiosensitive and resemble cutaneous melanomas elsewhere in their response. Radiotherapy is delivered either with a strontium eye applicator or by superficial x-rays with protection of the lens. Intraocular malignant melanoma is treated surgically.

The palliative value of radiotherapy for distant metastases in malignant melanoma is well established (Hilaris et al., 1963). Significant subjective relief can be achieved in over 50% of lesions irradiated. Palliative high-dose radiation can also be of great value to patients who have advanced disease for which surgery is not feasible. Combinations of systemic chemotherapy or immunotherapy with radiotherapy require further evaluation (Harmer, 1976; Currie and McElwain, 1975).

Biran et al. (1973) report a five-year survival rate of 45% in Stage I and II patients with malignant melanoma who were treated by wide excision of the primary lesion followed by radiation to the lymphatic pathway and to the regional lymph node drainage area even if no clinical evidence of lymph-node involvement was found. Similarly, Dickson (1958) reported a series of patients treated by wide excision of the primary lesion and immediate drainage areas followed by radiation therapy to all areas which showed disease on histologic examination. The five-year survival rate of this series was 41% and but 26% with radical surgery alone.

Barranco et al. (1971) studied the response to radiation of three cell lines *in vitro* from human malignant melanomas. These authors conclude: "The response of these malignant melanoma cells to X-ray *in vitro* does not correlate with a model of the classically radioresistant tumor cell that clinical experience might predict." Most likely the differences in sensitivity to ionizing radiation *in vivo* and *in vitro* are related to variations in the cell cycle and tumor growth fraction. Shirakawa et al. (1970) determined the median cell cycle time of human malignant melanoma *in vivo* to be three days. However, the growth fraction was only 20%. Terz et al. (1971) report a cell cycle of 21 hours and a 39–44% growth fraction. Therefore, radioresistance of this malignant melanoma *in vivo* as compared to the results *in vitro* may be accounted for by the fact that at any one time 55 to 80% of the tumor cells are in the non-dividing phase of the cell cycle and would not be responsive to radiation damage. It is also possible that malignancies *in vivo* contain large numbers of anoxic cells. Radiosensitivity diminishes as the availability of oxygen to tissues decreases.

We have recently submitted for publication a comprehensive review article on the present role and future prospects of radiotherapy in the treatment of malignant melanomas (Cooper et al., 1978). The reader is referred to this source for greater details concerning radiotherapy of primary and metastatic melanomas.

REFERENCES

Barranco, S. C., Romsdahl, M. M., and Humphrey, R. M. The radiation response of human malignant melanoma cells grown *in vitro*. Cancer Res. 31:830–833, 1971.

Biran, S., Hochman, A., and Walach, N. Malignant melanoma: a survey of 232 cases. Oncology 28:331–342, 1973.

Castro, J. R., Oliver, G. D., Withers, H. R., and Almond, P. R. Experience with Californium 252 in clinical radiotherapy. Am. J. Roentgenol. Radium Ther. Nucl. Med. 117:182–194, 1973.

Catterall, M. Fast neutrons in oncology. Br. J. Hosp. Med. 12:853–860, 1974.

Cooper, J. S., Kopf, A. W., and Bart, R. S. Present role and future prospects of radiotherapy in the treatment of malignant melanoma. J. Derm. Surg. Oncol. Submitted for publication, 1978.

Currie, G. A., and McElwain, T. J. Active immunotherapy as an adjunct to chemotherapy in the treatment of disseminated malignant melanoma: a pilot study. Br. J. Cancer 31:143–156, 1975.

Dewey, D. L. The radiosensitivity of melanoma cells in culture. Br. J. Radiol. 44:816, 1971.

Dickson, R. J. Malignant melanoma: a combined surgical and radiotherapeutic approach. Am. J. Roentgenol. Radium Ther. Nucl. Med. 79:1063–1070, 1958.

Edwards, J. M. Malignant melanoma: treatment by endolymphatic radio-isotope infusion. Ann. R. Coll. Surg. Engl. 44:237–254, 1969.

Gottlieb, J. A., Frei, E., and Luce, J. K. An evaluation of the management of patients with cerebral metastases from malignant melanoma. Cancer 29:701–705, 1972.

Habermalz, H. J., and Fischer, J. J. Radiation therapy of malignant melanoma: Experience with high individual treatment doses. Cancer 38:2258–2262, 1976.

Harmer, C. L. The radiotherapy of melanoma. Clin. Exp. Dermatol. 1:29–36, 1976.

Hellriegel, W. Radiation therapy of primary and metastatic melanoma. Ann. N.Y. Acad. Sci. 100:131–141, 1963.

Hilaris, B. S., Raben, M., Calabrese, A. S., Phillips, R. F., and Henschke, U. K. Value of radiation therapy for distant metastases from malignant melanoma. Cancer 16:765–773, 1963.

Hornsey, S. The radiosensitivity of melanoma cells in culture. Br. J. Radiol. 45:158, 1972.

Konecný, M., and Krenarová, V. A contribution to the radiotherapy of malignant melanoma. Neoplasma 16:335, 1969.

Kopf, A. W., Mintzis, M., and Bart, R. S. Diagnostic accuracy in malignant melanoma. Arch. Dermatol. 111:1291–1292, 1975.

Kopf, A. W., Bart, R. S., and Gladstein, A. H. Treatment of melanotic freckle with x-rays. Arch. Dermatol. 112:801–807, 1976.

Lederman, M. Radiotherapy of malignant melanomata of the eye. Br. J. Radiol. 34:21–42, 1961.

Levene, A. Moles and melanoma: the pathological basis of clinical management. Proc. R. Soc. Med. 65:137–140, 1972.

Lissner, J., and von Lieven, H. Die Strahlentherapie des malignen Melanoms. Chirurg. 45:362–365, 1974.

Pearson, D. Radiotherapy in malignant melanoma. Proc. R. Soc. Med. 67:96–97, 1974.

Petratos, M. A., Kopf, A. W., Bart, R. S., Grisewood, E. N., and Gladstein, A. H. Treatment of melanotic freckle with x-rays. Arch. Dermatol. 106:189–194, 1972.

Regnier, R. Role de la Radiotherapie dans le Traitement des Melanomes Malins du Tronc et des Membres. Brux. Med. 55:423–428, 1975.

Sealy, R., Hockly, J., and Shepstone, B. The treatment of malignant melanoma with cobalt and hyperbaric oxygen. Clin. Radiol. 25:211–215, 1974.

Scherer, R., and Makoski, H. B. Die Strahlentherapie des malignen Melanoms. Langenbechs Arch. Chir. 342:545–548, 1976.

Storck, H., and Ott, F. Zu Verlauf und Therapie der malignen Melanome. Schweiz. Med. Wschr. 106:1871–1877, 1976.

Terz, J. J., Curutchet, H. P., and Lawrence, W., Jr. Analysis of cell kinetics of human solid tumors. Cancer 28:1100–1110, 1971.

Wiskemann, A. Rontgentherapie der Praekanzerosen der Haut. Z. Hautkr. 8:461–462, 1977.

Withers, H. R., and Harter, D. Radiotherapy in the management of malignant melanoma. In Neoplasms of the Skin and Melanomas. Chicago, Year Book Publishers, 1976, pgs. 453–459.

Chapter 20

Survival Rates in Malignant Melanoma

The survival of patients who have malignant melanomas depends on many factors, some already discussed in the chapter on Prognostication of Behavior of Melanomas. Those factors may include (1) the type, level, thickness, size (diameter), clinical aspects (e.g., ulceration) of the primary lesion; (2) the type and extent of the surgical therapy; (3) the patient's immune status; (4) the use of any other forms of therapy (chemotherapy, immunotherapy); (5) the patient's general medical condition; (6) the patient's age and sex; (7) the stage of the tumor; (8) certain histologic characteristics, and (9) the location of the lesion.

McNeer and Das Gupta (1964) reported a five-year survival of 71% and a 10-year survival of 62% for 359 Stage I patients (localized melanoma without metastases). Five and ten-year survivals (19% and 17%, respectively) were markedly worse for 295 Stage II patients (regional nodal metastases).

McLeod and associates (1971) observed a death rate of 45% for men with malignant melanoma and a death rate of 19.3% for women. Jones et al. (1968) reported a five-year survival rate of 41% for women and 25% for men. Bodenham stated (1968) that females have a 15% advantage in five-year survival over males.

According to Bodenham (1968) the five-year survival for Stage I patients is 74% and 21% for Stage II patients. Booher (1969), in his review of the literature, also reported a markedly higher 10-year survival rate for Stage I patients: 62% for Stage I and 12% for Stage II.

A report from the National Cancer Institute (End Results in Cancer, 1972) substantiates a higher five-year survival rate for female patients, and also, differences in survival of both males and females, depending on the site of the primary melanoma. Survival rates are the same for malignant melanomas on upper and lower limbs, but were higher than those of malignancies on the face, head and neck. Survival rates are worst for primary malignant melanomas on the skin of the back.

Donnellan and co-workers (1972) reviewed 119 cases of melanoma of the head and neck and reported five-year survival rates for level II lesions of 94%; level III lesions, 76%; level IV lesions, 69%; and level V lesions, 57%. Clark et al. (1969) reported mortality rates correlated to depth of tumor invasion as follows: level II, 8.3%; level III, 35.2%; level IV, 46.1%; level V, 52%.

From Australia, Davis et al. (1976) review 1130 patients registered with the Queensland Melanoma Project who had their primary lesions examined for levels of invasion. They report the age-adjusted 5-year survival rate to be as follows: level I, 100%; levels II and III, 93.1%; level IV, 80.6%; and level V, 37.8%. They believe these high survival rates are due to public awareness of the potential danger of a "change in a mole" and physician alertness allowing for early diagnosis. These attitudes are the result of public and physican education programs conducted by the Queensland Anti-Cancer and Health Education Councils.

Conley and Pack (1974) found a five-year cure rate of only 15% for malignant melanomas of the mucous membranes of the head and neck. Salem and Travezan (1973) reported that of 18 patients treated for mucosal melanomas of the head and neck, only three survived (16.7%) though none of the patients had evidence of metastatic disease at the time of treatment. Mucosal lesions carry an ominous prognosis.

Whether or not elective lymph node dissections increase the survival rate in melanoma patients has been debated by many investigators and is discussed in detail in the chapter on Elective Lymph Node Dissection for Melanomas. Harris et al. (1972) report that of 26 patients with microscopically positive lymph nodes found at dissection, 15 were diagnosed preoperatively as having negative nodes, an error of 58%.

TABLE 16*
Survival After Regional Lymph Node Dissections in 185 Patients

Microscopic findings	Clinical findings	Survival at 5 years or more (%)
Nodes microscopically negative	Nodes clinically negative	56
	Nodes clinically positive	27
Nodes microscopically positive	Nodes clinically negative	30
	Nodes clinically positive	10

* Adapted from Gumport and Harris (1974).

Table 16, adapted from Gumport and Harris (1974), summarizes five-year survival data in 185 cases of malignant melanoma in which regional node dissections were done. Sinha et al. (1974) reported that though not statistically significant, the survival rate of patients who had undergone elective lymph node dissections was better than for those who had not (50% versus 44%). Cady et al. (1975) found no statistically significant increase in survival rate in patients who had elective lymph node dissections. Hansen and McCarten (1974) reported that for Stage I lesions, 1.5 mm or greater in thickness, the addition of elective lymph node dissection offered significantly improved rates of survival. Wanebo and associates (1975) reported that for level III melanomas the five-year survival was significantly higher in a group of patients who had lymph node dissections (93%) than in a group who were not so operated upon (67%). No difference in survival rate or in the incidence of tumor recurrence was found for 640 patients with Stage II or III disease treated with wide local resection alone as compared to those treated with wide resection and lymphadenectomy (Conrad, 1972).

Fortner and colleagues (1977) compared 10-year cure rates in 145 Stage I patients who had wide excision only of their primary melanomas followed by therapeutic lymphadenectomies when and if clinically positive nodes appeared to 259 Stage I patients who had wide excision of their primaries plus elective lymph node dissections. Tables 17A and 17B present the results of this study, which, the authors conclude, support the value of elective lymphadenectomies.

TABLE 17A*
Elective Node Dissection 1954–1964 in 259 Patients

Histologically	No. Pts.	Cure 5-year	10-year
Negative	219	83%	79%
Positive	40 (15%)	42%	42%
Microscopic focus	9	67%	67%
One node	18	50%	50%
Multiple nodes	13	15%	15%
Total	259	76%	73%

* From Fortner et al., 1977.

TABLE 17B*
Wide Excision Alone 1955–1964 in 145 Patients

	No. Pt.	Cure 5-year	10-year
No regional recurrence	119	82%	81%
Subsequent regional node recurrence	26 (18%)	12%	6%
Total	145	70%	66%

* From Fortner et al., 1977.

Simons (1972) found a five-year survival rate of 45% for 336 patients with malignant melanoma on the head and neck. For those patients treated with elective lymph node dissections the five-year survival was 64%. For patients with clinically positive nodes the survival rate at five-years was about 20%.

Not all studies support the value of elective lymph node dissections (see Chapter 17, Elective Lymph Node Dissections in the Management of Malignant Melanomas).

Lesions situated on the extremities have the best survival rates and lesions on the trunk the worst according to reports by Franklin et al. (1975), Hansen and McCarten (1974), Sinha et al. (1974) and Davis et al. (1976).

The 5-year survival rate for Stage I malignant melanomas of the hands and feet, according to a recent report concerning 283 patients from Memorial Hospital (Keyhani, 1977), is 60.5% for lesions on the hands and 45.3% for lesions on the feet. For Stage II lesions, the survival decreases to 31.2% and 23.1%, respectively.

Cady et al. (1975) correlated six-year survival rates for 176 patients with the size of the lesion and the depth of invasion. If the maximum diameter of malignant melanomas was under 0.49 cm, the six-year survival was 83%; for

TABLE 18
Outcome Related to Thickness

Author	Number of patients	Sites	Thickness (mm)	Free of disease* or survival† (%)
Breslow, 1970	98	All	0.0–0.75	100*
			0.76–1.50	74
			1.51–2.25	79
			2.26–3.00	44
			over 3.00	22
Breslow, 1975	138	All	0.0–0.75	100*
			0.76–1.50	70
			over 1.50	44‡
Hansen and McCarten, 1974	154	All	0.0–1.50	100†
			1.51–3.00	80
			over 3.00	45
Wanebo et al., 1975	151	Extremities	0.0–0.50	100†
			0.6–1.00	100
			1.1–1.50	89
			1.6–2.00	87
			2.1–3.00	58
			over 3.00	55

‡ Overall: 25/57 (44%); Node dissection: 14/22 (64%); No node dissection: 11/35 (31%).

TABLE 19*
Malignant Melanoma of the Extremities Stage I Disease (clinically negative nodes) Factors in Survival

Five-year survival (%)	Factors Clark level	Thickness (mm)	Incidence of microscopic nodal metastases (%)
100	II	<1.0	4
88†	III		7
83		1.0–2.0	6
66	IV		25
58		2.1–3.0	22
55		>3.0	39
48		>4.0	50
15	V		70

* After Wanebo et al., 1975.
† 93% with dissection; 67% without dissection.

lesions 2.0 cm or larger the six-year survival was 27%. With regard to the depth of invasion the six-year survival rate for level II melanomas was 86%; for level III and IV, 67%; and for level V, 11%. For lesions less than 2 cm in diameter Wanebo and associates (1975) found a five-year survival rate of 61% as compared to 16% for tumors greater than 2 cm. Breslow (1970, 1975) found better cure rates for tumors 0.76 mm or less in thickness and much poorer cure rates for those lesions greater than 1.5 mm in thickness (see Table 18). Wanebo et al. (1975) compared levels versus thickness of melanomas in relation to five-year survival rates in a retrospective study of 151 patients with melanomas of the extremities (see Table 19).

A summary of several factors involved in the survival of melanoma patients using data from over 1000 patients treated in Queensland, is given by Davis and associates (1976). The overall five-year survival was found to be 81.6%. For women the survival rate was higher than that for men (87.7% versus 73.6%). For both men and women, the five-year survival rate was highest for lesions of the upper limb, followed by lesions of the lower limbs, then those of the head and neck, and, finally lesions on the trunk. The five-year survival rates were 89%, 86%, 79%, and 73%, respectively. The depth of tumor invasion was shown to be inversely related to survival rate. For level I lesions, 100% of the patients survived for at least five years; for level V lesions the five-year survival rate was only 37.8%. The authors believe that what accounts for their better overall survival rates is public and professional education. Both groups have been alerted to the possibility of malignant melanoma in any pigmented lesion and consequently, the diagnosis is made and the disease is treated earlier than ordinarily.

In his patient material over the years Cady (1975) notes an increased 10-year disease-free survival rate of all primary cases (64%), a 50% decrease in maximum diameter, a reduction from 55% to 30% in the incidence of invasion to level V, and a 10% increase of level II (superficial papillary dermis) lesions, whereas such superficial lesions were "not seen" before in their experience. He attributes such improvements in clinical presentation to the advent in the United States of an intensive lay and professional educational effort by the American Cancer Society directed at the early detection of cancers.

REFERENCES

Axtell, L. M., Cutler, S. J., and Myers, M. H., eds. End results In Cancer: Report No. 4. (National Cancer Institute, Maryland) 1972.

Bodenham, D. C. A study of 650 observed malignant melanomas in the South-West region. Ann. R. Coll. Surg. 43:218–239, 1968.

Booher, R. J. Recognition and treatment of melanoma. Surg. Clin. North Am. 49:389–405, 1969.

Cady, B. Changing concepts in malignant melanoma. Med. Clin. North Am. 59:301–308, 1975.

Cady, B. Legg, M. A., and Redfern, A. B. Contemporary treatment of malignant melanoma. Am. J. Surg. 129:472–482, 1975.

Clark, W. H., Jr., From, L., Bernardino, E. A., and Mihm, M. C. The histogenesis and biologic behavior of primary human malignant melanomas of the skin. Cancer Res. 29:705–727, 1969.

Conley, J., and Pack, G. T. Melanoma of the mucous membranes of the head and neck. Arch. Otolaryngol. 99:315–319, 1974.

Conrad, F. G. Treatment of malignant melanoma. Wide excision alone vs. lymphadenectomy. Arch. Surg. 104:587–593, 1972.

Davis, N., McLeod, R., Beardmore, G., Little, J., Quinn, R., and Holt, J. The Henry Joseph Windsor Lecture: Melanoma is a word, not a sentence. Aust. N. Zealand J. Surg. 46:188–196, 1976.

Davis, N. C., McLeod, G. R., Beardmore, G. L., Little, J. H., Quinn, R. L., and Holt, J. Primary cutaneous melanoma: a report from the Queensland melanoma project. CA 26:80–107, 1976.

Donnellan, M. J., Seemayer, T., Huvos, A. G., Mike, V., and Strong, E. W. Clincopathologic study of cutaneous melanoma of the head and neck. Am. J. Surg. 124:450–455, 1972.

Fortner, J. G., Woodruff, J., Shottenfeld, D., and Maclean, B. Biostatistical basis of elective node dissection for malignant melanoma. Ann. Surg. 186:101–103, 1977.

Franklin, J. D., Reynolds, V. H., and Page, D. L. Cutaneous melanoma: a twenty-year retrospective study with clinicopathologic correlation. Plast. Reconstr. Surg. 56:277–285, 1975.

Gumport, S. L., and Harris, M. N. Results of regional lymph node dissection for melanoma. Ann. Surg. 179:105–108, 1974.

Hansen, M. G., and McCarten, A. B. Tumor thickness and lymphocytic infiltration in malignant melanoma of the head and neck. Am. J. Surg. 128:557–561, 1974.

Harris, M. N., Gumport, S. L., and Maiwandi, H. Auxillary lymph node dissection for melanoma. Surg. Gynecol. Obstet. 135:936–940, 1972.

Jones, W. M., Jones Williams, W., Roberts, M. M., and Davies, K. Malignant melanoma of the skin: prognostic value of clinical features and the role of treatment in 111 cases. Br. J. Cancer 22:437–451, 1968.

Keyhani, A. Comparison of clinical behavior of melanoma of the hands and feet. A Study of 283 patients. Cancer 40:3168–3176, 1977.

Knutson, C. O., Hori, J. M., Spratt, J. S., Jr. Melanoma. Curr. Probl. Surg. Dec:1–55, 1971.

Little, J. H. Histology and prognosis of cutaneous melanoma. Prog. Clin. Cancer 6:163–176, 1975.

McLeod, G. R., Beardmore, G. L., Little, J. H., Quinn, R. L., and Davis, N. C. Results of treatment of 361 patients with malignant melanoma in Queensland. Med. J. Aust. 1:1211–1216, 1971.

McNeer, G., and Das Gupta, T. Prognosis in malignant melanoma. Surgery 56:512–518, 1964.

Salem, L. E. and Travenzan, R. Malignant melanoma of the head and neck. Int. Surg. 58:790–792, 1973.

Simons, J. N. Malignant melanoma of the head and neck. Am. J. Surg. 124:485–488, 1972.

Sinha, B. K., and Buntine, D. W. Prognosis of cutaneous malignant melanoma: a clinicopathological study. Can. J. Surg. 17:328–334, 1974.

Stehlin, J. S. Malignant melanoma. An appraisal. Surgery 64:1149–1157, 1968.

Shaw, H. W., McCarthy, W. H., and Milton, G. W. Changing trends in mortality from malignant melanoma. Med. J. Aust. 2: 77–80, 1977.

Tonak, J., Hermanek, P., Hornstein, O. P., and Weidner, F. Therapie des malignen Melanomes der klinichen Stadien I und II. Dtsch. Med. Wochenschr. 101:435–440, 1976.

Wanebo, H. J., Woodruff, J., and Fortner, J. G. Malignant melanoma of the extremities: a clinicopathologic study using levels of invasion (micro-stage). Cancer 35:666–676, 1975.

Wanebo, H. J., Fortner, J. G., Woodruff, J., MacLean, B., and Binkowski, E. Selection of the optimum surgical treatment of stage I melanoma by depth of microinvasion: use of the combined microstage technique (Clark-Breslow). Ann. Surg. 182:302–315, 1975.

Chapter 21

Immunologic Aspects of Malignant Melanoma

A significant proportion of all articles currently published on malignant melanomas deals with some aspects of host-tumor immunologic interactions or with approaches to immunotherapy. Since these subjects have been recently reviewed (Kopf, 1971, 1975; Gutterman et al., 1975; Sober, 1976; Clark et al., 1977; Lewis, 1977; Milton et al., 1977), they will merely be summarized in this section. Some current conclusions based on the literature follow:

(1) A large body of literature has appeared which indicates that human malignant melanomas have specific antigenic components that differ from those of all other normal and cancerous cells. Such "melanoma-associated antigens" have been partially purified in both murine and human malignant melanoma (Bystryn and Smalley, 1977). Melanoma-associated antigens are recognized by the immune systems and call forth both humoral and cell-mediated immune responses. Some such responses are considered beneficial to the host whereas others (e.g., circulating blocking factors) are harmful.

(2) Most of the data for the above are based on testing procedures *in vitro* that utilize a wide variety of techniques to demonstrate immunologic reactivity to "melanoma-associated antigens." Despite the numerous reports that continuously appear in the literature, the reliability, specificity, reproducibility and interpretation of virtually all current procedures are open to question (Abel and Bystryn, 1976). Thus, there is a major need for the development of tests *in vitro* that may be used reliably to demonstrate and follow anti-melanoma immune responses in man.

(3) Most studies indicate that the general immunologic competence of patients who are afflicted with malignant melanoma is intact, although there may be some suppression of delayed hypersensitivity to dinitrochlorobenzene (DNCB). Unlike other malignant conditions, such as Hodgkin's disease in which there is a marked reduction in immune competence, patients who have malignant melanomas are probably better candidates for immunotherapy because they have the intact biologic mechanisms to react upon immunologic stimulation.

(4) It is possible to destroy some lesions of malignant melanoma purely by immunologic means. The greatest success has been achieved by the intratumoral injection into cutaneous metastases of a non-specific immunogen (e.g., BCG-Bacillus Calmette Guérin) for a patient who is able to mount an immune response to the immunogen (Rosenberg and Rapp, 1976). Visceral metastases rarely respond to specific or non-specific immunotherapy. It is the cutaneous lesions (satellite, in-transit and distant) that respond best to immunotherapy.

(5) Considerable interest has been expressed in combining procedures that reduce bulk of malignant tissue (e.g., surgery, chemotherapy, radiotherapy) with immunotherapy. The basic principle is that immunodestruction has many limitations, one of the most important being the bulk of the tumor burden. It does not seem possible for immune systems, no matter how maximally stimulated, to mount successful attacks to eliminate any but small amounts of tumor.

(6) Adjuvant immunotherapy (i.e., therapy administered in addition to definitive surgical treatment) is still experimental. For this purpose, the use of BCG, *Corynebacterium parvum,* levamisole, transfer factor, melanoma cells or subcellular "antigens," cross transplantation-cross transfusion techniques, immune RNA, etc. are currently under investigation. Many of these studies are plagued with serious faults in design, the most common of which is the lack of concurrent, randomized, untreated controls in adequate numbers.

(7) Although work in animal models using melanoma cell lines indicates that certain immunologic manipulations

favor the host and harm the tumor, such results may not be duplicable in man. It may be that the very promising results now being achieved in these laboratory models will never have much relevance to the management of human melanomas.

SUMMARY

Many findings indicate that human malignant melanomas contain antigens that are recognized by their hosts as "non-self" and induce humoral and cell-mediated responses. Much work needs to be done to develop reproducible and reliable testing procedures *in vitro*. The fact that man reacts immunologically to melanoma has spurred a massive effort to boost antimelanoma responses by both specific and non-specific immunotherapeutic procedures. Currently, with the exception of the destruction of cutaneous metastases of malignant melanomas by intratumoral injection of potent non-specific immunogens such as BCG, these attempts must be considered experimental. Immunotherapeutic procedures that are reasonably effective in treating visceral metastatic melanoma have not yet been developed.

REFERENCES

Abel, E. A., and Bystryn, J.-C. Reproducibility of the immunofluorescent test for antimelanoma antibodies. J. Invest. Derm. 66:117–121, 1976.

Bystryn, J.-C., Bart, R. S., Livingston, P., and Kopf, A. W. Growth and immunogenicity of murine B-16 melanoma. J. Invest. Dermatol. 63: 369–373, 1974.

Bystryn, J.-C., and Smalley, J. R. Identification and solubilization of iodinated cell surface human melanoma associated antigens. Int. J. Cancer 20:165–172, 1977.

Clark, W. H., Mastrangelo, M. J., Ainsworth, A. M., Berd, D., Bellet, R. E., and Bernardino, E. A. Current concepts of the biology of human cutaneous malignant melanoma. Adv. Cancer. Res. 24:267–338, 1977.

Gerner, R. E., and Moore, G. E. Feasibility study of active immunotherapy in patients with solid tumors. Cancer 38:131–143, 1976.

Gersten, M. J., Hadden, E. M., Kaplan, M. H., Pinsky, C. M., Armstrong, D., and Hadden, J. W. Immunologic defects in melanoma patients: Lack of effect of BCG therapy. Clin. Bulletin (Memorial Sloan-Kettering Cancer Center) 7:63–69, 1977.

Gutterman, J. U., Mavligit, G., Reed, R., Richman, S., McBride, C. E., and Hersh, E. M. Immunology and immunotherapy of human-malignant melanoma: historic review and perspectives for the future. Semin. Oncol. 2:155–174, 1975.

Kopf, A. W. Host defenses against malignant melanoma. Hosp. Practice 6:116–124, 1971.

Kopf, A. W. Immunotherapy for human malignant melanoma. South. Med. J. 68:495–503, 1975.

Lewis, M. G. In Milton, G. W., McGovern, V. J., and Lewis, M. G., eds. Malignant Melanoma of the Skin and Mucous Membrane. Edinburgh, London, and New York, Churchill Livingstone, 1977, pgs. 102–151.

Mastrangelo, M. J., Bird, D., and Bellet, R. E. Critical review of previously reported clinical trials of cancer immunotherapy with non-specific immunopotentiators. Ann. NY Acad. Sci. 277:94–123, 1976.

Milton, G. W., McGovern, V. J., and Lewis, M. G. Malignant Melanoma of the Skin and Mucous Membrane. Edinburgh, London and New York, Churchill Livingstone, 1977.

Morton, D. L., Eibler, F. R., Holmes, E. S., Sparks, F. C., and Ramming, K. BCG immunotherapy as a systemic adjunct to surgery in malignant melanoma. Med. Clin. North Am. 60:431–439, 1976.

Rosenberg, S. A., and Rapp, H. J. Intralesional immunotherapy of melanoma with BCG. Med. Clin. N. Am. 60:419–430, 1976.

Seigler, H. F., and Fetter, B. F. Current management of melanoma. Ann. Surg. 186:1–12, 1977.

Sober, A. J. Immunology and cutaneous malignant melanoma. Int. J. Dermatol. 15:1–18, 1976.

Chapter 22

Miscellaneous Aspects of Malignant Melanomas

As suggested by the title of this chapter, the material here presented is a pot pourri of reports dealing with subjects that are of interest but which do not fall easily into or which could not be elaborated on in any of the previous chapters. Some items concern human material, whose clinical significance has yet to be fully established, but which may be of interest to the clinician treating malignant melanomas. The emphasis has been on items of potential usefulness in diagnosis and evaluation for extent of disease. Such items include the use of gallium-67 whole-body scintigraphy in the detection of melanoma metastases, studies on urinary melanogens, and the use of thermography in the detection of metastases. A few items are already of immediate usefulness to some practicing clinicians. Examples would be the report concerning the use of an operating microscope in the clinical diagnosis of malignant melanoma and the use of computerized axial tomography. Certain studies may prove of eventual significance in prophylaxis or treatment of malignant melanomas, such as those relating a viral oncogene and malignant melanoma, studies on MSH-daunomycin conjugate homing in on MSH receptor sites of melanoma cells, and results of experiments with laser radiation.

DIAGNOSTIC ACCURACY IN MALIGNANT MELANOMA

Kopf, Mintzis and Bart (1976) reviewed 99 malignant melanomas that were recorded from 1955 to 1967 in the Oncology Section of the Skin and Cancer Unit of New York University Medical Center. The diagnostic accuracy of the physicians in the Oncology Section, where only one diagnosis is permitted per lesion, was determined to be 64%. Thus, when only one diagnosis was allowed per lesion, approximately one error was made in every three cases. The Index of Suspicion in relation to malignant melanoma in this study was 96%, so that physicians in the Oncology Section demonstrated an appropriate awareness of this tumor; however, coupled with the diagnostic accuracy of 64%, a problem exists in the clinical diagnosis of this serious cutaneous cancer.

Comment. This study indicated the importance of routine histologic verification prior to any definitive radical surgery in patients with suspected malignant melanomas.

REFERENCE

Kopf, A. W., Mintzis, M., and Bart, R. S. Diagnostic accuracy in malignant melanoma. Arch. Dermatol. 111:1291–1292, 1975.

MAGNIFICATION AS AN AID IN THE DIAGNOSIS OF MELANOMA

MacKie (1972) using a Zeiss operating microscope capable of magnifying from 6 to 40× examined 298 pigmented cutaneous lesions. She found that the overall degree of accuracy in diagnosing pigmented cutaneous lesions was 88%. The accuracy of the diagnosis of malignant melanomas was 85% in 74 cases. The lowest degree of accuracy (72%) was found in attempting to diagnose 11 cases of pigmented basal-cell carcinomas. The author described the features she found useful in distinguishing the various pigmented lesions, namely, malignant melanoma, junctional, intradermal, and compound nevi, blue nevi, angiomata, basal-cell papillomata and pigmented basal-cell carcinomas.

Comment. The report does not include a comparison of the degree of accuracy using the operating microscope as compared to that using the naked eye. It is also obvious that magnification will increase the diagnostic acumen of a physician with poor eyesight more than it will a physician with very good eyesight, everything else being equal.

REFERENCE

MacKie, R. Cutaneous microscopy *in vivo* as an aid to preoperative assessment of pigmented lesions of the skin. Br. J. Plast. Surg. 25:123–129, 1972.

EYE COLOR IN DARKLY PIGMENTED BASAL-CELL CARCINOMAS AND MALIGNANT MELANOMAS

Bart and Schnall (1973) reviewed clinical photographs in the Oncology Section of the Skin and Cancer Unit, New York University Medical Center. From about 3500 patients seen with basal-cell carcinomas from 1955 to 1971, 40 lesions were selected which were black or dark brown papules, nodules and plaques for inclusion in the study, because they could be mistaken for malignant melanomas. For a comparison, 50 malignant melanomas of similar appearance were selected. Eye colors of all types were found in patients with malignant melanomas. Forty percent had dark brown eyes, 16% had light brown eyes, and 44% had blue, gray, or green eyes. Of those patients who had solidly pigmented basal-cell carcinomas, 90% had dark brown eyes, 10% had light brown eyes and none had blue, gray or green eyes. It was concluded that light eyes are uncommon in patients with solidly pigmented black or dark brown basal-cell carcinomas. Therefore, a solidly pigmented black or dark brown malignant lesion in a patient with blue, gray or green eyes is more likely to be a malignant melanoma than a basal-cell carcinoma.

Comment. Since a solidly pigmented black or dark-brown malignant lesion in a blue-eyed patient is not likely to be a basal-cell carcinoma, it should tentatively be regarded as a malignant melanoma rather than a basal-cell carcinoma. Consequently, biopsy in toto if feasible would be more useful than a shave-type biopsy for typing, levelling, and measuring its greatest thickness should it be a malignant melanoma.

REFERENCE

Bart, R. S., and Schnall, S. Eye color in darkly pigmented basal-cell carcinomas and malignant melanomas: an aid in their clinical differentiation. Arch. Dermatol. 107:206–207, 1973.

FROZEN SECTION DIAGNOSIS OF SUSPECTED MALIGNANT MELANOMA OF THE SKIN

Little and Davis (1974) reviewed the experience at Princess Alexandra Hospital in Brisbane, Australia concerning the use of cryostat-prepared frozen sections of 329 pigmented skin lesions suspected of being malignant melanomas. Major changes in diagnosis between the frozen section and the paraffin sections occurred in four tumors, for a rate of error of 1.2% for the 329 lesions. In each case the error was one of overdiagnosis of malignancy. Two of these patients were overdiagnosed as melanoma on frozen sections, resulting in unnecessary surgery. For 19 of the lesions from which frozen sections were made, the pathologist did not have sufficient confidence in his ability to give a firm diagnosis on the cryostat sections because of some unusual features. Therefore, diagnosis had to await paraffin sections. Features which tended to obscure the diagnosis on frozen sections included superficial level of the tumor, heavy lymphocytic infiltration, partial tumor regression and unusual cell type and arrangement.

Excessively wide excision was done in 16 lesions or 5% of the total examined when diagnosed on clinical grounds alone prior to wide excision. Of these 16, there were six nevi, five pigmented basal-cell carcinomas, three vascular tumors and two tumors of other types. Some of these excisions were over 100 mm in diameter. Thus, the authors concluded that frozen-section diagnosis of malignant melanoma in experienced hands is reliable and is of considerable value to the surgeon.

Comment. The policy at New York University Medical Center has been that when possible, excisional biopsy of the entire lesion be carried out. Definitive surgery awaits the careful histologic study of paraffin step-sections of the excised specimen. In the event that total biopsy is not practical, biopsy of a part is done. If the biopsy confirms the diagnosis of malignant melanoma, wide local excision is carried out. If biopsy shows only superficial involvement, elective lymph node dissection is postponed until step sections of the excised specimen demonstrate that the lesion is of such thickness that in the opinion of the surgeon a node dissection is warranted. (See chapter on Elective Lymph-Node Dissections and section on Classification).

REFERENCES

Hughes, L. E. The place of frozen section in the practical management of melanoma. Brit. J. Surg. 62:840–844, 1975.

Little, J. H. and Davis, N. C. Frozen section diagnosis of suspected malignant melanoma of the skin. Cancer 34:1163–1172, 1974.

PSEUDOMELANOMA

Kornberg and Ackerman (1975) reviewed the cases of eight patients in whom a benign melanocytic nevus had been shaved off with recurrence of pigmentation. Biopsy of this pigmentation showed histologic features which might be confused with malignant melanoma. These pseudomelanomatous changes generally occurred in young adults within a few weeks following partial surgical shave excision of an intradermal melanocytic nevus. The histologic features that help separate psuedomelanoma from superficial spreading malignant melanoma are (1) sharp circumscriptions of the intraepidermal melanocytic component of the lesion, with no lateral spread of individual melanocytes at the periphery; (2) atypical melanocytes confined wholly to the epidermis; (3) few, if any, melanocytes in mitosis or tending to necrosis; and (4) fibrosis usually, but not invariably, present in the papillary and sometimes in the reticular dermis.

REFERENCE

Kornberg, R., and Ackerman, A. B. Pseudomelanoma: recurrent melanocytic nevus following partial surgical removal. Arch. Dermatol. 111:1588–1590, 1975.

DESMOPLASTIC MALIGNANT MELANOMA

In 1971, Conley, Lattes, and Orr published a report on an unusual type of malignant melanoma. The report was based on seven cases. Desmoplastic malignant melanoma arises from a superficial melanotic lesion and evolves into an aggressive infiltrating and potentially metastasizing tumor. The original skin lesions are usually flat and of a red or brown color. These initial lesions tend to appear innocous clinically, and microscopically may not be considered to be definitely malignant. Characteristically there is the subsequent development of a hard subcutaneous mass deep to the original lesion. This may take 6 months to 3 years to develop after treatment of the initial lesion. "In most cases they were believed to be fibromatosis or fibrosarcomas histologically and grossly by the pathologists who first studied them, although a number of other diagnoses were also suggested." There was a marked tendency for these tumors to recur locally, and regional lymph node and visceral metastases occurred. Microscopically, the initial pigmented skin lesions showed atypical junctional melanocytic proliferations, sometimes also involving the epidermis, and downward growth composed of atypical melanocytes and elongated spindle-shaped cells. Melanin was seen easily in association with the initial superficial lesions but not with the deep masses. The histology of lymph node and distant metastases varied from that of classic malignant melanoma to that of a spindle-cell desmoplastic tumor resembling fibrosarcoma. Both types of metastases might occur in the same patient.

In summary, the desmoplastic malignant melanoma tends to begin with a junctional lesion acceptable as a superficial malignant melanoma or lentigo maligna. This is followed by an invasive fibromatosis-like phase. The authors suggest that "it is most important for the practicing pathologist and surgeon to be aware of the fact that if in the history of a stubbornly recurrent fibroma or fibromatosis, there was an associated or antecedent inconspicuous pigmented lesion of the overlying skin, they may well be dealing with this rare variant of malignant melanoma."

Additional cases of desmoplastic melanoma have been reported by Frolow et al. (1975) and Valensi (1977).

REFERENCES

Conley, J., Lattes, R., and Orr, W. Desmoplastic malignant melanoma (A rare variant of spindle-cell melanoma). Cancer 28:914–936, 1971.
Frolow, G. R., Shapiro, L., and Brownstein, M. H. Desmoplastic malignant melanoma. Arch. Dermatol. 111: 753–754, 1975.
Valensi, Q. J.: Desmoplastic malignant melanoma: A report of two additional cases. Cancer 39:286–292, 1977.

THERMOGRAPHY IN MALIGNANT MELANOMA

Hessler and Maillard (1970) used thermography and found that melanomas were frequently hyperthermic whereas other pigmented lesions were usually isothermic. Other lesions found to be hyperthermic were angiomas and inflammatory lesions. They found thermography useful in detecting metastases or extensions of melanoma not obvious clinically.

Bodenham (1968) had observed previously that faster growing malignant melanomas were warmer than slower growing malignant melanomas.

In 1977 Tapernoux and Hessler reported on further studies concerning infrared thermography of malignant melanomas. They reviewed their experience with 44 primary melanomas, prior to any surgical procedures, and 9 secondary melanomas, i.e., local recurrences, satellite lesions, and metastases. They found hyperthermia in 68% of primary malignant melanomas and in 75% of secondary lesions. Hyperthermia was detectable less often with malignant melanomas of the face and neck than on other areas of the body. Correlation of hyperthermia with Clark's levels of invasion was attempted. The authors again stressed that benign angiomatous and inflammatory lesions can also be hyperthermic.

Comment. The usefulness of temperature measuring techniques for diagnostic purposes remains to be determined.

REFERENCES

Bodenham, D. C. A study of 650 observed malignant melanomas in the south-west region. Ann. R. Coll Surg. 43:218–239, 1968.

Hessler, C., and Maillard, G. F. Apport de la thermographie dans le diagnostic et le traitment du mélanome malin. Schweiz. Med. Wochenschr. 100:972–975, 1970.

Tapernoux, B., and Hessler, C. Thermography of malignant melanomas. J. Dermatol. Surg. Oncol. 3:299–302, 1977.

URINARY MELANOGENS IN MALIGNANT MELANOMA

Rorsman and co-workers (1973) demonstrated 5-S-cysteinyldopa in melanomas in mice and in humans, as well as in the urine of mice bearing melanomas and in humans with metastatic malignant melanoma. Urinary titers are normal in patients with clinically localized disease. Amelanotic melanoma metastases may not be detected by this determination, since the excretion of 5-S-cysteinyldopa may be normal in patients with metastases from amelanotic malignant melanomas. In some patients the urinary excretion of dopa and dopamine is normal whereas the excretion of 5-S-cysteinyldopa is elevated. 5-S-cysteinyldopa is considered a precursor of phaeomelanin. Patients with melanoma need not have red hair or freckles to show 5-S-cysteinyldopa in their urine and elevations are also found in Negroes with melanoma. Since this substance may be elevated in the urine of patients who have normal urinary levels of dopa and dopamine, it may prove to be useful in the detection of metastatic disease in patients with malignant melanoma.

Agrup and co-investigators (1975) reported two patients with metastatic malignant melanoma who had large amounts of 5-S-cysteinyldopa in the urine and lesser amounts in the blood plasma.

Morgan and co-workers (1974) studied the relationship of tumor tyrosinase (dopa oxidase) levels, urinary levels of homovanillic acid (a phenolic melanogen) and the stage of disease in 169 patients with malignant melanoma. The amount of homovanillic acid found in urine was found to correlate with the degree of tyrosinase activity within the tumor, but neither of these could be correlated with the stage of disease. As one might expect, these findings did correlate with the degree of pigmentation of the tumor, being much reduced in association with amelanotic malignant melanoma. Thus, normal homovanillic acid excretion may occur in a patient who has had elevated excretion when there is regression of malignant melanoma, or when the melanoma converts from pigmented to the amelanotic state.

Trapeznikov and his colleagues (1975) found a correlation between the stage of melanotic melanomas and urinary excretion of homovanillic acid. They reported that patients with primary malignant melanoma had normal levels, that patients with locally disseminated disease (e.g., regional node involvement) had approximately double the normal value, and that patients with disseminated melanotic disease in the skin had approximately triple the normal values. Excretion of homovanillic acid in patients with widely disseminated amelanotic melanoma in the skin was only very slightly elevated.

Gan and his co-workers (1975) described a procedure for determining phenolic compounds in urine. They reported that the amounts of phenols in 24-hour urine collections from patients with melanomas were higher than those for healthy persons and patients with other diseases. Unfortunately, these authors did not group their results according to stages of melanoma or according to degrees of pigmentation, so it is unclear whether a small volume of pigmented tumor is detectable by this means or if amelanotic melanoma, even in large volumes, is detectable.

Recently, Blois and Banda (1976) have reported their preliminary results on attempts to detect occult metastatic melanoma by ion-exchange column chromatography of urine. They demonstrated elevated levels of five peaks in the urines of patients with metastatic disease. These peaks include DOPA (3,4-dihydroxyphenylalanine), MOPA (3-methoxy-4-hydroxyphenylalanine), and 5-S-cysteinyldopa. Sustained levels of one or more peaks was considered evidence of recurrent or continuing tumor. This technique, according to the authors, provides earlier evidence of liver metastases than does liver scan, may detect occult metastases generally, and has predicted tumor in clinically enlarged lymph nodes.

Comment. If sufficient sensitivity without significant loss of specificity can be achieved, determination of urinary melanogens will become a useful method for detecting occult metastatic melanoma. The usefulness of any test would be somewhat reduced if it proves unable to detect amelanotic melanoma.

REFERENCES

Agrup, G., Andersson, T., Falck, B., Persson, K., Rorsman, H., Rosengren, A.-M., and Rosengren, E. 5-S-cysteinyldopa in the plasma of melanoma patients and the renal clearance of this amino acid. Acta Derm. Venereol. (Stockh.) 55:5–6, 1975.

Blois, M. S., and Banda, P. W. Detection of occult metastatic melanoma by urine chromatography. Cancer Res. 36:3317–3323, 1976.

Gan, E. V., Haberman, H. F., and Menon, I. A. A simple and sensitive test for the determination of phenolic compounds in urine and its application to melanoma. J. Invest. Dermatol. 64:139–144, 1975.

Morgan, L. R., Lolley, D., Maddox, B., Samuels, M., and Krementz, E. Urine homovanillic acid and tissue DOPA oxidase in patients with melanoma. Cancer 33:1601–1606, 1974.

Rorsman, H., Rosengren, A.-M., and Rosengren, E. Determination of 5-S-cysteinyldopa in melanomas with a fluoremetric method. Yale J. Biol. Med. 46:516–522, 1973.

Trapeznikov, N. N., Raushenbakh, M. O., Ivanova, V. D., and Yavorsky, V. V. Clinical evaluation of a method of quantitative determination of homovanillic acid for the estimation of degree of tumor dissemination process in melanoma of the skin. Cancer 36:2064–2068, 1975.

URINARY POLYAMINES IN MALIGNANT MELANOMA

Townsend and co-workers studied the urinary excretion of polyamines in 79 patients with malignant melanomas in various stages. They attempted to determine the relationship between the amounts of putrescine, spermidine, and spermine and the clinical extent and activity of disease. The data indicated that elevation of two or more of these polyamines occurred more frequently in patients with disseminated melanomas and at the time of active progression than in patients of localized stable disease. The mean values and percentage of patients with elevations increased as stage, activity, or both increased. Polyamines are increased in other cancers, in patients on birth-control pills, and in pregnancy. The authors suggest that to aid in the interpretation of urinary polyamine elevations, more information is needed concerning other conditions that may cause elevated polyamines, such as medications, thyroid disease, infectious processes, cardiovascular problems, heart failure, or coexisting common benign tumors such as prostatic hyperplasia and uterine leiomyoma. The authors suggest that serial determination of urinary polyamines during therapy may be useful in evaluating the response to therapy. One-half of the patients receiving chemotherapy who maintained multiple elevated values did not respond, whereas two patients who were stable under treatment had normal levels.

Comment. The study of the excretion of polyamines in the urine in patients with melanoma has the advantage, as compared to the study of urinary melanogens, that theoretically it should be able to detect amelanotic disseminated disease. Unfortunately, this reflects a nonspecificity which may cause great difficulties in interpreting the data.

REFERENCE

Townsend, R. N., Banda, P. W., and Marton, L. J. Polyamines in malignant melanoma: Urinary excretion and disease progress. Cancer 38: 2088–2092, 1976.

COMPUTERIZED AXIAL TOMOGRAPHY FOR DETECTION OF BRAIN METASTASES

Menzer and co-workers (1975) reported on the use of computerized axial tomography (CAT) in the diagnosis of dementia. One of the cases that they reported was found to have an amelanotic malignant melanoma metastasis in the brain with no primary site detectable. Computerized axial tomography carries little risk for the patient and should make possible the decreased use of more dangerous procedures such as arteriography, pneumoencephalography and radionuclide brain scanning. It will probably be found that CAT of the head is complementary to standard roentgenography of the skull. As pointed out by Twigg and associates (1975) optimal spacial and density resolution can only be achieved if the examined structure is ordinarily immobile or can be made so during the scanning cycle. Thus, axial tomography is good for examination of the head and neck, spine, retroperitoneal structures, pelvic organs and extremities, but is not as suited for mobile organs such as the liver, spleen, lungs, heart, gut and diaphragm.

REFERENCES

Menzer, L., Sabin, T., and Mark, V. H. Computerized axial tomography. Use in the diagnosis of dementia. J.A.M.A. 234:754–757, 1975.

Twigg, H. L., Axelbaum, S. P. and Schellinger, D. Computerized body tomography with the ACTA scanner. J.A.M.A. 234:314–317, 1975.

BLOOD LACTIC DEHYDROGENASE AND ALKALINE PHOSPHATASE IN HEPATIC METASTASES

Einhorn and co-workers (1974) studied patients with advanced metastatic malignant melanoma. They found that lactic dehydrogenase (LDH) correlated best with the finding of liver metastases on liver scan. They studied LDH levels on 282 patients with malignant melanomas and found normal levels in 134 and elevated levels in 148 (52%). Only three patients (2%) with normal LDH levels were found to have metastases on liver scan. However, there were 68 patients with elevated LDH levels (46%) that had normal liver scans and were presumed not to have liver metastases. The authors concluded that as compared to SGOT, alkaline phosphatase, and total bilirubin levels, LDH is the most sensitive blood test for liver metastases of malignant melanoma. Because the LDH is considered by the authors a sensitive indicator of hepatic metastases they consider that a liver scan is not needed as part of a routine evaluation of patients with malignant melanoma.

Stehlin and his associates (1974) found alkaline phosphatase the single most valuable blood test for detecting liver involvement from various malignancies, including malignant melanomas. It was elevated in 90% of such patients, but normal values were occasionally observed in patients whose livers had less than 75% cancerous involvement.

Blois (1975) considers the alkaline phosphatase the most sensitive chemical test for hepatic metastases.

REFERENCES

Blois, M. S. Cited in Arnold, H. L., and Rees, R. B. Meeting review: Pacific Dermatologic Association (1974). Arch. Dermatol. 112:396, 1975.

Einhorn, L., Burgess, M. A., Vallejos, C., Bodey, G. P. Sr., Gutterman, J., Mavliget, G., Hersh, E. M., Luce, J. K., Frei, E., III, Freireich, E. J., and Gottlieb, J. A. Prognostic correlations and response to treatment in advanced metastatic malignant melanoma. Cancer Res. 34:1995–2004, 1974.

Stehlin, J. S., Jr., Hafström, L., and Greeff, P. J. Experience with infusion and resection in cancer of the liver. Surg. Gynecol. Obstet. 138:855–863, 1974.

RADIONUCLIDE PHOTOSCANNING

Roth and his co-workers (1975) evaluated the usefulness of radionuclide scanning of liver, bone, brain and the whole body during the initial evaluation of Stage I and Stage II malignant melanomas. Because the scan results in this group of patients did not substantially influence the clinical decision-making process, the authors concluded that such routine screening in the initial evaluation of Stage I and Stage II melanoma patients was not justified, since scans represent a great expense to the patient and may delay initiation of therapy. Their scan results only prompted a change in staging or therapy in but one of 100 patients studied.

REFERENCE

Roth, J. A., Eilber, F. R., Bennett, L. R., and Morton, D. L. Radionuclide photoscanning: usefulness in preoperative evaluation of melanoma patients. Arch. Surg. 110:1211–1212, 1975.

GALLIUM-67 SCINTIGRAPHY IN MALIGNANT MELANOMA

Milder and his co-workers (1973) included whole body gallium-67 scintigraphy in the diagnostic workup of 44 consecutive patients with biopsy-proved malignant melanomas in order to study the uptake of this nuclide by known melanoma tissue and to assess its value in the detection of known and unknown metastatic disease. It is the only procedure capable of visualizing tumor in any organ of the body. If recent surgery or infection can be excluded, a positive finding carries great significance. False positives were only about 2%. However, lesions were missed about 45% of the time and therefore this technique must be combined with other screening methods such as liver and brain scans. Uptake is equally good in melanotic and amelanotic malignant melanomas. Masses larger than 2 cm were detected by gallium-67 scanning in 75% of instances, whereas tumors 2 cm or less were found only 17% of times. The authors concluded that although almost half of the metastases were not detected, positive scanning in the absence of inflammation is almost diagnostic of metastasis and that therefore gallium-67 whole body scintigraphy is a useful tool in evaluating patients with metastatic disease.

REFERENCE

Milder, M. S., Frankel, R. S., Bulkley, G. B., Ketcham, A. S., and Johnston, G. S. Gallium-67 scintigraphy in malignant melanoma. Cancer 32:1350–1356, 1973.

SPLEEN SCANS IN PATIENTS WITH MALIGNANT MELANOMA

Goldman, Braunstein and Song (1974) studied the liver scans of 63 consecutive patients with malignant melanomas for augmented splenic uptake of ^{99m}Tc-sulfur colloid in the absence of hepatic abnormalities. Of 22 patients with malignant melanoma but without hepatic abnormalities ten showed augmented splenic radioactivity. Sixty patients with carcinoma of various sites were used as controls. Of 54 such patients without hepatic abnormalities, only one had increased splenic uptake.

Comment. This phenomenon is not limited to melanoma in the human. Chandra et al. (1977) have demonstrated increased splenic uptake in C57 black mice bearing B16 melanomas as compared to control C57 mice bearing mammary carcinomas. Although one could assign many reasons for this increased splenic uptake in humans and mice bearing malignant melanomas, the cause is obscure.

REFERENCES

Chandra, R., Bart, R. S., Mintzis, M. M., Kopf, A. W., and Braunstein, P. Distribution of technetium-99m sulfur colloid in mice bearing melanomas and mammary carcinomas. Cancer Res. 37:3293–3296, 1977.

Goldman, A. B., Braunstein, P., and Song, C. Augmented splenic uptake of ^{99m}Tc-sulfur colloid in patients with malignant melanoma. Radiology 112:631–634, 1974.

LEVODOPA AND MALIGNANT MELANOMA

Lieberman and Shupack (1974) wrote on a possible relationship between levodopa therapy for Parkinson's disease and accelerated growth of malignant melanomas. They reported three patients and reviewed two more from the literature. They described a 70-year-old man who had a "pigmented flat nevus" on his right arm about 20 years prior to the initiation of levodopa treatment. About a year after the initiation of the levodopa therapy the "pigmented nevus" began to increase in size, and a biopsy substantiated the diagnosis of malignant melanoma. Of the five cases described in this review of the literature this is the only one that the authors thought had had a benign pigmented nevus which changed into a malignant melanoma after initiation of levodopa therapy. The other cases had proven malignant melanomas before levodopa therapy that worsened after the initiation of therapy. Although there is some suggestion from the reports given that levodopa was associated with a change in the behavior of malignant melanomas in the patients, the course in all cases was nevertheless consistent with the known natural history of malignant melanoma. Furthermore, it is quite possible that the lesion thought to have been a benign nevus and subsequently found to be a melanoma may have been malignant melanoma from the beginning. The authors adduced two mechanisms by which levodopa might stimulate the growth of melanoma. First, the drug might be incorporated into the tumor and stimulate its growth directly. Second, the increased growth of the tumor might be due to stimulation of growth hormone which in turn augmented tumor growth. The authors "sound a note of caution" about the use of levodopa in patients with known malignant melanomas and suggest that patients receiving the drug be observed for changes in pigmented lesions. Perhaps one should go under the assumption that their second suggested mechanism of increased tumor growth is pertinent. If this be so, then it is possible that increased growth of many different types of cancers could occur as a result of levodopa therapy. However, it should be emphasized that in the cases presented, evidence of increased tumor growth is entirely circumstantial; levodopa therapy and increased tumor growth in these patients could have been coincidental.

Sober and Wick (1978) concluded from their review of 1099 patients from the Melanoma Clinical Cooperative Group that levodopa, if a factor in the induction of melanoma, must be inconsequential.

REFERENCE

Lieberman, A. N., and Shupack, J. L. Levodopa and melanoma. Neurology 24:340–343, 1974.

Sober, A. J., and Wick, M. M. Levodopa therapy and malignant melanoma. J.A.M.A. 240: 554–555, 1978.

LASER RADIATION OF MALIGNANT MELANOMAS

Kozlov and co-workers (1973) reported on the anti-neoplastic effects of laser radiation. The studies were done on malignant melanoma and Ehrlich tumors in mice. As might be expected they found that tumors with a great deal of pigmentation responded better than those without significant pigmentation, although tumors of "soft" consistency also responded. An obligatory condition of successful laser therapy was exposure of the entire surface of the malignant growth to the laser beam. The authors suggested that at this time in the clinical situation, laser beam could only be of potential use for surface neoplasms. They considered that the laser beam might be useful for the treatment of localized forms of human tumors of a precancerous and benign character. The authors suggested that the applicability of the laser beam to the clinical situation would be increased with the development of appropriate fiber optics. They found in their animal experiments that high-speed electrons plus laser beam had a greater effect than either of these modalities used separately.

Gameleya and Polischuk (1977) reported on 420 cutaneous tumors treated with neodymium lasers and 139 tumors treated with carbon dioxide lasers. Of these there were 50 melanomas treated with the former and two with the latter. Most of the melanomas measured from 1 to 4 cm in largest diameter. In this study the lasers were used to irradiate normal-appearing skin bordering on the tumor before an attempt was made to eradicate the tumor itself with radiation. It is not clear if the two melanomas treated with carbon dioxide laser were both treated in this way or if the carbon dioxide laser was used as an "optical knife." Of the 48 patients with stage I malignant melanomas, twelve developed metastases to the regional nodes, one had metastases to the lungs, one had metastases to the brain, and one had distant metastases to the skin. These metastases developed from within 3 months to 3 years after treatment. Twelve of the patients with metastatic disease died subsequently following surgery. The authors point out that the laser is unique among therapeutic instruments in that it has a selective effect on pigmented structures.

Comment. It is still unclear what the exact role of lasers will be in the armamentarium against malignant melanomas. It is obvious that methods of therapy which depend on pigment production, such as the use of the laser or the use of antitumor substances which bind preferentially to melanin, have the significant limitation that they would be relatively ineffective for nonpigmented lesions and nonpigmented metastases.

Labandter and Kaplan (1977) reported on their preliminary evaluation of the treatment with the "continuous" carbon dioxide laser of 76 benign lesions and 79 malignant lesions, including 53 malignant melanomas. The laser beam was used exactly as a knife would be in the excision and the dissection of tissue, according to the authors. Since their study covered a period of only $2\frac{1}{2}$ years, their follow-ups were all short and on a limited number of patients. They had not yet analyzed the data nor compared it with other methods such as scalpel excision. It was the authors' impression, however, that there were no "startling differences" following excision by laser as compared to scalpel surgery for malignant melanomas, squamous-cell carcinomas, and basal-cell carcinomas.

REFERENCES

Gamaleya, N. F., and Polischuk, E. I. Treatment of skin tumors by pulsed neodymium and continuous wave carbon dioxide lasers. Dermatol. Digest 16:43–50, 1977.

Kozlov, A. P., Akimov, A. A., Moskalik, K. G., and Pertsov, O. L. Antitumour effect of laser radiation. Acta Radiol. [Ther] (Stockh) 12: 241–256, 1973.

Labandter, H., and Kaplan, I. Experience with a "continuous" laser in the treatment of suitable cutaneous conditions: preliminary report. J. Dermatol. Surg. Oncol. 3:5 527–530, 1977.

USE OF MSH RECEPTORS IN MELANOMA THERAPY

In 1977 Varga and co-workers reported on the use of MSH-daunomycin conjugate against murine melanoma cells and murine 3T3 fibroblasts in culture. It was found that the conjugate had toxic effects only on the melanoma cells in culture, not on the murine 3T3 fibroblasts in culture, presumably because only the melanoma cells have MSH receptors.

Comment. The use of MSH (melanotropin) receptors to attack melanoma cells is indeed intriguing. The questions that remain to be answered are whether such a conjugate will have an effect when used *in vivo;* what general toxic effects the conjugate will have in doses sufficient to inhibit tumor growth; what effect the conjugate will have on other melanocytic system (e.g., those in the eye); and, most importantly, what the effects of such a conjugate is on amelanotic malignant melanomas and amelanotic metastases. It is possible that some amelanotic melanoma cells, and indeed, some pigmented melanoma cells, may lack receptors for MSH.

REFERENCE

Varga, J. M., Asato, N., Lande, S., and Lerner, A. B. Melanotropin-daunomycin conjugate shows receptor-mediated cytotoxicity in cultured murine melanoma cells. Nature 267:56–58, 1977.

ACKNOWLEDGMENTS

We wish to thank the members of the Malignant Melanoma Clinical Cooperative Group (Harvard University, Temple University, New York University, and the University of California-San Francisco) for permission to use some of the statistical data presented in the text.

The Members of the Malignant Melanoma Clinical Cooperative Group at New York University School of Medicine are: A. Bernard Ackerman, M.D., Daniel Baker, M.D., Robert S. Bart, M.D., Jean-Claude Bystryn, M.D., Philip Casson, M.D., Neil Dubin, Ph.D., Frederick M. Golomb, M.D., W. Robson Grier, M.D., Stephen M. Gumport, M.D., Matthew N. Harris, M.D., Patrick Hennessey, M.D., Alfred W. Kopf, M.D., George Lipkin, M.D., Medwin M. Mintzis, M.D., Bernard Pasternack, Ph.D., Allen Postel, M.D., Geraldine Richards, Daniel Roses, M.D., Harold Sage, M.D., Ziporah Scheiner, Fred Valentine, M.D., Francois Viau, Elaine Waldo, M.D.

We are also indebted to Gilbert Clausman and Eleonor E. Pasmik, of the Medical Library of New York University School of Medicine, for their aid in obtaining the monthly computer readouts of the world's literature on malignant melanoma. Without their help many more hours would have been required on our search of the literature.

This work was supported, in part, by a grant (2 R10 CA 13662) from the National Cancer Institute, Institutes of Health, Public Health Service, Department of Health Education and Welfare as part of the Malignant Melanoma Clinical Cooperative Group and by a grant from the Rudolf L. Baer Foundation for Skin Diseases, Inc.

The American Society for Dermatologic Surgery, Inc., Barnes-Hind Pharmaceuticals, Inc., The Schering Corporation, E.R. Squibb & Sons, Inc., and Westwood Pharmaceuticals, Inc. generously provided funds to defray the cost of reproducing the color illustrations.

We thank the staff of the *Journal of Dermatologic Surgery* for their unending attention to details in processing our original manuscript. In particular, we appreciate the editorial skills of Dr. Morris Leider and Hiroko Kiffner.

Finally, we would like to thank the staff of Masson Publishing USA Inc. for their cooperation and advice in the preparation of this book.

Appendix

The following demographic data were gathered by the Malignant Melanoma Clinical Cooperative Group supported by a grant (2 RIO CA 13662) from the National Cancer Institute, Institutes of Health, Public Health Service, Department of Health, Education and Welfare.

These data were presented at the XV International Congress of Dermatology meeting held in Mexico City, October 16–21, 1977. An abstract of this work was submitted on page 81 in the Proceedings of this meeting by Drs. Arthur J. Sober, Thomas B. Fitzpatrick, Martin C. Mihm, M. Scott Blois, Wallace H. Clark, and Alfred W. Kopf.

The members of the Malignant Melanoma Clinical Cooperative Group include:

Boston (Harvard Medical School at Massachusetts General Hospital)
    Dr. Thomas B. Fitzpatrick, Group Chairman and Principal Investigator
    G. Octo Barnett, M.D.
    A. Benedict Cosimi, M.D.
    Robert Lew, Ph.D.
    Ronald A. Malt, M.D.
    Martin C. Mihm, Jr., M.D.
    Ms. Barbara Pearson
    John W. Raker, M.D.
    Arthur J. Sober, M.D.
    William Wood, M.D.

New York (New York University School of Medicine)
    Dr. Alfred W. Kopf, Principal Investigator
    A. Bernard Ackerman, M.D.
    Robert S. Bart, M.D.
    Daniel Baker, M.D.
    Jean-Claude Bystryn, M.D.
    Phillip Casson, M.D.
    Neil Dubin, Ph.D.
    Frederick M. Golomb, M.D.
    W. Robson Grier, M.D.
    Stephen M. Gumport, M.D.
    Matthew N. Harris, M.D.
    Patrick Hennessey, M.D.
    George Lipkin, M.D.
    Medwin M. Mintzis, M.D.
    Bernard Pasternack, Ph.D.
    Allen Postel, M.D.
    Mrs. Geraldine Richards
    Daniel Roses, M.D.
    Harold Sage, M.D.
    Ms. Ziporah Scheiner
    Elaine Waldo, M.D.
    Fred Valentine, M.D.
    Mr. Francois Viau

Philadelphia (Temple University)
    Dr. Wallace H. Clark, Jr., Principal Investigator
    Ann M. Ainsworth, M.D.
    Evelina Bernardino, M.D.
    David E. Elder, M.D.
    Leonard I. Goldman, M.D.
    Michael J. Mastrangelo, M.D.

San Francisco (University of California at San Francisco)
    Dr. M. Scott Blois, Principal Investigator
    Robert Allen, M.D.
    Richard Dakin, M.D.
    William L. Epstein, M.D.
    Douglas Kaufman, M.D.
    Richard W. Sagebiel, M.D.
    Lynn Spitler, M.D.

ABBREVIATIONS

LMM—Lentigo maligna melanoma
MCCG—Melanoma Clinical Cooperative Group
MGH—Massachusetts General Hospital
N—Number
NM—Nodular melanoma
NYU—New York University
SSM—Superficial spreading melanoma
UCSF—University of California, San Francisco

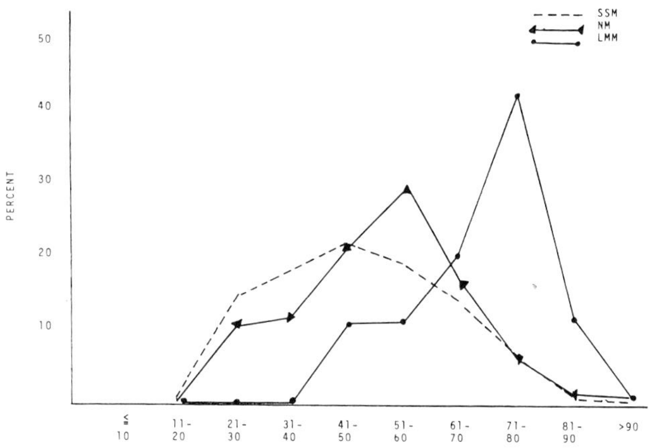

FIGURE 1A. *Percentage distribution for ages by type of melanoma.*

TABLE A1

Total number of MCCG patients	=	1130	
Patients with intact primaries	=	545	48.2%
Patients seen within 30 days of excision	=	585	51.8%

TABLE A2
Sex Distribution

	N	%
Males	577	51.1
Females	553	48.9

TABLE A3
Multiple Primaries

N	%
21/1130	1.9

TABLE A4
Familial Melanoma

N	%
69/1130	6.1

TABLE A5
Percentage Distribution by Type of Melanoma*

	N	%
SSM	777	69.6
NM	175	15.7
LMM	52	4.7
Unclassified	113	10.1

* N = 1117.

TABLE A6
Percentage Distribution by Clark Levels*

	N	%
II	309	27.3
III	349	30.9
IV	357	31.6
V	79	7.0
Unknown	36	3.2

* N = 1130.

TABLE A7
MCCG Patient Distribution by Type of Melanoma*

	LMM		SSM		NM		Unclassified		
	N	%	N	%	N	%	N	%	Total
MGH	9	3.8	168	71.2	44	18.6	15	6.4	236
UCSF	2	1.5	96	72.2	25	18.8	10	7.5	133
NYU	15	3.6	304	73.8	53	12.9	40	9.7	412
Temple	26	7.7	209	62.2	53	15.8	48	14.3	336
Total	52	4.7	777	69.6	175	15.7	113	10.1	1117

* N = 1117.

TABLE A8
Total Number and Percentage by Level and Type of Melanoma*

	LMM		SSM		NM		Unclassified	
	N	%	N	%	N	%	N	%
II	24	46.2	258	33.2	0	0	27	23.9
III	13	25.0	256	32.9	59	33.7	21	18.6
IV	9	17.3	230	29.6	77	44.0	41	36.3
V	4	7.7	28	3.6	36	20.6	11	9.7
Unknown	2	3.8	5	0.6	3	1.7	13	11.5

* $N = 1117$.

TABLE A9
Mean Age by Level for SSM, NM, and Unclassified Melanoma

	Average Age	Low	High
II	46.7	17	91
III	47.0	12	85
IV	51.1	12	91
V	55.0	18	83

TABLE A10
Mean Age by Type of Melanoma

	Average Age	Low	High
SSM	47.3	12	91
NM	50.5	18	91
LMM	69.4	47	94

TABLE A11
Distribution of Malignant Melanoma by Body Surface Area*

Region	Number of cases (males)	Number of cases (females)
Scalp	17	4
Head and Neck	48	44
Back	132	86
Buttocks	1	5
Anterior torso	79	24
Upper Extremities	60	60
Hand	7	8
Thigh	19	36
Leg	17	72
Foot	13	25
Genitalia	2	2
Total	395	366

* $N = 761$.

TABLE A12
Patients with Positive Elective Node Dissections by Type and Level

	LMM		SSM		NM		Unclassified	
	N	%	N	%	N	%	N	%
II	0	0	1/24	4.1	0/0	0	0/2	0
III	0.2	0	12/120	10.0	5/32	15.6	3/8	37.5
IV	0/1	0	23/154	14.9	12/44	27.2	3/22	13.6
V	1/1	100.0	3/8	37.5	12/20	60.0	2/4	50.0

TABLE A13
Patients with Positive Therapeutic Node Dissections by Type and Level

	LMM		SSM		NM		Unclassified	
	N	%	N	%	N	%	N	%
II	0/0	0	0/3	0	0/0	0	1/2	50.0
III	0/0	0	10/21	47.6	2/2	100.0	1/1	100.0
IV	0/0	0	13/17	76.5	7/9	77.8	3/3	100.0
V	0/0	0	6/7	85.7	6/8	75.0	2/2	100.0

General Bibliography*

Abel, E. A., and Bystryn, J.-C. Reproducibility of the immunofluorescent test for antimelanoma antibodies. J. Invest. Derm. 66:117-121, 1976. [21]

Ackerman, L. V. Malignant melanoma of the skin: Clinical and pathologic analysis of 75 cases. Am. J. Clin. Pathol. 18:602-624, 1948. [4]

Agrup, G., Andersson, T., Falck, B., Persson, K., Rorsman, H., Rosengren, A.-M., and Rosengren, E. 5-S-cysteinyldopa in the plasma of melanoma patients and the renal clearance of this amino acid. Acta Derm. Venereol. (Stockh.) 55:5-6, 1975. [22]

Ahman, D. L., Hahn, R. G., and Bisel, H. F. A comparative study of 1-(2-chlorolthyl)-3-cyclohexyl-1-nitrosourea (NSC 79037) and imidazole carboxamide (NSC 45388) with vincristine (NSC 67574) in the palliation of disseminated malignant melanoma. Cancer Res. 32:2432-2434, 1972. [18A]

Ahman, D. L., Hahn, R. G., and Bisel, H. F. Evaluation of 1-(2-chloroethyl-3-4-methylcyclohexyl)-1-nitrosourea (methyl-CCNU, NSC 95441) versus combined imidazole carboxamide (NSC 45388) and vincristine (NSC 67574) in palliation in disseminated malignant melanoma. Cancer 33:615-618, 1974. [18A]

Ahman, D. L., Hahn, R. G., Bisel, H. F., Eagan, R. T., and Edmonson, J. H. Comparative study of methyl-CCNU (NSC-95441) with cyclophosphomide (NSC-26271) and 5-(3,3-dimethyl 1-triazeno) imidazole-4-carboxamide (NSC-45388) with vincristine (NSC-67574) in patients with disseminated malignant melanoma. Cancer Chemother. Rep. 59:451-453, 1975. [18A]

Allen, A. C. Survey of pathologic studies of cutaneous disease during World War II. Arch. Dermat. Syph. 57:19-56, 1948 [4]

Allen, A. C. and Spitz, S. Malignant melanoma. A clinicopathological analysis of the criteria for diagnosis and prognosis. Cancer 6:1-45, 1953. [4, 8]

Allyn, B., Kopf, A. W., Kahn, M., and Witten, V. H. Incidence of pigmented nevi. J.A.M.A. 186:890-893, 1963. [9]

---

*References listed in the General Bibliography are arranged alphabetically by author. The number(s) that appears in bold-face at the end of each reference corresponds to the Chapter (see Table of Contents) in which the reference is cited.

Anaise, D., Steinitz, R., and Ben Hur, N. Solar radiations: A possible etiological factor in malignant melanoma in Israel. Cancer 42:499-504, 1978. [2]

Anderson, D. E. Clinical characteristics of the genetic variety of cutaneous melanoma in man. Cancer 21:721-25, 1971. [5]

Anderson, W. A. D., and Otti, T. M.: Synopsis of Pathology, 9th ed. St. Louis, C. V. Mosby Co., 1976. Chap. 24, p. 1019. [4]

Ariel, I. M. Results of treating malignant melanoma intralymphatically with radioactive isotopes. Surg. Gynecol. Obstet. 139:726-730, 1974. [18B]

Ariel, I. M., Resnick, M. I., and Galey, D. The intralymphatic administration of radioactive isotopes and cancer chemotherapeutic drugs. Surgery 55:355-363, 1964. [9]

Arao, T., Kuwahara, H., and Inone, S. Clinico-pathological and electronmicroscopical studies on melanotic freckle Hutchinson and malignant melanoma arising from the melanotic freckle. Jpn. J. Dermatol., Series B., 81:444-453, 1971. [4]

Arrington, J. H., III, Reed, R. J., Ichinose, H., and Krementz, E. T. Plantar lentiginous melanoma: A distinctive variant of human cutaneous malignant melanoma. Am. J. Surg. Path. 1:131-143, 1977. [4]

Axtell, L. M., Cutler, S. J., and Myers, M. H., eds. End Results In Cancer: Report No. 4. (National Cancer Institute, Maryland), 1972. [20]

Baab, G. H., and McBride, C. M. Malignant melanoma. The patient with an unknown site of primary origin. Arch. Surg. 110:896-900, 1975. [11]

Balch, C. M., Murad, T. M., Soong, S-j, Griffin, A. L., Halpern, N. B., and Maddox, W. A. A multifactorial analysis of melanoma: 1. Prognostic histopathological features comparing Clark's and Breslow's staging methods. Annals of Surgery, in press. [4, 14]

Balda, B.-R., and Birkmayer, G. D. Further evidence for viral etiology of human melanoma. Naturwissenschaften 60:304, 1973. [5]

Balda, B.-R., and Birkmayer, G. D. Drug effects in melanoma: Tumor-specific interactions of proflavine and ethidiumbromide. Yale J. Biol. Med. 46:464-470, 1973. [18A]

Balda, B.-R., Birkmayer, G. D., and Braun-Falco, O. Particle-associated RNA-directed DNA polymerase and 70S RNA in the hamster melanoma A Mel 3. Arch. Dermatol. Forsch. 248:229-36, 1973. [5]

Balda, B.-R., Hehlmann, K., Cho, J.-R., and Spiegelman, S. Oncornavirus-like particles in human skin cancers. Proc. Natl. Acad. Sci. 72:3697–3700, 1975. [5]

Barclay, T. L., Crockett, D. J., Eastwood, D. S., Eastwood, J., and Giles, G. R. Assessment or prognosis in cutaneous malignant melanoma. Br. J. Surg. 64:54–58, 1977. [14]

Barranco, S. C., Romsdahl, M. M., and Humphrey, R. M. The radiation response of human malignant melanoma cells grown in vitro. Cancer Res. 31:830–833. [19]

Bart, R. S., and Kopf, A. W. Tumor Conference #10. A darkly pigmented lesion of the great toe (Acral lentiginous melanoma). J. Derm. Surg. Oncol. 3:158–159, 1977. [3]

Bart, R. S., Lam, S., Cooper, J. S., and Kopf, A. W. Retention of antimelanoma effect of polyinosinic-polycytidylic acid in neonatally thymectomized, irradiated, leukopenic mice. J. Invest. Dermatol. 65:285–289, 1975. [18A]

Bart, R. S., and Schnall, S. Eye color in darkly pigmented basal-cell carcinomas and malignant melanomas: an aid in their clinical differentiation. Arch. Dermatol. 107:206–207, 1973. [3, 22]

Barton, R. T. Mucosal melanomas of the head and neck. Laryngoscope 85:93–99, 1975. [16]

Bauman, L. Melanoma in relatives. J.A.M.A. 218:1300–1301, 1971. [5]

Beardmore, G. L., and Davis, N. C. Multiple primary cutaneous melanomas. Arch. Dermatol. 111:603–609, 1975. [8]

Becker, S. W. Cutaneous melanoma. Arch. Dermat. Syph., 21:818–840, 1930. [4]

Becker, S. W. Critical evaluation of the so-called junction nevus. J. Invest. Dermat. 22:217–223, 1954. [4]

Bellet, R. E., Vaisman, I., Mastrangelo, M. J., and Lustbader, E. Multiple primary malignancies in patients with cutaneous melanoma. Cancer 40:1974–1981, 1977. [8]

Berg, J. W. The incidence of multiple primary cancers. Development of further cancers in patients with lymphomas, leukemias and myeloma. J. Natl. Cancer Inst. 38:741–752, 1967. [8]

Berg, O., and Gordon, M. Relationship of atypical pigment cell growth to gonadal development in hybrid fishes. In: Gordon, M. ed. Pigment Cell Growth, New York, Academic Press, 1953, pp. 43–72. [5]

Berger, R. S., and Voorhees, J. J. Multiple congenital giant nevocellular nevi with halos. Arch. Dermatol. 104:515–521, 1971. [10]

Berger, R., and LaCour, J. Estude chromosomique de Melanomes malins. Biomedicine [Express]. 19:22–27, 1973. [5]

Bergfeld, W., and Helwig, W. B. Exhibit at Academy of Dermatology, Miami Beach, December, 1972. [7]

Bernardino, V. B., Naidoff, M. A., and Clark, W. H. Malignant melanomas of the conjunctiva. Am. J. Ophthal. 82:383–394, 1976. [3]

Biran, S., Hochman, A., and Walach, N. Malignant melanoma: a survey of 232 cases. Oncology 28:331–342, 1973. [19]

Birkmayer, G. D., Balda, B. R., and Miller, F. The inhibitory effect of proflavine and ethidiumbromide on the cell-free transmission and the growth of the hamster melanoma A Mel 3. Eur. J. Cancer 9:859–864, 1973. [18A]

Birkmayer, G. D., Balda, B.-R., and Miller, F. Oncorna-viral information in human melanoma. Europ. J. Cancer 10:419–424, 1974. [5]

Birkmayer, G. D., Balda, B.-R., Miller, F., and Braun-Falco, O. Virus-like particles in metastases of human malignant melanoma. Naturwissenshaften, 59:369–370, 1972. [5]

Blois, M. S. Cited in Arnold, H. L., and Rees, R. B. Meeting review: Pacific Dermatologic Association (1974). Arch. Dermatol. 112:396, 1975. [22]

Blois, M. S., and Banda, P. W. Detection of occult metastatic melanoma by urine chromatography. Cancer Res. 36:3317–3323, 1976. [22]

Blum, R. H., Carter, S. K., and Agre, K. A clinical review of bleomycin—a new antineoplastic agent. Cancer 31:903–914, 1973. [18A]

Bodenham, D. C. A study of 650 observed malignant melanomas in the south-west region. Ann. R. Coll. Surg. Engl. 43:218–239, 1968. [2, 4, 11, 14, 17, 20, 22]

Bodenham, D. C. Malignant melanoma: the problem of lymph-node metastases. Proc. R. Soc. Med. 62:1090–1092, 1969. [4, 14, 17]

Bodurtha, A. J., Berkelhammer, J., Kim, Y. H., Laucius, J. F., and Mastrangelo, M. J. A clinical, histologic, and immunologic study of a case of metastatic malignant melanoma undergoing spontaneous remission. Cancer 37:735–742, 1976. [11]

Bondy, P. K., and Harwick, H. J. Longitudinal banded pigmentation of nails following adrenalectomy for Cushing's syndrome. N. Engl. J. Med. 281:1056–1057, 1969. [9]

Booher, R. J. Recognition and treatment of melanoma. Surg. Clin. North Am. 49:389–405, 1969. [8, 11, 16, 20]

Booher, R. J., and Pack, G. T. Malignant melanoma of the feet and hands. Surgery 42:1084–1121, 1957. [4, 9]

Booker, H. G., et al. Environmental Impact of Stratospheric Flight: Biological and Climatic Effects of Aircraft Emissions in the Stratosphere, National Academy of Sciences, 1975, pp. 177–221. [2]

Boyd, W. The Spontaneous Regression of Cancer. Springfield, Charles C. Thomas, 1966. [11]

Breslow, A. Thickness, cross-sectional areas and depth of invasion in the prognosis of cutaneous melanoma. Ann. Surg. 172:902–908, 1970. [3, 4, 14, 16, 17]

Breslow, A. Tumor thickness, level of invasion and node dissection in stage I cutaneous melanoma. Ann. Surg. 182:572–575, 1975. [3, 4, 14, 16, 17]

Breslow, A.: In search of thin lethal melanomas. Surg. Gynecol. and Obstet. 143:799, 1976. [3]

Breslow, A. Problems in the measurement of tumor thickness and level of invasion of cutaneous melanoma. Human Path. 8:1–2, 1977. [3]

Breslow, A. Melanoma thickness and elective node dissection. Arch. Dermatol. 114:1399, 1978. [17]

Breslow, A., Cascinelli, V., van der Esch, E. P., and Marabito, A. Stage I melanoma of the limbs: assessment of prognosis by levels of invasion and maximum thickness. In press. [4]

Breslow, A. and Macht, S. D. Optimal size of resection margin for thin cutaneous melanoma. Surg. Gynecol. Obstet. 145: 691–692, 1977. [4, 16]

Breslow, A. and Macht, S. D. Evaluation of prognosis in stage I cutaneous melanoma. Plas. Reconstr. Surg. 61:342–346, 1978. [4]

Brodkin, R. H., Kopf, A. W., and Andrade, R. Basal-cell epithelioma and elastosis: a comparison of distribution. In: Urbach, F., ed. The Biologic Effects of Ultraviolet Radiation: With Emphasis on the Skin. New York, Pergamon, 1969, pp. 581–618. [2]

Brown, A. S., Wallack, M. K., Horstmann, J. T., Hamilton, R. W., Johnson, J. L., and Rosato, F. E. Perfusion therapy for extremity melanoma. Arch. Surg. 111:961–963, 1976. [18B]

Brownstein, M. H., and Helwig, E. B. Patterns of cutaneous metastasis. Arch. Dermatol. 105:862–868, 1972. [11]

Bulkley, G. B., Cohen, M. H., Banks, P. M., Char, D. H., and Ketcham, A. S. Long-term spontaneous regression of malignant melanoma with visceral metastases. Report of a case with immunologic profile. Cancer 36:485–494, 1975. [11]

Bystryn, J.-C., Bart, R. S., Livingston, P., and Kopf, A. W. Growth and immunogenicity of murine B-16 melanoma. J. Invest. Dermatol. 63:369–373, 1974. [21]

Bystryn, J.-C., and Smalley, J. R. Identification and solubilization of iodinated cell surface human melanoma associated antigens. Int. J. Cancer 20:165–172, 1977. [21]

Cady, B. Changing concepts in malignant melanoma. Med. Clinics North Am. 59:301–308, 1975. [14, 15, 20]

Cady, B., Legg, M. A., and Redfern, A. B. Contemporary treatment of malignant melanoma. Am. J. Surg. 129:472–482, 1975. [1, 17, 20]

Callen, J. P., Chanda, J. J., and Stowiski, M. A. Malignant melanoma. Arch. Dermatol. 114:369–370, 1978. [4]

Caro, M. R.: Diagnostic pitfalls in dermal pathology. Arch. Derm 67:18–29, 1953. [4]

Carswell, R. Pathological Anatomy, Part 9, "Melanoma." London, Longman, 1838. [4]

Cascinelli, N., Fontana, V., Cataldo, I., and Balzarini, G. P. Multiple primary melanoma. Tumori 61:481–486, 1975. [8]

Castro, J. R., Oliver, G. D., Withers, H. R., and Almond, P. R. Experience with Californium 252 in clinical radiotherapy. Am. J. Roentgenol. Radium Ther. Nucl. Med. 117:182–194, 1973. [19]

Catterall, M. Fast neutrons in oncology. Br. J. Hosp. Med. 12: 853–860, 1974. [19]

Chandra, R., Bart, R. S., Mintzis, M. M., Kopf, A. W., and Braunstein, P. Distribution of technetium-99m sulfur colloid in mice bearing melanomas and mammary carcinomas. Cancer Res. 37:3293–3296, 1977. [22]

Chen, T. R., and Shaw, M. W. Stable chromosome changes in a human malignant melanoma. Cancer Res. 33:2042–2047, 1973. [5]

Chopra, D. P. Ultraviolet light carcinogenesis in hairless mice. J. Invest. Dermatol. 66:242–247, 1976. [2]

Chung, A. F., Woodruff, J. M., and Lewis, J. L. Malignant melanoma of the vulva. Obstet. Gynecol. 45:638–646, 1975. [3]

Clark, W. H. A classification of malignant melanoma in man correlated with histogenesis and biological behavior. In Montagna, W., and Hu, F., eds., Advances In Biology of Skin—Volume VIII. The Pigmentary System. Oxford and New York, Pergamon Press, 1967, pgs. 621–647. [3, 4]

Clark, W. H., Jr. Clinical diagnosis of cutaneous malignant melanoma. J.A.M.A. 236:484–485, 1976. [3]

Clark, W. H., Jr., From, L., Bernardino, E. A., and Mihm, M. C. The histogenesis and biologic behavior of primary human malignant melanomas of the skin. Cancer Res. 29:705–727, 1969. [3, 4, 14, 16, 20]

Clark, W. H., Jr., Ainsworth, A. M., Bernardino, E. A., Yang, C. H., Mihm, M. C., Jr., and Reed, R. J. The developmental biology of primary human malignant melanomas. Semin. Oncol. 2:83–103, 1975. [3, 4, 8, 9, 14]

Clark, W. H., Mastrangelo, M. J., Ainsworth, A. M., Berd, D., Bellet, R. E., and Bernardino, E. A. Current concepts of the biology of human cutaneous malignant melanoma. Adv. Cancer Res. 24:267–338, 1977. [3, 21]

Clark, W. H., and Mihm, M. C. Lentigo maligna and lentigo-maligna melanoma. Am. J. Patho. 55:39–67, 1969. [3]

Clark, W. H., Jr., Reimer, R. R., Greene, M., Ainsworth, A. M., and Mastrangelo, M. F. Origin of familial malignant melanomas from heritable melanocytic lesions: The B-K mole syndrome. Arch. Dermatol. In press. [4]

Claudy, A. L., Viac, J., Pelletier, N., Fouad-Wassef, N., Alario, A., and Thiovolet, J. Prognostic correlations in malignant melanoma. Europ. J. Cancer 2:821–827, 1975. [14]

Clinicopathologic conference: multiple malignancies: chronic lymphocytic leukemia, malignant melanoma, multiple myeloma, and acute myelomonocytic leukemia. Am. J. Med. 58: 408–416, 1975. [8]

Cochrane, A. J.: Histology and prognosis in malignant melanoma. J. Path. 97:459, 1969. [4]

Cohen, S. M., Greenspan, E. M., Weiner, M. J., and Kabakow, B. Triple combination chemotherapy of disseminated melanoma. Cancer 29:1489–1495, 1972. [18A]

Cohen, M. H., Ketcham, A. S., Felix, E. L., Li, S-H., Tomaszewski, M-M., Costa, J., Rabson, A. S., Simon, R. M., and

Rosenberg, S. A. Prognostic factors in patients undergoing lymphadenectomy for malignant melanoma. Ann. Surg. 186:635–642, 1977. [14]

Conley, J., Lattes, R. and Orr, W.: Desmoplastic malignant melanoma (a rare variant of spindle cell melanoma). Cancer 28:914–936, 1971. [4, 22]

Conley, J., and Pack, G. T. Melanoma of the mucous membranes of the head and neck. Arch. Otolaryngol. 99:315–319, 1974. [20]

Conrad, F. G. Treatment of malignant melanoma. Wide excision alone vs. lymphadenectomy. Arch. Surg. 104:587–593, 1972. [20]

Constanza, M. E., Nathanson, L., Lenhard, R., Wolter, J., Colsky, J., Oberfield, R. A., and Schilling, A. Therapy of malignant melanoma with an imidazole carboxamide and bis-chloroethyl nitrosourea. Cancer 30:1457–1461, 1972. [18A]

Constanzi, J. J., Vaitkevicius, V. K., Quagliana, J. M., Hoogstraten, B., Coltman, C. A., Jr., and Delaney, F. C. Combination chemotherapy for disseminated malignant melanoma. Cancer 35:342–346, 1975. [18A]

Cooper, J. S., Kopf, A. W., and Bart, R. S. Present and future prospects of radiotherapy in the treatment of malignant melanoma. J. Derm. Surg. Oncol. Submitted for publication, 1978. [19]

Copeman, P. W. M., and Elliott, P. G. Melanoma cytoplasmic humoral antibody test. Br. J. Dermatol. 94:565–568, 1976. [10]

Copeman, P. W. M., Lewis, M. G., Phillips, T. M., and Elliott, P. G. Immunological associations of the halo nevus with cutaneous malignant melanoma. Br. J. Dermatol. 88:127–137, 1973. [10]

Corsi, H. Three cases of melanose circonscrite precancereuse. Proc. Roy. Soc. Med. 32:261–263, 1938–1939. [4]

Cosman, B., Heddle, S. B., and Crikelair, G. F. The increasing incidence of melanoma. Plast. Reconstr. Surg. 57:50–56, 1976. [1]

Costello, M. J., Fisher, S. B., and DeFeo, C. P. Melanotic freckle: Lentigo maligna. A. M. A. Arch. Derm. 80:753, 1959. [4]

Couperus, M., and Rucker, R. C.: Histopathologic diagnosis of malignant melanoma. Arch. Dermat. 70:199–216, 1954. [4]

Cox, K. R. Survival after regional perfusion for limb melanoma. Aust. N.Z. J. Surg. 45:32–36, 1975. [18B]

Creech, O., Jr., Krementz, E. T., Ryan, R. F., and Winblad, J. N. Chemotherapy of cancer: regional perfusion utilizing an extracorporeal circuit. Ann. Surg. 148:616–632, 1958. [18B]

Currie, G. A., and McElwain, T. J. Active immunotherapy as an adjunct to chemotherapy in the treatment of disseminated malignant melanoma: a pilot study. Br. J. Cancer 31:143–156, 1975. [19]

Cutler, S. J., and Young, J. L. Third National Cancer Survey: Incidence Data, N.C.I. Monograph 41, DHEW Publication No. (NIH) 75-787, March, 1975. [1]

Cutler, S. J., Myers, M. H., and Green, S. B. Trends in survival rates of patients with cancer. N. Engl. J. Med. 293:122–124, 1975. [1]

Daniels, F. Sunlight. In: Schottenfeld, D., ed., Cancer Epidemiology and Prevention: Current Concepts. Springfield, Charles C. Thomas, 1975, pp. 126–152. [2]

Das Gupta, T. K. Results of treatment of 269 patients with primary cutaneous melanoma. Ann. Surg. 186:201–209, 1977. [14]

Das Gupta, T., and Brasfield, R. Metastatic melanoma; a clinicopathological study. Cancer 17:1323–1339, 1964. [12]

Das Gupta, T., and Brasfield, R. Subungual melanoma: 25-year review of cases. Ann. Surg. 161:545–552, 1965. [4, 9]

Das Gupta, T., and McNeer, G. The incidence of metastases to accessible lymph nodes from melanoma of the trunk and extremities: its therapeutic significance. Cancer 17:897–911, 1964. [16, 17]

Das Gupta, T., Bowden, L., and Berg, J. W. Malignant melanoma of unknown primary origin. Surg. Gynecol. Obstet. 117:341–345, 1963. [11, 16]

Davis, N. C. Elective lymph node dissection—Yes or No? In: McCarthy, W. H., ed. Melanoma and Skin Cancer. Sydney, V. C. N. Blight, 1972, pp. 407–416. [17]

Davis, N. C. Cutaneous Melanoma. The Queensland experience. Curr. Probl. Surg. 13:1–63, 1976. [1, 2, 5, 16]

Davis, N. C., and McLeod, G. R. The surgery of primary melanoma: problems and practice. Med. J. Aust. 2:778–782, 1972. [16, 17]

Davis, N. C., McLeod, G. R., Beardmore, G. L., Little, J. H., Quinn, R. L., and Holt, J. Primary cutaneous melanoma: a report from the Queensland melanoma project. CA 26:80–107, 1976. [3, 4, 14, 20]

Davis, N., McLeod, R., Beardmore, G., Little, J., Quinn, R., and Holt, J. The Henry Joseph Windsor Lecture: Melanoma is a word, not a sentence. Aust. N. Zealand J. Surg. 46:188–196, 1976. [20]

Davis, J., Pack, G. T., and Higgins, G. K. Melanotic freckle of Hutchinson. Am. J. Surg. 113:457–463, 1967. [4]

Decker, K. Zur Klinik der Melanome, Beitr. Klin. Chir. 154:159–166, 1931. [4]

Dellon, A. L., Edelson, R. L., and Chretien, P. B. Defining the malignant potential of the giant pigmented nevus. Plas. Reconstr. Surg. 57:611–618, 1976. [7]

Demian, S. D. E., Donnelly, W. H., Frias, J. L., and Monif, G. R. G. Placental lesions in congenital giant pigmented nevi. Am. J. Clin. Path. 61:438–442, 1974. [7]

Dewey, D. L. The radiosensitivity of melanoma cells in culture. Br. J. Radiol. 44:816, 1971. [19]

Dickson, R. J. Malignant melanoma: a combined surgical and radiotherapeutic approach. Am. J. Roentgenol. Radium Ther. Nucl. Med. 79:1063–1070, 1958. [19]

Donaldson, R. C., Canaan, S. A., McLean, R. B., and Ackerman, L. V. Uveitis and vitiligo associated with BCG treatment for malignant melanoma. Surgery 76:771–778, 1974. [10]

Donnellan, M. J., Seemayer, T., Huvos, A. G., Miké, V., and Strong, E. W. Clinicopathologic study of cutaneous melanoma of the head and neck. Am. J. Surg. 124:450–455, 1972. [20]

Dowell, K. E., Armstrong, D. M., Aust. J. B., Cruz, Jr., A. B. Systemic chemotherapy of advanced head and neck malignancies. Cancer 35:1116–1120, 1975. [18A]

Doyle, J. C., Bennett, R. C., and Newing, R. K. Spontaneous regression of malignant melanoma. Med. J. Aust. 2:551–552, 1973. [11]

Dubin, N., and Pasternack, B. S. Letter to the Editor. New Engl. J. Med. 298-223–224, 1978. [17]

Dubreuilh, M. W. De la mélanose circonscrite précancéreuse. Ann. Dermat. Syph. 3:129, 205, 1912. [4]

Dubreuilh, M. W. Lentigo malin des vieillards. Société de Dermatologie, 4 août, 1894. [4]

Duhring, L. A. A Practical Treatise on Diseases of the Skin. Philadelphia, J. B. Lippincott Co., 1882, pp. 559–560. [4]

Editorial: the halo naevus and malignant melanoma. Lancet 1:982, 1973. [10]

Edwards, J. M. Malignant melanoma: treatment by endolymphatic radio-isotope infusion. Ann. R. Coll. Surg. Eng. 44:237–254, 1969. [19]

Edwards, J. M. Treatment of melanoma by endolymphatic therapy. Proc. R. Soc. Med. 67:97–99, 1974. [18B]

Einhorn, L. H., McBride, C. M., Luce, J. K., Caoili, E., and Gottlieb, J. A. Intra-arterial infusion therapy with 5-(3,3-dimethyl-1-triazeno) imidazole-4-carboxamide (NSC 45388) for malignant melanoma. Cancer 32:749–755, 1973. [18B]

Einhorn, L. H., Burgess, M. A., Vallejos, C., Bodey, G. P., Gutterman, J., Mavligit, G., Hersh, E. M., Luce, J. K., Frei, E., Freireich, E. J., and Gottlieb, J. A. Prognostic correlations and response to treatment in advanced metastatic malignant melanoma. Cancer Res. 34:1995–2004, 1974. [**11, 12, 18A, 22**]

Eiselt, T. Ueber pigment Krebs. Viertegjahrsch. f. d. praktische Heilkunde, 70:87, 197, 1861; 76; 26, 1862. [4]

Elias, E. G., Didolkar, M. S., Goel, I. P., Formeister, J. F., Valenzuela, L. A., Pickren, J. L., and Moore, R. H. A clinicopathologic study of prognostic factors in cutaneous malignant melanoma. Surg. Gynecol. Obstet. 144:327–334, 1977. [14]

Elwood, J. M., and Lee, J. A. H. Recent data on the epidemiology of malignant melanoma. Semin. Oncol. 2:149–154, 1975. [1]

Elwood, J. M., Lee, J. A. H., Walters, S. D., Mo, T., and Green, A. E. S. Relationship of melanoma and other skin cancer mortality to latitude and ultraviolet radiation in the United States and Canada. Int. J. Epidemiology 3:325–332, 1974. [**1, 2**]

Epstein, E., Bragg, K., and Linden, G. Biopsy and prognosis of malignant melanoma. J.A.M.A. 208:1369–1371, 1969. [**4, 15**]

Epstein, J. H., Epstein, W. L., and Nakai, T. Production of melanomas from DMBA-induced "blue nevi" in hairless mice with ultraviolet light. J. Natl. Cancer Inst. 38:19–30, 1967. [2]

Epstein, J. H., Fukuyama, K., and Dobson, R. L. Ultraviolet light carcinogenesis. In: Urbach, F., ed. The Biologic Effects of Ultraviolet Radiation: With Emphasis on the Skin. New York, Pergamon, 1969, pp. 551–568. [2]

Epstein, W. L., Sagebeil, R., Spitler, L., Wybran, J., Reed, W. B., and Blois, M. S. Halo nevi and melanoma. J.A.M.A. 225:373–377, 1973. [10]

Everall, J. D., and Dowd, P. M. Diagnosis, prognosis, and treatment of melanoma. Lancet 2:286–289, 1977. [16]

Everson, T. C. Spontaneous regression of cancer. Ann. N.Y. Acad. Sci. 114-721–735, 1964. [10]

Everson, T. C., and Cole, W. H. Spontaneous Regression of Cancer. W. B. Saunders, Philadelphia, 1966. [10]

Falkson, G., van der Merwe, A. M., and Falkson, H. C. Clinical experience with 5-(3,3 bis (2-chloroethyl)-1-triazeno) imidazole-4-carboxamide (NSC-82196) in the treatment of metastatic malignant melanoma. Cancer Chemother. Rep. 56:671–677, 1972. [18A]

Fears, T. R., Scotto, J., and Schneiderman, M. A. Skin cancer, melanoma, and sunlight. Am. J. Public Health 66:461–464, 1976. [2]

Fish, J., Smith, E. B., and Canby, J. P. Malignant melanoma in childhood. Surgery 59:309–315, 1966. [7]

Fishman, H. C. Malignant melanoma arising with two halo nevi. Arch. Derm. 112:407–408, 1976. [10]

Fitzpatrick, P. J., Brown, T. C., and Reid, J. Malignant melanoma of the head and neck: a clinicopathological study. Can. J. Surg. 15:90–101, 1972. [**4, 14**]

Fitzpatrick, T. B., Sober, A., and Pearson, B. Early Diagnosis of Malignant Melanoma. Exhibit at the 1975 Meeting of the American Academy of Dermatology, San Francisco, December 6–11, 1975. [2]

Fletcher, W. S. In: Riley, V., ed. Pigment Cell: Mechanisms in Pigmentation. Vol. 1, Basel, Karger, 1973, pp. 255–260. [8]

Fodor, J., and Bodrogi, I. Vitiligo and malignant melanoma. Neoplasma 22:445–446, 1975. [10]

Fontaine, C. J., and Jamieson, C. W. Perfusion in limb melanoma: indications and results. Proc. R. Soc. Med. 67:99–100, 1974. [18B]

Fortner, J. G., Booher, R. J., and Pack, G. T. Results of groin dissection for malignant melanoma in 220 patients. Surgery 55:485–494, 1964. [16]

Fortner, J. G., Woodruff, J., Shottenfeld, D., and Maclean, B. Biostatistical basis of elective node dissection for malignant melanoma. Ann. Surg. 186:101–103, 1977 [**17, 20**]

Franklin, J. D., Reynolds, V. H., and Page, D. L. Cutaneous melanoma: a twenty-year retrospective study with clinicopathologic correlation. Plast. Reconstr. Surg. 56:277–285, 1975. [**4, 14, 20**]

Freckman, H. A. Results in 169 patients with cancer of the head and neck treated by intra-arterial infusion therapy. Am. J. Surg. 124:501–509, 1972. [18B]

Frenk, E. Depigmentations vitiligineuses chez des patients atteints de mélanomes malins. Dermatologica 139:84–91, 1969. [10]

Frolow, G. R., Englewood, N. J., Shaprio, L., and Brownstein, M. H. Desmoplastic malignant melanoma. Arch. Derm. 111: 753–754, 1975. [4]

Frolow, G. R., Shapiro, L., and Brownstein, M. H. Desmoplastic malignant melanoma. Arch. Dermatol. 111:753–754, 1975. [22]

Fraser, D. G., Bull, J. G., and Dunphy, J. E.: Malignant melanoma and coexisting malignant neoplasms. Am. J. Surg. 122:169–174, 1971. [8]

Frazier, T.-G.: Letter to the Editor. New Engl. J. Med. 298:223, 1978. [17]

Gamaleya, N. F., and Polischuk, E. I. Treatment of skin tumors by pulsed neodymium and continuous wave carbon dioxide lasers. Dermatol. Digest 16:43–50, 1977. [22]

Gams, R. A., and Carpenter, J. T. Central nervous system complications after combination treatment with adriamycin (NSC 123127) and 5-(3,3-dimethyl-1-triazeno) imidazole 4-carboxamide (NSC 45388). Cancer Chemother. Rep. 58:753–754, 1974. [18A]

Gan, E. V., Haberman, H. F., and Menon, I. A. A simple and sensitive test for the determination of phenolic compounds in urine and its application to melanoma. J. Invest. Dermatol. 64:139–144, 1975. [22]

Geehoed, G. W., Breslow, A., and McCune, W. S. Malignant melanoma: Correlation of long-term follow-up with clinical staging, level of invasion and thickness of the primary tumor. Am. Surgeon 43:77–85, 1977. [3, 17]

Gelfant, S. A new concept of tissue and tumor cell proliferation. Cancer Res. 37:3845–3862, 1977. [18A]

Gellin, G. A., Kopf, A. W., and Garfinkel, L. Basal cell epithelioma: a controlled study of associated factors. Arch. Dermatol. 91:38–45, 1965. [2]

Gellin, G. A., Kopf, A. W., and Garfinkel, L. Malignant melanoma: a controlled study of possible associated factors. Arch. Dermatol. 99:43–48, 1969. [2, 5]

Gerner, R. E., and Moore, G. E. Study of 5-(3,3-dimethyl-1-triazeno) imidazole-4-carboxamide (NSC 45388) in patients with disseminated melanoma. Cancer Chemother. Rep. 57:83–84, 1973. [18A]

Gerner, R. E., Moore, G. E., and Didolkhar, M. S. Chemotherapy of disseminated malignant melanoma with dimethyl triazeno imidazole carboxamide and dactinomycin. Cancer 32:756–760, 1973. [18A]

Gerner, R. E., Moore, G. E., and Dickey, C. Combination chemotherapy in disseminated melanoma and other solid tumors in adults. Oncology 31:22–30, 1975. [18A]

Gerner, R. E., and Moore, G. E. Feasibility study of active immunotherapy in patients with solid tumors. Cancer 38:131–143, 1976. [10, 21]

Gersten, M. J., Hadden, E. M., Kaplan, M. H., Pinsky, C. M., Armstrong, D., and Hadden, J. W. Immunologic defects in melanoma patients: Lack of effect of BCG therapy. Clin. Bulletin (Memorial Sloan-Kettering Cancer Center) 7:63–69, 1977. [21]

Gibson, S. H., Montgomery, H., Woolner, L. B., and Brunsting, L. A. Melanotic whitlow (subungual melanoma). J. Invest. Dermatol. 28:119–129, 1957. [4, 9]

Giovanella, G., et al. Human neoplastic and normal cells in tissue culture. I. Cell lines derived from malignant melanoma and normal melanocytes. J. Natl. Cancer Inst. 56:1131–1142, 1976. [18A]

Giraud, R. M. A., Rippey, E., and Rippey, J. J. Malignant melanoma of the skin in black africans. South Afr. Med. J. 49: 665–668, 1975. [3]

Goldman, A. B., Braunstein, P., and Song, C. Augmented splenic uptake of ^{99m}Tc-sulfur colloid in patients with malignant melanoma. Radiology 112:631–634, 1974. [22]

Goldsmith, H. S., Shah, J. P., and Kim, D. H. Prognostic significance of lymph node dissection in the treatment of malignant melanoma. Cancer 26:606–609, 1970. [13, 16, 17]

Golomb, F. Perfusion of melanoma; 105 isolated perfusions in 92 patients. Oncology 26:197–205, 1972. [18B]

Golomb, F. M. Perfusion therapy for skin cancer. J. Dermatol. Surg. 1(4):39–48, 1975. [18B]

Golomb, F. M., Solowey, A. C., Postel, A., Gumport, S. L., and Wright, J. C.: Induced remission of malignant melanoma with actinomycin D. Cancer 20:656–662, 1967. [18B]

Gordon, D., and Silverstone, H. Worldwide epidemiology of premalignant and malignant cutaneous lesions. In Cancer of the Skin, Andrade, R., et al., eds. Philadelphia, Saunders 1976, p. 423. [4]

Goss, P., and Parsons, P. G. The effect of hyperthermia and melphalan on survival of human fibroblast strains and melanoma cell lines. Cancer Res. 37:152–156, 1977. [18B]

Gottlieb, J. A., Frei, E., III, and Luce, J. K. Dose schedule studies with hydroxyurea (NSC-32065) in malignant melanoma. Cancer Chemother. Rep. 55:277–280, 1971. [18A]

Gottlieb, J. A., Frei, E., and Luce, J. K. An evaluation of the management of patients with cerebral metastases from malignant melanoma. Cancer 29:701–705, 1972 [19]

Graham, W. P. Subungual melanoma. Pennsylvania Med. 76:56, 1973. [4, 9]

Graham, G. F., and Stewart, R. Cryosurgery for unusual cutaneous neoplasms. J. Derm. Surg. Oncol. 3:437–444, 1977. [16]

Greeley, P. W., Middleton, A. G., and Curtin, J. W. Incidence of malignancy in giant pigmented nevi. Plast. Reconstr. Surg. 36:26–37, 1965. [7]

Greenhalgh, R. M., Talbot, I. C., and Calnan, J. S. Multiple malignant melanoma. Report of a patient with four primary malignant cutaneous melanomas. Br. J. Plast. Surg. 24:301-306, 1971. [8]

Gromet, M. A.: Treatment of lentigo maligna. Arch. Dermatol. 113:1128, 1977. [3]

Gromet, M. A., Sagebiel, R. W., and Epstein, W. L.: The regressing thin malignant melanoma: A distinctive lesion with metastatic potential. Cancer: 2282-2292, 1978. [3, 4]

Gromet, M.A., Sagebiel, R. W., and Epstein, W. L.: Clin. Res. 26: 103A, 1978. [4]

Gumport, S. L., and Harris, M. N. Results of regional node dissection for melanoma. Ann. Surg. 179:105-108, 1974. [**16, 17, 20**]

Gumport, S. L., and Harris, M. H.: Melanoma of the skin. In Cancer of the Skin, Andrade, R. et al. eds. Philadelphia, Saunders, 1976, pp. 950-971. [4]

Gumport, S. L., Harris, M. N., and Kopf, A. W. Diagnosis and management of common skin cancers. CA 24:218-228, 1974. [3]

Gumport, S. L., Lyall, D., and Zimany, A. A radical axillary lymph node dissection for malignancy. Arch. Surg. 83:227-230, 1961 [**16**]

Gumport, S. L., and Meyer, H. W.: An improved technique for an adequate radical groin dissection for malignancy. Surgery 38:660-66, 1955. [**16**]

Gumport, S. L., and Meyer, H. W. Treatment of 126 cases of malignant melanoma. Ann. Surg. 150:989-992, 1959. [**16**]

Gunz, F. W., and Angus, H. B. Leukemia and cancer in the same patient. Cancer 18:145-152, 1965. [8]

Gutterman, J. U., Mavligit, G., Gottlieb, J. A., Burgess, M. A., McBride, C. E., Einhorn, L., Freireich, E. J., and Hersh, E. M. Chemoimmunotherapy of disseminated malignant melanoma with dimethyl triazeno imidazole carboxamide and Bacillus Calmette-Guérin. N. Engl. J. Med 291:592-597, 1974, [**18A**]

Gutterman, J. U., Mavligit, G., Reed, R., Richman, S., McBride, C. M., and Hersh, E. M. Immunology and immunotherapy of human malignant melanoma: historic review and perspectives for the future. Semin. Oncol. 2:155-174, 1975. [**21**]

Habermalz, H. J., and Fischer, J. J. Radiation therapy of malignant melanoma: Experience with high individual treatment doses. Cancer 38:2258-2262, 1976. [**19**]

Hadwen, S. The melanomata of grey and white horses. Can. Med. Assoc. J. 25:519-530, 1931. [**5, 10**]

Hagemann, R. F., and Scbiffer, L. M. Cell kinetic analysis of a human melanoma *in vitro* and *in vivo-vitro*. J. Natl. Cancer Inst. 47:519-526, 1971. [**18A**]

Hansen, M. G., and McCarten, A. B. Tumor thickness and lymphocytic infiltration in malignant melanoma of the head and neck. Am. J. Surg. 128:557-561, 1974. [**3, 14, 16, 17, 20**]

Hansson, J. A., Simert, G., and Vang, J. The effect of regional perfusion treatment on recurrent melanoma of the extremities. Acta. Chir. Scand. 143:33-39, 1977. [**18B**]

Happle, R., Schotola, I., and Macher, E. Spontanregression and Leukoderm bein malignen Melanom. Der Hautarzt 26:120-123, 1975. [**10**]

Harmer, C. L. The radiotherapy of melanoma. Clin. Exp. Dermatol. 1:29-36, 1976. [**19**]

Harris, J. W. Effects of tumor-like assay conditions, ionizing radiation, and hyperthermia on immune lysis of tumor cells by cytotoxic T-lymphocytes. Cancer Res. 36:2733-2739, 1976. [**18B**]

Harris, M. N., and Gumport, S. L. Total excisional biopsy for primary malignant melanoma. J.A.M.A. 226:354-355, 1973. [**15**]

Harris, M. N., and Gumport, S. L. Biopsy technique for malignant melanoma. J. Dermatol. Surg. 1(1):24-27, 1975. [**15, 16**]

Harris, M. N., and Gumport, S. L. Present status of surgical management of malignant melanoma. J Dermatol. Surg. 2: 129-133, 1976. [**16**]

Harris, M. N., Gumport, S. L., and Maiwandi, H. Axillary lymph node dissection for melanoma. Surg. Gynecol. Obstet. 135: 936-940, 1972. [**20**]

Harris, M. N., Gumport, S. L., Berman, I. R., and Bernard, R. W. Ilioinguinal lymph node dissection for melanoma. Surg. Gynecol. Obstet. 136:33-39, 1973. [**16**]

Harris, M. N., Roses, D. F., Culliford, A. T., and Gumport, S. L. Melanoma of the head and neck. Ann. Surg. 182:86-91, 1975. [**16**]

Hazen, H. H. Malignant moles. South. M. J., 13:345, 1920. [4]

Hellriegel, W. Radiation therapy of primary and metastatic melanoma. Ann. N. Y. Acad. Sci. 100:131-141, 1963. [**19**]

Helwig, E. B.: Malignant melanoma of the skin of man. Natl. Cancer Inst., Monograph 10, 287:95, 1963. [4]

Helwig, E. B. In Neoplasms of the Skin and Malignant Melanoma, Chicago, Year Book Medical Publishers, Inc., 1975. [4]

Hermanek, P., Hornstein, O. P., Tonak, J., and Weidner, F.: Malignant melanoma: Depth of invasion and histologic typing. Beitr. Pathol., 157:269-282, 1976.[3, 4]

Hermann, W. P., Tritsch, H., and Gartmann, H. Rückbildung von Melanom-Metastasen nach Injektion von Freundschem Adjuvans. Hautarzt 21:181-183, 1970. [**10**]

Hersey, P., Morgan, G., Stone, D. E., McCarthy, W. H., and Milton, G. W. Previous pregnancy as a protective factor against death from melanoma. Lancet 1:451-452, 1977. [**14**]

Hersh, E. M., McBride, C. M., and Gschwind, C. Local and systemic immunologic effects of perfusion therapy for malignant melanoma. Surg. Gynecol. Obstet. 137:461-464, 1973. [**18B**]

Hertz, K. C., Gazze, L. A., Kirkpatrick, C. H., and Katz, S. I. Autoimmune vitiligo. New Engl. J. Med. 297:634–637, 1977. [10]

Hertzler, A. E. Melanoblastoma of the nail-bed (melanotic whitlow). Arch. Dermat. Syph, 6:701–708, 1922. [4]

Hessler, C., and Maillard, G. F. Apport de la thermographie dans le diagnostic et le traitment du mélanome malin. Schweiz. Med. Wochenschr. 100:972–975, 1970. [22]

Higashi, N. Melanocytes of nail matrix and nail pigmentation. Arch. Dermatol. 97:570–574, 1968. [9]

Hilaris, B. S., Raben, M., Calabrese, A. S., Phillips, R. F., and Henschke, U. K. Value of radiation therapy for distant metastases from malignant melanoma. Cancer 16:765–773, 1963. [19]

Hill, G. J., II, Ruess, R., Berris, R., Philpott, G. W., and Parkin, P. Chemotherapy of malignant melanoma with dimethyl triazeno imidazole carboxamide (DTIC) and nitrosourea derivatives (BCNU, CCNU). Ann. Surg. 180:167–174, 1974. [18A]

Hill, G. J., II, Johnson, R. O., Metter, G., Wilson, W. L., Davis, H. L., Grage, T., Fletcher, W. S., Golomb, F. M., and Cruz, A. B. Multimodal surgical adjuvant therapy for a broad spectrum of tumors in humans. Surg. Gynecol. Obstet. 1422:882–892, 1976. [18B]

Hirst, E., Cains, G. D., Bale, P. M., Palmer, A. A., and Hambly, C. K. Diagnosis by frozen section examination, II: Results in skin lesions. Aust. N. Z. J. Surg. 38:216–220, 1969. [4]

Hirst, E., McCarthy, S. W., and Bale, P. M. Frozen section diagnosis of cutaneous malignancy. In Melanoma and Skin Cancer (Proceedings of the International Cancer Conference, Sydney, 1972). McCarthy, W. H., ed. Sydney, V. C. N. Blight, 1972, pp. 185–192. [4]

Holmes, E. C., Clark, W., Morton, D. L., Eilber, F. R., and Bochow, A. J. Regional lymph node metastases and the level of invasion of primary melanoma. Cancer 37:199–201, 1976. [16, 17]

Holmes, E. C., Moseley, H. S., Morton, D. L., Clark, W., Robinson, D., and Urist, M. M. A rational approach to the surgical management of melanoma. Ann. Surg. 186:481–490, 1977. [16, 17]

Hornsey, S. The radiosensitivity of melanoma cells in culture. Br. J. Radiol. 45:158, 1972. [19]

Hornung, M. O., and Krementz, E. T. Specific tissue and tumor responses of chimpanzees following immunization against human melanoma. Surgery 75:477–486, 1974. [10]

Hughes, L. E. The place of frozen section in the practical management of melanoma. Br. J. Surg. 62:840–844, 1975. [22]

Husa, A., and Höckerstedt, K. Anorectal malignant melanoma. Acta Chir. Scand. 140:68–72, 1974. [3]

Hutchinson, J. Melanosis often not black: melanotic whitlow. Br. Med. J. 1:491, 1886. [4, 9]

Hutchinson, J. On cancer. Arch. Surg. 4:61–65, 1892. [4]

Hutchinson, J. On tissue dotage. Arch. Surg. (London) 3:315–322, 1892. [4]

Hutchinson, J. Lentigo-melanosis. A further report. Arch. Surg. (London) 5:253–256, 1894. [4]

Hutchinson, J. President's address at the Third International Congress of Dermatology. Arch. Surg. (London) 7:297–317, 1896. [4]

Huvos, A. G., Miké, V., Donnellan, M. J., Seemayer, T., and Strong, W. E. Prognostic factors in cutaneous melanoma of the head and neck. Am. J. Pathol. 71:33–48, 1973. [4, 14]

Huvos, A. G., Shah, J. P., and Goldsmith, H. S. A clinicopathologic study of amelanotic melanoma. Surg. Gynecol. Obstet. 135:917–920, 1972. [10, 14]

Huvos, A. G., Shah, J. P., and Miké, V. Prognostic factors in cutaneous malignant melanoma. Hum. Pathol. 5:347–357, 1974. [4, 14]

Hyde, J. N., and Montgomery, F. H. A Practical Treatise on Diseases of the Skin. Philadelphia and New York, Lea Brothers & Co., 1901, pp. 693–694, 711–712. [4]

Ironside, P., Pitt, T. T. E., and Rank, B. K. Malignant melanoma: Some aspects of pathology and prognosis. Aust. N. Z. J. Surg. 47:70–75, 1977. [14]

Jackson, G. T. The Ready Reference Handbook of Diseases of the Skin. New York and Philadelphia, Lea Brothers & Co., 1899, p. 487. [4]

Jackson, R. Myths of cutaneous malignant melanoma. Laval. Med. 42:921–925, 1971. [4]

Jackson, R., Williamson, G. S. and Beattie, W. G. Lentigo maligna and malignant melanoma. Can Med. Assoc. J., 95:846–851, 1966. [4]

Jochimsen, P. R., Pearlman, N. W., Lawton, R. L., and Platz, C. E. Melanoma of the skin of the breast: Therapeutic considerations based on six cases. Surgery 81:583–587, 1977. [16]

Johnson, F. D., and Jacobs, E. M. Chemotherapy of metastatic malignant melanoma. Experience with 73 patients. Cancer 27:1306–1312, 1971. [18A, 18B]

Jones, W. M., Jones Williams, W., Roberts, M. M., and Davies, K. Malignant melanoma of the skin: prognostic value of clinical features and the role of treatment in 111 cases. Br. J. Cancer 22:437–451, 1968. [4, 14, 15, 17, 20]

Jones Williams, W., Davies, K., Jones, W. M., and Roberts, M. M. Malignant melanoma of the skin: prognostic value of histology in 89 cases. Br. J. Cancer 22:452–460, 1968. [4, 14]

Jörgensen, G., and Lal, V. B. Serogenetic investigations on malignant melanomas with reference to the incidence of ABO system, Rh system, Gm, Inv, Hp and Gc systems. Humangenetik 15:227–231, 1972. [5]

Kahn, L. B., and Donaldson, R. C. Multiple primary melanoma. Case report and study of tumor growth in vitro. Cancer 25:1162–1169, 1970. [8]

Kakati, S., Song, S. Y., and Sandberg, A. A. Chromsomes and

causation of human cancer. XXII. Karyotypic changes in malignant melanoma. Cancer 40:1173-1181, 1977. [5]

Kaplan, A. M., Itabashi, H., Hanelin, L. G., and Lu, A. T. Neurocutaneous melanosis with malignant leptomeningeal melanoma. Arch. Neurol. 32:669-671, 1975. [7]

Kaplan, E. N. The risk of malignancy in large congenital nevi. Plast. Reconstr. Surg. 53:421-428, 1974. [7]

Kaposi, M. Pathologie und Therapie der Hautkrankheiten. Wein and Leipzig, Urban & Schwarzenberg, 1887, p. 881. [4]

Keyhani, A. Comparison of clinical behavior of melanoma of the hands and feet. A study of 283 patients. Cancer 40:3168-3176, 1977. [20]

Klauder, J. V., and Beerman, H.: Melanotic freckle (Hutchinson) Mélanose circonscrite précancéreuse (Dubreuilh). A. M. A. Arch. Derm. 71:2-10, 1955. [4]

Knutson, C. O., Hori, J. M., and Spratt, J. S., Jr. Melanoma. Curr. Probl. Surg., December 1971, pp. 1-55, [4, 5, 15, 20]

Konecný, M., and Krenarová, V. A contribution to the radiotherapy of malignant melanoma. Neoplasma 16:335, 1969. [19]

Konigsberg, H. A., and Gray, G. F.: Benign melanosis and malignant melanoma of penis and male urethra. Urology 7:323-326, 1976. [3]

Konrad, K., and Wolff, K. Pathogenesis of diffuse melanosis secondary to malignant melanoma. Br. J. Derm. 91:635-655, 1974. [4]

Koops, H. S., et al. Regional perfusion for recurrent malignant melanoma of the extremities. Am. J. Surg. 133:221-224, 1977. [18B]

Kopf, A. W. Host defenses against malignant melanoma. Hosp. Practice 6:116-124, 1971. [21]

Kopf, A. W. Immunotherapy for human malignant melanoma. South. Med. J. 68:495-503, 1975. [21]

Kopf, A. W., and Andrade, R. Benign juvenile melanoma. In: Year Book of Dermatology. Chicago, Year Book Medical Publishers, pp. 7-52, 1966. [6]

Kopf, A. W., Bart, R. S. and Rodriguez-Sains, R.: Malignant melanoma, a review. J. Dermat. Surg. Oncol., 3:41-125, 1977. [4, 17]

Kopf, A. W., Morrill, S. D., and Silberberg, I. Broad spectrum of leukoderma acquisitum centrifugum. Arch. Dermatol. 92:14-35, 1965. [10]

Kopf, A. W., Mintzis, M., and Bart, R. S. Diagnostic accuracy in malignant melanoma. Arch. Dermatol. 111:1291-1292, 1975. [3, 4, 15, 19, 22]

Kopf, A. W., Mintzis, M., Grier, W. R. N., Silvers, D. N., and Bart, R. S. Familial malignant melanoma. Cutis 17:873-876, 1976. [5]

Kopf, A. W., Bart, R. S., and Gladstein, A. H. Treatment of melanotic freckle with x-rays. Arch. Dermatol. 112:801-807, 1976. [19]

Kopf, A. W., et al. To do or not to do elective lymph-node dissections for certain malignant melanomas. J. Derm. Surg. Oncol. 4:493 and 497-498, 1978. [17]

Kornberg, R., and Ackerman, A. B. Pseudomelanoma: recurrent melanocytic nevus following partial surgical removal. Arch. Dermatol. 111:1588-1590, 1975. [4, 22]

Kornberg, R., Harris, M., and Ackerman, A. B. Epidermotropically metastatic malignant melanoma. Arch. Dermatol. 114:67-69, 1978. [4]

Korsch, A., Gartmann, H., and Steigleder, G. K. Primar multiple maligne Melanome mit ungewohnlich langem Verlauf. Z. Hautkr. 51:949-956, 1976. [8]

Kozlov, A. P., Akimov, A. A., Moskalik, K. G., and Perlsov, O. L. Antitumour effect of laser radiation. Acta Radiol. [Ther] (Stockh.) 12:241-256, 1973. [22]

Krebs, J. A., Roenigk, H. H., Deodhar, S. D., and Barna, B. Halo nevus: Competent surveillance of potential melanoma. Cleveland Clinic Quart. 43:11-15, 1976. [10]

Krementz, E. T. Node dissection for extremity melanoma? New Engl. J. Med. 297:627-730, 1977. [17]

Krementz, E. T., and Ryan, R. F. Chemotherapy of melanoma of the extremities by perfusion: fourteen years clinical experience. Ann. Surg. 175:900-917, 1972. [18B]

Kumer, L., and Lang, F. J. Die bösartigen Geschwulst der Haut. In Artz, L., and Zieler, K., eds. Die Haut- und Geschlechtskrankheiten, Vol. 2. Berlin, Urban & Schwarzenberg, 1935. [4]

Labandter, H., and Kaplan, I. Experience with a "continuous" laser in the treatment of suitable cutaneous conditions: Preliminary report. J. Dermatol. Surg. Oncol. 3(5):527-530, 1977. [22]

Labrecque, P. G., Hu, C. H., and Winkelmann, R. K. On the nature of desmoplastic melanoma. Cancer 38:1205-1213, 1976. [4]

Lamas, E., Lobato, R. D., Sotelo, T., Ricoy, J. R., and Castro, S. Neurocutaneous melanosis. Report of a case and review of the literature. Acta Neurochirurgica 36:93-105, 1977. [7]

Lamm, L. U., Kissmeyer-Nielsen, F., Kjerbye, K. E., et al. HL-A and ABO antigens and malignant melanoma. Cancer 33:1458-1461, 1974. [5]

Lancaster, H. O. Some geographical aspects of mortality from melanoma in europeans. Med. J. Aust. 1:1082-1087, 1956. [2]

Lane, N., Lattes, R., and Malm, J. Clinicopathological correlations in a series of 117 malignant melanomas of the skin of adults. Cancer 11:1025-1043, 1958. [4, 16, 17]

Lanier, V. C., Pickrell, K. L., and Georgiade, N. G. Congenital giant nevi: Clinical and pathological considerations. Plast. Reconstr. Surg. 58:48-54, 1976. [7]

Larsen, R. R., and Hill, G. J., II. Improved systemic chemotherapy for malignant melanoma. Am. J. Surg. 122:36-41, 1971. [18A]

Lederman, M. Radiotherapy of malignant melanomata of the eye. Br. J. Radiol. 34:21–42, 1961. [19]

Lee, J. A., and Merrill, J. M. Sunlight and the etiology of malignant melanomas: a synthesis. Med. J. Aust. 2:846–851, 1970. [2, 5]

Lee, J. A. H. The trend of mortality from primary malignant tumors of the skin. J. Invest. Dermatol. 59:445–448, 1973. [1]

Lee, J. A. H. Current evidence about the causes of malignant melanoma. Prog. Clin. Cancer 6:151–161, 1975. [1]

Lee, J. A. H., and Carter, A. P. Secular trends in mortality from malignant melanoma. J. Natl. Cancer Inst. 45:91–97, 1970. [1]

Lee, J. A. H., and Yongchaiyudha, S. Incidence of and mortality from malignant melanoma by anatomical site. J. Natl. Cancer Inst. 47:253–263, 1971. [5]

Lee, Y. T. N. Malignant melanoma: to biopsy or not to biopsy. CA 24:104–105, 1974. [15]

Lee, Y. N., Sparks, F. C., and Morton, D. L. Primary melanoma of the breast region. Ann. Surg. 185:17–22, 1977. [16]

Leppard, B., Sanderson, K. V., and Behan, F. Subungual malignant melanoma: difficulty in diagnosis. Br. Med. J. 1:310–312, 1974. [4, 9]

Lerman, R. I., Murray, D., O'Hara, J. M., Booher, R. J., and Foote, F. W., Jr. Malignant melanoma of childhood. A clinicopathologic study and a report of 12 cases. Cancer 25:436–449, 1970. [16]

Lerner, A. B., and Nordlund, J. J. Should vitiligo be induced in patients after resection of primary melanoma? Arch. Derm. 113:421, 1977.

Levene, A. Moles and melanoma: the pathological basis of clinical management. Proc. R. Soc. Med. 65:137–140, 1972. [19]

Lever, W. F. Histopathology of the Skin. Philadelphia, J. B. Lippincott Co., 1949, pp. 398–404. [4]

Lever, W. F. Pigmented nevi and malignant melanoma. In Histopathology of the Skin, 2d ed., Philadelphia, J. B. Lippincott Co., 1954, Chap. 25, p. 458. [4]

Lever, W. F. Histopathology of the Skin. Philadelphia, J. B. Lippincott Co., 3d ed., 1961, pp. 582–589. [4]

Lever, W. F. Histopathology of the Skin. Philadelphia, J. B. Lippincott Co., 4th ed., 1967, pp. 715–724. [4]

Lever, W. F. Histopathology of the Skin. Philadelphia, J. B. Lippincott Co., 5th ed., 1975, pp. 664–677. [4]

Lewin, K. Subungual epidermoid inclusions. Br. J. Dermatol. 81:671–675, 1969. [9]

Lewis, M. G. Malignant melanoma in Uganda. Br. J. Cancer 21:483–485, 1967. [2, 4]

Lewis, M. G. In Milton, G. W., McGovern, V. J., and Lewis, M. G. Malignant Melanoma of the Skin and Mucous Membrane. Edinburgh, London, and New York, Churchill Livingstone, 1977, pgs. 102–151. [21]

Lewis, M. G., and Copeman, P. W. M. Halo naevus—a frustrated malignant melanoma? Br. Med. J. 2:47–48, 1972. [10]

Lewis, M. G., and Kiryabwire, J. W. M. Aspects of behavior and natural history of malignant melanoma in Uganda. Cancer, 21:876–887, 1968. [4]

Leyden, J. J., Spott, D. A., and Goldschmidt, H. Diffuse and banded melanin pigmentation in nails. Arch. Dermatol. 105:548–550, 1972. [9]

Lieberman, A. N., and Shupack, J. L. Levodopa and melanoma. Neurology 24:340–343, 1974. [8, 22]

Lippman, M. M., Laster, W. R., Abbott, B. J., Venditti, J., and Baratta, M. Antitumor activity of macromomycin B (NSC 170105) against murine leukemias, melanoma, and lung carcinoma. Cancer Res. 35:939–945, 1975. [18A]

Lissner, J., and von Lieven, H. Die Strahlentherapie des malignen Melanoms. Chirurg. 45:362–365, 1974. [19]

Little, J. H. Histology and prognosis in cutaneous malignant melanoma. In: McCarthy, W. H., ed. Melanoma and Skin Cancer. Proceedings International Cancer Conference, Sydney, 1972, V.C.N., Blight, Government Printer, pp. 107–120. [3, 4, 10]

Little, J. H. Histology and prognosis of cutaneous melanoma. Prog. Clin. Cancer 6:163–176, 1975. [20]

Little, J. H., and Davis, N. C. Frozen section diagnosis of suspected malignant melanoma of the skin. Cancer 34:1163–1172, 1974. [4, 22]

Livingston, R. B., Einhorn, L. H., Bodey, G. P., Burgess, M. A., Freireich, E. J., and Gottlieb, J. A. COMB (cyclophosphamide, oncovin, methyl-CCNU, and bleomycin): a four-drug combination in solid tumors. Cancer 36:327–332, 1975. [18A]

London, D. A., Carter, D. M., and Condit, E. S. Effect of pigment on photomediated production of thymine dimers in cultured melanoma cells. J. Invest. Derm. 67:261–264, 1976. [2]

Lorenc, E., Wooldridge, W. E., and Huewe, D. A. The melanotic freckle of Hutchinson: Preliminary report. Cutis 16:485–486, 1975. [16]

Luce, J. K. Chemotherapy of malignant melanoma. Cancer 30:1604–1615, 1972. [18A, 18B]

Luce, J. K. Chemotherapy of melanoma. Semin. Oncol. 2:179–186, 1975. [18A]

Luce, J. K., McBride, C. M., and Frei, E. III. Melanoma. In: Holland, J. F. and Frei, E., eds. Cancer Medicine, Philadelphia, Lea & Febiger, 1973, pp. 1823–1843. [8, 13, 14]

Lund, R., and Ihned, M. Malignant melanoma, clinical and pathologic analysis of 93 cases—Is prophylactic lymph node dissection indicated? Surgery, 38:652, 1955. [3, 4]

Lupulescu, A., Pinkus, H., Birmingham, D. J., Usned, H. E., and Posch, J. L. Lentigo maligna of the fingertip. Arch. Derm. 107:717, 1973. [4, 9]

Lyall, D. Malignant melanoma in infancy. J.A.M.A. 202:1153, 1967. [6]

Lynch, H. T., Frichot, B. C., Lynch, P., Lynch, J., and Guirgis, H. A. Family studies of malignant melanoma and associated cancer. Surg. Gynecol. Obstet. 141:517–522, 1975. [5]

Macdonald, E. J. Epidemiology of melanoma. Prog. Clin. Cancer 6:139–149, 1975. [1]

MacKie, R. Cutaneous microscopy *in vivo* as an aid to preoperative assessment of pigmented lesions of the skin. Br. J. Plast. Surg. 25:123–129, 1972. [22]

MacKie, R. M., Carfrae, D. C., and Cochran, A. J. Assessment of prognosis in patients with malignant melanoma. Lancet 2: 455–456, 1972. [4, 14]

MacLeod, J. M. H., and Muende, I. Practical Handbook of the Pathology of the Skin: An Introduction to the Histology, Pathology, Bacteriology, and Mycology of the Skin with Special Reference to Technique. 2nd ed. Hagerstown, Maryland, Paul B. Hoeber, 1940, p. 321. [4]

Magnus, K. Incidence of malignant melanoma of the skin in Norway 1955–1970: variations in time and space and solar radiation. Cancer 32:1275–1286, 1973. [1, 2, 5]

Mark, G. J., Mihm, M. C., Liteplo, M. G., Reed, R. J. and Clark, W. H. Congenital melanocytic Nevi of the small and garment type: clinical, histologic and ultrastructural studies. Hum. Pathol. 4:395–418, 1973. [7]

Mason, T. J., et al. Atlas of Cancer Mortality for U.S. Counties: 1950–1969. DHEW Publication No. (NIH) 75-780, National Institutes of Health, Bethesda, Maryland, pp. 44–47 and 91–92. [1, 2]

Masson, P. My conception of cellular nevi. Cancer, 4:9–38, 1951. [4]

Mastrangelo, M. J., Bird, D., and Bellet, R. E. Critical review of previously reported clinical trials of cancer immunotherapy with non-specific immunopotentiators. Ann. NY Acad. Sci. 277: 94–123, 1976. [21]

Maurer, L. H., McIntyre, O. R., and Rueckert, F. Spontaneous regression of malignant melanoma: pathologic and immunologic study in a ten year survivor. Am. J. Surg. 127:397–403, 1974. [10, 11]

McBride, C. M., and Clark, R. L. Experience with 1-phenylalanine mustard dihydrochloride in isolation-perfusion of extremities for malignant melanoma. Cancer 28:1293–1296, 1972. [18B]

McBride, C. M., Sugarbaker, E. V., and Hickey, R. C. Prophylactic isolation-perfusion as the primary therapy for invasive malignant melanoma of the limbs. Ann. Surg. 182:316–324, 1975. [18B]

McCarthy, J. G., Haagensen, C. D., and Herter, F. P. The role of groin dissection in the management of melanoma of the lower extremity. Ann. Surg. 179:156–159, 1974. [16, 17]

McCarthy, L. Histopathology of Skin Diseases. St. Louis, C. V. Mosby Co., 1931, pp. 408–418. [4]

McCarthy, S. W., Palmer, A. A., Bale, P. M., and Hirst, E. Naevus cells in lymph nodes. Pathology 6:351–358, 1974. [11]

McGovern, V. J. The classification of melanoma and its relationship with prognosis. Pathology 2:85–98, 1970. [4, 14]

McGovern, V. J. Melanoma-growing patterns, multiplicity and regression. In: McCarthy, W. H., ed. Melanoma and Skin Cancer. Proceedings International Cancer Conference, Sydney, V.C.N. Blight, Government Printer, 1972, pp. 95–106. [10, 14]

McGovern, V. J. Spontaneous regression of melanoma. Pathology 7:91–99, 1975. [10, 11]

McGovern, V. J. Malignant Melanoma: Clinical and Histological Diagnosis. New York, Wiley, 1976. [3, 4]

McGovern, V. J., and Lane Brown, M. The Nature of Melanoma. Springfield, Illinois, C. C. Thomas, 1969. [3]

McGovern, V. J., Caldwell, R. A., Duncan, C. A., Finlay-Jones, L. R., Hardy, E. G., Hicks, J. D., Little, J. H., and Quinn, R. L. Moles and malignant melanoma: terminology and classification. Med. J. Aust. 1:123–125, 1967. [3, 4]

McGovern, V. J., Mihm, M. C., Jr., Bailly, C., Booth, J. C., Clark, W. H., Jr., Cochran, A. J., Hardy, E. G., Hicks, J. D., Levene, A., Lewis, M. G., Little, J. H., and Milton, G. W. The classification of malignant melanoma and its histologic reporting. Cancer 32:1446–1457, 1973. [3, 4, 14]

McKelvey, E. M., Luce, J. K., Talley, R. W., Hersh, E. M., Hewlett, J. S., and Moon, T. E. Combination chemotherapy with bis chloroethyl nitrosurca (BCNU), vincristine and dimethyl triazeno imidazole carboxamide (DTIC) in disseminated malignant melanoma. Cancer 39:1–4, 1977. [18A]

McLeod, G. R., Beardmore, G. L., Little, J. H., Quinn, R. L., and Davis, N. C. Results of treatment of 361 patients with malignant melanoma in Queensland. Med. J. Aust. 1:1211–1216, 1971. [4]

McLeod, G. R., Davis, N. C., Herron, J. et al. A retrospective survey of 498 patients with malignant melanoma. Surg. Gynecol. Obstet. 126:99–108, 1968. [17]

McLeod, G. R., Beardmore, G. L., Little, J. H., Quinn, R. L., and Davis, N. C. Results of treatment of 361 patients with malignant melanoma in Queensland. Med. J. Aust. 1:1211–1216, 1971. [2, 20]

McNeer, G., and Das Gupta, T. Prognosis in malignant melanoma. Surgery 56:512–518, 1964. [13, 20]

McPeak, C. J. Intralymphatic therapy with immune lymphocytes. Cancer 28:1126–1128, 1971. [10]

Mehnert, J. H. and Heard, J. L. Staging of malignant melanoma by depth of invasion: a proposed index to prognosis. Am. J. Surg. 110:168–176, 1965. [3, 4]

Menzer, L., Sabin, T., and Mark, V. H. Computerized axial tomography. Use in the diagnosis of dementia. J.A.M.A. 234: 754–757, 1975. [22]

Messeritsch, H. Multiple primäre melanome. Hautarzt 23:289, 1972. [10]

Meyer, H. W., and Gumport, S. L. Malignant melanoma: Appraisal of the disease and analysis of 105 cases. Surgery 138: 643–660, 1953. [16]

Miescher, G. Die Entstehung der bosartigen Melanome der Haut. Virchows Arch., 264:86, 1927. [4]

Miescher, G. Präanceröses Vorstadium des Melanoms, präcancerose Melanose. In Jadassohn, J., ed. Handbuch der Haut und Geschlechtskrankheiten, Vol. 12, Pt. 3, Berlin, Springer-Verlag, 1933, p. 1085. [4]

Miescher, G., Haberlin, L., and Guggenheim, L. Über fleckförmige Alterspigmentierungen: Ihre Beziehungen zur melanotischen Präcancerose und zur senilen Warze. Arch. Dermat. Syph., 174:105–125, 1936. [4]

Mihm, M. C., Jr. Melanoma cure possible if detected in its intraepidermal proliferative phase. Dermat. News 10(8)8, 1977. [4]

Mihm, M. C. Jr., Clark, W. H., Jr., and From, L. The clinical diagnosis, classification and histogenetic concepts of the early stages of cutaneous malignant melanoma. N. Engl. J. Med. 284:1078–1082, 1971. [3]

Mihm, M. C., Jr., Clark, W. H., and Reed, R. J. The clinical diagnosis of malignant melanoma. Semin. Oncol. 2:105–118, 1975. [4]

Mihm, M. C., Jr., and Fitzpatrick, T. B.: Early detection of malignant melanoma. Cancer 37:597–603, 1976. [3, 4]

Mihm, M. C., Jr., Fitzpatrick, T. B., Lane Brown, M. M., Raker, J. W., Malt, R. A., and Kaiser, J. S. Early detection of primary cutaneous malignant melanoma. A color atlas. N. Engl. J. Med. 289:989–996, 1973. [3, 4]

Mihm, M. C. Jr., Clark, W. H. Jr., and Reed, R. J. The clinical diagnosis of malignant melanoma. Semin. Oncol. 2:105–118, 1975. [3]

Milder, M. S., Frankel, R. S., Bulkley, G. B., Ketcham, A. S., and Johnston, G. S. Gallium-67 scintigraphy in malignant melanoma. Cancer 32:1350–1356, 1973. [22]

Millikan, L. E., Hook, R. R., and Manning, P. J. Gross and ultrastructural studies in a new melanoma model: the Sinclair swine. Yale J. Biol. Med. 46:631–645, 1973. [10]

Millikan, L. E., Boylon, J. L., Hook, R. R., and Manning, P. J. Melanoma in Sinclair swine: a new animal model. J. Invest. Dermatol. 62:20–30, 1974. [10]

Milne, J. A. An Introduction to the Diagnostic Histopathology of the Skin. Baltimore, The Williams and Wilkins Co., 1972, pp. 291–316. [4]

Milton, G. W., Lane Brown, M. M., and Gilder, M. Malignant melanoma with an occult primary lesion. Br. J. Surg. 54:651–658, 1967. [10, 11]

Mintzis, M. J., Berger, A. P., Greenwald, E., Greenwald, E., and Golomb, F. Malignant melanoma in spouses. Cancer 42:804–807, 1978. [5]

Mishima, Y. Melanosis circumscripta precancerose (Dubreuilh). A non-nevoid premelanoma distinct from junction nevus. J. Invest. Dermat. 34:361–375, 1960. [4]

Mishima, Y., and Matsunaka, M.: Pagetoid premalignant melanosis and melanoma: Differentiation from Hutchinson's melanotic freckle. J. Invest. Derm. 65:434–440, 1975. [3]

Mitchell, M. S., Mokyr, M. B., and Davis, J. M. Effect of chemotherapy and immunotherapy on tumor-specific immunity in melanoma. J. Clin. Invest. 59:1017–1026, 1977. [18A]

Milton, G. W., McGovern, V. J., and Lewis, M. G. Malignant Melanoma of the Skin and Mucous Membrane. Churchill Livingstone, Edinburgh, London, and New York, 1977. [1, 11, 14, 17, 21]

Moertel, C. G. Multiple Primary Malignant Neoplasms: Their Incidence and Significance. Recent Results in Cancer Research: (7) New York, Springer, 1966. [8]

Mohs, F. E. Chemosurgery for melanoma. Arch. Derm. 113:285–291, 1977. [17]

Moon, J. H., Gailani, S., Cooper, M. R., Hayes, D. M., Rege, V. E., Blom, J., Falkson, G., Maurice, P., Brunner, K., Glidewell, O., and Holland, J. F. Comparison of the combination of 1,3-bis(2-chloroethyl)-1-nitrosourea (BCNU) and vincristine with two dose schedules of 5-(3,3-dimethyl-1-triazeno) imidazole 4-carboxamide (DTIC) in the treatment of disseminated malignant melanoma. Cancer 35:368–371, 1975. [18A]

Moore, C., and Iverson, P. C. Xeroderma pigmentosum: showing common skin cancers plus melanocarcinoma controlled by surgery. Cancer 7:377–382, 1954. [2]

Morahan, P. S., Munson, J. A., Baird, L. G., Kaplan, A. M., and Ragelson, W. Antitumor action of pyran copolymer and tilorone against Lewis lung carcinoma and B-16 melanoma. Cancer Res. 34:506–511, 1974. [18A]

Morgan, L. R., Lolley, D., Maddox, B., Samuels, M., and Krementz, E. Urine homovanillic acid and tissue DOPA oxidase in patients with melanoma. Cancer 33:1601–1606, 1974. [22]

Morton, D. L., Eibler, F. R., Holmes, E. C., Sparks, F. C., and Ramming, K. BCG immunotherapy as a systemic adjunct to surgery in malignant melanoma. Med. Clin. North Am. 60:431–439, 1976. [21]

Movshovitz, M., and Modan, B. Role of sun exposure in the etiology of malignant melanoma: epidemiologic inference. J. Natl. Cancer Inst. 51:777–779, 1973. [2, 5]

Mukherji, B., Nathanson, L., and Clark, D. A. Studies of humoral and cell-mediated immunity in human melanoma. Yale J. Biol. Med. 46:681–692, 1973. [5]

Mundth, E. D., Guralnick, E. A., and Raker, J. W. Malignant melanoma: A clinical study of 427 cases. Ann. Surg. 162:15–28, 1965. [14]

Naidoff, M. A., Bernardino, V. B., and Clark, W. H. Melanocytic lesions of the eyelid skin. Am. J. Ophthal. 82:371–382, 1976. [3]

Nathanson, L. Spontaneous regression of malignant melanoma: A review of the literature on incidence, clinical features, and possible mechanisms. Natl. Cancer Inst. Monogr. 44:67–76, 1976. [11]

Nathanson, L., Wolter, J., Horton, J., Colsky, J., Schnider, B. I., and Schilling, A. Characteristics of prognosis and response to an imidazole carboxamide in malignant melanoma. Clin. Pharmacol. Ther. 12:955-962, 1971. [18A, 18B]

Nicholls, E. M. Development and elimination of pigmented moles and the anatomical distribution of primary malignant melanoma. Cancer 32:191-195, 1973. [7]

Niven, J., and Lubin, J. Pedunculated malignant melanoma. Arch. Derm. 111:755-856, 1975. [4]

Nordlund, J. J. Yale J. Biol. Med. 48:403-407, 1975. [3]

Norvell, S. T., McCleave, J. J., Bodurth, A. J., and Irwin, A. C. Prophylactic node dissection for malignant melanoma. Canad. J. Surg. 20:429-435, 1977. [17]

Oberfield, R. A. Current status of regional arterial infusion chemotherapy. Med. Clin. North Am. 59:411-424, 1975. [18B]

Ollstein, R. N., Kaplan, H. S., and Crikelair, G. F. Is there a malignant freckle? Cancer 19:767-775, 1966. [4]

Olsen, G. The Malignant Melanoma of the Skin: New Theories Based on a Study of 500 Cases. The Finsen Institute and Radium Centre. Copenhagen, Aarhuus Stiftsbogtrykkerie, 1966.

Orkin, M., Frichot, B. C., and Zelickson, A. S. Cerebriform intradermal nevus. Arch. Derm. 110:575-582, 1974. [7]

Ormsby, O. S., and Montgomery, H. Diseases of the Skin, 8th ed. Philadelphia, Lea and Febiger, 1954, pp. 864-898. [4]

Pack, G. T. End results in the treatment of malignant melanoma: a later report. Surgery 46:447-460, 1959. [8]

Pack, G. T. Functions and dysfunctions of the surgical pathologist. Surgery 52:752-755, 1962. [4]

Pack, G. T. The pigmented mole and the malignant melanoma. CA 12:11-26, 1962. [5]

Pack, G. T., and Davis, J. The pigmented mole. Post-Grad. Med. 27:370-382, 1960. [7]

Pack, G. T., Gerber, D. M., and Scharnagel, I. M. End results in the treatment of malignant melanoma: A Report of 1190 cases. Ann. Surg. 136:905-911, 1952. [4, 16]

Pack, G. T., and Oropeza, R. Subungual melanoma. Surg. Gynecol. Obstet. 124:571-582, 1967. [4, 9]

Papachristov, D., and Furtner, J. G. Comparison of lymphedema following incontinuity and discontinuity groin dissection. Ann. Surg. 185:13-16, 1977. [17]

Parsons, P. G., Klucis, E., Goss, P. D., Pope, J. H., Little, J. H., and Davis, N. C.: Oncornavirus-like particles in malignant melanoma and control biopsies. Int. J. Cancer 18:757-763, 1976. [5]

Pawelek, J. M. Factors regulating growth and pigmentation of melanoma cells. J. Invest. Dermatol. 66:201-209, 1976. [2]

Pearson, D. Radiotherapy in malignant melanoma. Proc. R. Soc. Med. 67:96-97, 1974. [19]

Pemberton, O. Observations on the History, Pathology and Treatment of Cancerous Disease, Part I, Melanosis. London, J. Churchill, 1858. [4]

Perlin, E., Engeler, J., Reid, J. W., Lokey, J. L., and Kostinas, J. Treatment of malignant melanoma with vinblastine (NSC-49842), procarbazine (NSC-77213), and actinomycin D (NSC-3053). Cancer Chemother. Rep. 59:767-768, 1975. [18A]

Perrot, H., Ortonne, J. P., and Schmitt, D. Vitiliginous achromia with malignant melanoma. Arch. Dermatol. Res. 257:247-253, 1977. [10]

Pers, M. Nevus pigmentosa giganticus. Indications for removal. Ugeskr. Laeger 125:613-619, 1963. [7]

Peterson, N. C., Bodenham, D. C., and Lloyd, O. C. Malignant melanomas of the skin. Br. J. Plast. Surg. 15, 45-94, 1962. [4]

Petratos, M. A., Kopf, A. W., Bart, R. S., Grisewood, E. N., and Gladstein, A. H. Treatment of melanotic freckle with x-rays. Arch. Dermatol. 106:189-194, 1972. [19]

Pinkus, H., and Mehregan, A. H. A Guide to Dermatohistopathology. New York, Appleton-Century-Crofts, Meredity Corp., 1969, pp. 362-366. [4]

Polk, H. C., Jr., and Linn, B. S. Selective regional lymphadenectomy for melanoma: a mathematical aid to clinical judgment. Ann. Surg. 174:402-413, 1971. [17]

Price, N. M., Rywlin, A. M., and Ackerman, A. B. Histologic criteria for the diagnosis of superficial spreading malignant melanoma: Formulated on the basis of proven metastatic lesions. Cancer 38:2434-2441, 1976. [4]

Reed, R. J. Acral lentiginous melanoma. In: New Concepts in Surgical Pathology of the Skin. New York, Wiley, 1976, pp. 89-90. [3, 4, 16]

Reed, W. B., Becker, S. W., Sr., Becker, S. W., Jr., and Nickel, W. R. Giant pigmented nevi, melanoma, and leptomeningeal melanocytosis. Arch. Dermatol. 91:100-119, 1965. [7]

Reese, A. B. Tumors of the Eye 2nd ed. New York, Harper and Row, 1963, pg. 335-345. [3]

Regnier, R. Role de la radiotherapie dans le traitment des melanomes malins du tronc et des membres. Brux. Med. 55:423-428, 1975. [19]

Reimer, R. R., Clark, W. H., Greene, M. H., Ainsworth, A. M., and Fraumeni, J. F. Precursor lesions in familial melanoma: A new genetic preneoplastic syndrome. J.A.M.A. 239:744-746, 1978. [4, 5, 8]

Resseguie, L. J., Marks, S. J., Winkelmann, R. K., and Kurtland, L. T. Malignant melanoma in the resident population of Rochester, Minnesota. Mayo Clin. Proc. 52:191-195, 1977. [1]

Ridley, C. M. Giant halo naevus with spontaneous resolution. Trans. St. Johns Hosp. Dermatol. Soc. 60:54-58, 1974. [10]

Ridolfi, R. L., Rosen, P. P., and Thaler, H. Nevus cell aggregates associated with lymph nodes: Estimated frequency and clinical significance. Cancer 39:164-171, 1977. [11]

Rippey, J. J., Rippey, E., and Giraud, R. M. A. Pathology of malignant melanoma of the skin in black Africans. South Afr. Med. J. 49:789–792, 1975. [3]

Robbins, J. H., Kraemer, K. H., Lutzner, M. A., Festoff, B. W., and Coon, H. G. Xeroderma pigmentosum: an inherited disease with sun sensitivity, multiple cutaneous neoplasms, and abnormal DNA repair. Ann. Intern. Med. 80:221–248, 1974. [2]

Robertson, M. G. Malignant melanoma in husband and wife. J.A.M.A. 217:1553, 1971. [5]

Robinson, E., Wajsbort, J., Hirshowitz, B. Levodopa and malignant melanoma. Arch. Pathol. 95:213, 1973. [8]

Robinson, M. J. Familial melanomas. J.A.M.A. 220:277, 1972. [5]

Rode, I. Clinical and Radiobiological Properties of Melanoblastoma. Budapest, Akademiai Kiado, 1968.

Roenigk, H. H., Doedhar, S., St. Jacques, R., and Burdick, K. Immunotherapy of malignant melanoma with vaccinia virus. Arch. Dermatol. 109:668–673, 1974. [10]

Rorsman, H., Rosengren, A.-M., and Rosengren, E. Determination of 5-S-cysteinyldopa in melanomas with a fluorometric method. Yale J. Biol. Med. 46:516–522, 1973. [22]

Rosenberg, S. A., and Rapp, H. J. Intralesional immunotherapy of melanoma with BCG. Med. Clin. N. Am. 60:419–430, 1976. [21]

Roses, D. F., Harris, M. N., and Gumport, S. L. Letter to the Editor. New Engl. J. Med. 298:223, 1978. [17]

Roses, D. F., Harris, M. N., Stern, J. S., and Gumport, S. L. Cutaneous melanoma of the breast (unpublished). [16]

Roth, J. A., Eilber, F. R., Bennett, L. R., and Morton, D. L. Radionuclide photoscanning: usefulness in preoperative evaluation of melanoma patients. Arch. Surg. 110:1211–1212, 1975. [22]

Roth, W. G. Vitiligo nach Röntgenbestrahlung Multipler Melanommetastasen. Hautzart 19:178–180, 1968. [10]

Sachs, W., MacKee, G. M., Schwartz, O. D., and Pierson, H. S. Junction nevus-nevocarcinoma (the so-called melanoma group). J.A.M.A. 135:216–218, 1947. [4]

Salem, L. E., and Travezan, R. Malignant melanoma of the head and neck. Int. Surg. 58:790–792, 1973. [20]

Savlov, E. D., Hall, T. C., and Oberfield, R. A. Intra-arterial therapy of melanoma with dimethyl triazeno imidazole carboxamide (NSC-45388). Cancer 28:1161–1164, 1971. [18B]

Schmoeckel, C., and Braun-Falco, O. The prognostic index in malignant melanoma, Arch. Dermatol. 114:871–873, 1978. [4,14]

SchraffordtKoops, H., Oldhoff, J., van der Ploeg, E., Vermey, A., Eibergen, R., and Beekhuis, H. Some aspects of the treatment of primary malignant melanoma of the extremities by isolated regional perfusion. Cancer 39:27–33, 1977. [18B]

Scherer, R., and Makoski, H. B. Die Strahlentherapie des malignen Melanoms. Langenbechs Arch. Chir. 342:545–548, 1976. [19]

Schultheis, W., Peter, H. H., Deicher, H. Gm(1) and Gm(2) immunoglobulin allotypes in patients with malignant melanoma. Humangenetik 28:177–181, 1975. [5]

Scotto, J., Kopf, A. W., and Urbach, F. Non-melanoma skin cancer among caucasians in four areas of the United States. Cancer 34:1333–1338, 1974. [1, 2]

Scotto, J., Fears, T. R., and Gori, G. B. Measurements of Ultraviolet Radiation in the United States and Comparisons with Skin Cancer Data. National Cancer Institute, Division of Cancer Cause and Prevention, National Institutes of Health, DHEW No. (NIH) 76-1039, 1976. [2]

Scotto, J., Fraumeni, J. F., and Lee, J. A. H. Melanomas of the eye and other noncutaneous sites: epidemiologic aspects. J. Natl. Cancer Inst. 56:489–491, 1976. [2]

Sealy, R., Hockly, J., and Shepstone, B. The treatment of malignant melanoma with cobalt and hyperbaric oxygen. Clin. Radiol. 25:211–215, 1974. [19]

Seigler, H. F., and Fetter, B. F.: Current management of melanoma. Ann. Surg. 186:1–12, 1977. [16, 21]

Shah, J. P., and Goldsmith, H. S. Incontinuity versus discontinuous lymph node dissection for malignant melanoma. Cancer 26:610–614, 1970. [16]

Shapiro, L., and Kopf, A. W. Leukoderma acquisitum centrifugum. Arch. Dermatol. 92:64–68, 1965. [10]

Shaw, H. W., McCarthy, W. H., and Milton, G. W. Changing trends in mortality from malignant melanoma. Med. J. Aust. 2:77–80, 1977. [20]

Shingleton, W. W. Perfusion chemotherapy for recurrent melanoma of extremity: a progress report. Ann. Surg. 169:969–973, 1969. [16, 18B]

Shingleton, W. W., Seigler, H. F., Stocks, L. H., and Downs, R. W. Management of recurrent melanoma of the extremity. Cancer 35:574–579, 1975. [16]

Shirakawa, S., Luce, J. K., Tannock, I., and Frei, E., III. Cell proliferation in human melanoma. J. Clin. Invest. 49:1188–1199, 1970. [18A]

Shiu, M. H., Schottenfeld, D., Maclean, B., and Fortner, J. G. Adverse effect of pregnancy on melanoma: a reappraisal. Cancer 37:181–187, 1976. [14]

Shoemaker, J. V. A Practical Treatise on Diseases of the Skin. Philadelphia, F. A. Davis Co., 1909, pp. 766–767. [4]

Siciliano, M. J., and Perlmutter, A. Maternal effect on development of melanoma in hybrid fish of the genus *Xiphophorous*. J. Natl. Cancer Inst. 49:415–421, 1972. [5]

Silberberg, I., Kopf, A. W., and Gumport, S. L. Diffuse melanosis in malignant melanoma. Arch. Derm. 97:671–677, 1968. [3, 4]

Sim, F. H., Taylor, W. F., Ivins, J. C., Pritchard, D. J., and Soule, E. H. A prospective randomized study of the efficacy of routine prophylactic lymphadenectomy in management of malignant melanoma: Preliminary results. Cancer. 41:948–956, 1978. [17]

Simons, J. N. Malignant melanoma of the head and neck. Am. J. Surg. 124:485–488, 1972. [20]

Singal, D. P., Bent, P. B., McCulloch, P. B., Blajchman, M. A., and MacLaren, R. G. C. HL-A antigens in malignant melanoma. Transplantation 18:186, 1974. [5]

Sinha, B. K., and Buntine, D. W. Prognosis of cutaneous malignant melanoma: a clinicopathological study. Can. J. Surg. 17:328–334 1974. [4, 14, 17, 20]

Skibba, J. L., Pinckley, J., Gilbert, E. F., and Johnson, R. O. Multiple primary melanoma following administration of levodopa. Arch. Pathol. 93:556–561, 1972. [8]

Skov-Jensen, T., Hastrup, J., and Lambrethsen, E. Malignant melanoma in children. Cancer 19:620–626, 1966. [6]

Smart, C. R., and Carle, B. N. Malignant melanoma in husband and wife. J.A.M.A. 232:705–706, 1975. [5]

Smith, J. L., and Stehlin, J. S. Spontaneous regression of primary malignant melanomas with regional metastases. Cancer 18:1399–1415, 1965. [10]

Snyder, D. S., and May, M. Ability of PABA to protect mammalian skin from ultraviolet light-induced skin tumors and actinic damage. J. Invest. Dermatol. 65:543–546, 1975. [2]

Sober, A. J. Immunology and cutaneous malignant melanoma. Int. J. Dermatol. 15:1–18, 1976. [21]

Sober, A. J., and Wick, M. M. Levodopa therapy and malignant melanoma. JAMA 240:554–555, 1978. [22]

Solly, E. Melanotic carcinoma and melanomata of doubtful character. Trans. Pathol. Soc. Lond. 41:315–319, 1890. [4]

Southwick, H. W. Malignant melanoma. Role of node dissection reappraisal. Cancer 37:202–205, 1976. [17]

Spitler, L. Personal communication, February, 1975. [5]

Spratt, J. S. Symposium on melanoma. Contemporary Surg. 9:45–72, 1976. [18A]

Stehlin, J. S., Jr. Malignant melanoma: an appraisal. Surgery 64:1149–1157, 1968. [16, 17, 20]

Stehlin, J. S., Smith, J. L., Jing, B. S., and Sherrin, D. Melanomas of the extremities complicated by in-transit metastases. Surg. Gynecol. Obstet. 122:314, 1966. [16]

Stehlin, J. S., Jr., Hafström, L., and Greeff, P. J. Experience with infusion and resection in cancer of the liver. Surg. Gynecol. Obstet. 138:855–863, 1974. [22]

Stehlin, J. S., Giovanella, B. C., Ipolyi, P. D., Muenz, L. R., and Anderson, R. F. Results of hyperthermic perfusion for melanoma of the extremities. Surg. Gynecol. Obstet. 140:339–348, 1975. [9, 18B]

Stevenson, H. E., Terry, C. W., Lukens, J. N., Shively, J. A., Busby, W. E., Stoeckle, H. E., and Esterly, N. A. Immunologic factors in human melanoma "metastatic" to products of gestation (with exchange transfusion of infant to mother). Surgery 69:515–522, 1971. [6]

Stolinsky, D. C., Jacobs, E. M., Braunwald, J., and Bateman, J. R. Further study of trimethylcolchicinic Acid, methyl ether, d-tartrate (TMCA: NSC-36354) in patients with malignant melanoma. Cancer Chemother. Rep. 56:263–265, 1972. [18A]

Storck, H., and Ott, F. Zu Verlauf und Therapie der malignen Melanome. Schweiz, Med. Wschr. 106:1871–1877, 1976. [19]

Stout, A. P.: Relationship of malignant melanoma (nevocarcinoma) to extramammary Paget's disease. Am. J. Cancer 33:196–204, 1938. [4]

Suffin, S. C., Waisman, J., and Clark, W. H., Jr. Congruence of diagnosis of malignant melanoma. Lab. Invest. 32:436, 1975. [4]

Suffin, S. C., Waisman, J., Clark, W. H., and Morton, D. L. Comparison of the classification by microscopic level (stage) of malignant melanoma by three independent groups of pathologists. Cancer 40:3112–3114, 1977. [3]

Sugarbaker, E. V., and McBride, C. M. Melanoma of the trunk: the results of surgical excision and anatomic guidelines for predicting nodal metastases. Surgery 80:22–30, 1976. [16, 17]

Sugarbaker, E. V. and McBride, C. M. Survival and regional disease control after isolation perfusion for invasive stage I melanoma of the extremities. Cancer 37:188–198, 1976. [18B]

Sulzberger, M. B., Kopf, A. W., and Witten, V. H. Pigmented nevi, benign juvenile melanoma and circumscribed precancerous melanosis. Postgrad. Med. 26:617–631, 1959. [3, 4]

Sumner, W. C. Spontaneous regression of melanoma. Cancer 6:1040–1043, 1953. [10]

Sumner, W. C., and Foraker, A. G. Spontaneous regression of human melanoma. Cancer 13:79–81, 1960. [10]

Sutherland, E. M., Klopfer, H. W., Mausell, P. W. A., and Krementz, E. T. Familial Melanoma. In: Proceedings of the IX International Pigment Cell Conference, Houston, 1975, p. 60. [5]

Sutton, R. L. Diseases of the Skin. St. Louis, the C. V. Mosby Co., 1928, pp. 828–832. [4]

Tapernoux, B., and Hessler, C. Thermography of malignant melanomas. J. Dermatol. Surg. Oncol. 3:299–302, 1977. [22]

Tarpley, J. L., Chretien, P. B., Rogentine, N., Twomey, P. L., and Dellon, A. L. Histocompatibility antigens and solid malignant neoplasms. Arch. Surg. 110:269–271, 1975. [5]

Terz, J. J., Curutchet, H. P., and Lawrence, W., Jr. Analysis of cell kinetics of human solid tumors. Cancer 28:1100–1110, 1971. [19]

Third National Cancer Survey: Incidence Data. National Cancer Institute Monograph 41. U.S. Department of Health, Education and Welfare, Public Health Service, National Institutes of Health, National Cancer Institute, Bethesda, Maryland. DHEW Publication No. (NIH) 75-787, 1975. [1, 2]

Tonak, J., Hermanek, P., Hornstein, O. P., and Weidner, F.

Therapie des malignen Melanomes der klinischen Stadien I und II. Dtsch. Med. Wochenschr. 101:435–440, 1976. [3, 20]

Townsend, R. N., Banda, P. W., and Marton, L. J. Polyamines in malignant melanoma: Urinary excretion and disease progress. Cancer 38:2088–2092, 1976. [22]

Trapeznikov, N. N., Raushenbakh, M. O., Ivanova, V. D., and Yavorsky, V. V. Clinical evaluation of a method of quantitative determination of homovanillic acid for the estimation of degree of tumor dissemination process in melanoma of the skin. Cancer 36:2064–2068, 1975. [22]

Trapl, J., Palecek, L., Ebel, J., and Kucara, M. Origin and development of skin melanoblastoma on the basis of 300 cases. Acta Derm. Venereol. 44:377–380, 1964. [4]

Trapl, J., Palecek, L., Ebel, J., and Kucera, M. Tentative new classification of melanoma of the skin. Acta. Derm. Venereol. 46:443–446, 1966. [4]

Trozak, D. J., Rowland, W. D., and Hu, F. Metastatic malignant melanoma in prepubertal children. Pediatr. Clinician 55: 191–204, 1975. [6]

Twigg, H. L., Axelbaum, S. P., and Schellinger, D. Computerized body tomography with the ACTA scanner. J.A.M.A. 234: 314–317, 1975. [22]

Unna, P. G. The Histopathology of the Disease of the Skin. New York, MacMillan and Co., 1896, pp. 745–755. [4]

Urteaga, B., and Pack, G. T. On the antiquity of melanoma. Cancer 19:607–619, 1966. [4]

Valensi, Q. J. Desmoplastic malignant melanoma: A report of two additional cases. Cancer 39:286–292, 1977. [22]

Varga, J. M., Asato, N., Lande, S., and Lerner, A. B. Melanotropindaunomycin conjugate shows receptor-mediated cytotoxicity in cultured murien melanoma cells. Nature 267:56–58, 1977. [22]

Veronesi, U., Cascinelli, N., and Preda, F. Prognosis of malignant melanoma according to regional metastases. Am. J. Roentgenol. Radium Ther. Nucl. Med. 111:301–309, 1971. [4, 13, 14]

Veronesi, V., et al. Inefficacy of immediate node dissection in Stage I melanoma of the limbs. New Engl. J. Med. 297:627–630, 1977. [16, 17]

Virchow, R. Die pathologischen pigmente. Arch. Pathol. Anat. Physiol. Virchows 1:379–404, 1847. [4]

Vogel, C. L., Comis, R. Ziegler, J. L., and Kiryabwire, J. W. M. Clinical trials of 5-(3,3-dimethyl-1-triazeno) imidazole-4-carboxamide (NSC-45388) given intravenously in the treatment of malignant melanoma in Uganda. Cancer Chemother. Rep. 55:143–149, 1971. [18A]

Voglino, A. La melanosi de Dubreuilh. Osservazioni su due casi a localizzazione rara. Chronica Dermatol. 2:728–730, 1971. [4]

Wagner, D. E. A retrospective study of regional perfusion for melanoma. Arch. Surg. 111:410–413, 1976. [18B]

Wallace, D. C., Beardmore, G. L., and Exton, L. A. Familial malignant melanoma. Ann. Surg. 177:15–20, 1973. [5, 8]

Wallace, D. C., Exton, L. A., and McLean, G. R. C. Genetic factors in malignant melanoma. Cancer 27:1262–1266, 1971. [5]

Walton, R. G., Jacobs, A. H., and Cox, A. J.: Pigmented lesions in newborn infants. Br. J. Derm. 95:389–396, 1976. [7]

Wanebo, H. J. Letter to the Editor. New Engl. J. Med. 298:222, 1978. [17]

Wanebo, H. J., Fortner, J. G., Woodruff, J., Maclean, B., and Binkowski, E. Selection of the optimum surgical treatment of stage I melanoma by depth of microinvasion: use of the combined microstage technique (Clark-Breslow). Ann. Surg. 182:302–315, 1975. [4]

Wanebo, H. J., Woodruff, J. and Fortner, J. G. Malignant melanoma of the extremities: a clinicopathologic study using levels of invasion (microstage). Cancer 35:666–676, 1975. [3, 4, 16, 17, 20]

Wanebo, H. J., Fortner, J. G., Woodruff, J., MacLean, B., and Binkowski, E. Selection of the optimum surgical treatment of stage I melanoma by depth of microinvasion: use of the combined microstage technique (Clark-Breslow). Ann. Surg. 182:302–315, 1975. [14, 20]

Wasserman, T. H., Slavik, M., and Carter, S. K. Clinical comparison of the nitrosoureas. Cancer 36:1258–1268, 1975. [18A]

Wayte, D. M., and Helwig, E. B. Melanotic freckle of Hutchinson. Cancer 21:892–911, 1968. [4]

Webster, J. P., Stevenson, T. W., and Stout, A. P. The surgical treatment of malignant melanomas of the skin. Surg. Clin. N. Am. 24:319, 1944. [4]

Wilkinson, T. S., and Paletta, F. X. Malignant melanoma: current concepts. Am. Surg. 35:301–309, 1969. [17]

Wiskemann, A. Rontgentherapie der Praekanzerosen der Haut. Z. Hautkr. 8:461–462, 1977. [19]

Withers, H. R., and Harter, D. Radiotherapy in the management of malignant melanoma. In Neoplasms of the Skin and Melanomas. Chicago, Year Book Publishers, 1976, pgs. 453–459. [19]

Wood, W. C., Cosimi, A. B., Carey, R. W., and Kaufman, S. D. Randomized trial of adjuvant therapy for "high risk" primary malignant melanoma. Surgery 83:677–681, 1978. [18A]

Young, R. C., Cavellos, G. P., Chabner, B. A., Schein, P. S., Brereton, H. D., and DeVita, V. T. Treatment of malignant melanoma with methyl CCNU. Clin. Pharmacol. Ther. 15: 617–622, 1974. [18A]

INDEX

(Page numbers in bold type indicate portions of book in which the subject is discussed in greatest detail. Page numbers in italics refer to sections of the book which deal with the histologic features.)

A

Acral-lentiginous malignant melanoma, **9**, *29, 39, 41,*
"Active" junction nevus, *115*
Adjuvant immunotherapy, 204
Age, 1
Alkaline phosphatase, 210
Amelanotic malignant melanoma, 19, 173
Analogies between cutaneous malignant melanoma and other neoplasms of the skin, *105*
Anatomical distribution, 5, 9, 16
Angiosarcoma, *84*
Animal melanomas, 149
Antigens, 204
Atypical melanocytic hyperplasia 9, *121*
Autopsy findings, 169

B

Balloon cells, *51*
Basal-cell carcinoma, 4, 5
BCG (Bacillus Calmette Guérin), 204
Benign juvenile melanoma (*see* Nevus of large spindle and/or epitheloid cells)
Bibliography, general, **218**
Biopsy
  excisional, **177**
  incisional, **177**
  of malignant melanoma, *135,* **177**
B-K moles, *53,* 148–149
Blacks, **1**, 20
Blue nevi, *26, 79, 86*
  cellular, *84*
"Borderline" malignant melanoma, *121*
Brain metastases, **210**

C

Carcinogens, 5
Caucasians, **1**, 4
Cerebriform intradermal nevi, 155
Chemotherapy
  by intravascular infusion, **193**
  by perfusion, **194**
  regional, **193**
  systemic, **187**
Childhood melanomas, **152**
Circumscribed precancerous melanosis, **7**, *27*
Classification of malignant melanomas, **7**
Clinical diagnosis, **7, 15**
Clinico-histologic types of malignant melanoma, **7**
Complexion, 5
Computerized axial tomography, **210**
Congenital nevi, *69, 79,* **154**
Congenital primary malignant melanoma, 153
Cure rates, 172
5-S-Cysteinyldopa, **209**

D

Deaths due to melanoma, 1, 2
Deaths from skin cancers other than malignant melanoma, 1
Definition
  "active junction nevus," *34*
  atypical melanocyte, *34*
  junctional "activity," *34*
  melanocyte, *34*
  melanophage, *34*
  nevus cell (nevocyte), *34*
Desmoplastic malignant melanoma, *51, 79,* **208**
Diagnostic accuracy in malignant melanoma, **177**, 206
Diameter of melanomas, 3, 173
Differential diagnosis, 22
Differentiation of primary from metastatic malignant melanomas, *81*

E

Early diagnosis, 3, 175
Elastosis, 4
Elective lymph node dissection, **183**
Elevation, *34*
Epidemiology, 4
Epidermotropically metastatic malignant melanoma, *79, 81*
Extramammary Paget's disease, *79, 113*
Extra-regional metastases, 21, **169**
Eye color, **5,** 23, **207**

F

Familial melanomas, **148**
Five-year survival rates, 2
Fontana-Masson stain *87, 138*
Frozen sections, 138
Frozen section diagnosis, **207**

G

Gallium-67 scintigraphy, **211**
Geographic aspects, 1
Giant nevocytic nevi, **154**

H

Hair color, 5
Hairless mouse, 4
Halo nevi, *69, 70, 79*
Hepatic metastases, **210**
Histologic criteria for the diagnosis of malignant melanoma, *68*
Histology, 25
Histopathology, 25
Historical review, 25
HL-A phenotypes, 148
Homovanillic acid, **209**
Horizontal-growth phase, 16, *39*

I

Immune responses, 204
Immunologic aspects, **204**
Immunotherapy, **204**
Incidence, **1**
Inflammatory-cell infiltrate in melanoma, *34, 51, 65, 70*

235

Intralesional transformation, 27
In-transit metastasis, 21
Invasion of blood vessels or lymphatics, 34
Irritated junction or compound melanocytic nevus, 69

J

Junction nevi, 79
Junctional "activity", *115*

L

Lactic dehydrogenase, 210
Large congenital melanocytic nevi, *71*
Laser radiation, 212
Lentigo maligna [*also see* Melanotic freckle (Hutchinson)], **18**, *79*
Lentigo maligna melanoma, **7**, *27*, **35**, *69*
Leukoderma and malignant melanomas, **162**
Levels of invasion, **12**, *33*, 87, 172, 173
Levodopa, 212
Local recurrence, 21
Lymphocytic infiltrate, *69*, 172

M

MSH receptors, **213**
Magnification as an aid in diagnosis, **206**
Malignant Melanoma Clinical Cooperative Group data (Appendix), **214**
Malignant melanoma metastatic to the skin, *81*
Melanocarcinoma, 25
Melanosarcoma, 25
Melanosis, 21, *86*
Melanotic freckle (Hutchinson) (*also see* Lentigo maligna), **7**
Minimal deviation melanoma, *121*
Mitoses, *34*, 172
Mole syndrome, 148–149, 157
Mortality rates, 1
Mucous membrane melanomas, **11**
Multinucleated melanocytic giant cells, *71*
Multiple primary malignant melanomas, **157**
Mycosis fungoides, *81*

N

Nevocytic nevi, 21, 22
  giant, 154
Nevus of large spindle and/or epitheloid cells (Spitz's nevus), *62, 69, 79*
Nodular malignant melanoma, **9, 19,** *32*, **39,** *45*

O

Occult primary malignant melanomas, **166**
Ocular melanoma, 5
Outdoor exposure, 5

P

Pagetoid Bowen's disease, *79*
Pagetoid cells, *51*
Pagetoid melanocytes, *45*
Palms and soles, 20
Pathology, **25**
Pautrier's microabscesses, *81*
Perl stain, *87*
Placental metastases, 153
Polyamines, **210**
Polyclonism, 27
Preexisting acquired melanocytic nevi, 53
Pregnancy, **175**
Prepubertal melanomas, **152**
Prognosis, 87, 172
  amelanotic melanoma, 173
  blood vessel invasion, 173
  diameter, 173
  level, 173
  lymph node metastases, 175
  lymphocytic infiltration, 173
  of primary cutaneous malignant melanoma, 33
  pregnancy, 175
  sex, 173
  site, 173
  type of melanoma, 173
  ulceration, 173
Prognostic index, 97
Prognostic score sheet, 173–174
Prognostication of behavior, **172**
Pseudomelanoma, 22, **207**
Pyogenic granuloma, 53

R

Radial-growth phase, 7, *27, 39*
Radical groin dissection, 180
Radionuclide photoscanning, **211**
Radiotherapy, **197**
Recurrent melanocytic nevi, *69*
Regional metastasis, 21
Regression in malignant melanoma, 65
"Ring" melanomas, 173

S

Satellitosis, **21,** *84*
Scalp, 21, 155
Scintigraphy, **211**
Sectioning and processing, *136*
Skin markings, 16
Small cells, *51*
"Solar circulating factor," 5
Solar elastosis, *41*
Soles, 20
Spitz's nevus (*see also* Nevus of large spindle and/or epithelioid cells), *69, 70*
Spleen scans, **211**
Spontaneous regression of malignant melanomas, **166**
Squamous-cell carcinomas, 4
  in situ, *105*
Staging melanomas, **170,** 173
Step-sections, **13**
Sunburn, 5
Sun-damaged skin, *39*
Subungual malignant melanoma, 20, **159**
Sunlight, 1, **4**
Superficial basal-cell carcinomas, *105*
Superficial spreading malignant melanoma, **8, 16,** *35, 45*
Surgical management, **179**
Survival rate, 1, **200**

T

Thermography, **208**
Thickness as prognostic guide, *98*
Thickness of malignant melanomas, **13,** *33*
Thickness plus number of mitotic figures as a prognostic guide, 97
Third National Cancer Survey, **1**
Traumatized junction or compound nevi, 79

Tumor-node-metastases (TNM) classification, 170
Types of malignant melanoma, *27*
Tyrosinase, **209**

U

Ulceration, 34
Ultraviolet light, **4**, 5

Urinary melanogens, **209**
Urinary polyamines, **210**

V

Verrucous malignant melanomas, *32,* 51
Vertical-growth phase, 7, *27, 39*
Vitiligo, **162**

W

Whites, **1**, 4
Work-up for malignant melanoma, 179

X

Xeroderma pigmentosum, 5
X-ray therapy, **197**